Neuropharmacology: A Case-Based Approach

Neuropharmacology: A Case-Based Approach

Editor: Sullivan Willis

AMERICAN
MEDICAL PUBLISHERS
www.americanmedicalpublishers.com

AMERICAN
MEDICAL PUBLISHERS
www.americanmedicalpublishers.com

Cataloging-in-Publication Data

Neuropharmacology : a case-based approach / edited by Sullivan Willis.
p. cm.
Includes bibliographical references and index.
ISBN 979-8-88740-315-1
1. Neuropharmacology. 2. Neuropharmacology--Case studies. 3. Pharmacology.
4. Neurosciences. I. Willis, Sullivan.
RM315 .N48 2023
615.78--dc23

American Medical Publishers,
41 Flatbush Avenue,
1st Floor, New York,
NY 11217, USA

ISBN 979-8-88740-315-1 (Hardback)

Contents

Preface

Neuropharmacology is the study of the manner in which medications alter the cellular function in the nervous system, and the neurological mechanisms by which they influence behavior. Behavioral neuropharmacology and molecular neuropharmacology are the two main branches of neuropharmacology. The study of the impact of drugs on human behavior is the focus of behavioral neuropharmacology. It also studies how drug dependency and addiction affect the human brain. The study of neurons and their neurochemical interactions is known as molecular neuropharmacology. It aims to discover the medications that improve brain function. Both these branches of neuropharmacology deal with the interplay of neurotransmitters, neuropeptides, neurohormones, neuromodulators, enzymes, second messengers, co-transporters, ion channels and receptor proteins in the central and peripheral nervous systems. Various researches are being conducted for studying these interactions with an aim to develop medications to treat various neurological problems, including pain, neurodegenerative diseases, psychiatric disorders and addiction. This book consists of contributions made by international experts. The various advancements in neuropharmacology along with their applications have also been explained in detail within this book. It will serve as an excellent reference for a broad spectrum of readers.

This book is a result of research of several months to collate the most relevant data in the field.

When I was approached with the idea of this book and the proposal to edit it, I was overwhelmed. It gave me an opportunity to reach out to all those who share a common interest with me in this field. I had 3 main parameters for editing this text:

1. Accuracy - The data and information provided in this book should be up-to-date and valuable to the readers.

2. Structure - The data must be presented in a structured format for easy understanding and better grasping of the readers.

3. Universal Approach - This book not only targets students but also experts and innovators in the field, thus my aim was to present topics which are of use to all.

Thus, it took me a couple of months to finish the editing of this book.

I would like to make a special mention of my publisher who considered me worthy of this opportunity and also supported me throughout the editing process. I would also like to thank the editing team at the back-end who extended their help whenever required.

Editor

1

Therapeutic Challenges of Post-Traumatic Stress Disorder: Focus on the Dopaminergic System

Sebastiano Alfio Torrisi, Gian Marco Leggio, Filippo Drago and Salvatore Salomone*

Department of Biomedical and Biotechnological Sciences, University of Catania, Catania, Italy

***Correspondence:**
Salvatore Salomone
salomone@unict.it

Post-traumatic stress disorder (PTSD) is a mental illness developed by vulnerable individuals exposed to life-threatening events. The pharmacological unresponsiveness displayed by the vast majority of PTSD patients has raised considerable interest in understanding the poorly known pathophysiological mechanisms underlying this disorder. Most studies in the field focused, so far, on noradrenergic mechanisms, because of their well-established role in either tuning arousal or in encoding emotional memories. However, less attention has been paid to other neural systems. Manipulations of the dopaminergic system alter behavioral responses to stressful situations and recent findings suggest that dopaminergic dysfunction might play an overriding role in the pathophysiology of PTSD. In the present review, dopaminergic mechanisms relevant for the pathogenesis of PTSD, as well as potential dopaminergic-based pharmacotherapies are discussed in the context of addressing the unmet medical need for new and effective drugs for treatment of PTSD.

Keywords: post-traumatic stress disorder, dopamine D_3 receptor, intrusive symptoms, mood and cognition, arousal, SSRI

INTRODUCTION

Post-traumatic stress disorder (PTSD) is the most prevalent neuropsychiatric disorder developed by vulnerable individuals exposed to life-threatening events (Benjet et al., 2016). The probability of developing PTSD ranges from 5 to 31% according to different factors such as social background, home country and kind of traumatic event experienced (Girgenti et al., 2017; Shalev et al., 2017). The complex diagnosis of PTSD relies on several criteria described in the Diagnostic and Statistical Manual of Mental Disorders, fifth edition (DSM-5): an individual, after exposure to death, threatened death, actual or threatened serious injury, or actual or threatened sexual violence (Criterion A), must exhibit ongoing intrusive re-experiencing symptoms (Criterion B, one required), avoidance symptoms (Criterion C, one required), negative alterations in mood and cognitions (Criterion D, two required) and symptoms of hyperarousal (Criterion E, two required). These symptoms must last for more than 1 month (Criterion F) and cause a functional impairment (Criterion G). It is also important to exclude that these symptoms are triggered by medications or other psychiatric disorders (Criterion H). Besides the classic PTSD, a cluster of patients may experience a dissociative subtype of PTSD, characterized by additional symptoms of depersonalization and derealization (Fenster et al., 2018). The first-line pharmacotherapy for PTSD consists of two selective serotonin reuptake inhibitors (SSRI), namely paroxetine and sertraline, which are the only medications approved by the U.S. Food and Drug Administration.

However, because among PTSD patients only a few (less than 30%) achieve full remission (Berger et al., 2009), there is an urgent need to discover and develop new effective medications. Several inconclusive approaches have been proposed to overcome this pharmacological unresponsiveness. The preventive therapy, which should be undertaken before the onset of the symptoms, indeed raises both economical and ethical issues, considering that some individuals are prone while others are resilient to develop PTSD after the trauma, and an univocal reliable method to identify the susceptible ones (those supposed to receive a preventive treatment) is still unavailable (Steckler and Risbrough, 2012). The results concerning the augmentation strategies with atypical antipsychotics for SSRI non-responders are also rather arguable (Krystal et al., 2011). One promising drug that could shed light on this issue is the non-competitive N-methyl-D-aspartate (NMDA) receptor antagonist ketamine. A key pilot randomized controlled trial demonstrated a rapid relief of PTSD symptoms after intravenous infusion of ketamine without the occurrence of dissociative symptoms (Feder et al., 2014). Despite these encouraging results, the efficacy and safety of repeated infusions of ketamine would need to be tested in further confirmatory clinical trials. Indeed, preclinical studies suggest that ketamine might promote the development of PTSD (Morena et al., 2017; Radford et al., 2018).

A promising, recently proposed, strategy is the combination of pharmacological treatment and cognitive behavioral therapy (CBT, Morena et al., 2018). In PTSD, CBT consists of repeated exposure of the patient to trauma-related reminders in a safe controlled situation. It is believed that this kind of exposure-based psychotherapy may trigger extinction learning processes, which could result effective in a subset of PTSD patients. However, a substantial number of PTSD patients drops out of CBT, while a high rate of relapse of PTSD symptoms has been observed after the end of CBT (Gutner et al., 2016). In this regard, either drugs able to counteract the excessive retrieval or drugs that can enhance the extinction of traumatic memories could increase the efficacy of CBT (Morena et al., 2018).

Increasing our understanding of the neurobiology of a given disease is essential for the development of new effective and safe medications (Everitt et al., 2018). The etiology and the pathophysiological mechanisms underlying PTSD remain poorly understood despite the numerous experimental studies carried out over the last 30 years. Although the vast majority of the research in the field is focused on noradrenergic mechanisms (Naegeli et al., 2018), growing evidence suggests that other neural systems may be involved in the etiology and pathophysiology of PTSD. Great attention in this respect has been given to the endocannabinoid system. This neuromodulatory system is altered in PTSD patients (Hauer et al., 2013; Hill et al., 2013, 2018) and represents a potential therapeutic target in the treatment of PTSD (Fidelman et al., 2018; Morena et al., 2018). Intriguingly, a valuable body of findings demonstrate that the dopaminergic (DAergic) system controls behavioral responses to stressful situations (Pruessner et al., 2004). Various coping strategies to stressful events are sustained by fluctuations of tonic dopamine (DA) levels in the nucleus accumbens (NAc) (Cabib and Puglisi-Allegra, 2012) and manipulations of midbrain DAergic transmission alter resilience to stress (Friedman et al., 2014). A prominent role of DA into the prefrontal cortex (PFC) in mediating responses to stressful events has been also proposed (Pascucci et al., 2007) and, more interestingly, increasing evidence suggests that DAergic dysfunction might play a pivotal role in PTSD (**Table 1**). In the present review, DAergic mechanisms relevant for the pathogenesis of PTSD, as well as potential DAergic-based pharmacotherapies are discussed in the context of addressing the unmet medical need for new and effective drugs for treatment of PTSD.

DAergic SYSTEM

In the late 1950s, Arvid Carlsson discovered that the catecholamine DA was not just the precursor of norepinephrine (NE) but also a neurotransmitter, *per se* (Carlsson, 1959). DA exerts profound influences over several physiological functions including reward, cognition and emotional processes through the activation of two classes of DA receptors, the D1-like receptors (D1R and D5R) and the D2-like receptors (D2R, D3R, and D4R), which are G-protein-coupled receptors coupled to G_s and G_i protein, respectively (Leggio et al., 2016). DA is synthesized and released by DAergic nuclei located in the midbrain, whose projections create four major DAergic pathways (Hillarp et al., 1966). DAergic neurons located in the ventral tegmental area (VTA) send projections mainly to the PFC (mesocortical pathway) and the ventral striatum (mesolimbic pathway). The nigrostriatal pathway consists of DAergic projections from the substantia nigra to the dorsal striatum. Lastly, the DAergic neurons of the tuberoinfundibular pathway originate in the arcuate nucleus of the hypothalamus and terminate in the median eminence. Besides these classic DAergic nuclei, relatively less-studied DAergic neurons in the ventral periaqueductal gray (vPAG) and dorsal raphe nucleus (DRN) finely modulate specific physiological functions, such as associative learning of fear, arousal states and social behavior (Matthews et al., 2016; Cho et al., 2017; Groessl et al., 2018), which are altered in several neuropsychiatric disorders including PTSD. In line with these observations, converging lines of evidence indicate that DAergic dysfunction may subserve the development of the pathophysiological processes underlying several symptoms of this disorder.

DA AND INTRUSION SYMPTOMS

Criterion B of the DSM-5 criteria for PTSD diagnosis refers to intrusion symptoms. Intrusive re-experiencing of traumatic events represents a hallmark symptom of PTSD. This re-experiencing may occur in several ways such as flashbacks, repetitive intrusive memories and distressing dreams (Brewin, 2015). Growing evidence indicates that a failure of the top-down inhibitory control exerted by the medial prefrontal cortex (mPFC) over the limbic regions and especially over the amygdala is responsible for these intrusion symptoms (**Figure 1**; Lanius et al., 2010). Particularly, the impairment of

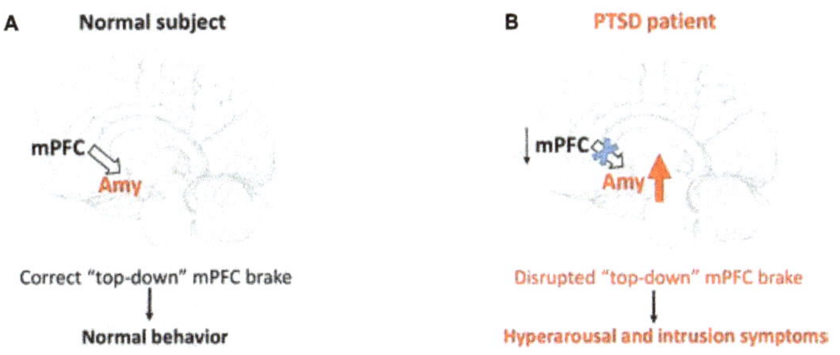

FIGURE 1 | The failure of the "top-down" inhibitory control exerted by the mPFC over the amygdala triggers hyperarousal and intrusion symptoms. In a normal subject **(A)**, the mPFC exerts a homeostatic inhibitory control over the amygdala (Amy). This "top-down" brake maintains appropriate behavior patterns under stressful conditions. In PTSD patients **(B)** the hypoactive mPFC removes the brake over the Amy, whose hyperactivity mainly generates hyperarousal and intrusion symptoms (Fenster et al., 2018, see also text).

cortical inhibitory control seems to be intimately related to a disrupted fear extinction (Milad et al., 2009), which contributes to exaggerated fear associated with the recurrence of traumatic memories. In the PFC, DA plays a pivotal role in regulating extinction memory consolidation (Hikind and Maroun, 2008; Mueller et al., 2010; Haaker et al., 2013; Gerlicher et al., 2018). Indeed, the pharmacological blockade of the D1R in the infralimbic cortex (IL) induced conditioned fear responses through a disruption of extinction consolidation in rats trained for auditory fear conditioning (Hikind and Maroun, 2008). On the other hand, a dietary zinc restriction-induced long-term rescue of deficient fear extinction has been associated with an enhancement of DAergic D1R and D2R receptor gene expression in the mPFC of a particular strain (129S1/SvImJ) of mice, which are basically characterized by deficient fear extinction acquisition and impaired fear extinction consolidation/retrieval (Whittle et al., 2016). This view is further substantiated by recent data showing that L-DOPA-induced burst of DAergic activity during extinction consolidation ameliorated extinction memory retrieval by increasing spontaneous ventromedial prefrontal cortex (vmPFC) reactivations (Gerlicher et al., 2018). The vmPFC has reciprocal connections with a key brain region involved in the acquisition and expression of conditioned fear, namely the amygdala (Phelps et al., 2004; Stevens et al., 2013). Hitora-Imamura et al. (2015) demonstrated a mesocortical DA-dependent modulation of fear extinction involving the

TABLE 1 | Findings from human studies demonstrating an impact of DAergic dysfunction on PTSD.

Dopaminergic dysfunction	Description	References
↑ Urinary DA levels	↑ Severity of PTSD symptoms (especially intrusion symptoms) CRITERION B	Yehuda et al., 1992
VNTR DAT SLC6A3 3′ polymorphism	Excess of nine repeat allele in PTSD patients	Segman et al., 2002
VNTR DRD4 exon III polymorphism	↑ Severity of PTSD symptoms on the Avoidance/Numbing scale. CRITERION C	Dragan and Oniszczenko, 2009
VNTR DAT SLC6A3 3′ polymorphism	↑ Arousal symptoms CRITERION E	Drury et al., 2009
COMT Val158Met polymorphism	↑ Risk of PTSD in Met/Met homozygotes	Kolassa et al., 2010
COMT Val158Met polymorphism	Attenuation of the effect of PTSD-related processes on right anterior cingulate cortex volume	Schulz-Heik et al., 2011
↑ DAT density	↑ Striatal DAT density in PTSD patients	Hoexter et al., 2012
COMT Val158Met polymorphism	↑ Fear to safety signal and impaired fear extinction in PTSD Met/Met homozygotes as compared to Val allele carrier CRITERION B	Norrholm et al., 2013
DRD3 single nucleotide polymorphisms (rs2134655, rs201252087, rs4646996, and rs9868039)	The minor alleles give resilience against PTSD	Wolf et al., 2014
COMT Val158Met polymorphism	Smaller left hippocampus in PTSD Val/Val homozygotes as compared to Met allele carriers	Hayes et al., 2017
COMT Val158Met polymorphism	Childhood trauma-dependent association between the Met/Met genotype and fear inhibition/extinction deficit CRITERION B	Deslauriers et al., 2018
COMT Val158Met polymorphism	Better working memory and executive functions in PTSD Met carriers as compared to Val/Val homozygotes CRITERION D	Havelka Mestrovic et al., 2018

interconnection between the IL and the central nucleus of the amygdala (CeA) (Hitora-Imamura et al., 2015). The shock reminder-induced release of DA within the IL dampens the activity of this cortical region, which in turn removes the "brake" on the CeA. This aberrant mechanism triggers the fear reinstatement. Among the amygdaloid nuclei, the CeA receives the most abundant DAergic fibers from the mesolimbic DA-containing neurons (de la Mora et al., 2010). These fibers release DA within the CeA under fear responses (Naylor et al., 2010). Notably, the DAergic vPAG/DRN neurons also represent a great source of DAergic fibers projecting to the CeA (Matthews et al., 2016). This DAergic vPAG/DRN – CeA circuitry has been recently proposed as a new pivotal participant of the Pavlovian fear conditioning processes. It couples a positive aversive prediction error signal (a central component of reinforcement learning, representing the mismatch between the actual outcome and the predicted outcome) to a DAergic reinforcement of an experience-dependent fear memory trace into the CeA (Groessl et al., 2018). Thus, a dysfunction of the DAergic vPAG/DRN – CeA circuitry together with a DA-dependent failure of the top-down inhibitory control exerted by the mPFC primarily over the hyperactive CeA might be responsible for the aberrant fear memory formation in PTSD patients.

At a clinical level, the severity of PTSD symptoms, particularly that of the intrusion symptoms, has been correlated to augmented urinary DA and NE levels (Yehuda et al., 1992). An inverse relationship between plasma DA and heart rate during fear inhibition has been also found in military service members with more severe subthreshold PTSD symptoms (Costanzo et al., 2016). Other human studies have found the Catechol-O-Methyltransferase (COMT) Val158/108Met (rs4680) polymorphism associated with fear inhibition and extinction deficits in PTSD. COMT is an enzyme that catalyzes the O-methylation and thereby the inactivation of catecholamines. Met/Met carriers exhibit a 40% reduction in COMT activity that leads to a heightened DAergic tone, especially in the cortex (Chen et al., 2004). In general, either enhanced fear memory consolidation or fear extinction resistance has been reported in Met/Met carriers (Lonsdorf et al., 2009, 2010). In a fear-potentiated startle study, PTSD patients with the Met/Met genotype showed higher fear to a safety signal as well as a more impaired fear extinction as compared to those patients carrying the Val allele (Norrholm et al., 2013). These findings have been further confirmed in a more recent study in which the authors discovered a childhood trauma-dependent association between the Met/Met genotype and a fear inhibition/extinction deficit (Deslauriers et al., 2018). Overall, these preclinical and clinical results indicate that DAergic mechanisms/dysfunctions may be deeply correlated to intrusion symptoms.

DA AND AVOIDANCE SYMPTOMS

Criterion C of the DSM-5 criteria for PTSD diagnosis concerns attempting to avoid distressing, trauma-related stimuli, including thoughts, people, places, conversations, objects and more in general attempting to avoid emotional experiences. These symptoms are closely related to fear extinction deficits showed by PTSD patients. Indeed, greater avoidance symptomatology has been associated with greater activation of fear circuits in a sample of veterans with PTSD (Sripada et al., 2013). In this respect, Stein and Paulus hypothesized that PTSD would represent a disorder originating from an altered homeostatic balance between the approach system and the avoidance system (Stein and Paulus, 2009). By definition, approach indicates the tendency to move toward positively valenced stimuli and it is closely linked to reward processes. Conversely, avoidance is the tendency to turn away from negatively valenced stimuli and, as mentioned before, is more connected to fear-related mechanisms. DA is the most important neurotransmitter regulating the reward-related learning of approach behavior (Contreras-Vidal and Schultz, 1999; Schultz, 1999, 2007). Moreover, animal studies demonstrate a key involvement of DA in avoidance behavior. DA in the PFC modulates top-down circuits involved in encoding aversive stimuli, able to trigger avoidance and escape-related defensive behaviors (Vander Weele et al., 2018). However, a more important role is played by subcortical DAergic mechanisms. Indeed, the photo-stimulation of DAergic neurons in the midbrain enhances active avoidance behavior and accelerates the extinction of passive avoidance behavior (e.g., freezing) under the presentation of a fear-conditioned cue. By contrast, the photo-inhibition of the same neurons, as well as the accumbal D1R antagonism, attenuate the active avoidance behavior (Wenzel et al., 2018). Worthy of note, optogenetic activation of the aforementioned DRN DAergic neurons increases place avoidance (Matthews et al., 2016).

A fundamental role of striatal DA in mediating avoidance behavior is also documented. Genetic deletion of the D2R on striatopallidal neurons increases avoidance behavior (LeBlanc et al., 2018) and activation of DAergic axons innervating the posterior tail of the striatum reinforces avoidance of threatening stimuli (Menegas et al., 2018).

The human neurobiological basis of avoidance symptoms has been less studied in PTSD. With regard to DA, one human genetic study has reported a significant association between the polymorphism of DRD4 exon III and the severity of PTSD symptoms on the Avoidance/Numbing scale (Dragan and Oniszczenko, 2009).

DA AND ALTERATION IN MOOD AND COGNITION

Criterion D of the DSM-5 criteria for PTSD diagnosis refers to the persistent negative changes in mood and cognition. PTSD patients may indeed experience cognitive dysfunctions such as dissociative amnesia (inability to recall crucial features of the traumatic event), impairment of executive functions (working memory and cognitive flexibility), but also enduring negative emotions (horror, anger, guilt, and shame), loss of interest in previously rewarding activities, social detachment, and incapacity to experience positive emotions (anhedonia). In this respect, a mutual interaction between emotions and cognition has been observed in PTSD. In PTSD patients, trauma-related memories and trauma-related cues generate negative emotions that may interfere with ongoing cognitive processes (Hayes et al., 2012). For instance, a reward deficiency has been described in PTSD (Elman et al., 2005). Some PTSD patients are less motivated to obtain positive rewards and because the decision-making process is highly influenced by the motivational state, these individuals show a disrupted decision-making capacity (Hayes et al., 2012). The mesolimbic DAergic pathway is the key player in reward-seeking behavior (Pessiglione et al., 2006, 2007) and, as suggested by Enman et al. (2015), striatal DAergic dysfunction may contribute to the occurrence of PTSD symptomatology, including anhedonia and emotional numbing, by altering reward processes (Enman et al., 2015). In line with these findings, a clinical study reported that PTSD patients showed an increased striatal dopamine transporter (DAT) density in comparison with traumatizing asymptomatic individuals (Hoexter et al., 2012). Because reward processes mainly rely on DA activity in the ventral striatum, this greater DAT density may underlie DA-dependent aberrant reward system in PTSD patients. It is important to point out that anhedonia is also a characteristic and severe symptom of major depressive disorder (MDD) (Keedwell et al., 2005) and a high rate of comorbidity between PTSD and MDD has been observed (Flory and Yehuda, 2015). In this latter condition, reduced striatal DAT density seems to reflect a compensatory mechanism aimed at counteracting a chronic hypodopaminergic tone (Meyer et al., 2001). Conversely, as mentioned before, increased striatal DAT density in PTSD may be related to hyperdopaminergia (van de Giessen et al., 2009; Hoexter et al., 2012). Thus, it seems that opposite striatal DAergic abnormalities may generate anhedonia, through the disruption of the reward processing. In an attempt to reveal the neural substrates of this decision-making/reward connection in PTSD, Sailer et al. found that PTSD patients exhibited hypoactivation of both the NAc and PFC during the processing of gains in the late learning phase of a decision-making task (Sailer et al., 2008). Hence, cortical DAergic mechanisms may also be involved in the decision-making/reward connection, and, more in general, in cognitive dysfunctions characterizing PTSD. Veterans PTSD patients carrying the COMT Val158Met polymorphism and homozygous for the Val allele displayed a volume of the anterior cingulate cortex smaller than controls non-PTSD (Schulz-Heik et al., 2011). In the PFC, DAT is low expressed and does not contribute to DA reuptake; COMT plays a more substantial role, being responsible for approximately one half of the total DA clearance (Kaenmaki et al., 2010). Remarkably, a significant association between the COMT Val158/108Met polymorphism and working memory performance has been found in PTSD patients. PTSD met carriers showed better working memory and executive functions than Val/Val homozygotes (Havelka Mestrovic et al., 2018). Considering that the met allele is associated with reduced COMT activity, which leads to a slower prefrontal DA degradation (Chen et al., 2004), it may maintain adequate level of DA in the PFC, associated to better cognitive performance. The critical impact of the COMT Val158/108Met polymorphism on PTSD symptoms, particularly on PTSD cognitive dysfunctions, is supported by the observation that a cluster of Val/Val homozygotes with severe PTSD symptomatology showed smaller left hippocampus compared to those patients carrying the met allele (Hayes et al., 2017). The hippocampus is highly enriched in COMT (Matsumoto et al., 2003), therefore, reduced hippocampal DA availability in Val carriers may impair crucial processes for memory formation such as, neurogenesis and long term potentiation.

Although these findings suggest that mood and cognitive alterations in PTSD patients may be triggered by dysregulation of the DAergic system, additional research would be relevant to better clarify the impact of this DAergic dysfunction.

DA AND HYPERAROUSAL SYMPTOMS

Criterion E of the DSM-5 criteria for PTSD diagnosis focuses on hyperarousal symptoms, including exaggerated startle, sleep disturbance, hypervigilance, impulsivity and aggressiveness. These symptoms often occur first (Bremner et al., 1996) and have a major impact in the natural course of the disease by influencing the development and onset of the other symptoms (Schell et al., 2004; Weston, 2014). Although NE is historically recognized as the key neurotransmitter in the modulation of arousal, DA is also involved in. DA fosters wakefulness (Monti and Monti, 2007) and VTA DAergic neurons play a central role in this effect. VTA DAergic neurons strongly fire during motivated waking (Dahan et al., 2007) and selective photo-stimulation of such DAergic neurons induces arousal on mice under isoflurane-induced continuous, steady-state general anesthesia (Taylor et al., 2016). Other studies further report a fluctuation of extracellular DA levels across different arousal states in the NAc and mPFC (Lena et al., 2005), the two main brain regions receiving DAergic projections from the VTA. However, VTA DAergic inputs to the NAc but not to the mPFC have the most fundamental role in mediating arousal states and ethologically relevant sleep-wake behaviors (Eban-Rothschild et al., 2016). VTA DAergic neurons are not the only DAergic neurons regulating arousal states. Lu et al. (2006) were able to label the vPAG DAergic neurons as wake-active DAergic neurons (Lu et al., 2006), showing that they project to several brain regions belonging to the wake–sleep regulatory system, including the mPFC. Thus, DA fluctuations within the mPFC (Lena et al., 2005) across different arousal states are likely triggered by vPAG DAergic neurons. A more recent study reveals that DRN DAergic neurons tune arousal and promote wakefulness upon the presentation of salient stimuli (Cho et al., 2017). All these observations prompt us to hypothesize that dysfunctional alterations of the midbrain DAergic neurons and their respective DAergic circuitries might underlie the sleep disturbances of PTSD patients, which may also explain the high contribution of hyperarousal symptoms on the occurrence of the other PTSD symptoms. For instance, a DA-dependent hyperarousal state could interfere with motivational processes, which are known to influence cognitive processes such as decision-making (**Figure 2**).

Relatively few studies have explored the role of DA in the startle reactivity. An increase of the DAergic signaling obtained by systemic administration of DA agonists is able

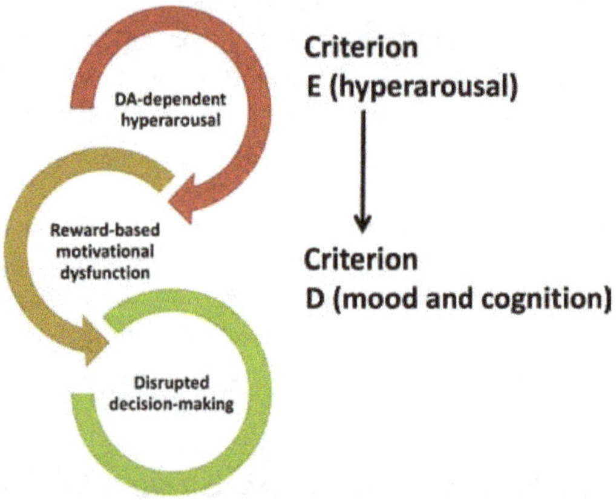

FIGURE 2 | Hypothetical influence of DA-induced hyperarousal (CRITERION E) on symptoms (CRITERION D) occurring in post-traumatic stress disorder.

to strengthen the startle reactivity (Davis et al., 1986; Meloni and Davis, 2000). Conversely, the genetic deletion of D2R and D3R produces an increase of startle habituation as well as a decrease of startle reactivity (Halberstadt and Geyer, 2009; Torrisi et al., 2017). These preclinical findings are substantiated by human studies reporting a connection between polymorphisms of genes implicated in DA metabolism and variable startle reactivity. The COMT Val158/108Met polymorphism is one of the polymorphisms affecting the startle reactivity. In a human genetic study, COMT Val carriers exhibited a heightened unpleasant stimuli-induced startle that was not modified by L-DOPA administration, while COMT Met/Met carriers did not show any change in startle under the presentation of unpleasant stimuli or neutral stimuli, but they displayed heightened unpleasant stimuli-induced startle after L- DOPA administration (Domschke et al., 2015).

Aggressive and/or dysfunctional impulsive behavior elicited by perceived threat is another common hyperarousal symptom characterizing PTSD. Aggressive and/or dysfunctional impulsive behavior has been linked to a deficient cortical brake over the limbic regions similarly to the disrupted fear extinction discussed above (**Figure 1**; Fenster et al., 2018). DA is also believed to be a key modulator of impulsive behavior (Dalley and Roiser, 2012; Besson et al., 2013). Intriguingly, a low prefrontal DAergic tone has been associated with high impulsivity, while increasing cortical levels of DA diminishes impulsive choice by varying corticostriatal connectivity (Kayser et al., 2012). Other studies provide clear evidence of a prominent contribution of subcortical DAergic mechanisms in aggressive and/or impulsive behavior. Optogenetic activation of VTA DAergic neurons raises aggressive behavior (Yu et al., 2014) and substantia nigra/VTA D2/D3 autoreceptor availability inversely and positively correlates with impulsivity and amphetamine-induced DA release in the striatum, respectively (Buckholtz et al., 2010). Hence, DAergic dysfunction might have a critical role in the development of aggressive and/or dysfunctional impulsive behavior exhibited by PTSD patients.

To our knowledge, only one clinical study (Drury et al., 2009) has provided direct evidence that DAergic dysfunction has a major influence on hyperarousal symptoms compared to other PTSD symptoms. Again, genetically induced variations of the DAergic system have a critical role in this regard. Genetic variants of the variable number tandem repeat element of 40 base pairs located in the 3′ UTR of the DAT gene have been related to variable transcription rate (Heinz et al., 2000; Michelhaugh et al., 2001). The nine repeat allele, whose excess has been found in a cluster of PTSD patients (Segman et al., 2002), has been specifically associated with hyperarousal symptoms (Drury et al., 2009).

THE POTENTIAL THERAPEUTIC VALUE OF TARGETING THE DAergic SYSTEM IN PTSD

The human and animal data discussed in this review suggest that DAergic dysfunction is implicated in the pathophysiology of PTSD and, as a consequence, drugs targeting the central DAergic system could have a therapeutic value for the management of this disorder. As mentioned above, the failure of the top-down inhibitory control exerted by the PFC over the limbic regions might be one of the key aberrant mechanisms subserving predominantly both the intrusion and the hyperarousal symptoms (Fenster et al., 2018). Because the reactivation of the PFC may restore the homeostatic inhibitory control over the subcortical regions and promote the consolidation of fear extinction, which is believed to subserve resilience against PTSD (Gerlicher et al., 2018), an effective strategy might be the administration of drugs known to boost the activity of this region via increasing the DAergic signaling. In this regard, a promising candidate drug might be methylphenidate, a NET and DAT blocker. Low doses of methylphenidate preferentially increase prefrontal catecholaminergic neurotransmission (Berridge et al., 2006). It dose-dependently increases extinction of contextual fear (Abraham et al., 2012) and, most importantly, has been shown to be effective on veterans suffering from PTSD and largely refractory to standard medications (Houlihan, 2011). As discussed above, L-DOPA increases spontaneous vmPFC reactivation via strengthening the DAergic signaling. In an ongoing clinical trial (NCT02560389), the investigators are testing the hypothesis that this commercially available drug may enhance fear extinction learning in PTSD women patients. In this respect, we speculate that a combination of these DAergic drugs able to promote the consolidation of fear extinction with CBT could be a successful strategy that can significantly diminish the relapse of PTSD symptoms. However, it is important to state that such drugs also affect the DAergic signaling in the subcortical regions and this effect may create issues because abrupt variation of the subcortical DAergic tone may facilitate the development of drug abuse (Volkow, 2006). One intriguing drug endowed with preferential activity on the PFC is the atypical stimulant atomoxetine.

This drug, which is a potent and selective blocker of NE re-uptake approved for the treatment of attention-deficit/hyperactivity disorder, selectively increases DA levels in the PFC without affecting the subcortical DAergic system (Bymaster et al., 2002). This peculiar effect is based on the fact that, in the PFC, the re-uptake of DA is carried out by the highly expressed NET instead of the low expressed DAT (Yamamoto and Novotney, 1998). Several studies demonstrate that atomoxetine is able to ameliorate impulsivity and executive function deficits, which are found across different neuropsychiatric disorders (Ansquer et al., 2014; Borchert et al., 2016). Thus, atomoxetine might be effective in PTSD patients mainly showing hyperarousal symptoms. COMT inhibitors are another class of compounds that could restore the proper functioning of the PFC by increasing the DAergic signaling. As extensively discussed above, COMT Val158/108Met polymorphism has been associated with PTSD. The Val allele, being linked to higher COMT activity, lowers synaptic DA availability and disrupts PFC function (Chen et al., 2004). Therefore, we speculate that COMT inhibitors could be effective on Val/Val homozygotes PTSD patients. It is important to remark that PFC presents a high sensitiveness to catecholamine levels (Cools and D'Esposito, 2011). Small changes of NE and DA levels can markedly affect PFC-dependent brain function. It is thus important to select the correct dose of a given DAergic drug to reach the optimal DA levels, adequate for the PFC.

It has been further suggested that D3R antagonists may be effective cognitive enhancers in individuals with neuropsychiatric disorders (Nakajima et al., 2013). The pro-cognitive effect of D3R antagonists has been linked to a facilitation of PFC top-down control of subcortical brain regions, implicated in the modulation of cognition (Millan et al., 2007; Loiseau and Millan, 2009). To date, only two studies have examined the interaction between D3R and PTSD.

In a candidate gene study, the minor alleles of four DRD3 single nucleotide polymorphisms (rs2134655, rs201252087, rs4646996, and rs9868039) have been found to be protective against the risk for PTSD (Wolf et al., 2014). Preclinical findings have also demonstrated that the selective blockade of D3R ameliorates the PTSD-like behavior of rats, previously exposed to the single-prolonged stress model (Song et al., 2018). These observations indicate that the D3R may be considered an interesting pharmacological target for the development of new effective drugs for the treatment of PTSD. From another perspective, commercially available drugs targeting the D3R might undergo a drug repositioning process. This process aims to discover new uses for already approved and commercialized medications and it offers great advantages over the long-lasting, risky and expensive, *de novo* drug discovery. In this context, two intriguing commercially available drugs are the antipsychotic aripiprazole and cariprazine, both endowed with D2R/D3R partial agonist activity and preferential binding to D3R (Leggio et al., 2016). By definition, partial agonists may act either as agonist or antagonist according to the surrounding levels of the neurotransmitter. Thus, these drugs may result effective on a wide range of PTSD patients characterized by a condition of DA imbalance, triggered by different genetic and epigenetic factors. This view is substantiated by a recent study showing that aripiprazole improved fear extinction retrieval via a normalization of the DA efflux in the amygdala (Lin et al., 2019). Finally, as mentioned above, ketamine, a drug candidate for PTSD, enhances DAergic neurotransmission in both humans and rodents (Lindefors et al., 1997; Kegeles et al., 2000; Can et al., 2016) and its activity on DAergic neurons relies on functional intact D3R (Cavalleri et al., 2018).

CONCLUSION

Currently available pharmacotherapies for PTSD are poorly effective on a substantial proportion of patients. Given this high rate of pharmacological unresponsiveness, further studies are needed to extend the knowledge of the basic mechanisms associated with the pathophysiology of this disorder. The findings discussed in this review suggest that DAergic dysfunction, especially genetic-dependent DAergic alteration, plays a prominent role in the pathophysiology of PTSD; as a consequence, drugs targeting the DAergic system might be therapeutically relevant. A better understanding of how and which DAergic dysfunction contributes to the symptoms of PTSD patients with different genetic background may lead to the development of effective drugs and more personalized treatments.

AUTHOR CONTRIBUTIONS

All authors listed have contributed to the work, by searching the literature, critical reading, and summarizing published data and writing this review. All authors listed have approved this review for publication.

FUNDING

This work was supported by Piano Triennale per la Ricerca – Linea Intervento 2, University of Catania, Italy.

REFERENCES

Abraham, A. D., Cunningham, C. L., and Lattal, K. M. (2012). Methylphenidate enhances extinction of contextual fear. *Learn. Mem.* 19, 67–72. doi: 10.1101/lm.024752.111

Ansquer, S., Belin-Rauscent, A., Dugast, E., Duran, T., Benatru, I., Mar, A. C., et al. (2014). Atomoxetine decreases vulnerability to develop compulsivity in high impulsive rats. *Biol. Psychiatry* 75, 825–832. doi: 10.1016/j.biopsych.2013.09.031

Benjet, C., Bromet, E., Karam, E. G., Kessler, R. C., Mclaughlin, K. A., Ruscio, A. M., et al. (2016). The epidemiology of traumatic event exposure worldwide: results from the World Mental Health Survey Consortium. *Psychol. Med.* 46, 327–343. doi: 10.1017/S0033291715001981

Berger, W., Mendlowicz, M. V., Marques-Portella, C., Kinrys, G., Fontenelle, L. F., Marmar, C. R., et al. (2009). Pharmacologic alternatives to antidepressants in posttraumatic stress disorder: a systematic review. *Prog. Neuropsychopharmacol. Biol. Psychiatry* 33, 169–180. doi: 10.1016/j.pnpbp.2008.12.004

Berridge, C. W., Devilbiss, D. M., Andrzejewski, M. E., Arnsten, A. F., Kelley, A. E., Schmeichel, B., et al. (2006). Methylphenidate preferentially increases catecholamine neurotransmission within the prefrontal cortex at low doses that enhance cognitive function. *Biol. Psychiatry* 60, 1111–1120. doi: 10.1016/j.biopsych.2006.04.022

Besson, M., Pelloux, Y., Dilleen, R., Theobald, D. E., Lyon, A., Belin-Rauscent, A., et al. (2013). Cocaine modulation of frontostriatal expression of Zif268, D2, and 5-HT2c receptors in high and low impulsive rats. *Neuropsychopharmacology* 38, 1963–1973. doi: 10.1038/npp.2013.95

Borchert, R. J., Rittman, T., Passamonti, L., Ye, Z., Sami, S., Jones, S. P., et al. (2016). Atomoxetine enhances connectivity of prefrontal networks in Parkinson's disease. *Neuropsychopharmacology* 41, 2171–2177. doi: 10.1038/npp.2016.18

Bremner, J. D., Southwick, S. M., Darnell, A., and Charney, D. S. (1996). Chronic PTSD in Vietnam combat veterans: course of illness and substance abuse. *Am. J. Psychiatry* 153, 369–375. doi: 10.1176/ajp.153.3.369

Brewin, C. R. (2015). Re-experiencing traumatic events in PTSD: new avenues in research on intrusive memories and flashbacks. *Eur. J. Psychotraumatol.* 6:27180. doi: 10.3402/ejpt.v6.27180

Buckholtz, J. W., Treadway, M. T., Cowan, R. L., Woodward, N. D., Li, R., Ansari, M. S., et al. (2010). Dopaminergic network differences in human impulsivity. *Science* 329:532. doi: 10.1126/science.1185778

Bymaster, F. P., Katner, J. S., Nelson, D. L., Hemrick-Luecke, S. K., Threlkeld, P. G., Heiligenstein, J. H., et al. (2002). Atomoxetine increases extracellular levels of norepinephrine and dopamine in prefrontal cortex of rat: a potential mechanism for efficacy in attention deficit/hyperactivity disorder. *Neuropsychopharmacology* 27, 699–711. doi: 10.1016/s0893-133x(02)00346-9

Cabib, S., and Puglisi-Allegra, S. (2012). The mesoaccumbens dopamine in coping with stress. *Neurosci. Biobehav. Rev.* 36, 79–89. doi: 10.1016/j.neubiorev.2011.04.012

Can, A., Zanos, P., Moaddel, R., Kang, H. J., Dossou, K. S., Wainer, I. W., et al. (2016). Effects of ketamine and ketamine metabolites on evoked striatal dopamine release, dopamine receptors, and monoamine transporters. *J. Pharmacol. Exp. Ther.* 359, 159–170. doi: 10.1124/jpet.116.235838

Carlsson, A. (1959). The occurrence, distribution and physiological role of catecholamines in the nervous system. *Pharmacol. Rev.* 11, 490–493.

Cavalleri, L., Merlo Pich, E., Millan, M. J., Chiamulera, C., Kunath, T., Spano, P. F., et al. (2018). Ketamine enhances structural plasticity in mouse mesencephalic and human iPSC-derived dopaminergic neurons via AMPAR-driven BDNF and mTOR signaling. *Mol. Psychiatry* 23, 812–823. doi: 10.1038/mp.2017.241

Chen, J., Lipska, B. K., Halim, N., Ma, Q. D., Matsumoto, M., Melhem, S., et al. (2004). Functional analysis of genetic variation in catechol-O-methyltransferase (COMT): effects on mRNA, protein, and enzyme activity in postmortem human brain. *Am. J. Hum. Genet.* 75, 807–821. doi: 10.1086/425589

Cho, J. R., Treweek, J. B., Robinson, J. E., Xiao, C., Bremner, L. R., Greenbaum, A., et al. (2017). Dorsal raphe dopamine neurons modulate arousal and promote wakefulness by salient stimuli. *Neuron* 94, 1205–1219.e8. doi: 10.1016/j.neuron.2017.05.020

Contreras-Vidal, J. L., and Schultz, W. (1999). A predictive reinforcement model of dopamine neurons for learning approach behavior. *J. Comput. Neurosci.* 6, 191–214.

Cools, R., and D'Esposito, M. (2011). Inverted-U-shaped dopamine actions on human working memory and cognitive control. *Biol. Psychiatry* 69, e113–e125. doi: 10.1016/j.biopsych.2011.03.028

Costanzo, M., Jovanovic, T., Norrholm, S. D., Ndiongue, R., Reinhardt, B., and Roy, M. J. (2016). Psychophysiological investigation of combat veterans with subthreshold post-traumatic stress disorder symptoms. *Mil. Med.* 181, 793–802. doi: 10.7205/MILMED-D-14-00671

Dahan, L., Astier, B., Vautrelle, N., Urbain, N., Kocsis, B., and Chouvet, G. (2007). Prominent burst firing of dopaminergic neurons in the ventral tegmental area during paradoxical sleep. *Neuropsychopharmacology* 32, 1232–1241. doi: 10.1038/sj.npp.1301251

Dalley, J. W., and Roiser, J. P. (2012). Dopamine, serotonin and impulsivity. *Neuroscience* 215, 42–58. doi: 10.1016/j.neuroscience.2012.03.065

Davis, M., Commissaris, R. L., Cassella, J. V., Yang, S., Dember, L., and Harty, T. P. (1986). Differential effects of dopamine agonists on acoustically and electrically elicited startle responses: comparison to effects of strychnine. *Brain Res.* 371, 58–69. doi: 10.1016/0006-8993(86)90810-3

de la Mora, M. P., Gallegos-Cari, A., Arizmendi-Garcia, Y., Marcellino, D., and Fuxe, K. (2010). Role of dopamine receptor mechanisms in the amygdaloid modulation of fear and anxiety: structural and functional analysis. *Prog. Neurobiol.* 90, 198–216. doi: 10.1016/j.pneurobio.2009.10.010

Deslauriers, J., Acheson, D. T., Maihofer, A. X., Nievergelt, C. M., Baker, D. G., Geyer, M. A., et al. (2018). COMT val158met polymorphism links to altered fear conditioning and extinction are modulated by PTSD and childhood trauma. *Depress. Anxiety* 35, 32–42. doi: 10.1002/da.22678

Domschke, K., Winter, B., Gajewska, A., Unterecker, S., Warrings, B., Dlugos, A., et al. (2015). Multilevel impact of the dopamine system on the emotion-potentiated startle reflex. *Psychopharmacology* 232, 1983–1993. doi: 10.1007/s00213-014-3830-9

Dragan, W. L., and Oniszczenko, W. (2009). The association between dopamine D4 receptor exon III polymorphism and intensity of PTSD symptoms among flood survivors. *Anxiety Stress Coping* 22, 483–495. doi: 10.1080/10615800802419407

Drury, S. S., Theall, K. P., Keats, B. J., and Scheeringa, M. (2009). The role of the dopamine transporter (DAT) in the development of PTSD in preschool children. *J. Trauma. Stress* 22, 534–539. doi: 10.1002/jts.20475

Eban-Rothschild, A., Rothschild, G., Giardino, W. J., Jones, J. R., and De Lecea, L. (2016). VTA dopaminergic neurons regulate ethologically relevant sleep-wake behaviors. *Nat. Neurosci.* 19, 1356–1366. doi: 10.1038/nn.4377

Elman, I., Ariely, D., Mazar, N., Aharon, I., Lasko, N. B., Macklin, M. L., et al. (2005). Probing reward function in post-traumatic stress disorder with beautiful facial images. *Psychiatry Res.* 135, 179–183. doi: 10.1016/j.psychres.2005.04.002

Enman, N. M., Arthur, K., Ward, S. J., Perrine, S. A., and Unterwald, E. M. (2015). Anhedonia, reduced cocaine reward, and dopamine dysfunction in a rat model of posttraumatic stress disorder. *Biol. Psychiatry* 78, 871–879. doi: 10.1016/j.biopsych.2015.04.024

Everitt, B. J., Giuliano, C., and Belin, D. (2018). Addictive behaviour in experimental animals: prospects for translation. *Philos. Trans. R. Soc. Lond. B Biol. Sci.* 373:20170027. doi: 10.1098/rstb.2017.0027

Feder, A., Parides, M. K., Murrough, J. W., Perez, A. M., Morgan, J. E., Saxena, S., et al. (2014). Efficacy of intravenous ketamine for treatment of chronic posttraumatic stress disorder: a randomized clinical trial. *JAMA Psychiatry* 71, 681–688. doi: 10.1001/jamapsychiatry.2014.62

Fenster, R. J., Lebois, L. A. M., Ressler, K. J., and Suh, J. (2018). Brain circuit dysfunction in post-traumatic stress disorder: from mouse to man. *Nat. Rev. Neurosci.* 19, 535–551. doi: 10.1038/s41583-018-0039-7

Fidelman, S., Mizrachi Zer-Aviv, T., Lange, R., Hillard, C. J., and Akirav, I. (2018). Chronic treatment with URB597 ameliorates post-stress symptoms in a rat model of PTSD. *Eur. Neuropsychopharmacol.* 28, 630–642. doi: 10.1016/j.euroneuro.2018.02.004

Flory, J. D., and Yehuda, R. (2015). Comorbidity between post-traumatic stress disorder and major depressive disorder: alternative explanations and treatment considerations. *Dialogues Clin. Neurosci.* 17, 141–150.

Friedman, A. K., Walsh, J. J., Juarez, B., Ku, S. M., Chaudhury, D., Wang, J., et al. (2014). Enhancing depression mechanisms in midbrain dopamine neurons achieves homeostatic resilience. *Science* 344, 313–319. doi: 10.1126/science.1249240

Gerlicher, A. M. V., Tuscher, O., and Kalisch, R. (2018). Dopamine-dependent prefrontal reactivations explain long-term benefit of fear extinction. *Nat. Commun.* 9:4294. doi: 10.1038/s41467-018-06785-y

Girgenti, M. J., Hare, B. D., Ghosal, S., and Duman, R. S. (2017). Molecular and cellular effects of traumatic stress: implications for PTSD. *Curr. Psychiatry Rep.* 19:85. doi: 10.1007/s11920-017-0841-3

Groessl, F., Munsch, T., Meis, S., Griessner, J., Kaczanowska, J., Pliota, P., et al. (2018). Dorsal tegmental dopamine neurons gate associative learning of fear. *Nat. Neurosci.* 21, 952–962. doi: 10.1038/s41593-018-0174-5

Gutner, C. A., Gallagher, M. W., Baker, A. S., Sloan, D. M., and Resick, P. A. (2016). Time course of treatment dropout in cognitive-behavioral therapies for posttraumatic stress disorder. *Psychol. Trauma* 8, 115–121. doi: 10.1037/tra0000062

Haaker, J., Gaburro, S., Sah, A., Gartmann, N., Lonsdorf, T. B., Meier, K., et al. (2013). Single dose of L-dopa makes extinction memories context-independent and prevents the return of fear. *Proc. Natl. Acad. Sci. U.S.A.* 110, E2428–E2436. doi: 10.1073/pnas.1303061110

Halberstadt, A. L., and Geyer, M. A. (2009). Habituation and sensitization of acoustic startle: opposite influences of dopamine D1 and D2-family receptors. *Neurobiol. Learn. Mem.* 92, 243–248. doi: 10.1016/j.nlm.2008.05.015

Hauer, D., Schelling, G., Gola, H., Campolongo, P., Morath, J., Roozendaal, B., et al. (2013). Plasma concentrations of endocannabinoids and related primary fatty acid amides in patients with post-traumatic stress disorder. *PLoS One* 7:e62741. doi: 10.1371/journal.pone.0062741

Havelka Mestrovic, A., Tudor, L., Nikolac Perkovic, M., Nedic Erjavec, G., Kovacic Petrovic, Z., Svob Strac, D., et al. (2018). Significant association between catechol-O-methyltransferase (COMT) Val(158/108)Met polymorphism and cognitive function in veterans with PTSD. *Neurosci. Lett.* 666, 38–43. doi: 10.1016/j.neulet.2017.12.033

Hayes, J. P., Logue, M. W., Reagan, A., Salat, D., Wolf, E. J., Sadeh, N., et al. (2017). COMT Val158Met polymorphism moderates the association between PTSD symptom severity and hippocampal volume. *J. Psychiatry Neurosci.* 42, 95–102. doi: 10.1503/jpn.150339

Hayes, J. P., Vanelzakker, M. B., and Shin, L. M. (2012). Emotion and cognition interactions in PTSD: a review of neurocognitive and neuroimaging studies. *Front. Integr. Neurosci.* 6:89. doi: 10.3389/fnint.2012.00089

Heinz, A., Goldman, D., Jones, D. W., Palmour, R., Hommer, D., Gorey, J. G., et al. (2000). Genotype influences in vivo dopamine transporter availability in human striatum. *Neuropsychopharmacology* 22, 133–139. doi: 10.1016/s0893-133x(99)00099-8

Hikind, N., and Maroun, M. (2008). Microinfusion of the D1 receptor antagonist, SCH23390 into the IL but not the BLA impairs consolidation of extinction of auditory fear conditioning. *Neurobiol. Learn. Mem.* 90, 217–222. doi: 10.1016/j.nlm.2008.03.003

Hill, M. N., Bierer, L. M., Makotkine, I., Golier, J. A., Galea, S., McEwen, B. S., et al. (2013). Reductions in circulating endocannabinoid levels in individuals with post-traumatic stress disorder following exposure to the World Trade Center attacks. *Psychoneuroendocrinology* 38, 2952–2961. doi: 10.1016/j.psyneuen.2013.08.004

Hill, M. N., Campolongo, P., Yehuda, R., and Patel, S. (2018). Integrating endocannabinoid signaling and cannabinoids into the biology and treatment of posttraumatic stress disorder. *Neuropsychopharmacology* 43, 80–102. doi: 10.1038/npp.2017.162

Hillarp, N. A., Fuxe, K., and Dahlstrom, A. (1966). Demonstration and mapping of central neurons containing dopamine, noradrenaline, and 5-hydroxytryptamine and their reactions to psychopharmaca. *Pharmacol. Rev.* 18, 727–741.

Hitora-Imamura, N., Miura, Y., Teshirogi, C., Ikegaya, Y., Matsuki, N., and Nomura, H. (2015). Prefrontal dopamine regulates fear reinstatement through the downregulation of extinction circuits. *eLife* 4:e08274. doi: 10.7554/eLife.08274

Hoexter, M. Q., Fadel, G., Felicio, A. C., Calzavara, M. B., Batista, I. R., Reis, M. A., et al. (2012). Higher striatal dopamine transporter density in PTSD: an in vivo SPECT study with [(99m)Tc]TRODAT-1. *Psychopharmacology* 224, 337–345. doi: 10.1007/s00213-012-2755-4

Houlihan, D. J. (2011). Psychostimulant treatment of combat-related posttraumatic stress disorder. *J. Psychopharmacol.* 25, 1568–1572. doi: 10.1177/0269881110385600

Kaenmaki, M., Tammimaki, A., Myohanen, T., Pakarinen, K., Amberg, C., Karayiorgou, M., et al. (2010). Quantitative role of COMT in dopamine clearance in the prefrontal cortex of freely moving mice. *J. Neurochem.* 114, 1745–1755. doi: 10.1111/j.1471-4159.2010.06889.x

Kayser, A. S., Allen, D. C., Navarro-Cebrian, A., Mitchell, J. M., and Fields, H. L. (2012). Dopamine, corticostriatal connectivity, and intertemporal choice. *J. Neurosci.* 32, 9402–9409. doi: 10.1523/JNEUROSCI.1180-12.2012

Keedwell, P. A., Andrew, C., Williams, S. C., Brammer, M. J., and Phillips, M. L. (2005). The neural correlates of anhedonia in major depressive disorder. *Biol. Psychiatry* 58, 843–853. doi: 10.1016/j.biopsych.2005.05.019

Kegeles, L. S., Abi-Dargham, A., Zea-Ponce, Y., Rodenhiser-Hill, J., Mann, J. J., Van Heertum, R. L., et al. (2000). Modulation of amphetamine-induced striatal dopamine release by ketamine in humans: implications for schizophrenia. *Biol. Psychiatry* 48, 627–640. doi: 10.1016/s0006-3223(00)00976-8

Kolassa, I. T., Kolassa, S., Ertl, V., Papassotiropoulos, A., and De Quervain, D. J. (2010). The risk of posttraumatic stress disorder after trauma depends on traumatic load and the catechol-o-methyltransferase Val(158)Met polymorphism. *Biol. Psychiatry* 67, 304–308. doi: 10.1016/j.biopsych.2009.10.009

Krystal, J. H., Rosenheck, R. A., Cramer, J. A., Vessicchio, J. C., Jones, K. M., Vertrees, J. E., et al. (2011). Adjunctive risperidone treatment for antidepressant-resistant symptoms of chronic military service-related PTSD: a randomized trial. *JAMA* 306, 493–502. doi: 10.1001/jama.2011.1080

Lanius, R. A., Vermetten, E., Loewenstein, R. J., Brand, B., Schmahl, C., Bremner, J. D., et al. (2010). Emotion modulation in PTSD: clinical and neurobiological evidence for a dissociative subtype. *Am. J. Psychiatry* 167, 640–647. doi: 10.1176/appi.ajp.2009.09081168

LeBlanc, K. H., London, T. D., Szczot, I., Bocarsly, M. E., Friend, D. M., Nguyen, K. P., et al. (2018). Striatopallidal neurons control avoidance behavior in exploratory tasks. *Mol. Psychiatry*

Leggio, G. M., Bucolo, C., Platania, C. B., Salomone, S., and Drago, F. (2016). Current drug treatments targeting dopamine D3 receptor. *Pharmacol. Ther.* 165, 164–177. doi: 10.1016/j.pharmthera.2016.06.007

Lena, I., Parrot, S., Deschaux, O., Muffat-Joly, S., Sauvinet, V., Renaud, B., et al. (2005). Variations in extracellular levels of dopamine, noradrenaline, glutamate, and aspartate across the sleep–wake cycle in the medial prefrontal cortex and nucleus accumbens of freely moving rats. *J. Neurosci. Res.* 81, 891–899. doi: 10.1002/jnr.20602

Lin, C. C., Chang, H. A., Tai, Y. M., Chen, T. Y., Wan, F. J., Chang, C. C., et al. (2019). Subchronic administration of aripiprazole improves fear extinction retrieval of Pavlovian conditioning paradigm in rats experiencing psychological trauma. *Behav. Brain Res.* 362, 181–187. doi: 10.1016/j.bbr.2018.12.051

Lindefors, N., Barati, S., and O'connor, W. T. (1997). Differential effects of single and repeated ketamine administration on dopamine, serotonin and GABA transmission in rat medial prefrontal cortex. *Brain Res.* 759, 205–212. doi: 10.1016/s0006-8993(97)00255-2

Loiseau, F., and Millan, M. J. (2009). Blockade of dopamine D(3) receptors in frontal cortex, but not in sub-cortical structures, enhances social recognition in rats: similar actions of D(1) receptor agonists, but not of D(2) antagonists. *Eur. Neuropsychopharmacol.* 19, 23–33. doi: 10.1016/j.euroneuro.2008.07.012

Lonsdorf, T. B., Ruck, C., Bergstrom, J., Andersson, G., Ohman, A., Lindefors, N., et al. (2010). The COMTval158met polymorphism is associated with symptom relief during exposure-based cognitive-behavioral treatment in panic disorder. *BMC Psychiatry* 10:99. doi: 10.1186/1471-244X-10-99

Lonsdorf, T. B., Weike, A. I., Nikamo, P., Schalling, M., Hamm, A. O., and Ohman, A. (2009). Genetic gating of human fear learning and extinction: possible implications for gene-environment interaction in anxiety disorder. *Psychol. Sci.* 20, 198–206. doi: 10.1111/j.1467-9280.2009.02280.x

Lu, J., Jhou, T. C., and Saper, C. B. (2006). Identification of wake-active dopaminergic neurons in the ventral periaqueductal gray matter. *J. Neurosci.* 26, 193–202. doi: 10.1523/jneurosci.2244-05.2006

Matsumoto, M., Weickert, C. S., Akil, M., Lipska, B. K., Hyde, T. M., Herman, M. M., et al. (2003). Catechol O-methyltransferase mRNA expression in human and rat brain: evidence for a role in cortical neuronal function. *Neuroscience* 116, 127–137. doi: 10.1016/s0306-4522(02)00556-0

Matthews, G. A., Nieh, E. H., Vander Weele, C. M., Halbert, S. A., Pradhan, R. V., Yosafat, A. S., et al. (2016). Dorsal raphe dopamine neurons represent the experience of social isolation. *Cell* 164, 617–631. doi: 10.1016/j.cell.2015.12.040

Meloni, E. G., and Davis, M. (2000). Synergistic enhancement of the acoustic startle reflex by dopamine D1 and 5-HT1A agonists and corresponding changes in c-Fos expression in the dorsal raphe of rats. *Psychopharmacology* 151, 359–367. doi: 10.1007/s002130000474

Menegas, W., Akiti, K., Amo, R., Uchida, N., and Watabe-Uchida, M. (2018). Dopamine neurons projecting to the posterior striatum reinforce avoidance of threatening stimuli. *Nat. Neurosci.* 21, 1421–1430. doi: 10.1038/s41593-018-0222-1

Meyer, J. H., Kruger, S., Wilson, A. A., Christensen, B. K., Goulding, V. S., Schaffer, A., et al. (2001). Lower dopamine transporter binding potential in striatum during depression. *Neuroreport* 12, 4121–4125. doi: 10.1097/00001756-200112210-00052

Michelhaugh, S. K., Fiskerstrand, C., Lovejoy, E., Bannon, M. J., and Quinn, J. P. (2001). The dopamine transporter gene (SLC6A3) variable number of tandem repeats domain enhances transcription in dopamine neurons. *J. Neurochem.* 79, 1033–1038. doi: 10.1046/j.1471-4159.2001.00647.x

Milad, M. R., Pitman, R. K., Ellis, C. B., Gold, A. L., Shin, L. M., Lasko, N. B., et al. (2009). Neurobiological basis of failure to recall extinction memory in posttraumatic stress disorder. *Biol. Psychiatry* 66, 1075–1082. doi: 10.1016/j.biopsych.2009.06.026

Millan, M. J., Di Cara, B., Dekeyne, A., Panayi, F., De Groote, L., Sicard, D., et al. (2007). Selective blockade of dopamine D(3) versus D(2) receptors enhances frontocortical cholinergic transmission and social memory in rats: a parallel neurochemical and behavioural analysis. *J. Neurochem.* 100, 1047–1061. doi: 10.1111/j.1471-4159.2006.04262.x

Monti, J. M., and Monti, D. (2007). The involvement of dopamine in the modulation of sleep and waking. *Sleep Med. Rev.* 11, 113–133. doi: 10.1016/j.smrv.2006.08.003

Morena, M., Berardi, A., Colucci, P., Palmery, M., Trezza, V., Hill, M. N., et al. (2018). Enhancing endocannabinoid neurotransmission augments the efficacy of extinction training and ameliorates traumatic stress-induced behavioral alterations in rats. *Neuropsychopharmacology* 43, 1284–1296. doi: 10.1038/npp.2017.305

Morena, M., Berardi, A., Peloso, A., Valeri, D., Palmery, M., Trezza, V., et al. (2017). Effects of ketamine, dexmedetomidine and propofol anesthesia on emotional memory consolidation in rats: consequences for the development of post-traumatic stress disorder. *Behav. Brain Res.* 329, 215–220. doi: 10.1016/j.bbr.2017.04.048

Mueller, D., Bravo-Rivera, C., and Quirk, G. J. (2010). Infralimbic D2 receptors are necessary for fear extinction and extinction-related tone responses. *Biol. Psychiatry* 68, 1055–1060. doi: 10.1016/j.biopsych.2010.08.014

Naegeli, C., Zeffiro, T., Piccirelli, M., Jaillard, A., Weilenmann, A., Hassanpour, K., et al. (2018). Locus coeruleus activity mediates hyperresponsiveness in posttraumatic stress disorder. *Biol. Psychiatry* 83, 254–262. doi: 10.1016/j.biopsych.2017.08.021

Nakajima, S., Gerretsen, P., Takeuchi, H., Caravaggio, F., Chow, T., Le Foll, B., et al. (2013). The potential role of dopamine D(3) receptor neurotransmission in cognition. *Eur. Neuropsychopharmacol.* 23, 799–813. doi: 10.1016/j.euroneuro.2013.05.006

Naylor, J. C., Li, Q., Kang-Park, M. H., Wilson, W. A., Kuhn, C., and Moore, S. D. (2010). Dopamine attenuates evoked inhibitory synaptic currents in central amygdala neurons. *Eur. J. Neurosci.* 32, 1836–1842. doi: 10.1111/j.1460-9568.2010.07457.x

Norrholm, S. D., Jovanovic, T., Smith, A. K., Binder, E., Klengel, T., Conneely, K., et al. (2013). Differential genetic and epigenetic regulation of catechol-O-methyltransferase is associated with impaired fear inhibition in posttraumatic stress disorder. *Front. Behav. Neurosci.* 7:30. doi: 10.3389/fnbeh.2013.00030

Pascucci, T., Ventura, R., Latagliata, E. C., Cabib, S., and Puglisi-Allegra, S. (2007). The medial prefrontal cortex determines the accumbens dopamine response to stress through the opposing influences of norepinephrine and dopamine. *Cereb. Cortex* 17, 2796–2804. doi: 10.1093/cercor/bhm008

Pessiglione, M., Schmidt, L., Draganski, B., Kalisch, R., Lau, H., Dolan, R. J., et al. (2007). How the brain translates money into force: a neuroimaging study of subliminal motivation. *Science* 316, 904–906. doi: 10.1126/science.1140459

Pessiglione, M., Seymour, B., Flandin, G., Dolan, R. J., and Frith, C. D. (2006). Dopamine-dependent prediction errors underpin reward-seeking behaviour in humans. *Nature* 442, 1042–1045. doi: 10.1038/nature05051

Phelps, E. A., Delgado, M. R., Nearing, K. I., and Ledoux, J. E. (2004). Extinction learning in humans: role of the amygdala and vmPFC. *Neuron* 43, 897–905.

Pruessner, J. C., Champagne, F., Meaney, M. J., and Dagher, A. (2004). Dopamine release in response to a psychological stress in humans and its relationship to early life maternal care: a positron emission tomography study using [11C]raclopride. *J. Neurosci.* 24, 2825–2831. doi: 10.1523/jneurosci.3422-03.2004

Radford, K. D., Park, T. Y., Jaiswal, S., Pan, H., Knutsen, A., Zhang, M., et al. (2018). Enhanced fear memories and brain glucose metabolism (18F-FDG-PET) following sub-anesthetic intravenous ketamine infusion in Sprague-Dawley rats. *Transl. Psychiatry* 8:263. doi: 10.1038/s41398-018-0310-8

Sailer, U., Robinson, S., Fischmeister, F. P., Konig, D., Oppenauer, C., Lueger-Schuster, B., et al. (2008). Altered reward processing in the nucleus accumbens and mesial prefrontal cortex of patients with posttraumatic stress disorder. *Neuropsychologia* 46, 2836–2844. doi: 10.1016/j.neuropsychologia.2008.05.022

Schell, T. L., Marshall, G. N., and Jaycox, L. H. (2004). All symptoms are not created equal: the prominent role of hyperarousal in the natural course of posttraumatic psychological distress. *J. Abnorm. Psychol.* 113, 189–197. doi: 10.1037/0021-843x.113.2.189

Schultz, W. (1999). The reward signal of midbrain dopamine neurons. *News Physiol. Sci.* 14, 249–255. doi: 10.1152/physiologyonline.1999.14.6.249

Schultz, W. (2007). Behavioral dopamine signals. *Trends Neurosci.* 30, 203–210. doi: 10.1016/j.tins.2007.03.007

Schulz-Heik, R. J., Schaer, M., Eliez, S., Hallmayer, J. F., Lin, X., Kaloupek, D. G., et al. (2011). Catechol-O-methyltransferase Val158Met polymorphism moderates anterior cingulate volume in posttraumatic stress disorder. *Biol. Psychiatry* 70, 1091–1096. doi: 10.1016/j.biopsych.2011.06.012

Segman, R. H., Cooper-Kazaz, R., Macciardi, F., Goltser, T., Halfon, Y., Dobroborski, T., et al. (2002). Association between the dopamine transporter gene and posttraumatic stress disorder. *Mol. Psychiatry* 7, 903–907. doi: 10.1038/sj.mp.4001085

Shalev, A., Liberzon, I., and Marmar, C. (2017). Post-traumatic stress disorder. *N. Engl. J. Med.* 376, 2459–2469.

Song, D., Ge, Y., Chen, Z., Shang, C., Guo, Y., Zhao, T., et al. (2018). Role of dopamine D3 receptor in alleviating behavioural deficits in animal models of post-traumatic stress disorder. *Prog. Neuropsychopharmacol. Biol. Psychiatry* 84, 190–200. doi: 10.1016/j.pnpbp.2018.03.001

Sripada, R. K., Garfinkel, S. N., and Liberzon, I. (2013). Avoidant symptoms in PTSD predict fear circuit activation during multimodal fear extinction. *Front. Hum. Neurosci.* 7:672. doi: 10.3389/fnhum.2013.00672

Steckler, T., and Risbrough, V. (2012). Pharmacological treatment of PTSD - established and new approaches. *Neuropharmacology* 62, 617–627. doi: 10.1016/j.neuropharm.2011.06.012

Stein, M. B., and Paulus, M. P. (2009). Imbalance of approach and avoidance: the yin and yang of anxiety disorders. *Biol. Psychiatry* 66, 1072–1074. doi: 10.1016/j.biopsych.2009.09.023

Stevens, J. S., Jovanovic, T., Fani, N., Ely, T. D., Glover, E. M., Bradley, B., et al. (2013). Disrupted amygdala-prefrontal functional connectivity in civilian women with posttraumatic stress disorder. *J. Psychiatr. Res.* 47, 1469–1478. doi: 10.1016/j.jpsychires.2013.05.031

Taylor, N. E., Van Dort, C. J., Kenny, J. D., Pei, J., Guidera, J. A., Vlasov, K. Y., et al. (2016). Optogenetic activation of dopamine neurons in the ventral tegmental area induces reanimation from general anesthesia. *Proc. Natl. Acad. Sci. U.S.A.* 113, 12826–12831. doi: 10.1073/pnas.1614340113

Torrisi, S. A., Salomone, S., Geraci, F., Caraci, F., Bucolo, C., Drago, F., et al. (2017). Buspirone counteracts MK-801-induced schizophrenia-like phenotypes through dopamine D3 receptor blockade. *Front. Pharmacol.* 8:710. doi: 10.3389/fphar.2017.00710

van de Giessen, E., De Win, M. M., Tanck, M. W., Van Den Brink, W., Baas, F., and Booij, J. (2009). Striatal dopamine transporter availability associated with polymorphisms in the dopamine transporter gene SLC6A3. *J. Nucl. Med.* 50, 45–52. doi: 10.2967/jnumed.108.053652

Vander Weele, C. M., Siciliano, C. A., Matthews, G. A., Namburi, P., Izadmehr, E. M., Espinel, I. C., et al. (2018). Dopamine enhances signal-to-noise ratio in cortical-brainstem encoding of aversive stimuli. *Nature* 563, 397–401. doi: 10.1038/s41586-018-0682-1

Volkow, N. D. (2006). Stimulant medications: how to minimize their reinforcing effects? *Am. J. Psychiatry* 163, 359–361. doi: 10.1176/appi.ajp.163.3.359

Wenzel, J. M., Oleson, E. B., Gove, W. N., Cole, A. B., Gyawali, U., Dantrassy, H. M., et al. (2018). Phasic dopamine signals in the nucleus accumbens that cause active avoidance require endocannabinoid mobilization in the midbrain. *Curr. Biol.* 28, 1392–1404.e5. doi: 10.1016/j.cub.2018.03.037

Weston, C. S. (2014). Posttraumatic stress disorder: a theoretical model of the hyperarousal subtype. *Front. Psychiatry* 5:37. doi: 10.3389/fpsyt.2014.00037

Whittle, N., Maurer, V., Murphy, C., Rainer, J., Bindreither, D., Hauschild, M., et al. (2016). Enhancing dopaminergic signaling and histone acetylation promotes long-term rescue of deficient fear extinction. *Transl. Psychiatry* 6:e974. doi: 10.1038/tp.2016.231

Wolf, E. J., Mitchell, K. S., Logue, M. W., Baldwin, C. T., Reardon, A. F., Aiello, A., et al. (2014). The dopamine D3 receptor gene and posttraumatic stress disorder. *J. Trauma. Stress* 27, 379–387. doi: 10.1002/jts.21937

Yamamoto, B. K., and Novotney, S. (1998). Regulation of extracellular dopamine by the norepinephrine transporter. *J. Neurochem.* 71, 274–280. doi: 10.1046/j.1471-4159.1998.71010274.x

Yehuda, R., Southwick, S., Giller, E. L., Ma, X., and Mason, J. W. (1992). Urinary catecholamine excretion and severity of PTSD symptoms in Vietnam combat veterans. *J. Nerv. Ment. Dis.* 180, 321–325. doi: 10.1097/00005053-199205000-00006

Yu, Q., Teixeira, C. M., Mahadevia, D., Huang, Y., Balsam, D., Mann, J. J., et al. (2014). Dopamine and serotonin signaling during two sensitive developmental periods differentially impact adult aggressive and affective behaviors in mice. *Mol. Psychiatry* 19, 688–698. doi: 10.1038/mp.2014.10

2

Harnessing Microglia and Macrophages for the Treatment of Glioblastoma

Ioanna Prionisti[1,2], Léo H. Bühler[1], Paul R. Walker[3†] and Renaud B. Jolivet[4,5†]*

[1] Division of Digestive and Transplantation Surgery, Geneva University Hospitals, Geneva, Switzerland, [2] Lemanic Neuroscience Doctoral School, Geneva, Switzerland, [3] Center for Translational Research in Onco-Hematology, Division of Oncology, Geneva University Hospitals – University of Geneva, Geneva, Switzerland, [4] Département de Physique Nucléaire et Corpusculaire (DPNC), University of Geneva, Geneva, Switzerland, [5] European Organization for Nuclear Research (CERN), Geneva, Switzerland

***Correspondence:**
Renaud B. Jolivet
renaud.jolivet@unige.ch

† These authors have contributed equally to this work

Glioblastoma multiforme (GBM) is the most malignant form of brain tumors, with a dismal prognosis. During the course of the disease, microglia and macrophages both infiltrate the tumor microenvironment and contribute considerably in glioma development. Thus, tumor-associated microglia and macrophages have recently emerged as potentially key therapeutic targets. Here, we review the physiology of microglia and their responses in brain cancer. We further discuss current treatment options for GBM using radiotherapy, and novel advances in our knowledge of microglia physiology, with emphasis on the recently discovered pathway that controls the baseline motility of microglia processes. We argue that the latter pathway is an interesting therapeutic avenue to pursue for the treatment of glioblastoma.

Keywords: macrophage, microglia, two-pore domain K^+ channels, glioblastoma, cancer

INTRODUCTION

As the resident immune cells of the Central Nervous System (CNS), microglia play key roles under both normal and pathological conditions. Microglia contribute to tissue homeostasis by actively surveying the brain, and by promoting the development of healthy neural networks by removing apoptotic cells, eliminating synapses and enhancing the production and survival of neuronal precursor cells (Wolf et al., 2017). However, when microglia are challenged, like for instance in the case of tumor formation, their immunological response can be strikingly suppressed, or maladapted (Kettenmann et al., 2011). Glioblastoma multiforme (GBM) is the most malignant form of primary brain tumor, characterized by significant infiltration of resident microglia and peripheral macrophages in the tumor, and by pervasive infiltration of tumor cells in the healthy surroundings of the tumor. Advances in our understanding of microglial physiology and in our understanding of the complex interactions between microglia and tumor cells in GBM can elucidate their role in glioma progression and indicate potentially interesting druggable targets. Here, we argue that the two-pore domain potassium channel THIK-1 (Tandem-pore domain Halothane-Inhibited K^+ channel; *Knck13*) might be such a target. THIK-1 was recently identified by some of us as a key "hub" mechanism regulating microglia ramification, baseline motility of processes and release of interleukin-1β (Madry et al., 2018; Kyrargyri et al., unpublished). In the following, we briefly review key aspects of microglia physiology before moving on to tumor-associated microglia and macrophages (TAMs). We then conclude by reviewing current and future treatment options for GBM, highlighting how targeting THIK-1 could be harnessed to complement these.

PHYSIOLOGY OF MICROGLIA

Microglia are the resident mononuclear macrophages of the CNS, and constitute ~5–20% of all glial cells in the CNS parenchyma (Saijo and Glass, 2011; Ginhoux et al., 2013; Sousa et al., 2017). These cells are heterogeneously distributed in non-overlapping regions throughout the brain and spinal cord (Lawson et al., 1990). In addition to parenchymal microglia, the CNS macrophage population includes non-parenchymal perivascular, meningeal and choroid plexus border-associated macrophages (BAMs) (Ransohoff and Cardona, 2010; Saijo and Glass, 2011; Goldmann et al., 2016; Mrdjen et al., 2018). The origin of microglia has been controversial since Pío del Río Hortega first introduced the concept of microglia and argued that these cells are of mesodermal origin and enter the brain during early development (Sierra et al., 2016). Recent studies have shown that microglia originate from primitive hematopoiesis in the fetal yolk sac and populate the brain during embryonic development (Ginhoux et al., 2010; Saijo and Glass, 2011; Prinz and Priller, 2014). Although microglia and brain macrophages were considered two ontogenetically distinct populations, new fate-mapping approaches have challenged this assumption (Prinz and Priller, 2014; Goldmann et al., 2016; Greter, 2016).

During development and in the adult brain, microglial cells play an important role, extensively interacting with neuronal circuits (Squarzoni et al., 2014; Miyamoto et al., 2016). They accommodate neuronal apoptosis, eliminate less active synaptic connections (synaptic pruning) and regulate neuronal activity (Paolicelli et al., 2011; Li et al., 2012). Interestingly, recent reports have indicated that microglia also promote synapse formation in the mature brain (Parkhurst et al., 2013; Miyamoto et al., 2016).

In the healthy adult CNS, microglia exhibit a not very aptly named "resting" phenotype, characterized by small cellular bodies from which thin ramified processes are extended. *In vivo* two-photon imaging studies have, however, demonstrated that these protrusions are highly motile, providing a kind of continuous surveillance of the extracellular space (Davalos et al., 2005; Nimmerjahn et al., 2005). Thus, microglia in their so-called "resting" state are not dormant, but instead actively scan their environment, ready to respond upon a threat on the CNS (Davalos et al., 2005; Kettenmann et al., 2011). The transition from the "resting" to the "activated" state under pathological conditions, such as inflammation or disease, implies not only functional but also morphological alterations. Highly "activated" microglia can take up an amoeboid shape, becoming morphologically indistinguishable from other macrophages (Boche et al., 2013). Depending on their state, microglia exhibit different types of motility (Kettenmann et al., 2011). Resting microglia survey the brain by constantly extending and retracting their ramified processes, without translocation of the cellular body (Nimmerjahn et al., 2005). Some of us have recently demonstrated that this baseline surveillance of the parenchyma by microglia is controlled by the two-pore domain potassium channel THIK-1 (see below) (Madry et al., 2018). The convergence of microglial processes toward a damaged area is triggered by "danger signals," like extracellular ATP and its derivatives, which target purinoreceptors of the P2Y family (Davalos et al., 2005; Burnstock and Verkhratsky, 2010). In particular, $P2Y_{12}$ receptors are highly expressed in resting microglia, but they are reduced after microglial activation (Haynes et al., 2006). The link between process outgrowth and ATP release is further reinforced by the observation that $P2Y_{12}$ proteins aggregate at the bulbous tips formed at the end of microglial branches upon ATP stimulation (Dissing-Olesen et al., 2014). In contrast with this baseline surveillance operated by resting, ramified, microglia, under pathological conditions, amoeboid microglia move in their entirety while migrating to the site of injury (Wolf et al., 2017).

In the diseased CNS, the blood brain barrier (BBB) is usually impaired, leading to an infiltration of peripheral macrophages (Hambardzumyan et al., 2016). Under tissue damage, macrophages can express two types of activation; the classical activation (M1) is a pro-inflammatory state, while the alternative activation (M2) is defined as the anti-inflammatory state. However, the concept of M1/M2 polarization is considered oversimplified in the case of microglia (Nakagawa and Chiba, 2014; Gabrusiewicz et al., 2016; Ransohoff, 2016; Broekman et al., 2018), with no clear dichotomy reported in GBM (Gabrusiewicz et al., 2016). Resident microglia express pattern recognition receptors (PRRs), which detect pathogen-associated molecular patterns (PAMPs), such as microbial pathogens, and damage-associated molecular patterns (DAMPs), like adenine nucleotides (ATP/ADP). PAMPs and DAMPs are though counteracted by glycans known as self-associated molecular patterns (SAMPs), which appear modified in tumor cells, inhibiting immune response in their surroundings (Rodriguez et al., 2018). The exploitation of glycans by cancer cells promotes immune suppression by controlling the differentiation of TAMs (Rodriguez et al., 2018). During an infection, the microglial immune response is mediated via several pathways, including transmembrane proteins known as Toll-like receptors (TLRs) (Lehnardt, 2010) and the cytoplasmic NOD-like receptors (NLRs). NLRP3 is a subset of the NLR family that, together with the adaptor protein ASC and Caspase-1, form the NLRP3 inflammasome (Walsh et al., 2014; Wolf et al., 2017). Activation of NLRP3, followed by activation of Caspase-1, results in the production and release of interleukin-1β (IL-1β) and interleukin-18 (IL-18) (Walsh et al., 2014; Wolf et al., 2017). High expression levels of NLRP3 in microglia (Zhang et al., 2014) and the contribution of IL-1β in the development and progression of malignant tumors (Voronov et al., 2003; Yuzhalin and Kutikhin, 2015) create new interesting directions for future cancer studies. Again, some of us have shown that NLRP3 activation and subsequent IL-1β release by microglia is also controlled by the same THIK-1-related pathway that controls baseline surveillance of the parenchyma by microglia (Madry et al., 2018).

A clear distinction between activated microglia and infiltrating macrophages is impeded due to their common myeloid lineage (Kettenmann et al., 2011). Nonetheless, several markers have been identified and are currently used to distinguish these two populations in the CNS. The ionized calcium-binding adaptor molecule 1 (Iba1) and the human fructose transporter 5 (GLUT5) are suggested as useful markers for both resting and activated microglia (Ito et al., 1998; Horikoshi et al., 2003; Sasaki, 2016).

Microglia, which are able to generate ATP by both glycolysis and oxidative phosphorylation, highly express GLUT5, which has a high affinity for fructose (Ghosh et al., 2018). However, since the brain shows low concentrations of fructose, the function of GLUT5 in microglia, and this is true in general for vast swaths of their metabolism, remains uncertain (Payne et al., 1997; Douard and Ferraris, 2008; Caruso et al., 2018). Moreover, the use of CD45 antibodies has shown low expression levels for resident microglia ($CD45^{low}$) and high expression levels for CNS macrophages ($CD45^{high}$) (Kettenmann et al., 2011), while CD49D was absent in microglia and can be used to distinguish them from CNS macrophages in mouse and human brain tumors (Bowman et al., 2016). Other microglia markers include the major histocompatibility complex (MHC) class II, the fractalkine receptor (CX_3CR1), and the recently identified Sall1, which can be used to discriminate parenchymal microglia from BAMs (Davalos et al., 2005; Buttgereit et al., 2016; Sasaki, 2016; Mrdjen et al., 2018).

Transcriptome analysis provides the tools to discriminate microglia not only from the peripheral macrophages, but also among the other cell populations of the nervous system (Gautier et al., 2012; Lavin et al., 2014; Zhang et al., 2014). Neurons, macroglia (astrocytes, oligodendrocytes) and vascular cells express no morphological resemblance with resting or activated microglia. However, gene expression profiles and immunophenotyping can provide insights into the functions of the different cell types of the CNS under normal and pathological conditions (Ginhoux et al., 2010; Gautier et al., 2012; Lavin et al., 2014; Zhang et al., 2014; Wieghofer et al., 2015). In particular, these genetic tools combined with imaging techniques can interpret the role of microglia and infiltrating macrophages in a number of diseases, such as brain cancer.

TUMOR-ASSOCIATED MICROGLIA AND MACROPHAGES IN GLIOBLASTOMA

While both resident microglia and macrophages are the main innate immune cells of the CNS, their role may be subverted in case of certain pathological insults. In brain cancer, these macrophage populations infiltrate the tumor area and can contribute to up to 50% of non-neoplastic cells, raising the possibility for new therapeutic strategies (Hambardzumyan et al., 2016). GBM (World Health Organization grade IV astrocytoma) is the most common type of malignant primary brain tumor, carrying a poor prognosis and high rate of recurrence (Louis et al., 2007) (**Figure 1**). It also contains cancer stem cells (CSCs), which contribute to tumor initiation and therapeutic resistance (Lathia et al., 2015). According to gene expression profiling based on data from The Cancer Genome Atlas (TCGA)[1], there are three molecular subtypes of GBM defined, including proneural, classical and mesenchymal (Verhaak et al., 2010; Sidaway, 2017). These subtypes are characterized by the patterns of alterations of the *EGFR*, *NF1*, *PDGFRA* and *IDH1* genes, in addition to their response to therapy (Crespo et al., 2015; Verhaak et al., 2010). However, phenotypic shifts are occurring upon treatment and relapse (Garnier et al., 2018). The implication of TAMs in several aspects of glioma development, including proliferation, angiogenesis and immunosuppression, contributes to the therapeutic resistance and the short survival rate of this malignant tumor (Schonberg et al., 2013; Hambardzumyan et al., 2016). Moreover, the gene-expression GBM subtype may be directly linked to microglia and TAM infiltration, with the mesenchymal subtype being associated with high infiltration, and even being driven by the presence of these infiltrating cells (Bhat et al., 2013; Wang et al., 2017). GBM is subdivided into primary GBM, which arises *de novo* without prior low-grade disease, and secondary GBM, deriving from previously detected low grade astrocytomas (Furnari et al., 2007). Genetic analysis of human GBM has shown frequent and diverse alterations in the *IDH1* gene among others, which lead to a reclassification of GBM as IDH-mutant or IDH-wild type, with IDH-mutant having better prognosis (Chin et al., 2008; Parsons et al., 2008; McFaline-Figueroa and Lee, 2018). IDH-mutant is further subdivided into two major types of glioma: astrocytoma (IDH-A) and oligodendroglioma (IDH-O), which differ genetically and histopathologically as shown by single-cell RNA sequencing analysis (Venteicher et al., 2017). Supplementary studies on genetic aberrations in GBM could provide more reliable diagnostic tools and patient-specific targeted therapies.

The recruitment of microglia and peripheral macrophages in the surroundings of the tumor is controlled via the release of several chemoattractants, including fractalkine (CX3CL1) whose receptor, CX3CR1, is mostly expressed by microglia in adults (Hambardzumyan et al., 2016). Chemoattraction by osteopontin was also recently reported in GBM, binding to macrophage-expressed integrin $\alpha v\beta 5$ (Wei et al., 2019). Upon accumulation to the glioma site, the functions of both microglia and macrophages are subverted and they can amplify tumor-mediated immunosuppression and promote tumor invasiveness (Reardon et al., 2017) (**Figure 2**). The expression of matrix metalloproteinases (MMPs), which degrade the extracellular matrix in the glioma microenvironment is associated with higher glioma invasion and angiogenesis (Poon et al., 2017). Notably, the activation of the CX3CL1/CX3CR1 system has been indicated to upregulate the expression of the gelatinases (MMP2, MMP9) and the membrane- associated MT1-MMP (or MMP14) (Held-Feindt et al., 2010). Further studies have highlighted the increased expression of MMP9 and MT1-MMP in TAMs via TLR2 signaling and p38 mitogen-activated protein kinase (MAPK) pathway (Charles et al., 2011; Vinnakota et al., 2013; Hu et al., 2014). TAMs release several anti-inflammatory factors such as transforming growth factor beta (TGF-β) and vascular endothelial growth factor (VEGF), that promote immune suppression and tumor angiogenesis (Watters et al., 2005). Results derived from the study of glioma stem-like cells (GSLCs) indicated that their invasiveness is enhanced following the release of TGF-β1 from TAMs, which increases MMP9 expression (Ye et al., 2012). Microglial MMP9 is suggested to promote glioma motility and enhance angiogenesis via VEGF regulation (Lee et al., 2005; Coniglio and Segall, 2013; Hu et al., 2014). Epidermal growth factor (EGF) and colony-stimulating

[1] http://cancergenome.nih.gov/

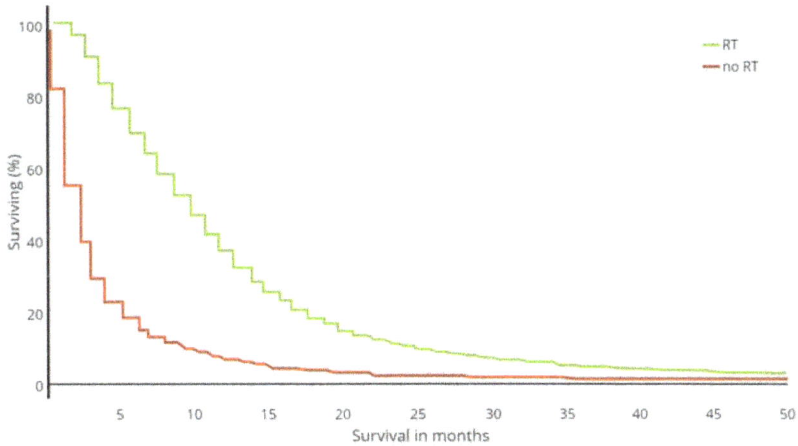

FIGURE 1 | Kaplan–Meier plot. Survival analysis of 21,783 GBM patients treated with radiotherapy (RT) versus no RT (1973–2007) [adapted from Zinn et al. (2013)].

factor-1 (CSF-1) have also been implicated in TAM glioma crosstalk. The microglial-released EGF increases tumor invasion by activating its receptors on GBM cells, while CSF-1 secreted by glioma acts as a chemoattractant for TAMs (Coniglio et al., 2012). Indeed, it was shown that CSF-1R inhibition alters macrophage polarization and blocks proneural glioma progression (Pyonteck et al., 2013; Quail et al., 2016). IL-1β is an isoform of the IL-1 cytokine superfamily secreted mainly by immune cells, including TAMs, while its receptor (IL-1R) has been found in glioma cells (Sasaki et al., 1998). Several studies have demonstrated that IL-1β is able to activate both MMP9 and VEGF, thus stimulating tumor invasiveness and angiogenesis (Sasaki et al., 1998; Voronov et al., 2003; Yuzhalin and Kutikhin, 2015). Moreover, IL-1β production has been shown to increase the expression of other cytokines in glioma microenvironment, such as IL-6 and IL-8, which also have crucial role in tumor development (Yeung et al., 2013). Microglial release of IL-1β can also be driven by the neuropeptide substance P (SP), which is expressed in both microglia and glioma cells, along with its receptor NK-1 (Rasley et al., 2002; Watters et al., 2005; Cordier et al., 2014). In the brain, microglia are the main source of IL-1β and the main K^+ channel they express at rest (THIK-1) plays an important role in IL-1β production (Madry et al., 2018), suggesting a potential role for this channel in GBM progression.

RADIOTHERAPY AND NEW APPROACHES IN GLIOBLASTOMA TREATMENT

The standard treatment for GBM is surgery, followed by adjuvant radiotherapy and chemotherapy. However, none of these treatments, alone or in combination, are effective enough to increase the median survival of 15 months. The use of ionizing radiation encounters considerable challenges in cancer treatment by the need to deliver sufficient energy to the tumor area without damaging the surrounding healthy tissue (Zhao et al., 2016). Furthermore, the antitumor effects of radiotherapy in tumor microenvironment are still controversial (Vatner and Formenti, 2015). It has been demonstrated that the recruitment of TAMs in glioma site is enhanced in response to radiotherapy (Vatner and Formenti, 2015). There is also a correlation between the presence of M2 glioma infiltrating macrophages and radiotherapy resistance (Wang et al., 2018). Glioma stem cells (GSCs) under temozolomide (TMZ) chemoradiation have been found to evolve from a TMZ-sensitive to a TMZ-resistant state (Garnier et al., 2018). Studies in prostate cancer indicated that the recruitment of myeloid cells results from the higher expression of CSF-1 in tumor cells following radiation (Xu et al., 2013). In addition, high doses of ionizing radiation upregulate the pro-inflammatory cytokines IL-1β and IL-6 (Betlazar et al., 2016). Despite the challenges, radiation therapy continues to be used for the treatment of malignant tumors. The efficacy of the treatment has been significantly enhanced with the development of image-guided techniques and the use of nanoparticle carriers as theranostic agents (Phillips et al., 2014).

In radiation therapy - external, internal and systemic - tumor cells are bombarded with ionizing radiation, such as α- and β-emitting radionuclides, X-rays, γ rays and Auger emitters. External beam radiotherapy (EBRT) has been the benchmark for radiation therapy for the last decades, delivering high energy X-rays from outside the body (Zhao et al., 2016). In stereotactic radiosurgery (SRS), a focused high radiation dose targets a well-defined tumor area, hence minimizing the effect of radiation in healthy tissue (Barani and Larson, 2015). Hadrontherapy is a form of radiotherapy that uses charged particles, such as protons and other ions, to irradiate the tumor. The use of particles instead of X-rays allows the precise definition of the tumor area, while minimizing the damage to the surrounding healthy tissue (Orecchia et al., 1998). In systemic radiation therapy, the radioactive sources are either ingested, infused or intravenously delivered (Zhang et al., 2010). Brachytherapy is a form of internal radiation where radioisotopes are placed inside or next to the tumor via craniotomy or stereotactic techniques (Vitaz et al., 2005). Image-guidance, such as positron emission tomography (PET) and single photon emission computed tomography

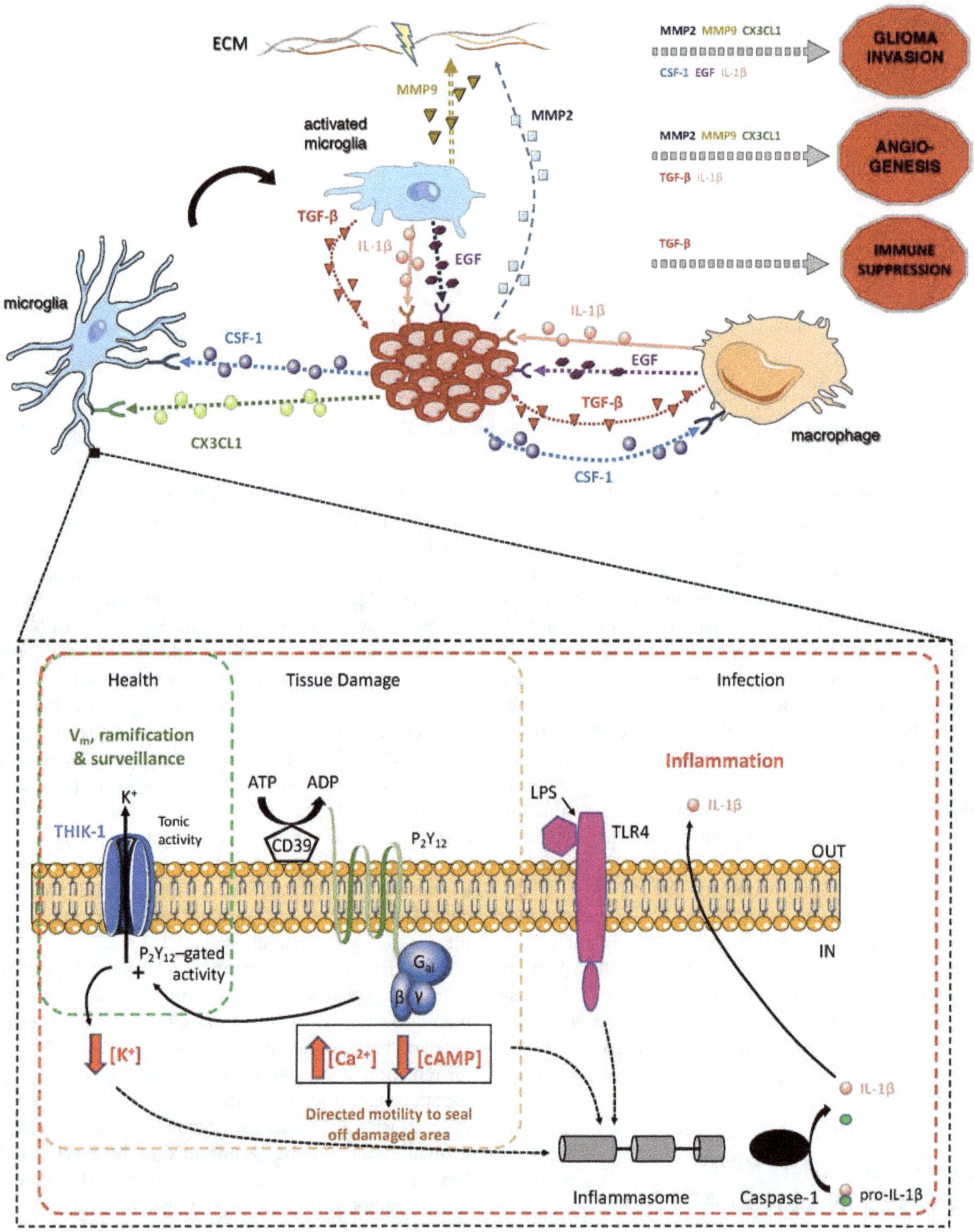

FIGURE 2 | Summary of the main pathways through which TAMs and glioma cells interact, and summary of the main pathways in microglia in which the two-pore domain potassium channel THIK-1 is involved [that second part adapted from Madry et al. (2018)].

(SPECT), is often used in combination with brachytherapy to monitor the tumor area and direct the nanoparticles accordingly (Phillips et al., 2014).

Nanoparticles have been a significant boost in glioma diagnosis and treatment (Glaser et al., 2017). The ability of nanoparticles to be conjugated with biological molecules or other receptor ligands potentiate their affinity to the tumor microenvironment and the delivery of tumor-targeted radioisotopes. Since the cellular expression between normal and tumor cells differs, the engineering of nanoparticles with molecules that target highly expressed tumor receptors is a promising area of nanomedicine research (Hernandez-Pedro et al., 2013). Both glioma cells and TAMs have become targets of radionuclide carriers but without any promising outcome so far. On the other hand, labeling nanoparticles with substance P (SP) antagonist is a promising method, though it will require further investigations (Cordier et al., 2014). Further research is also needed to determine the appropriate radioisotopes for each tumor type radiotherapy, also taking into account the chemical and physical properties of the selected isotope. It has been speculated that the recruitment of TAMs by tumor cells could be a potential approach for drug delivery (Phillips et al., 2014; Poon et al., 2017).

Immunotherapies and immunotherapy combinations have lately emerged as having the potential to offer benefit in brain cancer (Dutoit et al., 2016; Reardon et al., 2017). There are also 4 types of gene therapy currently being studied for GBM treatment by targeting the tumor area with minimum effects in the surrounding healthy tissue; suicide genes, immunomodulatory genes, tumor-suppressor genes and oncolytic virotherapy (Kane et al., 2015). Oncolytic viruses (OVs) can be engineered for tumor cell specificity and injected directly into the glioma site during surgery (Lawler et al., 2017). Several clinical studies for GBM and recurrent GBM tested oncolytic viruses, such as adenovirus and polio virus, as cancer therapeutics, but the challenge is to avoid early clearance of the OVs from the patient's immune system (Desjardins et al., 2016; Lawler et al., 2017). Nevertheless, the field is advancing rapidly, with macrophages considered to be a critical element that can dictate resistance or responsiveness to virotherapy (Saha et al., 2017; Delwar et al., 2018).

Another medical approach that is gaining increasing consideration is drug repositioning, which is defined as the investigation and use of already approved drugs for different therapeutic indications, including cancer. In this direction, several drugs are proposed for GBM treatment in combination with temozolomide (TMZ), such as *disulfiram*, which can cross the blood-brain barrier (BBB) and *metformin*, which has been shown to inhibit CSCs proliferation (Gritti et al., 2014; Wurth et al., 2016). A further approach has employed tricyclic antidepressants with the anticoagulant ticlopidine to induce cell-lethal autophagy in human and mouse glioma cells, and in mouse models *in vivo* (Shchors et al., 2015). Moreover, a new method for recurrent GBM called "coordinated undermining of survival paths with nine repurposed drugs," or CUSP9*, has been suggested in combination with TMZ (Kast et al., 2014).

In the context highlighted above, we argue that targeting the two-pore domain channel THIK-1 in microglia is an interesting therapeutic route to follow. THIK-1 was recently demonstrated to be the main K^+ channel in resting microglia, tonically active regardless of the state of $P2Y_{12}$ receptors, and the largest contributor to microglia's resting membrane potential (Madry et al., 2018). We have also established that THIK-1 activity determines microglial ramification, surveillance and is involved in IL-1β release. The contribution of IL-1β, whose receptors are expressed by glioma cells, in the development and progression of GBM has been extensively documented (Voronov et al., 2003; Feng et al., 2015). Additionally, targeting THIK-1 will impact microglia motility and the cellular machinery that supports it, which is intricately linked to the structure of the extracellular matrix, while it has been shown that diverse soluble factors released by glioma cells promote the degradation of the extracellular matrix by microglia, increasing the invasiveness of glioma cells. We believe that the fact that THIK-1 controls both IL-1β production and cellular motility in microglia makes this channel a very interesting target for the treatment of GBM, with the potential to impact both the tumor growth and its invasiveness. Microglia express two distinct motility modes, but only microglial ramification and surveillance depend on the tonic activity of THIK-1 (the convergence of microglial processes toward a damaged area is independent from THIK-1). Thus, THIK-1 inhibition could repress the capability of resting microglia close to glioma site to expand their processes during surveillance, preventing them from being recruited by cancer cells, but it would also limit IL-1β production, which, as we discussed above, is involved in glioma progression. Given that GBM growth relies on TAM recruitment, THIK-1 blockade could severely limit microglial involvement. Unfortunately, it is for now very difficult to target THIK-1 pharmacologically as this channel has not yet been extensively studied. Preclinical trials can of course be performed in THIK-1 knockout animals. SiRNA therapeutics have been studied in cancer clinical trials (Shen et al., 2012) and could be a potential approach for the treatment of glioblastoma in that context. The use of nanoparticles can be a means to direct these gene modulators in inhibiting THIK-1 (Es-Salah-Lamoureux et al., 2010). Whether the removal of this specific channel will also have negative consequences for different cell functions remains an open question. Interestingly, blocking other members of the two-pore-domain potassium channel family, like TASK-3 or TREK-1, has shown significant reduction in cell proliferation in some ovarian cancer cell lines (Comes et al., 2015), which appears to be a promising path for other cancer cells, like gliomas.

CONCLUSION

Since the advent of the current standard therapy for newly diagnosed GBM consisting of surgical resection and chemoradiotherapy, there have been no major treatment advances, with the possible exception of mitosis-disrupting tumor-treating fields (TTFields) (Geraldo et al., 2019). New insights into the inter- and intra-tumoral genetic heterogeneity of GBM (Patel et al., 2014; Sidaway, 2017) highlight the likely futility of discovering tumor cell-targeted therapies with therapeutic impact on sufficient patients, or on sufficient tumor cells within the tumor mass. Nevertheless, we argue that there is one common feature of GBM that can be potentially targeted: the massive infiltrate of microglia and macrophages. Non-mutated, widely expressed microglial cell targets such as the THIK-1 K^+ channel offer an opportunity to modulate the GBM stroma and to potentially tilt the balance of the multiple factors in the tumor microenvironment away from tumor promotion (Broekman et al., 2018). The future for treating highly aggressive, heterogenous, and therapy resistant malignancies such as GBM will likely be a rational combination of different therapeutic modalities. Critically, microglia and macrophages have been shown to influence efficacy (positively or negatively) of many treatments including chemotherapy, radiotherapy, virotherapy and immunotherapy. Consequently, we envisage that harnessing these cells for therapeutic advantage will be at the center of future, more potent, GBM therapies.

AUTHOR CONTRIBUTIONS

All authors listed have made a substantial, direct and intellectual contribution to the work, and approved it for publication.

FUNDING

This work was supported by MEDICIS-PROMED, a project of the European Commission (642889) with additional support from SEFRI (REF-1131-52107), and by grants Fondation Boninchi to RJ, from the Frédéric Fellay Association to PW, and Ligue Genevoise Contre Le Cancer to LB (1314).

ACKNOWLEDGMENTS

The authors wish to thank Dr. Vasiliki Kyrargyri for comments on earlier versions of this manuscript.

REFERENCES

Barani, I. J., and Larson, D. A. (2015). Radiation therapy of glioblastoma. *Cancer Treat. Res.* 163, 49–73. doi: 10.1007/978-3-319-12048-5_4

Betlazar, C., Middleton, R. J., Banati, R. B., and Liu, G. J. (2016). The impact of high and low dose ionising radiation on the central nervous system. *Redox Biol.* 9, 144–156. doi: 10.1016/j.redox.2016.08.002

Bhat, K. P. L., Balasubramaniyan, V., Vaillant, B., Ezhilarasan, R., Hummelink, K., Hollingsworth, F., et al. (2013). Mesenchymal differentiation mediated by NF-kappaB promotes radiation resistance in glioblastoma. *Cancer Cell* 24, 331–346. doi: 10.1016/j.ccr.2013.08.001

Boche, D., Perry, V. H., and Nicoll, J. A. R. (2013). Review: activation patterns of microglia and their identification in the human brain. *Neuropathol. Appl. Neurobiol.* 39, 3–18. doi: 10.1111/nan.12011

Bowman, R. L., Klemm, F., Akkari, L., Pyonteck, S. M., Sevenich, L., Quail, D. F., et al. (2016). Macrophage ontogeny underlies differences in tumor-specific education in brain malignancies. *Cell Rep.* 17, 2445–2459. doi: 10.1016/j.celrep.2016.10.052

Broekman, M. L., Maas, S. L. N., Abels, E. R., Mempel, T. R., Krichevsky, A. M., and Breakefield, X. O. (2018). Multidimensional communication in the microenvirons of glioblastoma. *Nat. Rev. Neurol.* 14, 482–495. doi: 10.1038/s41582-018-0025-8

Burnstock, G., and Verkhratsky, A. (2010). Long-term (trophic) purinergic signalling: purinoceptors control cell proliferation, differentiation and death. *Cell Death Dis.* 1:e9. doi: 10.1038/cddis.2009.11

Buttgereit, A., Lelios, I., Yu, X. Y., Vrohlings, M., Krakoski, N. R., Gautier, E. L., et al. (2016). Sall1 is a transcriptional regulator defining microglia identity and function. *Nat. Immunol.* 17, 1397–1406. doi: 10.1038/ni.3585

Caruso, G., Caraci, F., and Jolivet, R. B. (2018). Pivotal role of carnosine in the modulation of brain cells activity: multimodal mechanism of action and therapeutic potential in neurodegenerative disorders. *Prog. Neurobiol.* 175, 35–53. doi: 10.1016/j.pneurobio.2018.12.004

Charles, N. A., Holland, E. C., Gilbertson, R., Glass, R., and Kettenmann, H. (2011). The brain tumor microenvironment. *Glia* 59, 1169–1180. doi: 10.1002/glia.21136

Chin, L., Meyerson, M., Aldape, K., Bigner, D., Mikkelsen, T., VandenBerg, S., et al. (2008). Comprehensive genomic characterization defines human glioblastoma genes and core pathways. *Nature* 455, 1061–1068. doi: 10.1038/nature07385

Comes, N., Serrano-Albarras, A., Capera, J., Serrano-Novillo, C., Condom, E., Ramon, Y. C. S., et al. (2015). Involvement of potassium channels in the progression of cancer to a more malignant phenotype. *Biochim. Biophys. Acta* 1848(10 Pt B), 2477–2492. doi: 10.1016/j.bbamem.2014.12.008

Coniglio, S. J., Eugenin, E., Dobrenis, K., Stanley, E. R., West, B. L., Symons, M. H., et al. (2012). Microglial stimulation of glioblastoma invasion involves epidermal growth factor receptor (EGFR) and colony stimulating factor 1 receptor (CSF-1R) signaling. *Mol. Med.* 18, 519–527. doi: 10.2119/molmed.2011.00217

Coniglio, S. J., and Segall, J. E. (2013). Review: molecular mechanism of microglia stimulated glioblastoma invasion. *Matrix Biol.* 32, 372–380. doi: 10.1016/j.matbio.2013.07.008

Cordier, D., Gerber, A., Kluba, C., Bauman, A., Hutter, G., Mindt, T. L., et al. (2014). Expression of different neurokinin-1 receptor (NK1R) isoforms in glioblastoma multiforme: potential implications for targeted therapy. *Cancer Biother. Radiopharm.* 29, 221–226. doi: 10.1089/cbr.2013.1588

Crespo, I., Vital, A. L., Gonzalez-Tablas, M., Patino Mdel, C., Otero, A., Lopes, M. C., et al. (2015). Molecular and genomic alterations in glioblastoma multiforme. *Am. J. Pathol.* 185, 1820–1833. doi: 10.1016/j.ajpath.2015.02.023

Davalos, D., Grutzendler, J., Yang, G., Kim, J. V., Zuo, Y., Jung, S., et al. (2005). ATP mediates rapid microglial response to local brain injury in vivo. *Nat. Neurosci.* 8, 752–758. doi: 10.1038/nn1472

Delwar, Z. M., Kuo, Y., Wen, Y. H., Rennie, P. S., and Jia, W. (2018). Oncolytic virotherapy blockade by microglia and macrophages requires STAT1/3. *Cancer Res.* 78, 718–730. doi: 10.1158/0008-5472.CAN-17-0599

Desjardins, A., Sampson, J. H., Peters, K. B., Vlahovic, G., Randazzo, D., Threatt, S., et al. (2016). Patient survival on the dose escalation phase of the oncolytic polio/rhinovirus recombinant (PVSRIPO) against WHO grade IV malignant glioma (MG) clinical trial compared to historical controls. *J. Clin. Oncol.* 34:2061. doi: 10.1200/JCO.2016.34.15_suppl.2061

Dissing-Olesen, L., LeDue, J. M., Rungta, R. L., Hefendehl, J. K., Choi, H. B., and MacVicar, B. A. (2014). Activation of neuronal NMDA receptors triggers transient ATP-mediated microglial process outgrowth. *J. Neurosci.* 34, 10511–10527. doi: 10.1523/Jneurosci.0405-14.2014

Douard, V., and Ferraris, R. P. (2008). Regulation of the fructose transporter GLUT5 in health and disease. *Am. J. Physiol. Endocrinol. Metab.* 295, E227–E237. doi: 10.1152/ajpendo.90245.2008

Dutoit, V., Migliorini, D., Dietrich, P. Y., and Walker, P. R. (2016). Immunotherapy of malignant tumors in the brain: how different from other sites? *Front. Immunol.* 6:256. doi: 10.3389/fonc.2016.00256

Es-Salah-Lamoureux, Z., Steele, D. F., and Fedida, D. (2010). Research into the therapeutic roles of two-pore-domain potassium channels. *Trends Pharmacol. Sci.* 31, 587–595. doi: 10.1016/j.tips.2010.09.001

Feng, X., Szulzewsky, F., Yerevanian, A., Chen, Z., Heinzmann, D., Rasmussen, R. D., et al. (2015). Loss of CX3CR1 increases accumulation of inflammatory monocytes and promotes gliomagenesis. *Oncotarget* 6, 15077–15094. doi: 10.18632/oncotarget.3730

Furnari, F. B., Fenton, T., Bachoo, R. M., Mukasa, A., Stommel, J. M., Stegh, A., et al. (2007). Malignant astrocytic glioma: genetics, biology, and paths to treatment. *Genes Dev.* 21, 2683–2710. doi: 10.1101/gad.1596707

Gabrusiewicz, K., Rodriguez, B., Wei, J., Hashimoto, Y., Healy, L. M., Maiti, S. N., et al. (2016). Glioblastoma-infiltrated innate immune cells resemble M0 macrophage phenotype. *JCI Insight* 1:85841. doi: 10.1172/jci.insight.85841

Garnier, D., Meehan, B., Kislinger, T., Daniel, P., Sinha, A., Abdulkarim, B., et al. (2018). Divergent evolution of temozolomide resistance in glioblastoma stem cells is reflected in extracellular vesicles and coupled with radiosensitization. *Neuro. Oncol.* 20, 236–248. doi: 10.1093/neuonc/nox142

Gautier, E. L., Shay, T., Miller, J., Greter, M., Jakubzick, C., Ivanov, S., et al. (2012). Gene-expression profiles and transcriptional regulatory pathways that underlie the identity and diversity of mouse tissue macrophages. *Nat. Immunol.* 13, 1118–1128. doi: 10.1038/ni.2419

Geraldo, L. H. M., Garcia, C., da Fonseca, A. C. C., Dubois, L. G. F., de Sampaio, E. S. T. C. L., Matias, D., et al. (2019). Glioblastoma therapy in the age of molecular medicine. *Trends Cancer* 5, 46–65. doi: 10.1016/j.trecan.2018.11.002

Ghosh, S., Castillo, E., Frias, E. S., and Swanson, R. A. (2018). Bioenergetic regulation of microglia. *Glia* 66, 1200–1212. doi: 10.1002/glia.23271

Ginhoux, F., Greter, M., Leboeuf, M., Nandi, S., See, P., Gokhan, S., et al. (2010). Fate mapping analysis reveals that adult microglia derive from primitive macrophages. *Science* 330, 841–845. doi: 10.1126/science.1194637

Ginhoux, F., Lim, S., Hoeffel, G., Low, D., and Huber, T. (2013). Origin and differentiation of microglia. *Front. Cell Neurosci.* 7:45. doi: 10.3389/fncel.2013.00045

Glaser, T., Han, I., Wu, L., and Zeng, X. (2017). Targeted nanotechnology in glioblastoma multiforme. *Front. Pharmacol.* 8:166. doi: 10.3389/fphar.2017.00166

Goldmann, T., Wieghofer, P., Jordao, M. J. C., Prutek, F., Hagemeyer, N., Frenzel, K., et al. (2016). Origin, fate and dynamics of macrophages at central nervous system interfaces. *Nat. Immunol.* 17, 797–805. doi: 10.1038/ni.3423

Greter, M. (2016). Family ties among CNS macrophages. *Nat. Immunol.* 17, 742–743. doi: 10.1038/ni.3490

Gritti, M., Wurth, R., Angelini, M., Barbieri, F., Peretti, M., Pizzi, E., et al. (2014). Metformin repositioning as antitumoral agent: selective antiproliferative effects in human glioblastoma stem cells, via inhibition of CLIC1-mediated ion current. *Oncotarget* 5, 11252–11268. doi: 10.18632/oncotarget.2617

Hambardzumyan, D., Gutmann, D. H., and Kettenmann, H. (2016). The role of microglia and macrophages in glioma maintenance and progression. *Nat. Neurosci.* 19, 20–27. doi: 10.1038/nn.4185

Haynes, S. E., Hollopeter, G., Yang, G., Kurpius, D., Dailey, M. E., Gan, W. B., et al. (2006). The P2Y12 receptor regulates microglial activation by extracellular nucleotides. *Nat. Neurosci.* 9, 1512–1519. doi: 10.1038/nn1805

Held-Feindt, J., Hattermann, K., Muerkoster, S. S., Wedderkopp, H., Knerlich-Lukoschus, F., Ungefroren, H., et al. (2010). CX3CR1 promotes recruitment of human glioma-infiltrating microglia/macrophages (GIMs). *Exp. Cell Res.* 316, 1553–1566. doi: 10.1016/j.yexcr.2010.02.018

Hernandez-Pedro, N. Y., Rangel-Lopez, E., Magana-Maldonado, R., de la Cruz, V. P., del Angel, A. S., Pineda, B., et al. (2013). Application of nanoparticles on diagnosis and therapy in gliomas. *Biomed. Res. Int.* 2013:351031. doi: 10.1155/2013/351031

Horikoshi, Y., Sasaki, A., Taguchi, N., Maeda, M., Tsukagoshi, H., Sato, K., et al. (2003). Human GLUT5 immunolabeling is useful for evaluating microglial status in neuropathological study using paraffin sections. *Acta Neuropathol.* 105, 157–162. doi: 10.1007/s00401-002-0627-4

Hu, F., Ku, M. C., Markovic, D. A., Dzaye, O. D., Lehnardt, S., Synowitz, M., et al. (2014). Glioma-associated microglial MMP9 expression is upregulated by TLR2 signaling and sensitive to minocycline. *Int. J. Cancer* 135, 2569–2578. doi: 10.1002/ijc.28908

Ito, D., Imai, Y., Ohsawa, K., Nakajima, K., Fukuuchi, Y., and Kohsaka, S. (1998). Microglia-specific localisation of a novel calcium binding protein, Iba1. *Brain Res. Mol. Brain Res.* 57, 1–9.

Kane, J. R., Miska, J., Young, J. S., Kanojia, D., Kim, J. W., and Lesniak, M. S. (2015). Sui generis: gene therapy and delivery systems for the treatment of glioblastoma. *Neuro. Oncol.* 17(Suppl. 2), ii24–ii36. doi: 10.1093/neuonc/nou355

Kast, R. E., Karpel-Massler, G., and Halatsch, M. E. (2014). CUSP9* treatment protocol for recurrent glioblastoma: aprepitant, artesunate, auranofin, captopril, celecoxib, disulfiram, itraconazole, ritonavir, sertraline augmenting continuous low dose temozolomide. *Oncotarget* 5, 8052–8082. doi: 10.18632/oncotarget.2408

Kettenmann, H., Hanisch, U. K., Noda, M., and Verkhratsky, A. (2011). Physiology of microglia. *Physiol. Rev.* 91, 461–553. doi: 10.1152/physrev.00011.2010

Lathia, J. D., Mack, S. C., Mulkearns-Hubert, E. E., Valentim, C. L., and Rich, J. N. (2015). Cancer stem cells in glioblastoma. *Genes Dev.* 29, 1203–1217. doi: 10.1101/gad.261982.115

Lavin, Y., Winter, D., Blecher-Gonen, R., David, E., Keren-Shaul, H., Merad, M., et al. (2014). Tissue-resident macrophage enhancer landscapes are shaped by the local microenvironment. *Cell* 159, 1312–1326. doi: 10.1016/j.cell.2014.11.018

Lawler, S. E., Speranza, M. C., Cho, C. F., and Chiocca, E. A. (2017). Oncolytic viruses in cancer treatment: a review. *JAMA Oncol.* 3, 841–849. doi: 10.1001/jamaoncol.2016.2064

Lawson, L. J., Perry, V. H., Dri, P., and Gordon, S. (1990). Heterogeneity in the distribution and morphology of microglia in the normal adult mouse brain. *Neuroscience* 39, 151–170.

Lee, S., Jilani, S. M., Nikolova, G. V., Carpizo, D., and Iruela-Arispe, M. L. (2005). Processing of VEGF-A by matrix metalloproteinases regulates bioavailability and vascular patterning in tumors. *J. Cell Biol.* 169, 681–691. doi: 10.1083/jcb.200409115

Lehnardt, S. (2010). Innate immunity and neuroinflammation in the CNS: the role of microglia in Toll-like receptor-mediated neuronal injury. *Glia* 58, 253–263. doi: 10.1002/glia.20928

Li, Y., Du, X. F., Liu, C. S., Wen, Z. L., and Du, J. L. (2012). Reciprocal regulation between resting microglial dynamics and neuronal activity in vivo. *Dev. Cell* 23, 1189–1202. doi: 10.1016/j.devcel.2012.10.027

Louis, D. N., Ohgaki, H., Wiestler, O. D., Cavenee, W. K., Burger, P. C., Jouvet, A., et al. (2007). The 2007 WHO classification of tumours of the central nervous system. *Acta Neuropathol.* 114, 97–109. doi: 10.1007/s00401-007-0243-4

Madry, C., Kyrargyri, V., Arancibia-Carcamo, I. L., Jolivet, R., Kohsaka, S., Bryan, R. M., et al. (2018). Microglial ramification, surveillance, and interleukin-1beta release are regulated by the two-pore domain K(+) Channel THIK-1. *Neuron* 97, 299.e6–312.e6. doi: 10.1016/j.neuron.2017.12.002

McFaline-Figueroa, J. R., and Lee, E. Q. (2018). Brain tumors. *Am. J. Med.* 131, 874–882. doi: 10.1016/j.amjmed.2017.12.039

Miyamoto, A., Wake, H., Ishikawa, A. W., Eto, K., Shibata, K., Murakoshi, H., et al. (2016). Microglia contact induces synapse formation in developing somatosensory cortex. *Nat. Commun.* 7:12540. doi: 10.1038/ncomms12540

Mrdjen, D., Pavlovic, A., Hartmann, F. J., Schreiner, B., Utz, S. G., Leung, B. P., et al. (2018). High-dimensional single-cell mapping of central nervous system immune cells reveals distinct myeloid subsets in health, aging, and disease. *Immunity* 48, 380.e6-395.e6. doi: 10.1016/j.immuni.2018.02.014

Nakagawa, Y., and Chiba, K. (2014). Role of microglial m1/m2 polarization in relapse and remission of psychiatric disorders and diseases. *Pharmaceuticals* 7, 1028–1048. doi: 10.3390/ph7121028

Nimmerjahn, A., Kirchhoff, F., and Helmchen, F. (2005). Resting microglial cells are highly dynamic surveillants of brain parenchyma in vivo. *Science* 308, 1314–1318. doi: 10.1126/science.1110647

Orecchia, R., Zurlo, A., Loasses, A., Krengli, M., Tosi, G., Zurrida, S., et al. (1998). Particle beam therapy (hadrontherapy): basis for interest and clinical experience. *Eur. J. Cancer* 34, 459–468. doi: 10.1016/S0959-8049(97)10044-2

Paolicelli, R. C., Bolasco, G., Pagani, F., Maggi, L., Scianni, M., Panzanelli, P., et al. (2011). Synaptic pruning by microglia is necessary for normal brain development. *Science* 333, 1456–1458. doi: 10.1126/science.1202529

Parkhurst, C. N., Yang, G., Ninan, I., Savas, J. N., Yates, J. R., Lafaille, J. J., et al. (2013). Microglia promote learning-dependent synapse formation through brain-derived neurotrophic factor. *Cell* 155, 1596–1609. doi: 10.1016/j.cell.2013.11.030

Parsons, D. W., Jones, S., Zhang, X. S., Lin, J. C. H., Leary, R. J., Angenendt, P., et al. (2008). An integrated genomic analysis of human glioblastoma Multiforme. *Science* 321, 1807–1812. doi: 10.1126/science.1164382

Patel, A. P., Tirosh, I., Trombetta, J. J., Shalek, A. K., Gillespie, S. M., Wakimoto, H., et al. (2014). Single-cell RNA-seq highlights intratumoral heterogeneity in primary glioblastoma. *Science* 344, 1396–1401. doi: 10.1126/science.1254257

Payne, J., Maher, F., Simpson, I., Mattice, L., and Davies, P. (1997). Glucose transporter Glut 5 expression in microglial cells. *Glia* 21, 327–331.

Phillips, W. T., Bao, A. D., Brenner, A. J., and Goins, B. A. (2014). Image-guided interventional therapy for cancer with radiotherapeutic nanoparticles. *Adv. Drug Deliv. Rev.* 76, 39–59. doi: 10.1016/j.addr.2014.07.001

Poon, C. C., Sarkar, S., Yong, V. W., and Kelly, J. J. (2017). Glioblastoma-associated microglia and macrophages: targets for therapies to improve prognosis. *Brain* 140, 1548–1560. doi: 10.1093/brain/aww355

Prinz, M., and Priller, J. (2014). Microglia and brain macrophages in the molecular age: from origin to neuropsychiatric disease. *Nat. Rev. Neurosci.* 15, 300–312. doi: 10.1038/nrn3722

Pyonteck, S. M., Akkari, L., Schuhmacher, A. J., Bowman, R. L., Sevenich, L., Quail, D. F., et al. (2013). CSF-1R inhibition alters macrophage polarization and blocks glioma progression. *Nat. Med.* 19, 1264–1272. doi: 10.1038/nm.3337

Quail, D. F., Bowman, R. L., Akkari, L., Quick, M. L., Schuhmacher, A. J., Huse, J. T., et al. (2016). The tumor microenvironment underlies acquired resistance to CSF-1R inhibition in gliomas. *Science* 352:aad3018. doi: 10.1126/science.aad3018

Ransohoff, R. M. (2016). A polarizing question: do M1 and M2 microglia exist? *Nat. Neurosci.* 19, 987–991. doi: 10.1038/nn.4338

Ransohoff, R. M., and Cardona, A. E. (2010). The myeloid cells of the central nervous system parenchyma. *Nature* 468, 253–262. doi: 10.1038/nature09615

Rasley, A., Bost, K. L., Olson, J. K., Miller, S. D., and Marriott, I. (2002). Expression of functional NK-1 receptors in murine microglia. *Glia* 37, 258–267.

Reardon, D. A., Wucherpfennig, K., and Chiocca, E. A. (2017). Immunotherapy for glioblastoma: on the sidelines or in the game? *Discov. Med.* 24, 201–208.

Rodriguez, E., Schetters, S. T. T., and van Kooyk, Y. (2018). The tumour glyco-code as a novel immune checkpoint for immunotherapy. *Nat. Rev. Immunol.* 18, 204–211. doi: 10.1038/nri.2018.3

Saha, D., Martuza, R. L., and Rabkin, S. D. (2017). Macrophage polarization contributes to glioblastoma eradication by combination immunovirotherapy and immune checkpoint blockade. *Cancer Cell*, 32, 253.e5–267.e5. doi: 10.1016/j.ccell.2017.07.006

Saijo, K., and Glass, C. K. (2011). Microglial cell origin and phenotypes in health and disease. *Nat. Rev. Immunol.* 11, 775–787. doi: 10.1038/nri3086

Sasaki, A. (2016). Microglia and brain macrophages: an update. *Neuropathology* 37, 452–464. doi: 10.1111/neup.12354

Sasaki, K., Hattori, T., Fujisawa, T., Takahashi, K., Inoue, H., and Takigawa, M. (1998). Nitric oxide mediates interleukin-1-induced gene expression of matrix metalloproteinases and basic fibroblast growth factor in cultured rabbit articular chondrocytes. *J. Biochem.* 123, 431–439.

Schonberg, D. L., Bao, S., and Rich, J. N. (2013). Genomics informs glioblastoma biology. *Nat. Genet.* 45, 1105–1107. doi: 10.1038/ng.2775

Shchors, K., Massaras, A., and Hanahan, D. (2015). Dual targeting of the autophagic regulatory circuitry in gliomas with repurposed drugs elicits cell-lethal autophagy and therapeutic benefit. *Cancer Cell* 28, 456–471. doi: 10.1016/j.ccell.2015.08.012

Shen, H., Sun, T., and Ferrari, M. (2012). Nanovector delivery of siRNA for cancer therapy. *Cancer Gene Ther.* 19, 367–373. doi: 10.1038/cgt.2012.22

Sidaway, P. (2017). CNS cancer: glioblastoma subtypes revisited. *Nat. Rev. Clin. Oncol.* 14:587. doi: 10.1038/nrclinonc.2017.122

Sierra, A., de Castro, F., Del Rio-Hortega, J., Rafael Iglesias-Rozas, J., Garrosa, M., and Kettenmann, H. (2016). The "Big-Bang" for modern glial biology: translation and comments on Pio del Rio-Hortega 1919 series of papers on microglia. *Glia* 64, 1801–1840. doi: 10.1002/glia.23046

Sousa, C., Biber, K., and Michelucci, A. (2017). Cellular and molecular characterization of microglia: a unique immune cell population. *Front. Immunol.* 8:198. doi: 10.3389/fimmu.2017.00198

Squarzoni, P., Oller, G., Hoeffel, G., Pont-Lezica, L., Rostaing, P., Low, D., et al. (2014). Microglia modulate wiring of the embryonic forebrain. *Cell Rep.* 8, 1271–1279. doi: 10.1016/j.celrep.2014.07.042

Vatner, R. E., and Formenti, S. C. (2015). Myeloid-derived cells in tumors: effects of radiation. *Semin. Radiat. Oncol.* 25, 18–27. doi: 10.1016/j.semradonc.2014.07.008

Venteicher, A. S., Tirosh, I., Hebert, C., Yizhak, K., Neftel, C., Filbin, M. G., et al. (2017). Decoupling genetics, lineages, and microenvironment in IDH-mutant gliomas by single-cell RNA-seq. *Science* 355:eaai8478. doi: 10.1126/science.aai8478

Verhaak, R. G., Hoadley, K. A., Purdom, E., Wang, V., Qi, Y., Wilkerson, M. D., et al. (2010). Integrated genomic analysis identifies clinically relevant subtypes of glioblastoma characterized by abnormalities in PDGFRA, IDH1, EGFR, and NF1. *Cancer Cell* 17, 98–110. doi: 10.1016/j.ccr.2009.12.020

Vinnakota, K., Hu, F., Ku, M. C., Georgieva, P. B., Szulzewsky, F., Pohlmann, A., et al. (2013). Toll-like receptor 2 mediates microglia/brain macrophage MT1-MMP expression and glioma expansion. *Neuro Oncol.* 15, 1457–1468. doi: 10.1093/neuonc/not115

Vitaz, T. W., Warnke, P. C., Tabar, V., and Gutin, P. H. (2005). Brachytherapy for brain tumors. *J. Neurooncol.* 73, 71–86. doi: 10.1007/s11060-004-2352-4

Voronov, E., Shouval, D. S., Krelin, Y., Cagnano, E., Benharroch, D., Iwakura, Y., et al. (2003). IL-1 is required for tumor invasiveness and angiogenesis. *Proc. Natl. Acad. Sci. U.S.A.* 100, 2645–2650. doi: 10.1073/pnas.0437939100

Walsh, J. G., Muruve, D. A., and Power, C. (2014). Inflammasomes in the CNS. *Nat. Rev. Neurosci.* 15, 84–97. doi: 10.1038/nrn3638

Wang, Q., Hu, B., Hu, X., Kim, H., Squatrito, M., Scarpace, L., et al. (2017). Tumor evolution of glioma-intrinsic gene expression subtypes associates with immunological changes in the microenvironment. *Cancer Cell* 32, 42.e6–56.e6. doi: 10.1016/j.ccell.2017.06.003

Wang, Q., Hu, B., Hu, X., Kim, H., Squatrito, M., Scarpace, L., et al. (2018). Tumor evolution of glioma-intrinsic gene expression subtypes associates with immunological changes in the microenvironment. *Cancer Cell* 33:152. doi: 10.1016/j.ccell.2017.12.012

Watters, J. J., Schartner, J. M., and Badie, B. (2005). Microglia function in brain tumors. *J. Neurosci. Res.* 81, 447–455. doi: 10.1002/jnr.20485

Wei, J., Marisetty, A., Schrand, B., Gabrusiewicz, K., Hashimoto, Y., Ott, M., et al. (2019). Osteopontin mediates glioblastoma-associated macrophage infiltration and is a potential therapeutic target. *J. Clin. Invest.* 129, 137–149. doi: 10.1172/JCI121266

Wieghofer, P., Knobeloch, K. P., and Prinz, M. (2015). Genetic targeting of microglia. *Glia* 63, 1–22. doi: 10.1002/glia.22727

Wolf, S. A., Boddeke, H. W., and Kettenmann, H. (2017). Microglia in physiology and disease. *Annu. Rev. Physiol.* 79, 619–643. doi: 10.1146/annurev-physiol-022516-034406

Wurth, R., Thellung, S., Bajetto, A., Mazzanti, M., Florio, T., and Barbieri, F. (2016). Drug-repositioning opportunities for cancer therapy: novel molecular targets for known compounds. *Drug Discov. Today* 21, 190–199. doi: 10.1016/j.drudis.2015.09.017

Xu, J., Escamilla, J., Mok, S., David, J., Priceman, S., West, B., et al. (2013). CSF1R signaling blockade stanches tumor-infiltrating myeloid cells and improves the efficacy of radiotherapy in prostate cancer. *Cancer Res.* 73, 2782–2794. doi: 10.1158/0008-5472.CAN-12-3981

Ye, X. Z., Xu, S. L., Xin, Y. H., Yu, S. C., Ping, Y. F., Chen, L., et al. (2012). Tumor-associated microglia/macrophages enhance the invasion of glioma stem-like cells via TGF-beta1 signaling pathway. *J. Immunol.* 189, 444–453. doi: 10.4049/jimmunol.1103248

Yeung, Y. T., McDonald, K. L., Grewal, T., and Munoz, L. (2013). Interleukins in glioblastoma pathophysiology: implications for therapy. *Br. J. Pharmacol.* 168, 591–606. doi: 10.1111/bph.12008

Yuzhalin, A. E., and Kutikhin, A. G. (2015). *Interleukins in Cancer Biology*. Cambridge: Academic Press, 356. doi: 10.1002/cmdc.2015 00253

Zhang, L., Chen, H., Wang, L., Liu, T., Yeh, J., Lu, G., et al. (2010). Delivery of therapeutic radioisotopes using nanoparticle platforms: potential benefit in systemic radiation therapy. *Nanotechnol. Sci. Appl.* 3, 159–170. doi: 10.2147/NSA.S7462

Zhang, Y., Chen, K., Sloan, S. A., Bennett, M. L., Scholze, A. R., O'Keeffe, S., et al. (2014). An RNA-sequencing transcriptome and splicing database of glia, neurons, and vascular cells of the cerebral cortex. *J. Neurosci.* 34, 11929–11947. doi: 10.1523/JNEUROSCI.1860-14.2014

Zhao, J., Zhou, M., and Li, C. (2016). Synthetic nanoparticles for delivery of radioisotopes and radiosensitizers in cancer therapy. *Cancer Nanotechnol.* 7:9. doi: 10.1186/s12645-016-0022-9

Zinn, P. O., Colen, R. R., Kasper, E. M., and Burkhardt, J. K. (2013). Extent of resection and radiotherapy in GBM: A 1973 to 2007 surveillance, epidemiology and end results analysis of 21,783 patients. *Int. J. Oncol.* 42, 929–934. doi: 10.3892/ijo.2013.1770

3

Sodium Dichloroacetate Stimulates Angiogenesis by Improving Endothelial Precursor Cell Function in an AKT/GSK-3β/Nrf2 Dependent Pathway in Vascular Dementia Rats

Hui Zhao[1,2†], Junqin Mao[3†], Yuan Yuan[2], Jingjing Feng[2], Hao Cheng[2], Guorong Fan[4], Yuefan Zhang[4,5] and Tiejun Li[1,2]**

[1] *Department of Pharmacy, Punan Hospital, Shanghai, China,* [2] *College of Pharmacology, Anhui University of Chinese Medicine, Hefei, China,* [3] *Department of Pharmacy, Shanghai Pudong New Area People's Hospital, Shanghai, China,*
[4] *Department of Clinical Pharmacy, Shanghai General Hospital, Shanghai JiaoTong University School of Medicine, Shanghai, China,* [5] *Department of Pharmacology, College of Pharmacy, Second Military Medical University, Shanghai, China*

***Correspondence:**
Yuefan Zhang
zhangyuefan@126.com
Tiejun Li
Ltj204@163.com

† *These authors have contributed equally to this work*

Sodium dichloroacetate (DCA) is a mitochondrial pyruvate dehydrogenase kinase inhibitor, and has been shown to display vasoprotective effects in chronic ischemic stroke. The purpose of this study was to evaluate the therapeutic effect of DCA on vascular dementia (VD) and endothelial progenitor cell (EPC)-mediated angiogenesis. After cerebral ischemia-reperfusion in rats, DCA was administered continuously for 21 days; following which, histological analysis, and cognitive functional tests were conducted. Rat bone marrow-derived EPCs were isolated, their function and quantity were measured, and the effects of long-term administration of DCA on EPCs in a rat model of VD was studied. We found that long-term DCA administration improved cognitive function in VD rats, reduced brain infarct size and brain atrophy, increased VEGF and bFGF levels *in vivo*, promoted angiogenesis in damaged areas, and significantly improved EPC function in VD rats. Compared with the VD group, AKT, Nrf2, eNOS expression, and intracellular NO levels were elevated in EPCs of DCA-treated VD rats. In addition, GSK3β and intracellular ROS levels were decreased. Simultaneously, it was found that DCA directly acted on EPCs, and improved EPC functional behavior. Taken together, these findings suggested that long-term DCA administration improved cognitive function in a rat model of VD, and did so in part, by improving EPC function. Observations suggest that prolonged DCA administration might be beneficial in treating VD.

Keywords: sodium dichloroacetate, endothelial progenitor cells, reactive oxygen species, angiogenesis, vascular dementia

INTRODUCTION

Vascular dementia (VD) is a very frequently seen form of dementia that is recognized as a neurocognitive disorder, caused by stroke and other types of cerebrovascular disorders, which accounts for 15 percent of all dementias seen at the clinic. The risk of VD increases exponentially with age (O'Brien and Thomas, 2015). In fact, VD caused by cerebral vascular injury or vascular circulatory injury might lead to mental disability (Yew et al., 2017), including apathy, depression, agitation, and delusion, which are prevalent and gradually worsen over time (Jin et al., 2015).

A growing body of evidence suggests that following tissue ischemia or vascular endothelial injury, blood vessels can be repaired by bone marrow-derived endothelial progenitor cells (EPCs). EPCs contribute to the formation and recovery of new blood vessels, and are mobilized from the bone marrow to the blood circulation, and can reach sites of vascular injury, at which time they can proliferate and differentiate into endothelial cells to repair damaged blood vessels (Williamson et al., 2012). Recent reports indicate that EPCs encouraged therapeutic effects on long-term stroke prognosis in mice (Fan et al., 2010), and do so by enhancing EPCs function (migration, adhesion, and tube formation), and play protective roles in ischemic stroke (Xin et al., 2016). This suggests that improving EPC function might have therapeutic utility in treating brain damage caused by stroke.

Sodium dichloroacetate (DCA) is a mitochondrial pyruvate dehydrogenase kinase inhibitor, and is an orally absorbable small molecular compound for MELAS syndrome, and children with congenital lactic acidosis and other diseases that are treated in the clinic (Michelakis et al., 2008, 2010). Recent studies had found that DCA acts as a potential vasoprotective agent by inhibiting PDK2 and reducing coronary endarterium proliferation (Deuse et al., 2014). Further, DCA promotes brain regeneration after cerebral ischemia (Hong et al., 2018), which indicates that DCA might play an important role in VD.

Thus, the aim of this study was to validate the hypothesis that DCA could improve cognitive function by promoting EPC function and angiogenesis in VD rats.

MATERIALS AND METHODS

Animals

Adult male SD (Sprague-Dawley) rats (220–230 g) were purchased from the Changzhou CAVENS Laboratory Animal Co., Ltd (Changzhou, China). Food and water were available *ad libitum* under constant temperature (23 ± 2°C) and controlled light conditions (12 h light/dark cycle).

This study was carried out in accordance with the recommendations of "The Care and Use of Laboratory Animals, the Animal Committee of the Second Military Medical University." The protocol was approved by the "Animal Committee of the Second Military Medical University." All works were done to prevent animal suffering and to minimize the number of animals used in keeping with the 3R's principles of animal research.

Reagents

DCA was purchased from Sigma-Aldrich (St. Louis, MO, United States). Primary antibodies against eNOS (1: 1000), AKT (1: 1000), GSK-3β (1: 1000), and Nrf2 (1:1000) were purchased from Abcam (Cambridge, MA, United States).

Vascular Dementia (VD) Model

Cerebral ischemia-reperfusion was induced by middle cerebral artery occlusion (MCAO), resulting in a similar pathology to VD (Li et al., 2013). Left middle cerebral arterial occlusion was performed as previously described (Zhou et al., 2010; Zhang et al., 2012). Concisely, anesthesia was induced with 2 percent sodium pentobarbital (50 mg/kg, i.p.). Surgery exposed the left common carotid artery, which isolated, and permitted ligation of the external carotid artery (ECA) with 4-0 silk thread. After an ECA incision, a 4-0 single monofilament coated with poly L-lysine (Beijing Cinontech Co. Ltd, China) was gently introduced (18 ± 20 mm) into the internal carotid artery (ICA), thereby occluding the middle cerebral artery (MCA) origin. After 120 min, the thread was removed to allow for reperfusion, following which, rats were placed in a thermostat at 37 ± 0.5°C prior to recovery. Sham rats were undergone the exact same procedure without arterial ligation and monofilament insertion.

Experimental Groups and Drug Treatment

Rat behavior was examined at 24 h after reperfusion, and animals showing contralateral forelimb dysfunction were included for further experimentation (Longa et al., 1989). A total of 40 MCAO rats were randomly separated into five groups by lottery drawing: (1) sham group (sham, $N = 8$); (2) VD group (treated with 0.9%NaCl, $N = 8$); (3) 50 mg/kg DCA group (VD treated with 50 mg/kg/day DCA, $N = 8$); (4) 100 mg/kg DCA group (VD treated with 100 mg/kg/day DCA, $N = 8$); and (5) 200 mg/kg DCA group (VD treated with 200 mg/kg/day DCA, $N = 8$). DCA and normal saline were orally administered (by gastric gavage) for 21 consecutive days. After 21 days, the Morris water maze test was performed, and rat bone marrow-derived EPCs were isolated and cultured. In addition, pathological changes and angiogenesis in damaged parts of the brain were assessed.

Morris Water Maze (MWM)

Morris water maze experiments were performed based on experimental references and appropriate improvements (Morris, 1984; Cantarella et al., 2015). The Morris water maze (MWM) consisted of a black tank filled with black water (Black food additive) (24–25°C), which was divided into four quadrants (I, II, III, and IV). Spatial cues were presented in each quadrant, and a transparent platform with a diameter of 10 cm in the middle of the four-quadrant area was placed with 1–2 cm below the water surface. The MWM study consisted of two parts: (1) positioning navigation test and (2) space exploration test. The experimenter conducted this study without having any knowledge of animal grouping.

In the positioning navigation test, rats started from a random quadrant (except number four-quadrant), and recorded the time required to reach the hidden platform (latency). The maximum time of rats finding the platform was 60 s, Once the rats reached the platform within 60 s and stayed in place for 5 s on the platform, the timer automatically stopped, and allowed the rat to stay for 10 s. If the platform could not be found, then those failed rats were manually moved to the platform and allowed to

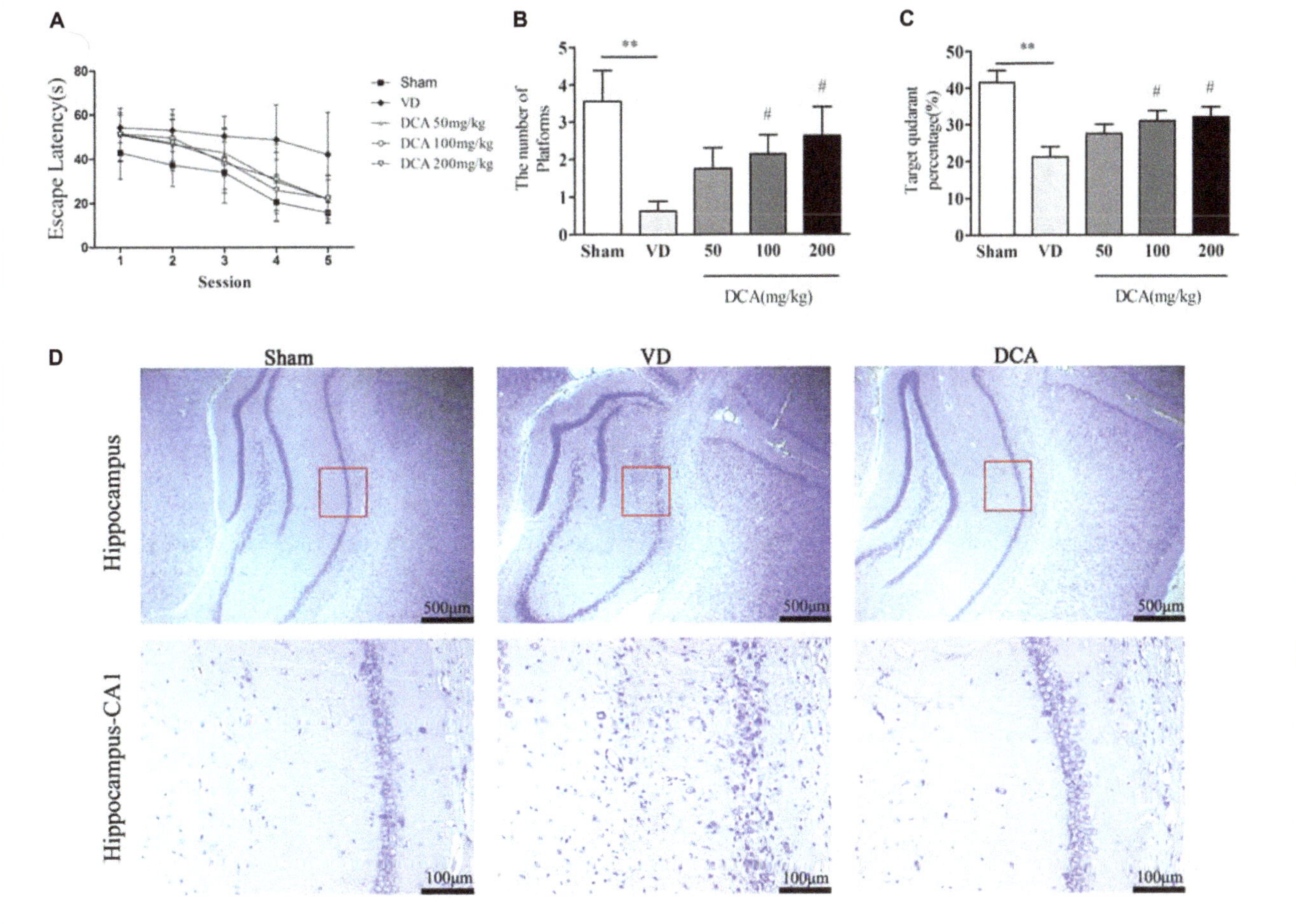

FIGURE 1 | Sodium dichloroacetate (DCA) improves cognitive function of vascular dementia (VD) and attenuates histopathological Characteristics in rats. Morris water maze test procedure determined the spatial learning ability in SD rats, 21 days after MCAO surgery. The escape latency of the learning trajectory, and the percentage time spent in the target quadrant and the number of passes through the platform in the spatial exploration test were calculated. **(A)** The escape latency of the learning trajectory. **(B)** The percentage time spent in the target quadrant (the position of the platform during training). **(C)** The number of passes through the platform within 60 s of commencing the test. $^{**}P < 0.01$ vs. Sham, $^{\#}P < 0.05$ vs. VD (n = 7–8). **(D)** Nissl staining of the rat hippocampus. Scale bar: 500 μm (up); 100 μm (below). Analyses were statistically tested by two-way ANOVA, followed by *post hoc* multiple comparisons analysis by the Scheffe test.

capillary density of DCA-treated VD rats was significantly increased as compared with the VD group ($P < 0.01$; **Figure 3B**), which indicates that DCA promoted angiogenesis in the cortex of the rat brain.

We further examined the levels of VEGF and bFGF in rat serum to elucidate the mechanism by which DCA promotes angiogenesis. As shown in **Figures 3C,D**, serum levels of VEGF and bFGF were elevated in the VD model group as compared with the sham group ($P < 0.01$). Interestingly, DCA (100 mg/kg) treatment significantly increased VEGF and bFGF levels as compared with the VD group ($P < 0.01$).

Characterization of EPCs

MNCs that were isolated from the rat bone marrow were seeded in vitronectin-coated six-well plates. Three days after seeding, central round cells and elongated peripheral cells appeared (**Supplementary Figure 1A**). By 7 days, spindle-shaped adherent EPCs were observed (**Supplementary Figure 1A**). After 14 days of culture, endothelial-like EPCs with a pebbled morphological character were found (**Supplementary Figure 1A**). EPCs also stained positive with DiI-acLDL and UEA-1 (**Supplementary Figure 1B**). Flow cytometry demonstrated that EPCs highly expressed both CD34 and VEGFR2 (**Supplementary Figure 1C**). These characteristics are consistent with those previously reported in EPCs (Dai et al., 2017).

DCA Promotes BM-EPC Function

For cell adhesion experiments, results showed that DCA (200 mM) treated cells were more potent than control cells ($p < 0.01$; **Figure 4A**), and bFGF was used as the positive control. Furthermore, tube forming ability was evaluated through an *in vitro* angiogenesis assay. As shown in **Figure 4B**, after incubation on Matrigel for 6 h, tubule numbers in the DCA-treated groups were significantly increased as compared with controls ($P < 0.01$). Thus, DCA potently enhanced the *in vitro* tube forming ability of BM-EPCs. Transwell experiments were used to investigate cell migration that was influenced by DCA (200 mM). When treated with DCA, BM-EPCs showed enhanced

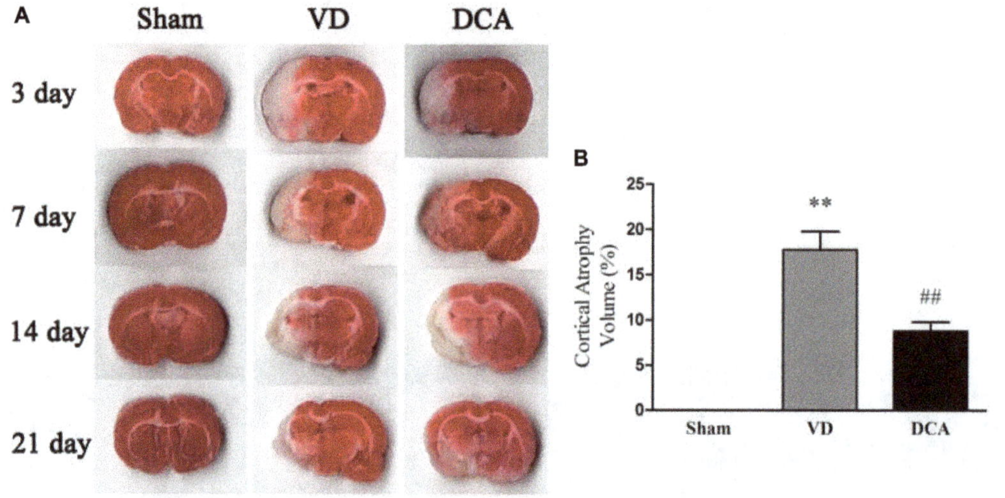

FIGURE 2 | DCA treatment reduces cerebral cortical atrophy in VD rats. TTC staining was used to detect cerebral cortex atrophy in rats, and the degree of brain atrophy in each group was compared. **(A)** Rat brain TTC staining on the 3rd, 7th, 14th, and 21st day (n = 5). **(B)** The degree of cerebral cortex atrophy in rats at 21st day. $^{**}P$ < 0.01 vs. Sham, $^{\#\#}P$ < 0.01 vs. VD (n = 5). Analyses were statistically tested by one-way ANOVA.

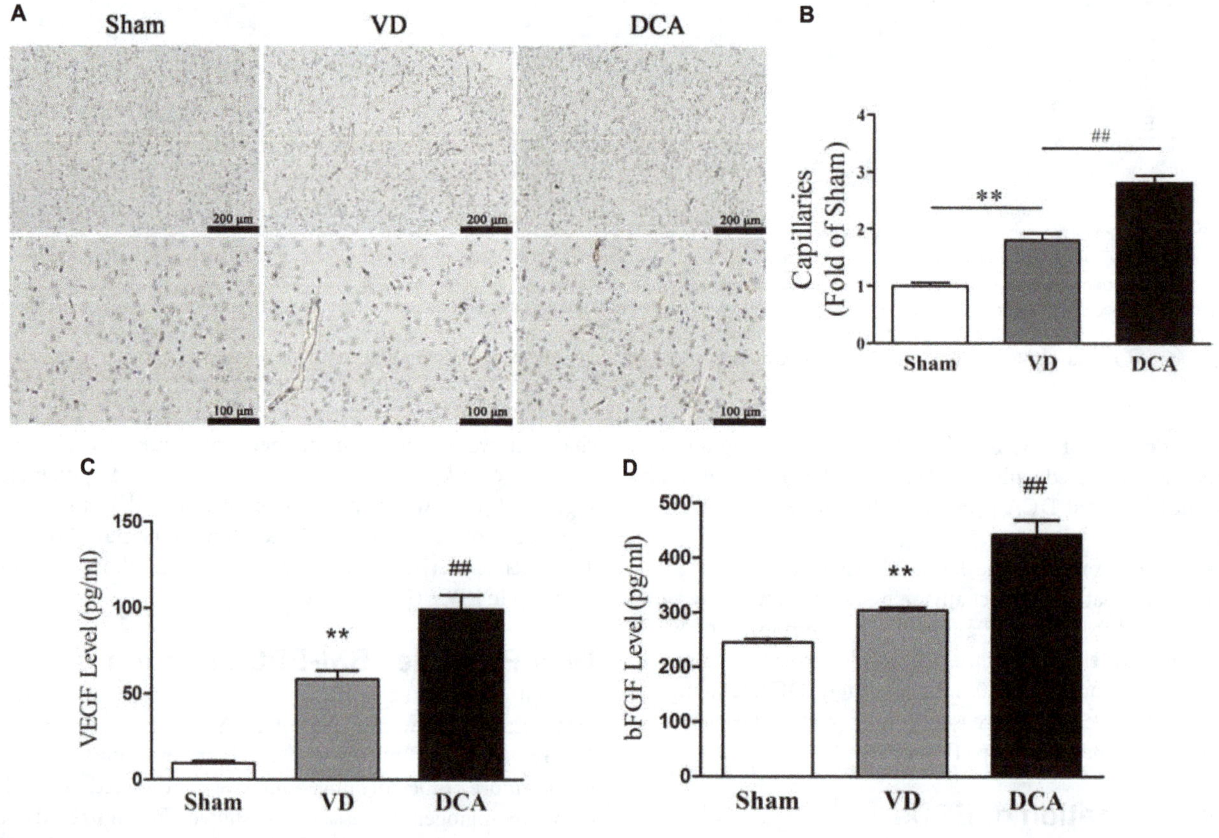

FIGURE 3 | DCA treatment increases angiogenesis in the cortex of VD rats. Immunohistochemistry was used to detect angiogenesis in the rat brain, and ELISA was used to detect the levels of VEGF and bFGF in the serum. **(A)** CD31 immunostaining of cerebral microvessels in rats. **(B)** The bar graph of the number of microvessels in the rats. $^{**}P$ < 0.01 vs. Sham,$^{\#\#}P$ < 0.01 vs. VD (n = 5). Scale bar: 100 μm (up), 50 μm (below). **(C)** Levels of VEGF in rat serum. **(D)** The levels of bFGF in rat serum. $^{**}P$ < 0.01 vs. Sham, $^{\#\#}P$ < 0.01 vs. VD (n = 6). Analyses were statistically tested by one-way ANOVA.

migration (**Figure 4C**), and increased numbers of migrating BM-EPCs were found as compared with controls ($p < 0.01$). In general, DCA enhances BM-EPC functionality.

DCA Increases Peripheral Blood EPC Numbers and Enhances Their Function in VD Rats

After DCA administration for 21 days, the number of peripheral blood EPCs and the functional activity of BM-EPCs in rats were measured. The number of peripheral blood $CD34^+/VEGFR2^+$ EPCs was significantly lower in the VD group as compared with the sham group ($P < 0.05$). Interestingly, DCA administration for 21 days significantly increased the number of peripheral blood $CD34^+/VEGFR2^+$ EPCs ($P < 0.01$; **Figure 5A**).

Bone marrow-derived EPCs culture adhesion ability decreased in VD rats ($P < 0.01$). By contrast, the adhesion of BM-EPCs in DCA-treated VD rats increased significantly ($P < 0.05$; **Figure 5B**). BM-EPC tube-forming ability of VD rats was decreased ($P < 0.01$), while the tube-forming ability of BM-EPCs was significantly increased in DCA-treated VD rats ($P < 0.01$; **Figure 5C**). BM-EPC migration was analyzed by the transwell chamber assay, which showed that BM-EPC migration ability was decreased in VD rats ($P < 0.01$). By contrast, the migration ability of BM-EPCs in DCA-treated VD rats increased significantly ($P < 0.01$; **Figure 5D**). In general, DCA enhanced endothelial progenitor function in VD rats.

DCA Treatment Increased NO Levels and Decreased ROS Levels in BM-EPCs

To determine the underlying mechanism of DCA in EPC protection, we evaluated intracellular ROS and NO levels in rat BM-EPCs (**Figures 6A,B**). Intracellular NO levels were significantly lower in BM-EPCs of VD rats as compared with sham controls ($P < 0.01$), while ROS levels were comparatively higher ($P < 0.05$). However, in the DCA-treated group, the NO levels in EPCs of DCA rats were significantly increased ($P < 0.01$), and the ROS levels were decreased ($P < 0.05$) as compared with the VD group. The results showed that DCA treatment increased NO levels and reduced levels of ROS in EPCs of VD rats.

DCA Improves EPC Function Through an AKT/GSK-3β/Nrf2-Dependent Pathway

We wished to further research the molecular mechanism of VD-induced increases in ROS synthesis by EPCs. We evaluated the expression of AKT, GSK-3β, Nrf2, and eNOS in EPCs. By Western blot analysis, the protein expression of GSK-3β in the VD group was significantly increased compared with controls ($P < 0.01$ and $P < 0.05$, respectively), while the protein expression levels of AKT, Nrf2, and eNOS were comparatively decreased as compared with the control group ($P < 0.05$). In the DCA-treated group, GSK-3β protein expression was significantly decreased as compared with the VD group ($P < 0.01$ and

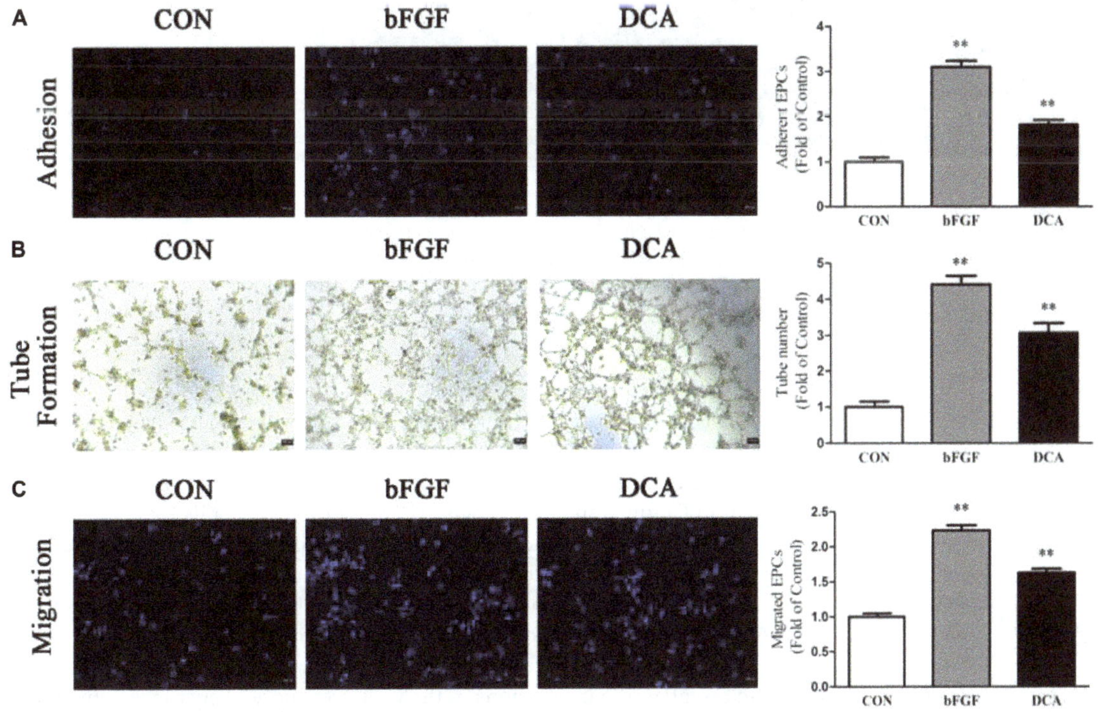

FIGURE 4 | DCA enhances BM-EPC functions. EPC function in each group was compared. **(A)** Adhesion assay for BM-EPC by staining with Hoechst 33258. **(B)** Tube formation of BM-EPC. **(C)** EPCs were cultured in EGM-2 media using transwell chambers at a density of 5×10^4 cells. After migration was permitted for 24 h, the EPCs were stained with Hochest 33258. Migration assay for BM-EPC was determined by counting the number of adherent cells. $^{**}P < 0.01$ vs. Control ($n = 4$). Scale bar: 200 μm. Analyses were statistically tested by one-way ANOVA.

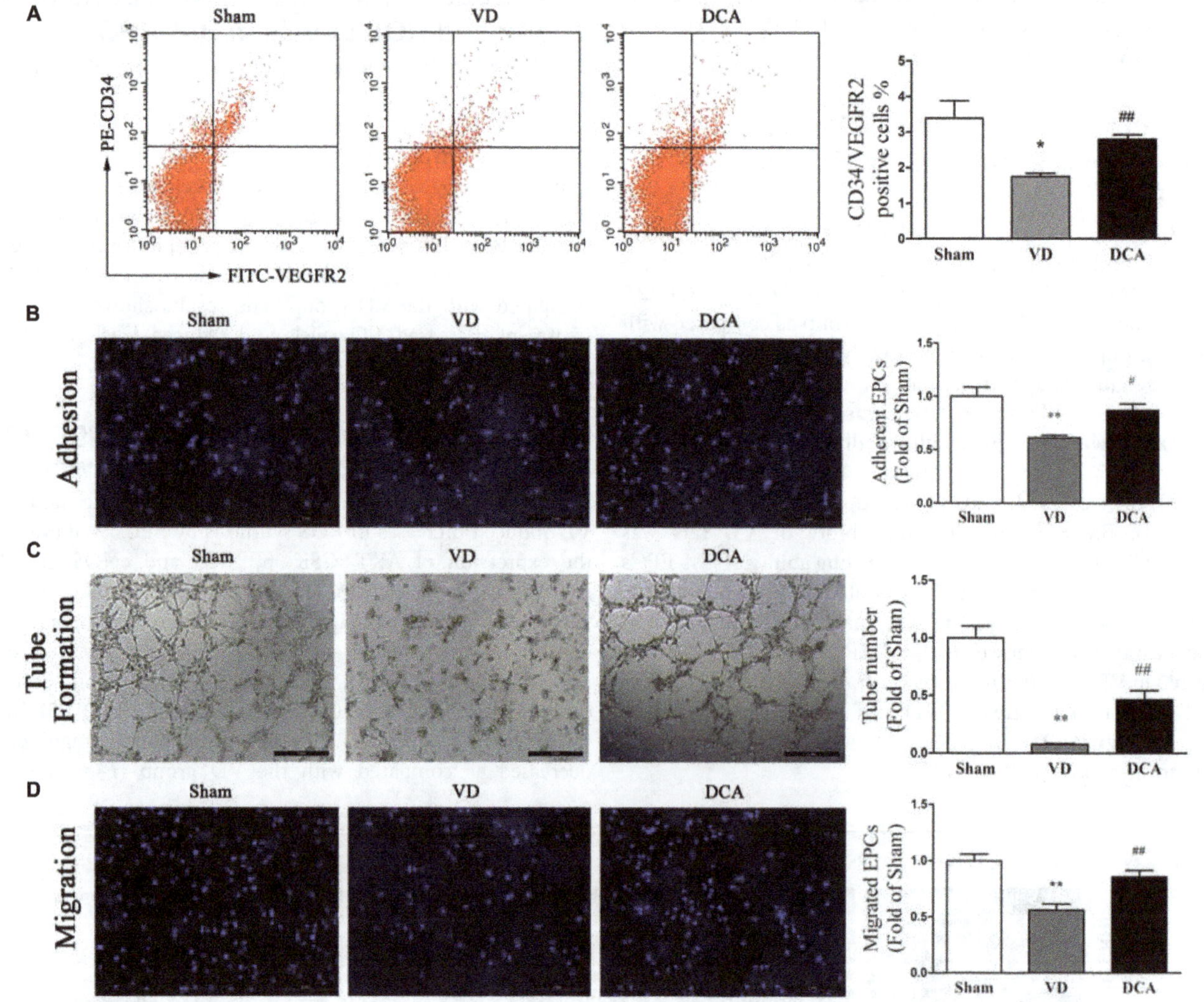

FIGURE 5 | DCA increases peripheral blood endothelial progenitor cells (EPCs) and enhances BM-EPC function in VD rats. **(A)** The number of EPCs in the peripheral blood was detected by flow cytometry (n = 5–6). **(B)** EPC function in each group was compared. EPCs were uniformly seeded in culture plates that were pre-coated with rat vitronectin. Adhesion assay for BM-EPC by staining with Hoechst 33258. **(C)** Tube formation of BM-EPC. **(D)** EPCs were cultured in EGM-2 media using transwell chambers at a density of 5×10^4 cells. After migration was permitted for 24 h, the EPCs were stained with Hochest 33258. Migration assay for BM-EPC was determined by counting the number of adherent cells. $^{*}P < 0.05$, $^{**}P < 0.01$ vs. Sham. $^{\#}P < 0.05$, $^{\#\#}P < 0.01$ vs. VD (n = 4). Scale bar: 200 μm. Analyses were statistically tested by one-way ANOVA.

$P < 0.05$, respectively; **Figure 6D**). Protein expression levels of AKT, Nrf2, and eNOS were all significantly increased ($P < 0.05$; **Figures 6C,D**). These results indicated that the AKT/GSK-3β signaling pathways are involved in improved EPC function following treatment with DCA.

DISCUSSION

Previous studies have shown that DCA plays an essential role in vascular protection and in promoting revascularization of blood vessels (Deuse et al., 2014; Hong et al., 2018) and improves vascular calcification in patients with atherosclerosis (Yang Y. et al., 2018). DCA might also have therapeutic effects in the context of vascular-related diseases.

In the current study, we first evaluated the effect of DCA on VD rats. The cognitive ability of rats tested by the MWM procedure found that an improvement was clearly seen in the cognitive ability of VD rats at 100 mg/kg/day DCA administration, and this dose of DCA could improve the cognitive function in this model and reduce brain damage and brain atrophy in VD rats. The hippocampus is highly sensitive to brain damage, and hippocampal lesions are one of the main causes of dementia (De Leon et al., 1989). The hippocampal lesions in the CA1 area more likely cause dementia with deficits in memory. Reducing lesions in this area of the brain is conducive to improving cognitive function (Ihara et al., 2018). Thus, improved cognitive function following DCA treatment can be partly attributed to reduced hippocampal damage. In this study, Nissl staining of the brain in VD rats showed that

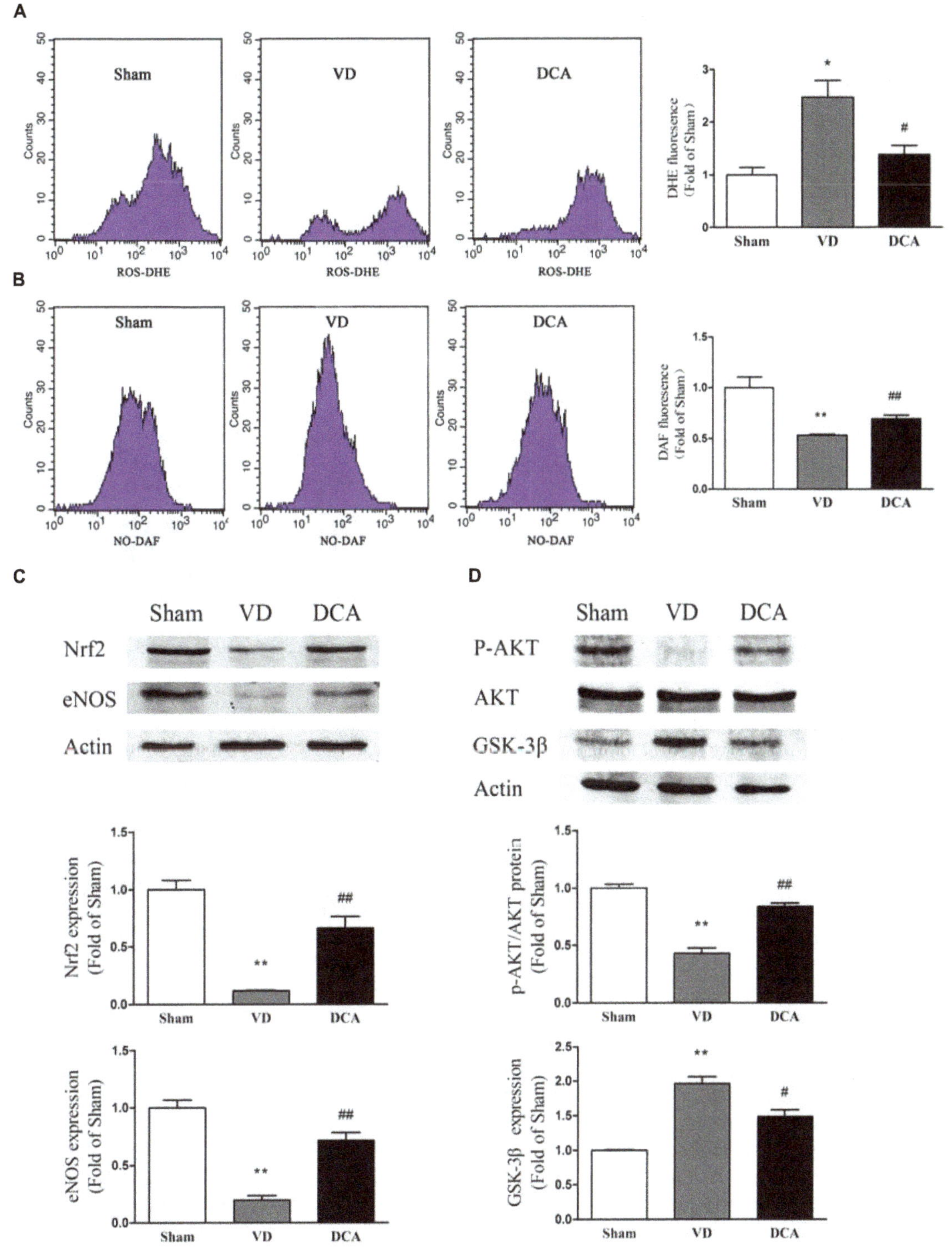

FIGURE 6 | DCA increased NO levels and decreased ROS levels in BM-EPC. Flow cytometry was used to detect the intracellular levels of ROS **(A)** and NO **(B)** in BM-EPCs, $n = 3$. Western Blot assay was used to detect the protein expression of Nrf2 and eNOS **(C)** and P-Akt, eNOS, and GSK-3β **(D)** in BM-EPCs ($n = 3$). $^*P < 0.05$, $^{**}P < 0.01$ vs. Sham. $^{\#}P < 0.05$, $^{\#\#}P < 0.01$ vs. VD. Analyses were statistically tested by one-way ANOVA.

the integrity of hippocampal formation was impaired and the number of necrotic neurons was also increased. DCA treatment significantly increased the number of Nissl bodies and reduced neuronal necrosis. This indicates that DCA has therapeutic effects on VD rats. However, its molecular mechanism needs further exploration.

We found that DCA administration promoted the levels of VEGF and bFGF in the serum of VD rats to increase.

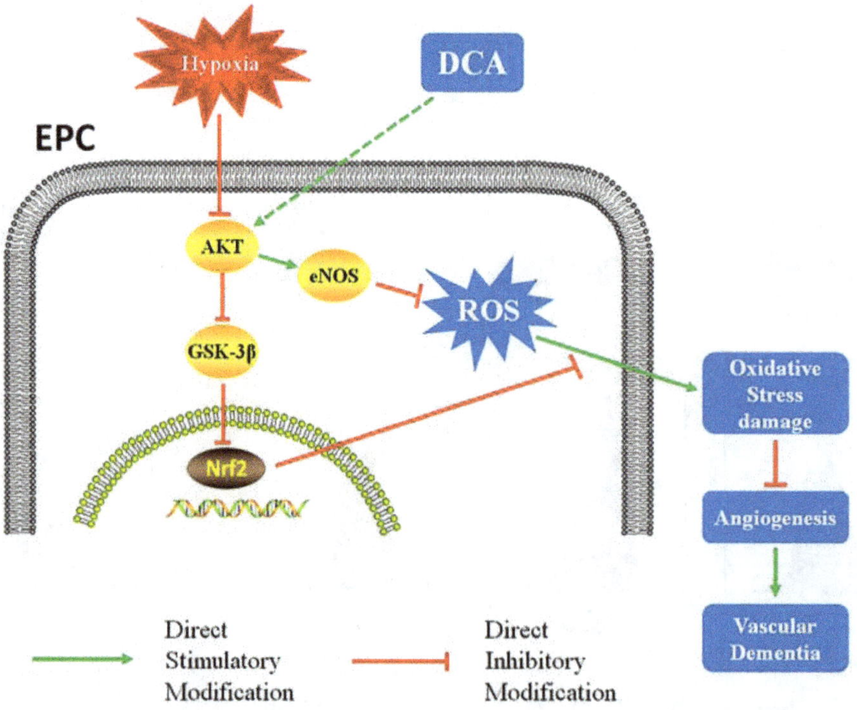

FIGURE 7 | DCA might reduces oxidative stress damage through the AKT/Nrf2 pathway and enhances EPCs function, resulting in faster vessel formation in rats.

VEGF is a potential angiogenic promoter that stimulates the recruitment, proliferation and differentiation of endothelial cells and increases vascular permeability through the VEGF signaling pathway. In addition, VEGF enhances endothelial PDGF-B expression, whereas bFGF, as a crucial vascular growth factor can enhance neural PDGF receptor-β (PDGFR-β) expression. The synergistic effect of VEGF and bFGF promotes mature blood vessel formation and mitosis (Kano et al., 2005; Dashnyam et al., 2017), indicating that the proangiogenic effects of DCA might be related to the release of these cytokines.

DCA treatment significantly improves EPC function (i.e., migration, adhesion, and tube formation) in VD rats. EPC play a vital role in ischemic vascular repair and angiogenesis, which had been previously shown to be a new target cell for the treatment of vascular-related diseases (Asahara et al., 1997). Recent reports have shown that increasing the function of BM-EPCs promotes wound healing and wound neovascularization in diabetic mice (Zhuge et al., 2018). Studies have shown that peripheral blood EPC levels, as biomarkers of vascular function, and homing to vascular injury sites in response to ischemic stimuli, promotes the restoration of endothelial integrity of damaged blood vessels and actively participates in neovascularization (Asahara et al., 1999; Li et al., 2012). Although the number of circulating EPCs peaked within 7 days after ischemic stroke, it was found that ischemic injury resulted in a gradual decrease in the number of circulating EPCs (Martí-Fàbregas et al., 2015), which is insufficient to promote vascular remodeling and regeneration, and an increasement in the number of circulating EPCs was associated with an improved recovery of brain function, and decreased infarct growth (Sobrino et al., 2007). Thus, it is important to improve the number of circulating EPCs after stroke to recover brain function.

We found that DCA treatment significantly increased circulating EPCs levels in VD rats. Consistent with DCA-enhanced EPC functions, DCA intervention also significantly increased local angiogenesis in the rat cerebral cortex. We found that DCA improved the function of EPCs in VD rats. Thus, in order to further verify whether DCA acts directly on EPCs *in vivo* to play a role in the treatment of VD, we performed *in vitro* experiments with DCA, to directly interfere with EPCs. The results showed that DCA significantly improved EPC function.

Several studies have shown that protein kinases including AKT, mTOR and eNOS kinase, regulate angiogenesis (Saraswati et al., 2013), and that the AKT /eNOS pathway is generally considered to be the most important pathway. The expression of Akt and endothelial nitric oxide synthase (eNOS) is thought to enhance EPC and endothelial cell migration and angiogenesis (Huang et al., 2018). GSK3β is a ubiquitously expressed serine/threonine protein kinase (Ma et al., 2010). In EPCs, small molecule inhibition of GSK3β increases the function of EPCs, and does so by increasing angiogenesis in the ischemic model and by improving arterial vascular injury after the repair process has been signaled (Werner et al., 2003). GSK3β expression was elevated in BM-EPCs that were harvested from VD rats, and GSK-3β was significantly reduced in BM-EPC in DCA rats. Studies have shown that decreased expression of eNOS and decreased levels of intracellular NO might be associated with EPC dysfunction (Marrotte et al., 2010), and increased production of ROS in EPCs might provoke apoptosis (Cui et al., 2015).

Nrf2 is a key redox sensor and one of the major regulators of antioxidant response. Nrf2 binds to regulatory antioxidant elements and activates transcription of many antioxidant genes (e.g., HO-1, NQO-1, etc.) to counter ROS accumulation and the potential for subsequent ROS-mediated cellular and DNA damage (Murakami, 2015). In the present study, we found that the expression of Nrf2 was significantly reduced in EPCs of VD rats and that the expression of Nrf2 was elevated in EPCs after DCA treatment. This result indicates that the antioxidant capacity of EPCs can be improved by activating Nrf2 expression. The important role of Nrf2 in endothelial function has also been widely recognized. Florczyk et al. (2014) reported that the lack of Nrf2 attenuates endothelial cell survival, proliferation and angiogenesis both *in vitro* and *in vivo*. Vascular endothelial growth factor increases the nuclear localization of Nrf2 and the expression of its target genes HO-1 and NQO-1, which stimulates the lumen formation of endothelial cells. Our studies in EPCs are consistent with these findings in endothelial cells, and these findings demonstrate that up-regulation of Nrf2 functional expression plays an important role in enhancing EPC function.

In the present study, we observed a significant increasement in AKT, eNOS, and Nrf2 expression in DCA-treated VD rat EPCs, and an increasement in intracellular NO levels with concordant decreases in intracellular ROS. Thus, increasing NO bioavailability by reducing GSK3β expression and increasing both eNOS and Nrf2 expression might partially contribute to enhanced EPC function following DCA treatment.

In conclusion, DCA intervention significantly improved EPC function, increased angiogenesis in the injured area, and improved cognitive function in a rat model of VD (**Figure 7**). These results serve as a new finding for the use of DCA in the setting of VD – providing a potential treatment for patients with vascular-related diseases.

This study demonstrates for the first time that DCA can improve cognitive and EPC functions in a rat model of VD.

AUTHOR CONTRIBUTIONS

TL and YZ conceived and designed the study. YY, JF, and HC constructed the animal model. HZ and JM performed the cell experiments and Western Blot experiment, analyzed the data, and wrote the manuscript. TL, GF, and YZ revised the manuscript.

FUNDING

This work was supported by the Project of Shanghai Science and Technology Transformation and Industrialization (Nos. 15431908500 and 16431901600), the Research project of Shanghai Municipal Commission of Health and Family Planning (Grant No. 201640404), Important Weak Subject Construction Project of shanghai Health and Family Planning Commission (No. 2016ZB0302), and Important Weak Subject Construction Project of Pudong Health and Family Planning Commission of Shanghai (Grant No. PWZbr2017-16).

REFERENCES

Asahara, T., Masuda, H., Takahashi, T., Kalka, C., Pastore, C., Silver, M., et al. (1999). Bone marrow origin of endothelial progenitor cells responsible for postnatal vasculogenesis in physiological and pathological neovascularization. *Circ. Res.* 85, 221–228. doi: 10.1161/01.res.85.3.221

Asahara, T., Murohara, T., Sullivan, A., Silver, M., van der Zee, R., Li, T., et al. (1997). Isolation of putative progenitor endothelial cells for angiogenesis. *Science* 275, 964–967.

Bianconi, V., Sahebkar, A., Kovanen, P., Bagaglia, F., Ricciuti, B., Calabro, P., et al. (2018). Endothelial and cardiac progenitor cells for cardiovascular repair: a controversial paradigm in cell therapy. *Pharmacol. Ther.* 181, 156–168. doi: 10.1016/j.pharmthera.2017.08.004

Cantarella, G., Di Benedetto, G., Puzzo, D., Privitera, L., Loreto, C., Saccone, S., et al. (2015). Neutralization of TNFSF10 ameliorates functional outcome in a murine model of Alzheimer's disease. *Brain* 138, 203–216. doi: 10.1093/brain/awu318

Cui, Y., Xie, X., Jia, F., He, J., Li, Z., Fu, M., et al. (2015). Ambient fine particulate matter induces apoptosis of endothelial progenitor cells through reactive oxygen species formation. *Cell Physiol. Biochem.* 35, 353–363. doi: 10.1159/000369701

Dai, X., Yan, X., Zeng, J., Chen, J., Wang, Y., Chen, J., et al. (2017). Elevating CXCR7 improves angiogenic function of EPCs via Akt/GSK-3beta/Fyn-mediated Nrf2 activation in diabetic limb ischemia. *Circ. Res.* 120, 7–23. doi: 10.1161/CIRCRESAHA.117.310619

Dashnyam, K., Jin, G. Z., Kim, J. H., Perez, R., Jang, J. H., and Kim, H. W. (2017). Promoting angiogenesis with mesoporous microcarriers through a synergistic action of delivered silicon ion and VEGF. *Biomaterials* 116, 145–157. doi: 10.1016/j.biomaterials.2016.11.053

De Leon, M. J., George, A. E., Stylopoulos, L. A., Smith, G., and Miller, D. C. (1989). Early marker for Alzheimer's disease: the atrophic hippocampus. *Lancet* 2, 672–673. doi: 10.1016/s0140-6736(89)90911-2

Deuse, T., Hua, X., Wang, D., Maegdefessel, L., Heeren, J., Scheja, L., et al. (2014). Dichloroacetate prevents restenosis in preclinical animal models of vessel injury. *Nature* 509, 641–644. doi: 10.1038/nature13232

Fan, Y., Shen, F., Frenzel, T., Zhu, W., Ye, J., and Liu, J. (2010). Endothelial progenitor cell transplantation improves long-term stroke outcome in mice. *Ann. Neurol.* 67, 488–497. doi: 10.1002/ana.21919

Florczyk, U., Jazwa, A., Maleszewska, M., Mendel, M., Szade, K., Kozakowska, M., et al. (2014). Nrf2 regulates angiogenesis: effect on endothelial cells, bone marrow-derived proangiogenic cells and hind limb ischemia. *Antioxid. Redox Signal.* 20, 1693–1708. doi: 10.1089/ars.2013.5219

Hong, D. K., Kho, A. R., Choi, B. Y., Lee, S. H., Jeong, J. H., Lee, S. H., et al. (2018). Combined treatment with dichloroacetic acid and pyruvate reduces hippocampal neuronal death after transient cerebral ischemia. *Front. Neurol.* 9:137. doi: 10.3389/fneur.2018.00137

Huang, H., Jin, C. Y., Bi, X. K., Zhao, Y. B., Xu, S. J., Wang, M. H., et al. (2018). Green tea polyphenol epigallocatechin-3-gallate promotes reendothelialization in carotid artery of diabetic rabbits by reactivating Akt/eNOS pathway. *Front. Pharmacol.* 9:1305. doi: 10.3389/fphar.2018.01305

Ihara, R., Vincent, B. D., Baxter, M. R., Franklin, E. E., Hassenstab, J. J., Xiong, C., et al. (2018). Relative neuron loss in hippocampal sclerosis of aging and Alzheimer's disease. *Ann. Neurol.* 84, 741–753. doi: 10.1002/ana.25344

Jin, Y. L., Zhang, H., Gao, Y. Z., Shu, M., Xu, Y., Liu, X., et al. (2015). Neuropsychiatric symptoms in patients with vascular dementia in mainland China. *Transl. Neurosci.* 6, 157–161.

Kano, M. R., Morishita, Y., Iwata, C., Iwasaka, S., Watabe, T., Ouchi, Y., et al. (2005). VEGF-A and FGF-2 synergistically promote neoangiogenesis through enhancement of endogenous PDGF-B-PDGFRbeta signaling. *J. Cell Sci.* 118, 3759–3768. doi: 10.1242/jcs.02483

Li, D. W., Liu, Z. Q., Wei, J., Liu, Y., and Hu, L. S. (2012). Contribution of endothelial progenitor cells to neovascularization (Review). *Int. J. Mol. Med.* 30, 1000–1006. doi: 10.3892/ijmm.2012.1108

Li, W., Huang, R., Shetty, R. A., Thangthaeng, N., Liu, R., Chen, Z., et al. (2013). Transient focal cerebral ischemia induces long-term cognitive function deficit in an experimental ischemic stroke model. *Neurobiol. Dis.* 59, 18–25. doi: 10. 1016/j.nbd.2013.06.014

Longa, E. Z., Weinstein, P. R., Carlson, S., and Cummins, R. (1989). Reversible middle cerebral artery occlusion without craniectomy in rats. *Stroke* 20, 84–91. doi: 10.1161/01.str.20.1.84

Ma, X., Hibbert, B., Dhaliwal, B., Seibert, T., Chen, Y. X., Zhao, X., et al. (2010). Delayed re- endothelialization with rapamycin-coated stents is rescued by the addition of a glycogen synthase kinase-3beta inhibitor. *Cardiovasc. Res.* 86, 338–345. doi: 10.1093/cvr/cvq047

Marrotte, E. J., Chen, D. D., Hakim, J. S., and Chen, A. F. (2010). Manganese superoxide dismutase expression in endothelial progenitor cells accelerates wound healing in diabetic mice. *J. Clin. Invest.* 120, 4207–4219. doi: 10.1172/ JCI36858

Martí-Fàbregas, J., Delgado-Mederos, R., Crespo, J., Peña, E., Marín, R., Jiménez-Xarrié, E., et al. (2015). Circulating endothelial progenitor cells and the risk of vascular events after ischemic stroke. *PLoS One* 10:e0124895. doi: 10.1371/ journal.pone.0124895

Michelakis, E. D., Sutendra, G., Dromparis, P., Webster, L., Haromy, A., Niven, E., et al. (2010). Metabolic modulation of glioblastoma with dichloroacetate. *Sci. Transl. Med.* 2, 31–34.

Michelakis, E. D., Webster, L., and Mackey, J. R. (2008). Dichloroacetate (DCA) as a potential metabolic-targeting therapy for cancer. *Br. J. Cancer* 99, 989–994. doi: 10.1038/sj.bjc.6604554

Morris, R. (1984). Developments of a water-maze procedure for studying spatial learning in the rat. *J. Neurosci. Methods* 11, 47–60. doi: 10.1016/0165-0270(84) 90007-4

Murakami, S. (2015). Roles of nrf2 in cell proliferation and differentiation. *Free Radic. Biol. Med.* 88, 168–178. doi: 10.1016/j.freeradbiomed.2015.06.030

O'Brien, J. T., and Thomas, A. (2015). Vascular dementia. *Lancet* 386, 1698–1706. doi: 10.1016/S0140-6736(15)00463-8

Patel, J., Seppanen, E. J., Rodero, M. P., Wong, H. Y., Donovan, P., Neufeld, Z., et al. (2017). Functional definition of progenitors versus mature endothelial cells reveals key SoxF-dependent differentiation process. *Circulation* 135, 786–805. doi: 10.1161/CIRCULATIONAHA.116.024754

Peng, C., Wang, L. P., Tao, X., Dong, X. H., Xu, C. F., Jiang, Y., et al. (2018). Preventive cold acclimation augments the reparative function of endothelial progenitor cells in mice. *Cell Physiol. Biochem.* 45, 175–191. doi: 10.1159/ 000486356

Rehman, J., Li, J., Orschell, C. M., and March, K. L. (2003). Peripheral blood "endothelial progenitor cells" are derived from monocyte/macrophages and secrete angiogenic growth factors. *Circulation* 107, 1164–1169. doi: 10.1161/ 01.cir.0000058702.69484.a0

Saraswati, S., Kumar, S., and Alhaider, A. A. (2013). alpha-santalol inhibits the angiogenesis and growth of human prostate tumor growth by targeting vascular endothelial growth factor receptor 2-mediated AKT/mTOR/P70S6K signaling pathway. *Mol. Cancer* 12:147. doi: 10.1186/1476-4598-12-147

Sobrino, T., Hurtado, O., Moro, M. A., Rodríguez-Yáñez, M., Castellanos, M., Brea, D., et al. (2007). The increase of circulating endothelial progenitor cells after acute ischemic stroke is associated with good outcome. *Stroke* 38, 2759–2764. doi: 10.1161/strokeaha.107.484386

Werner, N., Junk, S., Laufs, U., Link, A., Walenta, K., and Bohm, M. (2003). Intravenous transfusion of endothelial progenitor cells reduces neointima formation after vascular injury. *Circ. Res.* 93, 17–24.

Williamson, K., Stringer, S. E., and Alexander, M. Y. (2012). Endothelial progenitor cells enter the aging arena. *Front. Physiol.* 3:30. doi: 10.3389/fphys.2012.00030

Xin, B., Liu, C. L., Yang, H., Peng, C., Dong, X. H., Zhang, C., et al. (2016). Prolonged fasting improves endothelial progenitor cell-mediated ischemic angiogenesis in mice. *Cell Physiol. Biochem.* 40, 693–706. doi: 10.1159/ 000452581

Yang, J. X., Pan, Y. Y., Chen, B., Qiu, Y. G., Mao, W., and Hu, S. J. (2018). The role of RhoA in neovascular-related functions of endothelial progenitor cells induced by angiotensin. *Cell Physiol. Biochem.* 47, 2498–2510. doi: 10.1159/000491623

Yang, Y., Sun, Y., Chen, J., Bradley, W. E., Dell'Italia, L. J., Wu, H., et al. (2018). AKT-independent activation of p38 MAP kinase promotes vascular calcification. *Redox Biol.* 16, 97–103. doi: 10.1016/j.redox.2018.02.009

Yew, B., Nation, D. A., and Neuroimaging ASD (2017). Cerebrovascular resistance: effects on cognitive decline, cortical atrophy, and progression to dementia. *Brain* 140, 1987–2001. doi: 10.1093/brain/awx112

Zhang, Y., Chen, J., Li, F., Li, D., Xiong, Q., Lin, Y., et al. (2012). A pentapeptide monocyte locomotion inhibitory factor protects brain ischemia injury by targeting the eEF1A1/endothelial nitric oxide synthase pathway. *Stroke* 43, 2764–2773. doi: 10.1161/strokeaha.112.657908

Zhou, L., Li, F., Xu, H. B., Luo, C. X., Wu, H. Y., and Zhu, M. M. (2010). Treatment of cerebral ischemia by disrupting ischemia-induced interaction of nNOS with PSD-95. *Nat. Med.* 16, 1439–1443. doi: 10.1038/nm.2245

Zhu, Q., Zhang, Y., Liu, Y., Cheng, H., Wang, J., Zhang, Y., et al. (2016). MLIF Alleviates SH-SY5Y neuroblastoma injury induced by oxygen-glucose deprivation by targeting eukaryotic translation elongation factor 1A2. *PLoS One* 11:e0149965. doi: 10.1371/journal.pone.0149965

Zhuge, Y., Regueiro, M. M., Tian, R., Li, Y., Xia, X., Vazquez-Padron, R., et al. (2018). The effect of estrogen on diabetic wound healing is mediated through increasing the function of various bone marrow-derived progenitor cells. *J. Vasc. Surg.* 68, 127–135. doi: 10.1016/j.jvs.2018.04.069

4

Adiponectin Protects Against Cerebral Ischemic Injury Through AdipoR1/AMPK Pathways

Bin Liu†, Jing Liu†, Jiangong Wang, Fengjiao Sun, Shujun Jiang, Fengai Hu, Dan Wang, Dunjiang Liu, Cuilan Liu and Haijing Yan*

Institute for Metabolic and Neuropsychiatric Disorders, Binzhou Medical University Hospital, Binzhou, China

***Correspondence:**
Haijing Yan
hjyan211@163.com

†These authors have contributed equally to this work.

Excitotoxicity induced by excessive N-methyl-D-aspartate (NMDA) receptor activation underlies the pathology of ischemic injury. Adiponectin (APN) is an adipocyte-derived protein hormone that modulates a number of metabolic processes. APN exerts a wide range of biological functions in the central nervous system. However, the role of APN and its receptors in cerebral ischemia/reperfusion (I/R)-induced injury and the related mechanisms remain to be clarified. Here, we found that APN and APN receptor agonist AdipoRon (APR) were protective against excitotoxicity induced by oxygen and glucose deprivation/reperfusion (OGD/R) and NMDA in primary neurons. Adiponectin receptor 1 (AdipoR1) knockdown reversed the protection conferred by either APN or APR. Moreover, the protective effects offered by both APN and APR were compromised by compound C, an inhibitor of amp-activated protein kinase (AMPK) phosphorylation. Both APN and APR protected the dissipation of the $\Delta\Psi m$ caused by OGD/R. They also up-regulated the PGC-1α expression, which was reversed by compound C. Furthermore, both APN and APR ameliorated but APN knockout aggravated the infarct volume and neurological deficient induced by transient middle cerebral artery occlusion (tMCAO) *in vivo*. Taken together, these findings show that APN and APR protect against ischemic injury *in vitro* and *in vivo*. The protective mechanism is mainly related to AdipoR1-dependent AMPK phosphorylation and PGC-1α up-regulation.

Keywords: adiponectin, AdipoRon, ischemia, adiponectin receptor 1, amp-activated protein kinase, PGC-1α, mitochondrial

INTRODUCTION

Under physiological condition, glutamate mainly involves in synaptic plasticity, learning, and memory physiological process; however in pathological condition, it tends to show neuronal excitotoxicity (Wu and Tymianski, 2018), which is caused by overactivated NMDA receptor by excessive extracellular glutamate (Rothman and Olney, 1995). Abnormal function of the glutamatergic system has been implicated in the pathophysiology of stroke (Dirnagl et al., 1999).

Adiponectin (APN) is a fat-derived secreted protein negatively associated with fat accumulation (Hu et al., 1996; Diez and Iglesias, 2003). APN is able to cross the blood–brain barrier (BBB) (Kubota et al., 2007; Kusminski et al., 2007), and binds with its receptors (AdipoR1 and AdipoR2) to activate numerous signaling pathways, including amp-activated protein kinase (AMPK) and p38 mitogen-activated protein kinase (p38 MAPK), to regulate cell functions (Scherer et al., 1995; Mao et al., 2006;

Thundyil et al., 2012). AdipoR1 is widely expressed in the brain, whereas AdipoR2 is barely expressed in the brain (Hug et al., 2004). In the central nervous system (CNS), AdipoR1 is mainly expressed in neurons and is involved in the regulation of energy metabolism (Thundyil et al., 2012).

APN was primarily regarded important in regulating the functions, such as body weight, endothelial function, insulin-sensitization, anti-atherogenic, and anti-inflammatory actions (Ouchi et al., 1999; Yamauchi et al., 2001; Diez and Iglesias, 2003). Recently, many studies indicate that APN plays an important role in the regulation of CNS pathologies, such as depression, AD, epilepsy, and stroke. The APN peripheral levels were significantly lower in major depressive disorder patients (Carvalho et al., 2014), and administration of APN elicited antidepressant-like behavioral effects in mice through the inhibition of GSK-3β (Liu et al., 2012). The serum APN also significantly decreased in AD patients (Teixeira et al., 2013), and APN was protective against amyloid β-induced neurotoxicity in Alzheimer's disease through AMPK activation and NF-κB suppression (Chan et al., 2012). Decreased serum APN and increased hippocampal AdipoR1 were found in the hippocampus of KA-treated seizure mice (Jeon et al., 2009). APN was neuroprotective against seizures through preserving the integrity of the BBB (Jeon et al., 2009). However, APN deficiency exacerbated seizure-related brain injury (Lee et al., 2011). Thus, APN plays an important role in neurological disorders.

APN level is significantly reduced, and APN reversed the decreased cerebral blood flow (CBF) during cerebral ischemia (Nishimura et al., 2008). APN protects against glutamate-induced excitotoxicity in HT22 hippocampal neurons (Yue et al., 2016; Wang et al., 2018). APN also protects against ischemia in diabetic mice (Song et al., 2015). However, the protective mechanism of APN on cerebral ischemic injury remains to be studied in the neurons of cortex, which is the main damage area of ischemia. In this article, we will study the effects of APN and APN receptor agonist AdipoRon (APR) on OGD/R-induced excitotoxicity the further investigate the related mechanisms in primary neurons.

MATERIALS AND METHODS

Cell Culture

For primary neuronal cell culture, pregnant C57BL6J mice were anesthetized by intraperitoneal injection of chloral hydrate, and the cortex was isolated from embryos (18 days). Cells (800–1,000 cells/mm^2) were seeded on coverslips coated with 30 mg/ml poly-D-lysine. Cells were placed in fresh serum-free neurobasal medium (21103, Gibco) plus 2% B27 and fed every 4 days with fresh medium and used after 7 days (DIV7).

Oxygen-Glucose Deprivation and Drug Administration

Cells were rinsed twice with warm glucose-free dulbecco's modified eagle medium (DMEM) (Gibco), and refreshed with O_2- and glucose-free DMEM (pre-balanced in an O_2-free chamber at 37°C). Cells were then immediately placed in a sealed chamber (Billups Rothenburg, MIC-101) loaded with mixed gas containing 5% CO_2 and 95% N_2 for 5 min at 25 L/min. The primary neurons were then incubated at 37°C for 2 h before reperfusion. For reperfusion, cells were refreshed with normal culture medium. The indicated concentrations of APN was dissolved in PBS, whereas APR and compound C were dissolved in dimethyl sulfoxide. APN and APR were administrated 0.5 h, whereas compound C was administrated 1 h before OGD treatment. Control cells were given equal refreshment but were incubated in glucose-containing DMEM for 2 h for OGD/R. The indicated concentrations of the chemicals were administrated on the basis of previous studies (Zhang et al., 2011; Domise et al., 2016; Zhang et al., 2017).

MTT Assay

Cell viability was determined by 3-(4,5-dimethylthiazol-2-yl)-2,5-diphenyltetrazolium bromide (MTT) assay. Briefly, neurons were incubated with 0.5 mg/ml MTT for 2 h at 37°C after OGD/R treatment. The supernatant layer was removed, and 100 μl of dimethyl sulfoxide was added into each well. MTT metabolism was quantitated spectrophotometrically at 570 nm in a Biorad microplate reader. Results were expressed as the percentage of MTT reduction, taking the absorbance of control cells as 100%.

Apoptosis Determined by TUNEL Assay

Apoptotic cells were determined by terminal deoxynucleotidyl transferase dUTP nick-end labeling (TUNEL) assay (Roche), and the total cell number was counted after DAPI staining. Five random fields were observed on each coverslip, and the experiments were repeated independently three times. The results were expressed as the percentage of TUNEL$^+$/DAPI$^+$ cells in the sections.

Immunohistochemistry

Immunostaining was also performed in cultured neurons. Neurons seeded on coverslips were fixed in cold methanol for 10 min, and then incubated in 5% Bovine serum albumin (BSA) for 2 h to block nonspecific binding of IgG. Then the cells were reacted with antibody at 4°C overnight. The primary antibodies used in this experiment were MAP2 (MAB2418, Millipore, 1:300). After repeated washes in phosphate-buffered saline (PBS), cells were incubated with secondary antibody in 3% BSA for 2 h at 25°C. The secondary antibodies used in this experiment were goat anti-mouse IgG-AlexaFluo 594 (1:300, A11005; Invitrogen). After further washing in PBS, cultures were dried, coverslipped, and mounted on glass slides. The stained cells were observed under a fluorescence microscope (Olympus BX51, Japan). Total dendritic length and neuronal complexity were quantified by using ImageJ software and the Fiji plugins Simple Neurite Tracer Analysis as well as Sholl Analysis.

Western Blot

Cultured neurons were lysed in ice-cold lysis buffer containing (in mmol/L): 50 Tris-HCl, 150 NaCl, 1% NP-40, 2 EDTA, 1 Na_3VO_4, pH 7.4) after 24 h of reperfusion. Mice were anesthetized by intraperitoneal injection of chloral hydrate (400 mg/kg), sacrificed 24 h after tMCAO or sham operation, and the brain was quickly removed and was immediately put in −40°C for 5 min. The separated tissue was lysed in ice-cold lysis buffer. After clearing debris by centrifugation at 14,000×*g* at 4°C, the protein concentration in the extracts was determined by the Bradford assay (Thermo, Hercules, CA). The precipitates were denatured with SDS sample loading buffer and separated on 10% SDS-PAGE. Proteins were transferred onto nitrocellulose membranes using a Bio-Rad mini-protein-III wet transfer unit overnight at 4°C. Transfer membranes were then incubated with blocking solution (5% nonfat dried milk dissolved in tris buffered saline tween (TBST) buffer (in mM): 10 Tris-HCl, 150 NaCl, and 0.1% Tween-20) for 1 h at room temperature, washed three times, and incubated with primary antibody for 2 h at room temperature. The primary antibodies used in this experiment were AdipoR1 (ab70362; Abcam, 1:1,000), AdipoR2 (ab77612, Abcam; 1:1,000), β-Actin (4970, Cell Signaling Technology, 1:1,000), Phospho-AMPK (2535, Cell Signaling Technology, 1:1,000), AMPK (2532, Cell Signaling Technology, 1:1,000), PGC-1α (ab54481; Abcam, 1:1,000), GAPDH (1:3,000; KC-5G4, KangChen Bio-tech, Shanghai). Membranes were washed three times in TBST buffer and incubated with the appropriate secondary antibodies (Odyssey, LI-COR, 1:5,000 dilution) for 2 h. Images were acquired with the Odyssey infrared imaging system and analyzed as specified in the Odyssey software manual. The results were expressed as the target protein/GAPDH or β-actin ratio and then normalized to the values measured in the control groups (presented as 100%).

RNA Interference

Small-interfering RNA (siRNA) targeting mouse AdipoR1 were synthesized by corporation (GenePharm, Shanghai) as follows: negativecontrol(sense:5′-UUCUCCGAACGUGUCACGUTT-3′, antisense: 3′-ACGUGACACGUUCGGAGAATT-5′); sequence 1: (sense: 5′-AGGAGUUCGUGUAUAAGGUTT-3′, antisense: 5′-ACCU UAUACACGAACUCCUTT-3′); sequence 2: (sense: 5′-ACCAAAUAUGUACUU CAUGTT-3′, antisense: 5′-CAUG AAGUACAUAUUUGGUTT-3′); sequence 3: (sense: 5′-GGCUC UAUUACUCCUUCUATT-3′, antisense: 5′-UA GAAGGAGUAA UAGAGCCTT-3′). Primary neurons were transfected on DIV5, with 20 nmol AdipoR1 or negative control siRNA using Lipofectamine RNAiMAX (Invitrogen). After transfection in antibiotic-free medium for 8 h, cells were refreshed with normal medium. Experiments were performed 72 h after transfection.

Mitochondrial Membrane Potential Assessment

The changes in relative mitochondrial membrane potential (ΔΨm) were assessed by using the lipophilic cationic probe 5,5′,6,6′-tetrachloro-1,1′,3,3′-tetraethylbenzamid azolocarbocyanine iodide (JC-1; Molecular Probes). The dye JC-1 undergoes a reversible change in fluorescence emission from green to greenish orange as ΔΨm increases. Cells with high ΔΨm form JC-1 aggregates and fluoresce red; those with low ΔΨm contain monomeric JC-1 and fluoresce green. After 2-h OGD and 24-h reperfusion, culture medium was removed and the cells, grown on coverslips, were incubated in the dark with JC-1 at a final concentration of 1.5 μM for 20 min. The cells were rinsed with PBS and excited at 488 nm with an Olympus BX-51 fluorescence microscope.

Animals

Adult male WT and APN-KO mice (all C57BL/6 strain) were purchased from Shanghai Biomodel Organism Science & Technology Development Co. Ltd (Shanghai, China). Male WT mice and APN-KO mice weighing 22 to 25 g were used. For primary cortical neuronal culture, pregnant mice with embryonic (E18) fetuses were used. Mice were housed in separate cages under standard conditions, with a 12 h light/dark cycle (lights on at 9:00 AM), and with *ad libitum* access to food and water. All experiments and protocols were approved by and conducted in accordance with the ethical guidelines of the Bin Zhou Medical University Animal Experimentation Committee and were in complete compliance with the National Institutes of Health Guide for the Care and Use of Laboratory Animals. Efforts were made to minimize any pain or discomfort, and the minimum number of animals was used.

Transient MCAO Models and Drug Treatment

Mice were fasted overnight and anesthetized by intraperitoneal injection of chloral hydrate (400 mg/kg). Transient focal cerebral ischemia was induced by transient middle cerebral artery occlusion (tMCAO) (Yan et al., 2014). Briefly, a 6-0 nylon monofilament suture, blunted at the tip and coated with 1% poly-l-lysine, was advanced ~10 mm into the internal carotid to occlude the origin of the middle cerebral artery (MCA). Reperfusion was allowed after 1 h by monofilament removal. Body temperature was maintained at 37°C with a heat lamp (FHC; Bowdoinham, ME, USA) during surgery and for 2 h after the start of reperfusion. CBF was determined in the territory of the MCA by laser Doppler flowmetry (Moor Instruments Ltd). A flexible fiber-optic probe was affixed to the skull over the cortex supplied by the proximal part of the right MCA (2 mm caudal to bregma and 6 mm lateral to midline). Animals with <80% reduction in CBF in the core of the MCA territory were excluded from the study. WT mice were randomly divided into separate four groups of four to five mice. Mice were given an intracerebroventricular injection of APN (1 μl of 0.3 mg/ml dissolved in saline) and APR (1 μl of 1 mg/ml dissolved in dimethyl sulfoxide) at 0.5 h before tMCAO, whereas compound C (1 μl of 40 mg/ml dissolved in dimethyl sulfoxide) at 1 h before tMCAO. Mice in control group were given equal saline or dimethyl sulfoxide. The indicated concentrations of the chemicals were administrated on the basis of previous studies (Wen et al., 2012; Zhang et al., 2016; Zhang et al., 2017).

Neurologic deficit scores were evaluated at 24 h of reperfusion as follows: 0, no deficit; 1, flexion of the contralateral forelimb on lifting of the whole animal by the tail; 2, circling to the contralateral side; 3, falling to the contralateral side; and 4, no spontaneous motor activity (Longa et al., 1989).

The infarct volume was determined at 24 h of reperfusion. The brains were quickly removed, sectioned coronally at 2-mm intervals and stained by immersion in the vital dye 2,3,5-triphenyltetrazolium hydrochloride (0.25%) at 37°C for 30 min. The extents of the normal and infarcted areas were analyzed using ImageJ (National Institutes of Health, Bethesda, MD, USA) and determined by the indirect method, which corrects for edema (contralateral hemisphere volume minus non-ischemic ipsilateral hemisphere volume). The percentage of the corrected infarct volume was calculated by dividing the infarct volume by the total contralateral hemispheric volume, and this ratio was then multiplied by 100.

Statistical Analyses

Results are expressed as mean ± SEM. Statistical analysis was performed by one-way ANOVAs, followed by Tukey's *post hoc* comparisons, using Prism software. P value <0.05 was considered statistically significant.

RESULTS

Effects of APN and APR on Neuronal Viability on OGD/R- and NMDA-Induced Injury

Studies have shown that APN levels are significantly down-regulated in the brains of ischemic stroke victims (Pera et al., 2013), suggesting that low levels of APN might increase the risk of stroke. To figure out whether APN is protective against ischemic injury, two *in vitro* ischemic models on primary neurons were used. To investigate the role of APN on OGD/R-induced injury in primary neurons, various doses of APN on cell viability were detected by MTT. The results indicated that under OGD/R, the cell viability declined to 71.00 ± 3.32% of control (P <0.001, **Figure 1A**). APN could rescue neurons from OGD/R-induced cell viability impairment, as cell viability increased significantly to 88.47 ± 3.38% (P <0.01, **Figure 1A**) when APN (1 μg/ml) was administrated. However, no significant difference in cell viability was observed between vehicle (0 μg/ml) and low dose of APN (0.03, 0.3 μg/ml) groups (P > 0.05). Therefore, a dose of 1 μg/ml APN is selected for the later study. APR is an

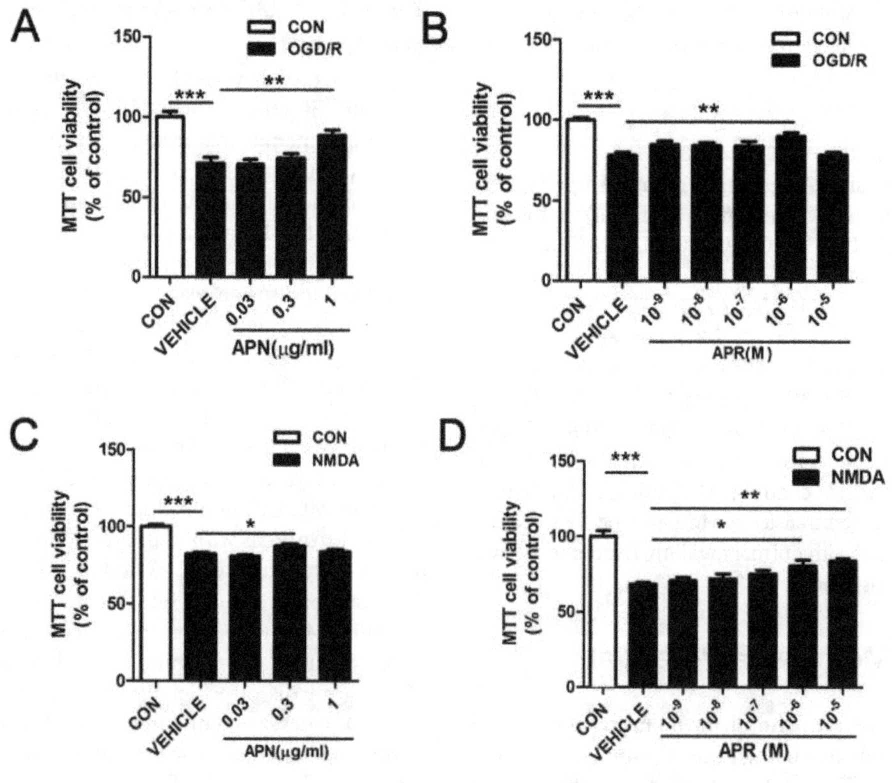

FIGURE 1 | Effects of APN and APR on OGD/R-induced and NMDA-induced cell viability in promary neurons. **(A)** When APN (0.5 h before OGD treatment) was administered, cell viability was tested in primary neurons by MTT assay after OGD/R-induced injury (n = 6 per condition; **P <0.01, ***P <0.001 with ANOVAs followed by Tukey's *post hoc* test). Data are presented as mean ± SEM. **(B)** When APR (0.5 h before OGD treatment) was administered, cell viability was tested in primary neurons by MTT assay after OGD/R-induced injury (n = 8-14 per condition; **P <0.01, ***P <0.001 with ANOVAs followed by Tukey's *post hoc* test). Data are presented as mean ± SEM. **(C)** When APN (0.5 h before NMDA treatment) was administered, cell viability was tested in primary neurons by MTT assay after NMDA-induced (200 μM, 2 h) (n = 9-14 per condition; *P < 0.05, ***P < 0.001 with ANOVAs followed by Tukey's *post hoc* test). Data are presented as mean ± SEM. **(D)** When APR (0.5 h before NMDA treatment) was administered, cell viability was tested in primary neurons by MTT assay after NMDA-induced (200 μM, 2 h) injury (n = 7 per condition; *P <0.05, **P <0.01, ***P <0.001 with ANOVAs followed by Tukey's *post hoc* test). Data are presented as mean ± SEM.

agonist of APN receptors, and then we also assessed the role of APR in OGD/R-induced injury. The results showed that the cell viability increased significantly from 78.11 ± 1.81% to 89.96 ± 2.34% (P <0.01, **Figure 1B**) when APR (10^{-6} M) was administrated, suggesting the APR was also protective against OGD/R-induced injury. Above all, these results told us that APN and APR protected neurons against OGD/R-induced injury in primary neurons.

Studies have demonstrated that excitotoxicity plays an important role in the pathological processes of ischemic brain injury (Rothman and Olney, 1995). To study the effects of APN and its receptors on neuronal excitotoxicity, an NMDA-induced excitotoxic model on primary neurons were used. The results showed that primary neurons exposed to NMDA exhibited a decreased cell viability of 80.20 ± 0.74% (P <0.001, **Figure 1C**), and APN (0.3 μg/ml) rescued the viability to 87.35 ± 1.29% (P <0.05, **Figure 1C**). Moreover, APR (10^{-6} M) rescued the viability from 78.34 ± 1.93% to 95.98 ± 3.58% (P <0.05, **Figure 1D**), and APR (10^{-5} M) rescued the viability to 98.16 ± 2.76% (P <0.01, **Figure 1D**). Above all, these results suggested that APN and APR were protective against NMDA-induced excitotoxicity in primary neurons.

Effects of APN and APR on Apoptosis and Neuronal Morphology on OGD/R

It is reported that ischemic injury induces neuronal apoptosis and morphological changes of dendrite (Kanazawa et al., 2017). Thus, we investigated the roles of APN and APR on apoptosis by TUNEL. The results indicated that the percentage of TUNEL-positive apoptotic cells was 10.61 ± 0.90% in the control group, and OGD/R induced an increase of the percentage to 83.46 ± 2.16% (P <0.001). APR (1 μM) and APN (1 μg/ml) rescued the apoptotic cells to 23.66 ± 2.50% (P <0.001, **Figure 2A**, **B**) and 24.36 ± 1.80%, respectively (P <0.001, **Figure 2A**, **B**).

Moreover, we investigated the roles of APN and APR on morphological changes of dendrite. The MAP-2 staining results showed that the total dendritic length was 436.3 ± 39.9 μm in the OGD/R group compared with 1,048 ± 84.91 μm in the control group (P <0.001, **Figure 2C**, **D**). APN (1 μg/ml) and APR (1 μM) rescued the total dendritic length to 840.3 ± 74.83% (P <0.01, **Figure 2C**, **D**) and 830.3 ± 59.25%, respectively (P <0.01, **Figure 2C**, **D**). We further analyzed the effects of APN and APR on dendritic complexity. The Sholl analysis showed that the dendritic intersections significantly reduced between 60 μand 80 μm from the soma in OGD/R group compared with the control group (P <0.01, **Figure 2C**, **E**). Both APN and APR significantly increased the dendritic intersections between 60 and 80 μm from the soma compared with the OGD/R group (P <0.01, **Figure 2C**, **E**). Taken together, the above results suggested that APN and APR reduced the apoptosis and increased either total dendritic length and dendritic complexity on OGD/R-induced injury in primary neurons.

Involvement of AdipoR1 in the Protective Effects of APN and APR Against OGD/R-Induced Injury

Reports show that AdipoR1 is widely expressed in the brain, whereas AdipoR2 is barely expressed in the brain (Hug et al., 2004). To investigate the role of APN receptors in ischemia, we examined their expression by Western blot. Results indicated that AdipoR1 was extensively expressed in the brain cortex, hippocampus, striatum, and thalamus (**Figure 3A**). Interestingly, the expression of AdipoR1 increased dramatically in the cortex and striatum, regions that are highly vulnerable to ischemia (Hammond et al., 1994; Miladinovic et al., 2015) (**Figure 3A**). This might be an endogenous protection against ischemic injury and implicated an important role of AdipoR1 in ischemia. We also examined the expression of AdipoR2 in the brain. Results showed that AdipoR2 is highly expressed in the liver, but barely expressed in brain regions including cortex, hippocampus, striatum, and thalamus (**Figure 3B**). These results reminded us that AdipoR1 but not AdipoR2 might play an important role in the CNS.

To further investigate the role of AdipoR1 in ischemia, AdipoR1 siRNA was transfected in primary neurons. Three siRNA fragments were applied, and the results showed that the effective siRNA fragment is sequence 2 (reduced to 32.71± 2.28% of negative control, P <0.01, **Figure 3C**). Thus, sequence 2 was selected for the later study. The results indicated that the protective effects of APN against OGD/R was reversed completely by AdipoR1 siRNA (from 94.94 ± 1.96% to 70.88 ± 4.04%, P <0.01, **Figure 3D**). In addition, the protection of APR against OGD/R was also reversed by AdipoR1 silencing (from 90.03 ± 12.48% to 66.93 ± 1.41%, P <0.05, **Figure 3D**). Moreover, we also observed similar effects of APN (from 105.3 ± 1.86% to 73.03 ± 3.18%, P <0.01, **Figure 3E**) and APR (from 103.1 ± 9.14% to 69.07 ± 3.62%, P <0.01, **Figure 3E**) in NMDA-induced excitotoxicity.

Involvement of AMPK Pathway in the Protective Effects of APN and APR on OGD/R-Induced Injury

Studies show that APN binds with AdipoR1 to activate AMPK pathway (Thundyil et al., 2012). APN improves numerous neurological diseases through AMPK signaling (Chan et al., 2012; Yan et al., 2013; Xu et al., 2018). To investigate the signaling pathway of the protective effects offered by APN and APR, we analyzed the AMPK phosphorylation. The Western blot results showed that the expressions of p-AMPK was significantly lower in the OGD/R group in primary neurons compared with the control group (reduced to 43.16 ± 9.36% of control, P <0.01, **Figure 4A**), suggesting OGD/R inactivated AMPK pathway. However, the expression of p-AMPK was significantly higher in APN group (increased to 92.27 ± 6.78% of control, P <0.05, **Figure 4A**) and APR group (increased to 94.63 ± 5.90% of control, P <0.05, **Figure 4A**) compared with the vehicle group, suggesting APN and APR promoted the activation AMPK pathway. Moreover, compound C, an inhibitor of p-AMPK, reversed the p-AMPK level offered by both APN (reduced to 36.87 ± 3.34% of control, P <0.05, **Figure 4A**) and APR (reduced to 43.55 ± 5.11% of control, P <0.05, **Figure 4A**), suggesting the effectiveness of compound C.

To further investigate the involvement of AMPK in the protections of APN and APR on OGD/R-induced injury, the cell viability was assessed when the inhibitor of p-AMPK (compound C) was administrated. The results showed that the cell viability markedly decreased both in the APN+ compound C group compared with the APN group (from 89.78 ± 2.09% to 63.99 ± 3.02% of control, P <0.001, **Figure 4B**) and in the APR+ compound C group compared with the APR group (from

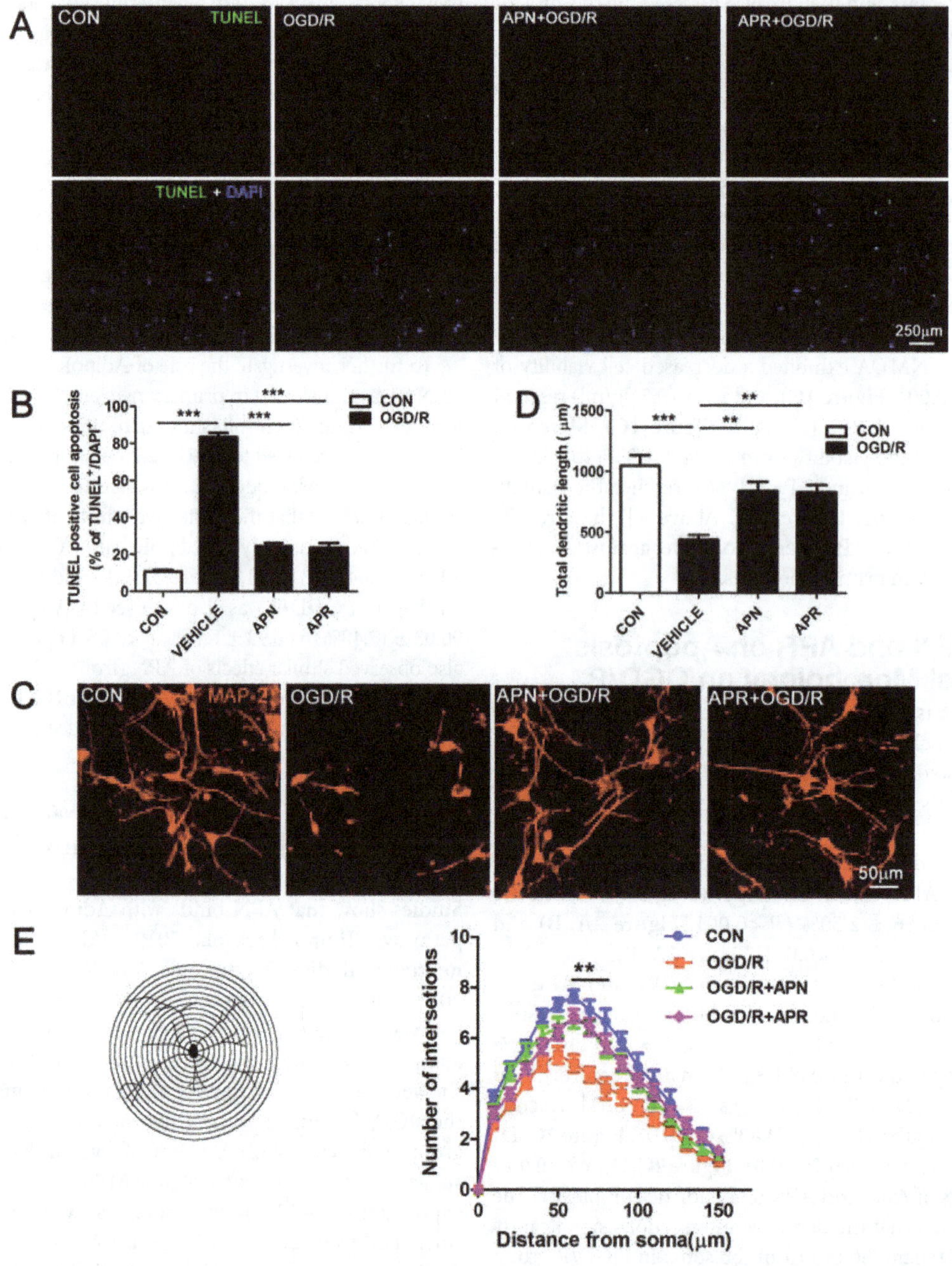

FIGURE 2 | Effects of APN and APR on OGD/R-induced apoptosis and dendritic morphology in promary neurons. **(A)** Effects of APN (1 μg/ml) and APR (1 μM) on apoptotic cells stained by TUNEL in primary neurons under OGD/R. TUNEL-positive cells are green, and all cells are stained with DAPI (blue). Scale bar: 250 μm. **(B)** The bar graph indicated the effects of APN and APR on the percentage of TUNEL-positive apoptotic neurons under OGD/R (n = 4 per condition; ****P* <0.001 with ANOVAs followed by Tukey's *post hoc* test). Data are presented as mean ± SEM. **(C)** Effects of APN (1 μg/ml) and APR(1 μM) on MAP-2-positive (red) neuronal morphology under OGD/R. Scale bar: 50 μm. **(D)** The bar graph indicated the effects of APN and APR on the total dendritic length under OGD/R in primary neurons. (n = 4 per condition; ***P* <0.01, ****P* <0.001 with ANOVAs followed by Tukey's *post hoc* test). Data are presented as mean ± SEM. **(E)** Sholl analysis of the effects of APN and APR on the dendritic intersections under OGD/R in primary neurons (n = 9 per condition; ***P* <0.01 with ANOVAs followed by Tukey's *post hoc* test). Data are presented as mean ± SEM.

90.18 ± 2.01% to 65.97 ± 1.91% of control, *P* <0.001, **Figure 4B**), suggesting an important role of AMPK pathway in the protective effects of APN and APR on OGD/R-induced injury in primary neurons. Results above revealed that the protective effects of APN and APR on OGD/R-induced injury might be at least in part via AMPK pathway.

Effects of APN and APR on Mitochondrial Dysfunction on OGD/R-Induced Injury

It is reported that impaired mitochondrial function occurred in ischemia (Galluzzi et al., 2009; Yang et al., 2018), and AMPK plays an important role in the maintenance of mitochondrial function (Rabinovitch et al., 2017). To reveal the effects of APN

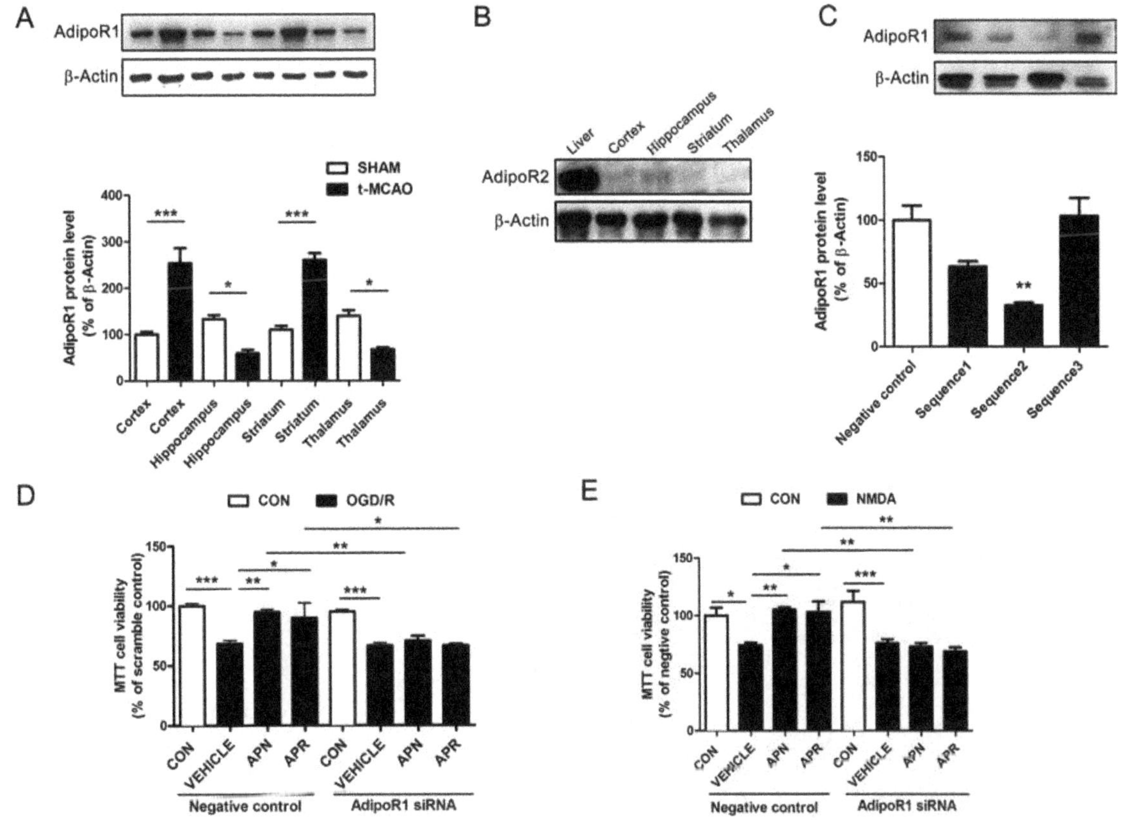

FIGURE 3 | Involvement of AdipoR1 in the protective effects of APN and APR against OGD/R-induced injury in primary neurons. **(A)** Representative Western blots and the bar graph showing the AdipoR1 expression in different brain regions under tMCAO-induced cerebral injury (n = 3 per condition; *P <0.05, ***P <0.001 with ANOVAs followed by Tukey's *post hoc* test). Data are presented as mean ± SEM. **(B)** Representative Western blots showing the AdipoR2 expression in the liver and brain. **(C)** Representative Western blots and the bar graph showing the AdipoR1 expression interfered by three different siRNA sequences cultured cortical neurons (n = 3 per condition; **P <0.01 vs. negative control group with ANOVAs followed by Tukey's *post hoc* test). Data are presented as mean ± SEM. **(D)** The cell viability tested by MTT assay showing the effect of AdipoR1 siRNA on the protections of APN and APR against OGD/R in primary neurons (n = 8–9 per condition; *P <0.05, **P <0.01, ***P <0.001 with ANOVAs followed by Tukey's *post hoc* test). Data are presented as mean ± SEM. **(E)** The cell viability tested by MTT assay showing the effect of AdipoR1 siRNA on the protection of APN and APR against NMDA in primary neurons (n = 9 per condition; *P <0.05, **P <0.01, ***P <0.001 with ANOVAs followed by Tukey's *post hoc* test). Data are presented as mean ± SEM.

and APR on mitochondrial function, we examined the ΔΨm on OGD/R-induced injury in primary neurons. The results indicated that OGD/R induced a significant dissipation of the ΔΨm (**Figure 4C**); however, both APN and APR reversed the dissipation of the ΔΨm on OGD/R-induced injury (**Figure 4C**). Moreover, to investigate the role of AMPK in the maintenance of mitochondrial function offered by APN and APR, the inhibitor of p-AMPK (compound C) was administrated. The results showed that compound C completely reversed the ΔΨm in the APN+ compound C group compared with the APN group, and similar results was observed in the APR+ compound C group compared with the APR group (**Figure 4C**). Above all, these results showed that APN and APR maintained the mitochondrial function through AMPK pathway.

Effects of APN and APR on the Expression of PGC-1α

Studies show that decreased levels of APN causes mitochondrial dysfunction by decreasing the PGC-1α expression in diabetic mice (Iwabu et al., 2010; Yan et al., 2013). To investigate whether APN and APR protect the mitochondrial function through up-regulation of PGC-1α, we assessed the expression of PGC-1α by Western blot. The results indicated that the PGC-1α expression was significantly increased in both APN group (326.2 ± 16.93% of control, P <0.01, **Figure 4D**) and APR group (346.2 ± 41.32% of control, P <0.01, **Figure 4D**) compared with the vehicle group (204.8 ± 12.84% of control, P <0.05, **Figure 4D**). Moreover, to study the role of AMPK in the up-regulation of PGC-1α offered by APN and APR, we inhibited the p-AMPK by compound C. The results showed that the PGC-1α protein level decreased significantly in the APN+ compound C group (115.3 ± 9.99% of control, P <0.001, **Figure 4D**) compared with the APN group and in the APN+ compound C group (90.12 ± 17.63% of control, P <0.001, **Figure 4D**) compared with the APR group. Taken together, these results indicated that with OGD/R-induced injury, APN and APR up-regulated PGC-1α level is through AMPK pathway.

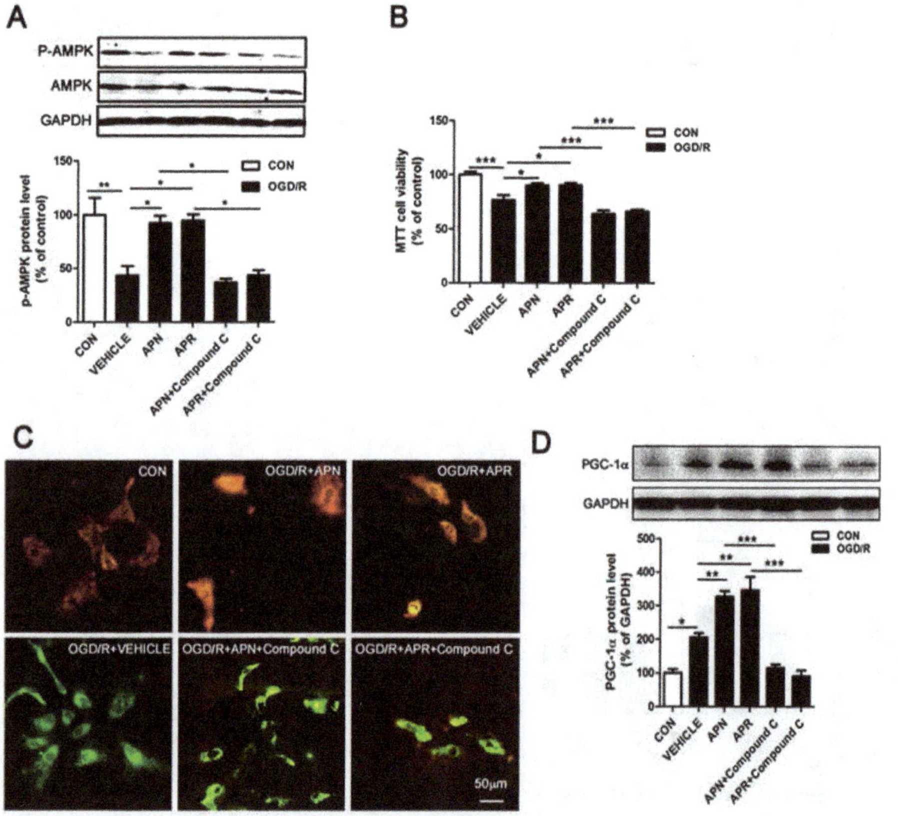

FIGURE 4 | Involvement of AMPK pathway in the protective effects of APN and APR against OGD/R-induced injury. **(A)** Representative Western blots and bar graph showing the effects of APN (1 μg/ml, 0.5 h before OGD), APR (1 μM, 0.5 h before OGD) and compound C (10 μM, 1 h before OGD) on AMPK phosphorylation under OGD/R in primary neurons (n = 3 per condition; **P* <0.05, ***P* <0.01 with ANOVAs followed by Tukey's *post hoc* test). Data are presented as mean ± SEM. **(B)** Effects of compound C (10 μM, 1 h before OGD) on the protections of APN (1 μg/ml, 0.5 h before OGD) and APR (1 μM, 0.5 h before OGD) against OGD/R-induced injury in primary neurons by MTT assay (n = 8 per condition; **P* <0.05, ****P* <0.001 with ANOVAs followed by Tukey's *post hoc* test). Data are presented as mean ± SEM. **(C)** Representative JC-1 fluorescence images showing the effects of APN (1 μg/ml, 0.5 h before OGD) and APR (1 μM, 0.5 h before OGD) on OGD/R-induced injury in primary neurons. Red fluorescence indicates a polarized state and green fluorescence indicates a depolarized state. Scale bar: 50 μm. **(D)** Representative Western blots and the bar graph showing the PGC-1α expression treated by compound C (10 μM, 1 h before OGD), APN (1 μg/ml, 0.5 h before OGD), and APR (1 μM, 0.5 h before OGD) in primary neurons under OGD/R-induced injury (n = 4 per condition; **P* <0.05, ***P* <0.01,****P* <0.001 with ANOVAs followed by Tukey's post *hoc test*). Data are presented as mean ± SEM.

APN and APR Alleviates the Cerebral Ischemia/Reperfusion (I/R)-Induced Injury Through AMPK Pathway *In Vivo*

As it was reported that APN is protective against cerebral I/R-induced injury in diabetic mice in a AdipoR1-dependent way (Song et al., 2015). However, the role of APN and APR on I/R-induced injury in mice remain to be clarified. To investigate the role of APN in cerebral I/R injury, the APN knockout (APN-KO) mice was used. The results indicated that the infarct volume increased significantly in the APN-KO group (49.18 ± 1.81%, *P* <0.001, **Figure 5A**, **B**) compared with the vehicle group (30.25 ± 2.07%, **Figure 5A**, **B**). The infarct volume increased significantly in the APN-KO group (49.18 ± 1.81%, *P* <0.001, **Figure 5A**, **B**) compared with the vehicle group (30.25 ± 2.07%, **Figure 5A**, **B**). The neurological deficit scores increased in the APN-KO group (3.25 ± 0.25, *P* <0.05, **Figure 5C**) compared with the vehicle group (2.20 ± 0.2, **Figure 5C**). To further study the role of APN and APR in ischemia, we assessed the effects of APN and APR on I/R-induced injury. The I/R-induced infarct volume reduced to 13.13 ± 1.43% in the APN group and 13.86 ± 0.83% in the APR group compared with the vehicle group (*P* <0.001, **Figure 5A**, **B**). The I/R-induced neurological deficient scores reduced to 1.20 ± 0.20 in the APN group and 1.17 ± 0.17 in the APR group compared with the vehicle group (*P* <0.05, **Figure 5C**). Moreover, to investigate the role of AMPK in the protective effects of APN and APR, compound C was administrated. The infarct volume increased significantly in both the APN+ compound C group compared with the APN group. (37.18 ± 1.63%, *P* <0.001, **Figure 5A**, **B**) and the APR+ compound C group (33.45 ± 2.26%, *P* <0.001, **Figure 5A**, **B**) compared with the APR group. The neurological deficit scores increased in both the APN+ compound C group (2.8 ± 0.2, *P* <0.01, **Figure 5C**) compared with the APN group and the APR+ compound C group (2.60 ± 0.24, *P* <0.001, **Figure 5C**) compared with the APR group. Above all, these results showed that APN and APR alleviated the tMCAO-induced injury no matter on infarct volume or neurological deficiency through AMPK pathway.

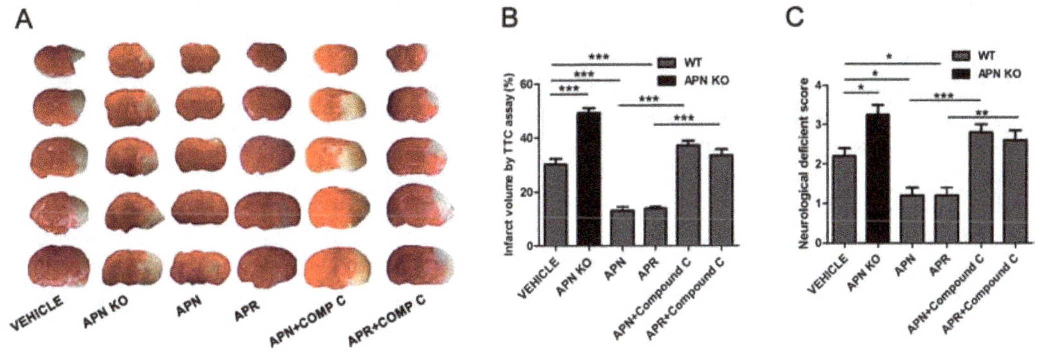

FIGURE 5 | APN and APR alleviate the tMCAO-induced injury through AMPK pathway. **(A)** Brain sections stained by 2,3,5-Triphenyltetrazolium chloride (TTC) from WT and APN-/- mice showing the infarct area in those receiving saline, APN (*i.c.v.,* 0.3 μg/mouse, 0.5 h before tMCAO), APR (i.c.v., 1 μg/mouse, 0.5 h before tMCAO), and compound C (*i.c.v.,* 40 μg/mouse, 1 h before tMCAO). The bar graph showing the infarct volume **(B)** and neurological scores **(C)** (n = 4–5 per condition; *P <0.05, **P <0.01, ***P <0.001 with ANOVAs followed by Tukey's *post hoc* test). Data are presented as mean ± SEM.

DISCUSSION

APN has been known to regard to glucose regulation and fatty acid oxidation (Diez and Iglesias, 2003). APN binds with its receptors (AdipoR1 and AdipoR2) to regulate cell functions (Scherer et al., 1995; Mao et al., 2006; Thundyil et al., 2012). Studies show that APN protects against glutamate-induced excitotoxicity in HT22 hippocampal neurons (Wang et al., 2018; Yue et al., 2016). APN also protects against ischemia in diabetic mice (Song et al., 2015). It is known that cortex and striatum are highly vulnerable to ischemia (Hammond et al., 1994; Miladinovic et al., 2015); thus, we investigated that role of APN and APR on primary cortical neurons. In this study, our findings suggested that APN and APR were all protective against OGD/R-induced injury in primary cortical neurons. In addition, we found that APN and APR were also protective against tMCAO-induced ischemic injury in adult mice, and APN-KO aggravated the tMCAO-induced injury. Therefore, our findings suggested that APN might protect neurons against OGD/R-induced injury *in vitro* and tMCAO-induced injury *in vivo*.

It had been reported that AdipoR1 is widely expressed in the brain, whereas AdipoR2 is barely expressed in the brain (Hug et al., 2004), and AdipoR1 is important for neuronal survival under pathological conditions (Thundyil et al., 2012). We also found that AdipoR1 level increased in cortex and striatum, a region that is vulnerable in ischemia, suggesting it might be an endogenous protective mechanism through AdipoR1. Moreover, the finding of the study also showed that AdipoR2 is highly expressed in the liver, but barely expressed in brain regions including cortex, hippocampus, striatum, and thalamus. Osmotin, as an APN homolog, protects H9c2 cells against I/R through AdipoR1-dependent PI3K/AKT signaling (Liu et al., 2017). APN attenuates neuronal apoptosis induced by hypoxia-ischemia via AdipoR1/APPL1 pathway in neonatal rats (Xu et al., 2018). Based on these results, we investigated the role of AdipoR1 in OGD/R-induced injury in primary neurons. This study showed that the protection of APN and APR against OGD/R- and NMDA-induced injury were compromised by siRNA of AdipoR1, suggesting that the protective effects were AdipoR1-dependent.

AMPK is a major downstream component of APN signaling that acts as the cellular energy sensor (Thundyil et al., 2012). Studies have shown that metabolic effects mediated by APN in peripheral tissues such as skeletal muscle and liver through activation of AMPK (Yamauchi et al., 2002). APN is protective against Parkinson's disease (PD) through AMPK activating (Li et al., 2014). AMPK activation is also involved in APN mediated protection against cardiovascular diseases (Kobayashi et al., 2004). APN protects neurons against hypoxia-ischemia induced injury via AMPK pathway *in vivo* (Xu et al., 2018). However, further studies are required to determine whether APN and APR protect against ischemic injury through AMPK pathway. As expected, this study showed that compound C, an AMPK activity inhibitor, reversed the protective effects offered by APN and APR on OGD/R-induced and NMDA-induced injury *in vitro*, and tMCAO-induced injury *in vivo*. Above all, the study showed that the abovementioned results revealed that the protective effects of APN and APR on I/R-induced injury might be at least in part via AMPK pathway.

Two early hallmarks of neuronal excitotoxicity are mitochondrial dysfunction and the formation of focal swellings along the length of the dendrites (Greenwood and Connolly, 2007). APN deficiency induces mitochondrial dysfunction and oxidative stress (Lin et al., 2014). Lacking AdipoR1 induces myocardial mitochondrial dysfunction (Koentges et al., 2015), and AMPK is a critical regulator involved in initiating mitochondrial biogenesis (Zong et al., 2002). These reports indicated that APN and downstream signaling AdipoR1/AMPK is beneficial to mitochondrial dysfunction. APN treatment activates AMPK and PGC-1α, increases mitochondrial biogenesis, and attenuates mitochondrial disorders in the heart (Yan et al., 2013). APN also induces PGC-1α up-regulation and increased mitochondria content in myocytes through AdipoR1/AMPK (Iwabu et al., 2010). Based on the abovementioned studies, we investigated the effects of APN and APR on mitochondrial function and PGC-1α expression on OGD/R-induced injury in primary neurons. This study indicated that APN and APR maintained the mitochondrial function through AMPK pathway. Moreover, APN and APR also up-regulated the PGC-1α level through AMPK pathway. Taken together, our results showed that APN and APR might enhance the PGC-1α level and repair the mitochondrial dysfunction through AMPK signaling.

CONCLUSION

The finding of this study showed that APN and APR were all protective against OGD/R-induced injury in primary neurons *in vitro*. This protective effect was mainly related to anti-apoptosis properties, increased either total dendritic length or dendritic complexity and repaired mitochondrial dysfunction. In addition, AdipoR1 and the downstream AMPK/PGC-1α signaling were related to the protection against OGD/R-induced injury. Moreover, APN and APR alleviated the tMCAO-induced injury on infarct volume and neurological deficiency through AMPK pathway *in vivo*.

AUTHOR CONTRIBUTIONS

HY designed the experiments and analyzed the data. HY and BL wrote the article. HY, BL, JL, JW, FS, SJ, FH, DW, DL, and CL performed the experiments.

FUNDING

Work of the authors was supported by grants from the National Natural Science Foundation of China (81500930), the Natural Science Foundation of Shandong Province (ZR2014HQ014 and ZR2017BC047), and University Science and Technology Plan of Shandong Province (J13LL06).

REFERENCES

Carvalho, A. F., Rocha, D. Q., McIntyre, R. S., Mesquita, L. M., Kohler, C. A., Hyphantis, T. N., et al. (2014). Adipokines as emerging depression biomarkers: a systematic review and meta-analysis. *J. Psychiatr. Res.* 59, 28–37. doi: 10.1016/j.jpsychires.2014.08.002

Chan, K. H., Lam, K. S., Cheng, O. Y., Kwan, J. S., Ho, P. W., Cheng, K. K., et al. (2012). Adiponectin is protective against oxidative stress induced cytotoxicity in amyloid-beta neurotoxicity. *PLoS One* 7, e52354. doi: 10.1371/journal.pone.0052354

Diez, J. J., and Iglesias, P. (2003). The role of the novel adipocyte-derived hormone adiponectin in human disease. *Eur. J. Endocrinol.* 148, 293–300. http://www.ncbi.nlm.nih.gov/pubmed/12611609. doi: 10.1530/eje.0.1480293

Dirnagl, U., Iadecola, C., and Moskowitz, M. A. (1999). Pathobiology of ischaemic stroke: an integrated view. *Trends Neurosci.* 22, 391–397. doi: 10.1016/S0166-2236(99)01401-0

Domise, M., Didier, S., Marinangeli, C., Zhao, H., Chandakkar, P., Buee, L., et al. (2016). AMP-activated protein kinase modulates tau phosphorylation and tau pathology in vivo. *Sci. Rep.* 6, 26758. doi: 10.1038/srep26758

Galluzzi, L., Blomgren, K., and Kroemer, G. (2009). Mitochondrial membrane permeabilization in neuronal injury. *Nat. Rev. Neurosci.* 10, 481–494. doi: 10.1038/nrn2665

Greenwood, S. M., and Connolly, C. N. (2007). Dendritic and mitochondrial changes during glutamate excitotoxicity. *Neuropharmacology* 53, 891–898. doi: 10.1016/j.neuropharm.2007.10.003

Hammond, C., Crepel, V., Gozlan, H., and Ben-Ari, Y. (1994). Anoxic LTP sheds light on the multiple facets of NMDA receptors. *Trends Neurosci.* 17, 497–503. http://www.ncbi.nlm.nih.gov/pubmed/7531893. doi: 10.1016/0166-2236(94)90140-6

Hu, E., Liang, P., and Spiegelman, B. M. (1996). AdipoQ is a novel adipose-specific gene dysregulated in obesity. *J. Biol. Chem.* 271, 10697–10703. http://www.ncbi.nlm.nih.gov/pubmed/8631877. doi: 10.1074/jbc.271.18.10697

Hug, C., Wang, J., Ahmad, N. S., Bogan, J. S., Tsao, T. S., and Lodish, H. F. (2004). T-cadherin is a receptor for hexameric and high-molecular-weight forms of Acrp30/adiponectin. *Proc. Natl. Acad. Sci. U. S. A.* 101, 10308–10313. doi: 10.1073/pnas.0403382101

Iwabu, M., Yamauchi, T., Okada-Iwabu, M., Sato, K., Nakagawa, T., Funata, M., et al. (2010). Adiponectin and AdipoR1 regulate PGC-1alpha and mitochondria by Ca(2+) and AMPK/SIRT1. *Nature* 464, 1313–9. doi: 10.1038/nature08991

Jeon, B. T., Shin, H. J., Kim, J. B., Kim, Y. K., Lee, D. H., Kim, K. H., et al. (2009). Adiponectin protects hippocampal neurons against kainic acid-induced excitotoxicity. *Brain Res. Rev.* 61, 81–88. doi: 10.1016/j.brainresrev.2009.05.002

Kanazawa, M., Miura, M., Toriyabe, M., Koyama, M., Hatakeyama, M., Ishikawa, M., et al. (2017). Microglia preconditioned by oxygen-glucose deprivation promote functional recovery in ischemic rats. *Sci. Rep.* 7, 42582. doi: 10.1038/srep42582

Kobayashi, H., Ouchi, N., Kihara, S., Walsh, K., Kumada, M., Abe, Y., et al. (2004). Selective suppression of endothelial cell apoptosis by the high molecular weight form of adiponectin. *Circ. Res.* 94, e27–31. doi: 10.1161/01.RES.0000119921.86460.37

Koentges, C., Konig, A., Pfeil, K., Holscher, M. E., Schnick, T., Wende, A. R., et al. (2015). Myocardial mitochondrial dysfunction in mice lacking adiponectin receptor 1. *Basic Res. Cardiol.* 110, 495. doi: 10.1007/s00395-015-0495-4

Kubota, N., Yano, W., Kubota, T., Yamauchi, T., Itoh, S., Kumagai, H., et al. (2007). Adiponectin stimulates AMP-activated protein kinase in the hypothalamus and increases food intake. *Cell Metab.* 6, 55–68. doi: 10.1016/j.cmet.2007.06.003

Kusminski, C. M., McTernan, P. G., Schraw, T., Kos, K., O'Hare, J. P., Ahima, R., et al. (2007). Adiponectin complexes in human cerebrospinal fluid: distinct complex distribution from serum. *Diabetologia* 50, 634–642. doi: 10.1007/s00125-006-0577-9

Lee, E. B., Warmann, G., Dhir, R., and Ahima, R. S. (2011). Metabolic dysfunction associated with adiponectin deficiency enhances kainic acid-induced seizure severity. *J. Neurosci.* 31, 14361–14366. doi: 10.1523/JNEUROSCI.3171-11.2011

Li, X., Geng, J., and Liu, J. (2014). Adiponectin offers protection against L166P mutant DJ-1-induced neuronal cytotoxicity mediated by APPL1-dependent AMPK activation. *Int. J. Neurosci.* 124, 350–361. doi: 10.3109/00207454.2013.846340

Lin, Z., Wu, F., Lin, S., Pan, X., Jin, L., Lu, T., et al. (2014). Adiponectin protects against acetaminophen-induced mitochondrial dysfunction and acute liver injury by promoting autophagy in mice. *J. Hepatol.* 61, 825–831. doi: 10.1016/j.jhep.2014.05.033

Liu, J., Guo, M., Zhang, D., Cheng, S. Y., Liu, M., Ding, J., et al. (2012). Adiponectin is critical in determining susceptibility to depressive behaviors and has antidepressant-like activity. *Proc. Natl. Acad. Sci. U. S. A.* 109, 12248–12253. doi: 10.1073/pnas.1202835109

Liu, J., Sui, H., Zhao, J., and Wang, Y. (2017). Osmotin protects H9c2 cells from simulated ischemia-reperfusion injury through AdipoR1/PI3K/AKT signaling pathway. *Front. Physiol.* 8, 611. doi: 10.3389/fphys.2017.00611

Longa, E. Z., Weinstein, P. R., Carlson, S., and Cummins, R. (1989). Reversible middle cerebral artery occlusion without craniectomy in rats. *Stroke* 20, 84–91. http://www.ncbi.nlm.nih.gov/pubmed/2643202. doi: 10.1161/01.STR.20.1.84

Mao, X., Kikani, C. K., Riojas, R. A., Langlais, P., Wang, L., Ramos, F. J., et al. (2006). APPL1 binds to adiponectin receptors and mediates adiponectin signalling and function. *Nat. Cell Biol.* 8, 516–523. doi: 10.1038/ncb1404

Miladinovic, T., Nashed, M. G., and Singh, G. (2015). Overview of glutamatergic dysregulation in central pathologies. *Biomolecules* 5, 3112–3141. doi: 10.3390/biom5043112

Nishimura, M., Izumiya, Y., Higuchi, A., Shibata, R., Qiu, J., Kudo, C., et al. (2008). Adiponectin prevents cerebral ischemic injury through endothelial nitric oxide synthase dependent mechanisms. *Circulation* 117, 216–223. doi: 10.1161/CIRCULATIONAHA.107.725044

Ouchi, N., Kihara, S., Arita, Y., Maeda, K., Kuriyama, H., Okamoto, Y., et al. (1999). Novel modulator for endothelial adhesion molecules: adipocyte-derived plasma protein adiponectin. *Circulation* 100, 2473–2476. http://www.ncbi.nlm.nih.gov/pubmed/10604883. doi: 10.1161/01.CIR.100.25.2473

Pera, J., Dziedzic, T., Szczudlik, A., and Slowik, A. (2013). Temporal changes of adiponectin plasma levels in patients with acute ischemic stroke. *Neurol. Res.* 35, 988–991. doi: 10.1179/1743132813Y.0000000241

Rabinovitch, R. C., Samborska, B., Faubert, B., Ma, E. H., Gravel, S. P., Andrzejewski, S., et al. (2017). AMPK maintains cellular metabolic homeostasis through regulation of mitochondrial reactive oxygen species. *Cell Rep.* 21, 1–9. doi: 10.1016/j.celrep.2017.09.026

Rothman, S. M., and Olney, J. W. (1995). Excitotoxicity and the NMDA receptor—still lethal after eight years. *Trends Neurosci.* 18, 57–58. http://www.ncbi.nlm.nih.gov/pubmed/7537407. doi: 10.1016/0166-2236(95)93869-Y

Scherer, P. E., Williams, S., Fogliano, M., Baldini, G., and Lodish, H. F. (1995). A novel serum protein similar to C1q, produced exclusively in adipocytes. *J. Biol. Chem.* 270, 26746–26749. http://www.ncbi.nlm.nih.gov/pubmed/7592907. doi: 10.1074/jbc.270.45.26746

Song, W., Guo, F., Zhong, H., Liu, L., Yang, R., Wang, Q., et al. (2015). Therapeutic window of globular adiponectin against cerebral ischemia in diabetic mice: the role of dynamic alteration of adiponectin/adiponectin receptor expression. *Sci. Rep.* 5, 17310. doi: 10.1038/srep17310

Teixeira, A. L., Diniz, B. S., Campos, A. C., Miranda, A. S., Rocha, N. P., Talib, L. L., et al. (2013). Decreased levels of circulating adiponectin in mild cognitive impairment and Alzheimer's disease. *Neuromolecular. Med.* 15, 115–121. doi: 10.1007/s12017-012-8201-2

Thundyil, J., Pavlovski, D., Sobey, C. G., and Arumugam, T. V. (2012). Adiponectin receptor signalling in the brain. *Br. J. Pharmacol.* 165, 313–327. doi: 10.1111/j.1476-5381.2011.01560.x

Wang, B., Guo, H., Li, X., Yue, L., Liu, H., Zhao, L., et al. (2018). Adiponectin attenuates oxygen-glucose deprivation-induced mitochondrial oxidative injury and apoptosis in hippocampal HT22 cells via the JAK2/STAT3 pathway. *Cell Transplant.* 27, 1731–1743. doi: 10.1177/0963689718779364

Wen, J. P., Liu, C., Bi, W. K., Hu, Y. T., Chen, Q., Huang, H., et al. (2012). Adiponectin inhibits KISS1 gene transcription through AMPK and specificity protein-1 in the hypothalamic GT1-7 neurons. *J. Endocrinol.* 214, 177–189. doi: 10.1530/JOE-12-0054

Wu, Q. J., and Tymianski, M. (2018). Targeting NMDA receptors in stroke: new hope in neuroprotection. *Mol. Brain* 11, 15. doi: 10.1186/s13041-018-0357-8

Xu, N., Zhang, Y., Doycheva, D. M., Ding, Y., Zhang, Y., Tang, J., et al. (2018). Adiponectin attenuates neuronal apoptosis induced by hypoxia-ischemia via the activation of AdipoR1/APPL1/LKB1/AMPK pathway in neonatal rats. *Neuropharmacology* 133, 415–428. doi: 10.1016/j.neuropharm.2018.02.024

Yamauchi, T., Kamon, J., Waki, H., Terauchi, Y., Kubota, N., Hara, K., et al. (2001). The fat-derived hormone adiponectin reverses insulin resistance associated with both lipoatrophy and obesity. *Nat. Med.* 7, 941–946. doi: 10.1038/90984

Yamauchi, T., Kamon, J., Minokoshi, Y., Ito, Y., Waki, H., Uchida, S., et al. (2002). Adiponectin stimulates glucose utilization and fatty-acid oxidation by activating AMP-activated protein kinase. *Nat. Med.* 8, 1288–1295. doi: 10.1038/nm788

Yan, H., Zhang, X., Hu, W., Ma, J., Hou, W., Zhang, X., et al. (2014). Histamine H3 receptors aggravate cerebral ischaemic injury by histamine-independent mechanisms. *Nat. Commun.* 5, 3334. doi: 10.1038/ncomms4334

Yan, W., Zhang, H., Liu, P., Wang, H., Liu, J., Gao, C., et al. (2013). Impaired mitochondrial biogenesis due to dysfunctional adiponectin-AMPK-PGC-1alpha signaling contributing to increased vulnerability in diabetic heart. *Basic Res. Cardiol.* 108, 329. doi: 10.1007/s00395-013-0329-1

Yang, J.-L., Mukda, S., and Chen, S.-D. (2018). Diverse roles of mitochondria in ischemic stroke. *Redox Biol.* 16, 263–275. doi: 10.1016/j.redox.2018.03.002

Yue, L., Zhao, L., Liu, H., Li, X., Wang, B., Guo, H., et al. (2016). Adiponectin protects against glutamate-induced excitotoxicity via activating SIRT1-dependent PGC-1alpha expression in HT22 hippocampal neurons. *Oxid. Med. Cell Longev.* 2016, 2957354. doi: 10.1155/2016/2957354

Zhang, D., Guo, M., Zhang, W., and Lu, X. Y. (2011). Adiponectin stimulates proliferation of adult hippocampal neural stem/progenitor cells through activation of p38 mitogen-activated protein kinase (p38MAPK)/glycogen synthase kinase 3beta (GSK-3beta)/beta-catenin signaling cascade. *J. Biol. Chem.* 286, 44913–44920. doi: 10.1074/jbc.M111.310052

Zhang, D., Wang, X., and Lu, X. Y. (2016). Adiponectin exerts neurotrophic effects on dendritic arborization, spinogenesis, and neurogenesis of the dentate gyrus of male mice. *Endocrinology* 157, 2853–2869. doi: 10.1210/en.2015-2078

Zhang, D., Wang, X., Wang, B., Garza, J. C., Fang, X., Wang, J., et al. (2017). Adiponectin regulates contextual fear extinction and intrinsic excitability of dentate gyrus granule neurons through AdipoR2 receptors. *Mol. Psychiatry* 22, 1044–1055. doi: 10.1038/mp.2016.58

Zong, H., Ren, J. M., Young, L. H., Pypaert, M., Mu, J., Birnbaum, M. J., et al. (2002). AMP kinase is required for mitochondrial biogenesis in skeletal muscle in response to chronic energy deprivation. *Proc. Natl. Acad. Sci. U. S. A.* 99, 15983–15987. doi: 10.1073/pnas.252625599

5

The Insula: A Brain Stimulation Target for the Treatment of Addiction

Christine Ibrahim[1,2†], *Dafna S. Rubin-Kahana*[1,3†], *Abhiram Pushparaj*[4,5], *Martin Musiol*[5], *Daniel M. Blumberger*[3,6], *Zafiris J. Daskalakis*[3,6], *Abraham Zangen*[7] *and Bernard Le Foll*[1,2,3,8,9,10,11]*

[1] *Translational Addiction Research Laboratory, Centre for Addiction and Mental Health, Toronto, ON, Canada,* [2] *Department of Pharmacology, University of Toronto, Toronto, ON, Canada,* [3] *Department of Psychiatry, Faculty of Medicine, University of Toronto, Toronto, ON, Canada,* [4] *Qunuba Sciences, Toronto, ON, Canada,* [5] *Ironstone Product Development, Toronto, ON, Canada,* [6] *Temerty Centre for Therapeutic Brain Intervention, Campbell Family Mental Health Research Institute, Centre for Addiction and Mental Health, Toronto, ON, Canada,* [7] *Department of Life Sciences and the Zlotowski Center for Neuroscience, Ben-Gurion University of the Negev, Beer-Sheva, Israel,* [8] *Addictions Division, Campbell Family Mental Health Research Institute, Centre for Addiction and Mental Health, Toronto, ON, Canada,* [9] *Institute of Medical Sciences, University of Toronto, Toronto, ON, Canada,* [10] *Alcohol Research and Treatment Clinic, Centre for Addiction and Mental Health, Toronto, ON, Canada,* [11] *Department of Family and Community Medicine, University of Toronto, Toronto, ON, Canada*

Correspondence:
Bernard Le Foll
bernard.lefoll@camh.ca

[†]*These authors have contributed equally to this work.*

Substance use disorders (SUDs) are a growing public health concern with only a limited number of approved treatments. However, even approved treatments are subject to limited efficacy with high long-term relapse rates. Current treatment approaches are typically a combination of pharmacotherapies and behavioral counselling. Growing evidence and technological advances suggest the potential of brain stimulation techniques for the treatment of SUDs. There are three main brain stimulation techniques that are outlined in this review: transcranial magnetic stimulation (TMS), transcranial direct current stimulation (tDCS), and deep brain stimulation (DBS). The insula, a region of the cerebral cortex, is known to be involved in critical aspects underlying SUDs, such as interoception, decision making, anxiety, pain perception, cognition, mood, threat recognition, and conscious urges. This review focuses on both the preclinical and clinical evidence demonstrating the role of the insula in addiction, thereby demonstrating its promise as a target for brain stimulation. Future research should evaluate the optimal parameters for brain stimulation of the insula, through the use of relevant biomarkers and clinical outcomes for SUDs.

Keywords: insula, addiction, brain stimulation, transcranial magnetic stimulation (TMS), transcranial direct current stimulation (tDCS), deep brain stimulation (DBS)

INTRODUCTION

Substance use disorders (SUDs) are chronic relapsing brain disorders, characterized by seeking a drug where use becomes compulsive or difficult to control, despite harmful consequences (American Psychiatric Association, 2013). They are complex diseases, characterized by a cycle of intake, withdrawal, craving, and relapse. As a result of drug use and abuse, different neuronal circuits, such as the circuits involved in reward and fear processing, are co-opted to each stage of the addictive cycle and continue to function to maintain addiction (Naqvi et al., 2014; Koob and Volkow, 2016; Chawla and Garrison, 2018). Despite the enormous efforts to find an effective treatment, there are only a handful of approved treatments for these disorders, with limited efficacy as demonstrated by high long-term relapse rates (O'Brien, 2008; Chiamulera et al., 2017).

Given considerable growth in understanding the brain mechanisms underlying addiction, there is an obvious potential to target specific neural regions with brain stimulation techniques. This has fueled a mounting body of research supporting brain stimulation's efficacy and safety in manipulating underlying neuronal processes and reducing addictive behaviors (for recent reviews see Coles et al., 2018; Hanlon et al., 2018b)[1]. To date, the majority of brain stimulation studies have targeted the dorsolateral prefrontal cortex (dlPFC) (Coles et al., 2018; Hanlon et al., 2018b).

However, in recent years, there is a better understanding of the insula's critical role in addiction and technological advances enabling stimulation of deeper brain structures (such as the insula) through non-invasive modalities. In fact, up until 2007, the role of the insular cortex in addiction was largely overlooked. In a seminal work, Naqvi et al. (2007) showed that insular damage was correlated with quitting smoking successfully, easily, and without relapse. As a result, the insula (also known as insular cortex, Island of Reil, and insular lobe) became a subject of interest for research on novel addictions treatments.

In this paper we describe brain stimulation techniques that could target the insula and review the insula and its addiction related functions through an examination of both preclinical and clinical evidence. We also discuss possible limitations of the body of knowledge, as well as future directions.

OVERVIEW OF BRAIN STIMULATION TECHNIQUES

In this section we discuss three main brain stimulation techniques: transcranial magnetic stimulation (TMS), transcranial direct current stimulation (tDCS), and deep brain stimulation (DBS). Although they are each unique in many ways, they share the principle idea of attempting to induce a behavioral change by stimulating a brain region *via* primary and secondary activations. The effect produced by the stimulation is mainly dependent on the parameters used, which will be briefly discussed below.

Transcranial Magnetic Stimulation

TMS is a non-invasive brain stimulation technique used to alter magnetic fields to generate electrical currents in a targeted brain area (Barker et al., 1985). The basis of this technique stems from Faraday's law of induction which states that a time-varying magnetic field drives an electric field of the same magnitude (Daskalakis et al., 2002; Rossi et al., 2009; Lefaucheur et al., 2014). There are many variations of TMS, but the fundamental idea is that of a magnetic coil placed over the scalp, whereby the discharge passes through the scalp, skull, and meninges (unattenuated), allowing the facilitation or suppression of neurons located beneath the coil (Barker et al., 1985; Lefaucheur et al., 2014; Diana et al., 2017).

The first generation of magnetic coils was round coils; they were powerful and easy to use, but less focal (Barker et al., 1985; Deng et al., 2013). Now, there are a number of different coil configurations, such as the figure-8 coil, and more recently, the H-coil. The figure-8 coil, which is the most commonly studied coil, consists of two round coils attached together, leading it to be more focal, yet it can only reach superficial areas (Ueno et al., 1988; Feil and Zangen, 2010), whereas the H-coil is able to reach deeper brain areas (Zangen et al., 2005), such as the insula, though it is less focal.

The parameters that are used during the administration of TMS are of great importance because they can produce differential effects. These settings include the frequency of stimulation, the intensity, the number and type of pulses, and the area being stimulated. The frequency affects the cortical excitability; low-frequency TMS (usually 1 Hz) is generally shown to inhibit cortical excitability, whereas high-frequency TMS (5–20 Hz) is shown to enhance cortical excitability (Gorelick et al., 2014). However, there is debate on whether or not that is always the case (de Jesus et al., 2014), and it seems that the baseline cortical activation state modulates the effect of the magnetic stimulation (Silvanto and Pascual-Leone, 2008). One can administer a single pulse, a paired pulse or if longer lasting changes are required several pulses can be delivered using repetitive TMS (rTMS). One form of rTMS is theta burst stimulation (TBS), whereby pulses are delivered in bursts of three at a frequency of 50 Hz and repeated every 200 ms (Huang et al., 2005). An advantage of this technique is that a session only lasts a few minutes.

As previously mentioned, TMS is a non-invasive form of brain stimulation. Treatment is usually well tolerated and presents no serious side effects. The most common side effects reported are transient headaches and local pain. More serious side effects, most notably seizures, are extremely rare and are unlikely when the proper safety guidelines are followed (Rossi et al., 2009).

Transcranial Direct Current Stimulation

Transcranial direct current stimulation is another non-invasive brain stimulation technique. However, unlike TMS, tDCS emits a weak current (usually 1–2 mA) *via* two or more electrodes in direct contact with the scalp (Priori et al., 1998; Nitsche and Paulus, 2000). tDCS does not directly result in neuron firing as it does not produce action potentials. Rather, it produces a subthreshold change in neuronal membrane potentials (Purpura and McMurtry, 1965; Nitsche et al., 2008). This brain stimulation technique is not able to reach deep brain areas; however, secondary activations are possible (see Secondary Activation below).

Similar to TMS, parameters can be adjusted to elicit different responses. For instance, the size and placement of the electrodes affect the site being stimulated, current distribution, and focality (Nitsche et al., 2007). Typically, two electrodes are placed on the scalp, one anode and one cathode. The current passes from one electrode, through the skull and through the brain, and then reaches the second electrode (Nitsche et al., 2008). Anodal stimulation usually results in cortical excitability, whereas cathodal stimulation usually results in cortical inhibition (Nitsche et al., 2008). The duration of stimulation

[1] Of note, there are currently no brain stimulation techniques approved by Health Canada or the U.S. Food and Drug Administration (FDA) for the treatment of addiction.

is also an important factor; it plays a role in the determination of the aftereffects (i.e., the continued effects after stimulation has stopped). It has been shown that to produce aftereffects of 1 h or more, there needs to be stimulation for at least 9 min (Nitsche and Paulus, 2001). It should be noted that longer or more intense stimulation does not always equate to increased effects. In fact, it can result in an excitatory effect becoming inhibitory and vice versa (Batsikadze et al., 2013). tDCS outcomes have also been shown to be subject to inter-individual variability, possibly due to a number of factors (Wiethoff et al., 2014), one of them being anatomical brain differences (Kim et al., 2014).

Side effects from tDCS are typically mild, such as tingling sensation and light itching under the electrode, and usually dissipate after stimulation. Afterward headaches and, occasionally, nausea are reported. In general, tDCS is well tolerated and presents no serious side effects (Matsumoto and Ugawa, 2016).

Deep Brain Stimulation

Deep brain stimulation is an invasive brain stimulation technique that requires neurosurgical implantation of bipolar electrodes attached to a permanently implanted pulse generator (usually subcutaneously in the chest) (Greenberg and Rezai, 2014). This technique has the ability to reach deep brain regions, more than any other stimulation technique, and it is highly focal. Currently, DBS is mainly used for movement disorders such as Parkinson's disease (Kringelbach et al., 2007); however, it has been approved by the U.S. FDA for treatment-resistant obsessive-compulsive disorder. The exact mechanism of DBS is not completely understood, it seems to elicit multiple mechanisms of action (see review by Herrington et al., 2016).

As described for the two previous stimulation techniques, the parameters used can determine to a large extent the neurophysiological response. These include the brain region targeted (to the degree of the precise location in which the electrode is implanted on the target region), intensity and frequency of stimulation, and pulse width (i.e., length of pulses). The combination of all these parameters leads to different outcomes of stimulation. The parameters used are decided on the basis of the treatment intended and can be changed and modified by external programmer devices (Kringelbach et al., 2007).

Although DBS has the capacity to target deeper areas in the brain that might be needed for addiction-related treatments, it should be noted that the risk of adverse events is much higher with this technique. Other than the adverse events that can occur from brain stimulation, this technique requires surgery, hence the added risks that can occur. Although not as common as when DBS first came into practice, hardware failure can still occur (Breit et al., 2004).

STRUCTURAL AND CONNECTIVITY OVERVIEW OF THE INSULA

The insular cortex is part of the cerebral cortex, folded in the lateral sulcus. It is commonly divided into anterior and posterior parts, based on the cytoarchitectonic and functional connectivity (Mesulam and Mufson, 1982; Deen et al., 2011; Kelly et al., 2012). It is also composed of three distinct subregions known as the granular, dysgranular, and agranular (Paxinos and Watson, 1986). The insula has major bidirectional connections with the orbitofrontal cortex (OFC), anterior cingulate cortex (ACC), supplementary motor areas, parietal (primary and secondary somatosensory areas), and temporal cortices and with subcortical structures that include the amygdala, globus pallidus, and thalamus. The anterior insular cortex (aIC) sends projections to the caudate-putamen, nucleus accumbens (NAcc), and extended amygdala (McGeorge and Faull, 1989; Wright and Groenewegen, 1996; Shi and Cassell, 1998b; McDonald et al., 1999) while having reciprocal connections with the basolateral amygdala (BLA) and the prelimbic cortex (Gerfen and Clavier, 1979; Saper, 1982; Vertes, 2004). The aIC receives inputs from the medial subdivision of the mediodorsal thalamic nucleus and other various medial thalamic nuclei involved in motivational/affective aspects of nocioception (Krettek and Price, 1977; Van der Werf et al., 2002). The posterior insular cortex (pIC) receives general viscerosensory unimodal inputs (Cechetto and Saper, 1987), nociceptive thalamic inputs (Gauriau and Bernard, 2004) and somatosensory cortex inputs. The pIC also sends projections to the caudate-putamen, thalamus, and somatosensory cortex (Shi and Cassell, 1998a). In general, the aIC has greater connectivity with the frontal lobe, and the pIC has greater connectivity with the parietal lobe (Gasquoine, 2014). Many of the insula's connectivity constitute areas known to be involved in addiction (**Figure 1**) (Naqvi and Bechara, 2010; Naqvi et al., 2014; Koob and Volkow, 2016).

Dopaminergic neuron terminals of the insula originating in the ventral tegmental area (VTA) and substantia nigra are believed to influence dopamine neuronal reactivity and dopamine release in the NAcc, critical for addictive behavior (Kalivas and Volkow, 2005). The entire granular subregion has notably high dopamine utilization (Gaspar et al., 1989) with the aIC having high density D1-subtype receptors surrounding dopaminergic terminals from the VTA and substantia nigra. These terminals project to the agranular subregion containing large pyramidal neurons with gamma-Aminobutyric acid (GABA) B-subtype receptors (Margeta-Mitrovic et al., 1999) which project to the amygdala and NAcc (Ohara et al., 2003).

Corticotropin-releasing factor (CRF) plays a role in the motivation to consume drugs in human subjects with substance dependence and distress during withdrawal and stress-induced relapse (Contoreggi et al., 2003). The agranular subregion contains a high density of CRF subtype 1 receptors (Sánchez et al., 1999). Furthermore, the insula has a high level of endogenous opioids (Gaspar et al., 1989), high density of μ-subtype opioid receptors (Baumgartner et al., 2006), high density of hypocretin subtype-1 receptors (Hollander et al., 2008), and a high level of nicotinic acetylcholine receptors (nAChRs) containing the β2 subunit (Rubboli et al., 1994), the major subtype of nAChR implicated in nicotine reward (Maskos et al., 2005; Grabus et al., 2006).

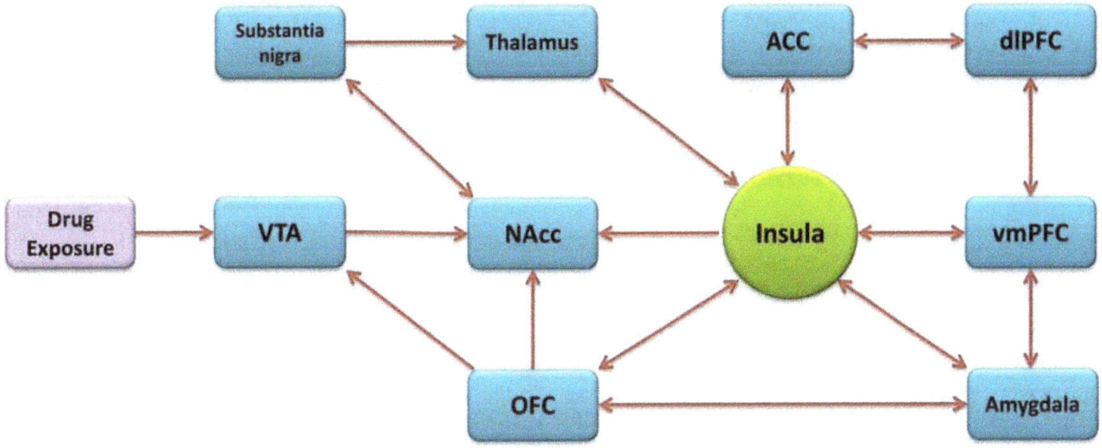

FIGURE 1 | Addiction-related neural circuitry of the insula.

FUNCTIONAL ROLE OF THE INSULA

The insular cortex is involved in feelings of anxiety, pain, cognition, mood, threat recognition, and conscious urges (Hardy, 1985; Suhara et al., 1992; Craig, 2002; Paulus and Stein, 2006). Although it is involved in a multitude of behaviors, the insular cortex was rarely studied in depth and was believed to be the "primary taste cortex" for decades (Penfield and Faulk, 1955; Pritchard et al., 1999). Since then, several studies have demonstrated the insula's primary role in sensations of taste and disgust (Ragozzino and Kesner, 1999; Fresquet et al., 2004; Isnard et al., 2004) and the integration of a wide variety of visceral sensations from the airways, gut, and cardiovascular systems (Cechetto and Saper, 1987; Allen et al., 1991), indicating the insula is heavily involved in the integration of internal and external stimuli to guide behavior toward or away from said stimuli for the purposes of maintaining homeostasis.

Studies of epileptic seizures in the insula (Isnard et al., 2004), stroke-induced lesions to the insula (Pritchard et al., 1999), lesioning studies in rats (DeCoteau et al., 1997; Ragozzino and Kesner, 1999; Fresquet et al., 2004), and direct electrical stimulation studies in primates (Verhagen et al., 2004) have shown the insula is critical for perception, recognition, and working memory in taste. The importance of visceral perception in addiction was first noted in the late 1980s, as dopaminergic innervation of the insular cortex was found to play an important role in the conditioning of the aversive aspects of opiate withdrawal (Zito et al., 1988) and the active avoidance of withdrawal. The insular cortex is critical for experiencing disgust and recognizing it in others, causing learning and memory of disgust to play a critical evolutionary role in mammals (Woolley et al., 2015).

Beyond acting as the primary taste cortex, the insula's critical thalamic connections allow it to integrate a range of visceral sensations, including inputs from the airways, gut, and cardiovascular systems (Cechetto and Saper, 1987), all known to be relevant with regard to bodily responses to the performance of addictive behaviors (Verdejo-Garcia et al., 2007). AD Craig first recognized the insula as the critical brain region underlying "interoception" (Craig, 2002), a process that integrates internal signals and external stimuli to maintain homeostasis (Craig, 2003). The pIC keeps a constant account of the current state of the body; this information is then relayed through the thalamus and dysgranular insular cortex, which appears to integrate salient external stimuli (Craig, 2004). The aIC compares the current state of the body and environment to prior states and environments to maintain homeostasis (Craig, 2009); such influence from representations of all bodily signals, and integration with external stimuli to guide behavior toward or away from said stimuli, indicates the aIC plays a significant role in drug seeking behavior. Through a study measuring skin conductance, anxiety ratings, and blood oxygenation level-dependent (BOLD) functional magnetic resonance imaging (fMRI) were used to assess responses to simulated threats, Alvarez et al. (2015) found that exaggerated insula activation during the threat of unpredictable shock is directly related to low perceived control in anxiety-prone individuals, supporting prior evidence that individuals prone to anxiety may have exaggerated activity in the anterior insula and altered activity in the cingulate cortex during anticipation of aversive events. Interestingly, individuals with methamphetamine dependence have a reduced emotional response to threatening scenes, empathy for another's pain, and fearful or angry face, all of which correlate with hypoactivation of the insula (Kim et al., 2011).

In addition to important interoceptive and homeostatic functions, the insula plays a major role in all aspects of decision making (Droutman et al., 2015). Bechara and Domasio's "Somatic Marker Hypothesis (SMH)" theory is one of several that offers an explanation of the insula's involvement in decision making, postulating that somatic markers of feelings in the body (e.g., rapid heartbeat in response to anxiety) influence decision-making, and highlighted the insula's role in decision making through its reactivation alongside the ventral medial prefrontal cortex (vmPFC) and amygdala as part of somatic state patterns previously learned by subjects evaluating a familiar stimulus (i.e., interoception) (Bechara and Damasio, 2005). Evidence from electroencephalogram (EEG) studies (Wiese et al., 2005; Mueller et al., 2007) has shown the insula's activation when "intentional" actions are initiated when faced with multiple external options. Intentional acts result from internal motivation and planning, versus automatic acts that are triggered by external stimuli (Brass and Haggard, 2010).

LARGE-SCALE BRAIN NETWORKS IN ADDICTION

Current neuroscience approaches investigate communication between brain regions in addition to the investigation of specific brain areas. fMRI allows exploration of fluctuations of BOLD signals in different brain regions which in turn allow the exploration of internetwork as well as intranetwork connectivity (Menon, 2011; Lu and Stein, 2014). In addictions, the main focus is on three well-established intrinsic networks: the default mode network (DMN) which includes the vmPFC and posterior cingulate cortex (PCC), the executive control network (ECN) hooked in the dlPFC and posterior parietal cortex (PPC), and the salience network (SN) which includes the aIC and ACC. The DMN is active when an individual is not focused on external tasks, and it is related to activities like day dreaming. In the context of addictions, it can be related to rumination about drug use. The ECN is active when an individual is focused on external tasks that demand cognitive functioning (e.g., working memory). The SN dynamically switches between the ECN and DMN, which are generally anticorrelated, following detection of relevant stimulation or condition (Menon and Uddin, 2010).

Sutherland et al. proposed a framework to understand the large-scale brain networks dynamics in addictions. They showed that under nicotine deprivation, the SN would switch to DMN, hence, direct attention resources toward internal withdrawal symptoms, while under nicotine administration, the SN would switch to ECN, hence direct attentional resources toward external stimuli and executive functions (Sutherland et al., 2012; Lerman et al., 2014; Sutherland and Stein, 2018). Therefore, an aberrant function of the SN (including the insula) may lead to an aberrant brain function, such as addiction. The activation of the insula and large-scale brain networks in addicted individuals is further demonstrated in the Neuroimaging Studies section below.

PRECLINICAL EVIDENCE FOR THE INSULA

As the critical brain region underpinning interoception, it is not surprising to see the insula involved in all major aspects of addiction. For simplicity sake, we provide here a short review of the preclinical literature examining the roles of various cytoarchitectural subregions of the insula in animal models representing each stage of the addictive cycle, as proposed by Koob and Volkow (2010): 1) Binge/Intoxication, 2) Withdrawal/Negative Affect, and 3) Preoccupation/Anticipation. The anterior agranular subregion (aAgIC) or posterior granular subregion (pGIC) is typically targeted in rodent models, as specific targeting of the dysgranular subregion is difficult with local infusions.

Binge/Intoxication Stage

Since the seminal findings of Naqvi and colleagues in human smokers (Naqvi et al., 2007), the majority of preclinical research on the IC's role in addiction has utilized nicotine. Noncontingent nicotine exposure has been demonstrated to induce a lasting increase in dendritic complexity (length/bifurcations) in the aAgIC (Ehlinger et al., 2012) while noncontingent nicotine pyrrolidine methiodide, which does not penetrate the blood–brain barrier, activates the aAgIC (Dehkordi et al., 2015). The acquisition of nicotine-induced conditioned place preference (CPP) is blocked by lesions to the aIC (Scott and Hiroi, 2011). Our own laboratory demonstrated that aAgIC or pGIC chemical inactivation attenuates nicotine taking, under various ratio schedules of reinforcement (Forget et al., 2010; Pushparaj et al., 2015), with similar attenuation observed when the pGIC was electrically inactivated (Pushparaj et al., 2013). These methods of inactivation demonstrated no effect on food taking in rats under a moderately restricted diet. Similar attenuation of nicotine, but not food, taking has been demonstrated by blockade of hypocretin-1 receptors in the pGIC, which is densely innervated by hypocretin-1 peptide-containing neurons (Hollander et al., 2008). Attenuation of nicotine taking is also observed following blockade dopamine D1, but not D2, receptors in the aAgIC (Kutlu et al., 2013), though high doses of D1 antagonists also attenuate food taking (Di Pietro et al., 2008).

Noncontingent alcohol exposure has been demonstrated to inhibit aIC activity (Jaramillo et al., 2016), which is unsurprising given it produces global cortical inhibition. *In vitro* ethanol inhibits electrically-evoked N-methyl-D-aspartate (NMDA) receptor-mediated excitatory post-synaptic currents (EPSCs) in brain slices of the aAgIC (Shillinglaw et al., 2018). Long-term synaptic depression (LTD) in the dorsolateral striatum also occurs exclusively at inputs from the aIC and is selectively disrupted by *in vivo* alcohol exposure (Muñoz et al., 2018). Inactivation of the aAgIC (Jaramillo et al., 2016) or chemogenic silencing of the aIC projections to the nucleus accumbens core (NAccCore) (Jaramillo et al., 2017), both produce sensitivity to the interoceptive effects of alcohol. Optogenetic inhibition of aIC glutamatergic input to the NAccCore attenuates aversion-resistant alcohol taking, but not alcohol taking in the absence of aversive stimuli (Seif et al., 2013). Contrarily, a recent study utilizing chemogenic partial inhibition demonstrated an increase in alcohol taking when the aIC was inhibited, but an attenuation in alcohol taking when aIC projections to the NAccCore were silenced, with the latter having no effect on sucrose taking (Jaramillo et al., 2018a; Jaramillo et al., 2018b). Our own laboratory has demonstrated that inactivation of the pGIC produces an attenuation of alcohol taking (Pushparaj and Le Foll, 2015).

Contrarily, aAgIC lesions have no effect on the acquisition of cocaine taking (Pelloux et al., 2013), nor does inactivation of the aAgIC affect established cocaine-taking (Pietro et al., 2006). In fact, lesions facilitate the escalation of cocaine intake, yet post-escalation lesions still reduce intake (Rotge et al., 2017). Interestingly, extended access self-administration, but not noncontingent exposure, to cocaine has also demonstrated effects on aAgIC-dependent learning (Kantak et al., 2005) and self-administration has also been shown to reduce glucose utilization in the aAgIC in primates (Porrino et al., 2002). Blockade of dopamine D1 receptors in the aAgIC does reduce cocaine intake; however, it also disrupts food intake, suggesting a global disruption of behavior (Di Pietro et al., 2008).

Finally, inactivation of the pGIC, but not the aAgIC, prevents the acquisition of CPP induced by morphine, without producing any effect on general motor and/or spatial learning (Li et al., 2013). Lesions of the aIC or pIC both produce no effect on the acquisition of morphine-induced CPP (Mackey et al., 1986; Sun et al., 2018).

Though the IC appears to play a greater role in the binge/intoxication stage for some addictive drugs (e.g., nicotine, alcohol) over others (e.g., cocaine), the region does appear to play some role in the neurocircuitry underlying this stage of addiction for all addictive drugs examined.

Withdrawal/Negative Affect

Inactivation of the aAgIC or pGIC prevents the acquisition of conditioned place aversion (CPA) induced acute morphine withdrawal (Li et al., 2013). Similarly, lesions of the aIC prevent the acquisition of CPA from morphine withdrawal (Wang et al., 2016). There is greater activation of glutamatergic neurons and signaling protein expression in the medial IC during protracted withdrawal, as compared to acute withdrawal from morphine (Ma et al., 2018). The anxiety-like behavior observed during protracted withdrawal is alleviated by lesions of the medial IC. The cannabinoid system has also been implicated, with the inhibition of monoacylglycerol lipase (causing elevation of the endocannabinoid 2-arachidonyl glycerol; 2-AG) in the pGIC preventing the acquisition of CPA from morphine withdrawal, which was reversed by the blockade of cannabinoid-1 receptors (Wills et al., 2016).

Contrary to the findings with morphine, lesions of the aIC had no effect on the acquisition of CPA induced by acute nicotine withdrawal (Scott and Hiroi, 2011). Though the studies on morphine withdrawal strongly support a critical role of the IC in the neurocircuitry underlying this stage of addiction, further work should be conducted to explore the role of the IC in other addictive drugs for which withdrawal is a major barrier to abstinence (e.g., alcohol).

Preoccupation/Anticipation

Our own laboratory demonstrated that aAgIC or pGIC inactivation attenuates nicotine seeking (Forget et al., 2010; Pushparaj et al., 2015), with similar attenuation observed when the pGIC was electrically inactivated (Pushparaj et al., 2013). The incubation of nicotine seeking (i.e., greater seeking after 7 days vs. 1 day of abstinence) is associated with higher levels of dopamine (DA)- and cyclic adenosine monophosphate (cAMP)-regulated phosphoprotein of 32 kDa (DARPP-32), enriched in DA neurons containing DA D1 receptors, in both the aAgIC and pGIC (Abdolahi et al., 2010).

Inactivation of the aAgIC, but not the pGIC, attenuates cue-induced cocaine seeking, while having no effect on drug priming-induced cocaine seeking or food seeking induced by either cues and/or priming (Cosme et al., 2015). Corticotropin-releasing factor (CRF) receptor-1 blockade of the aAgIC was also found to attenuate cue-induced cocaine seeking. Inactivation of the aAgIC attenuates context-induced reinstatement of cocaine seeking without altering locomotor activity; however, inactivation immediately following re-exposure to drug context has no effect on memory reconsolidation (Arguello et al., 2017). Interestingly, lidocaine inactivation of the aAgIC attenuates cue+context-induced cocaine seeking when the context was established by odor but not by sound (Pietro et al., 2006), which may be because gustation is influenced by odor, with the aAgIC being part of the gustatory cortex (Pritchard et al., 1999). In contrast to these studies, one study demonstrated an increase in cocaine seeking in aAgIC-lesioned rats (Pelloux et al., 2013); however, that effect is likely due to the rats having been lesioned prior to the acquisition of cocaine taking, as lesions post-acquisition result in an attenuation of drug-induced cocaine seeking (Rotge et al., 2017).

The presentation of amphetamine-induced CPP activates the pGIC and inactivation of the subregion prevents the presentation of said place preference (Contreras et al., 2007). Subsequent work from the same research group demonstrated a similar effect on the presentation of CPP when the protein synthesis inhibitor anisomycin was infused into the pGIC immediately following reactivation of CPP, and that this effect was longer lasting when anisomycin was infused into the higher-order aAgIC (Contreras et al., 2012). *In vivo* microdialysis of the aAgIC has also shown decreased depolarization-evoked GABA release in rats previously chronically exposed to methamphetamine (Mizoguchi et al., 2015). Inactivation of the aIC is capable of attenuating relapse to methamphetamine taking following the removal of contingency management (i.e., palatable food pellets mutually-exclusive from drug) (Venniro et al., 2017). The presentation of morphine-induced CPP is also abolished by lesions to the pIC (Sun et al., 2018) or the inhibition of nitric oxide in the pIC (Ma et al., 2014).

The IC appears to play various roles in the neurocircuitry underlying this stage of addiction, though differentially depending on the addictive drugs examined and the type of intervention (i.e., types of inactivation, lesions, etc.). Overall, there is evidence of some role for the IC in the neurocircuitry underlying all stages of the addictive cycle, clearly implicating the IC as a fundamental region in the maintenance and relapse to addictive drugs. Though this may seem contradictory to the idea of the IC as simply a part of the salience detection system, it is not unreasonable to posit that its interoceptive functions should play some role in drug intake, withdrawal, and anticipation. Future work should continue to evaluate the differential roles of the aAgIC and pGIC in various models of the stages of addiction.

CLINICAL EVIDENCE FOR THE INSULA

In this section, we provide the clinical evidence implicating the insula in addiction. Unlike the preclinical evidence which distinguishes between the addiction stages, clinical work does not always do so. For that reason, we present the clinical data based on study design: lesion, neuroimaging, and brain stimulation.

Lesion Studies

Despite the fact that the relevance of the insula for addiction had been observed in studies before, Naqvi et al. (2007) brought attention to its fundamental role in addiction. They found that smokers with damage to the insula experienced disruption of smoking addiction more so than those with damage not involving the insula. These smokers were able to quit smoking easily, immediately after damage onset, without relapse, and without any urge to smoke since quitting (Naqvi et al., 2007). Since then, other lesion studies have emerged, indicating that lesion to the insula best predicts smoking cessation and the probability of quitting smoking is five folds greater than when there is not damage to the insula (Suñer-Soler et al., 2012). Although, insular damage is associated with increased odds of smoking cessation, those that do relapse tend to remain abstinent for longer periods than those with non-insular damage (Abdolahi et al., 2015a). It has also been shown that smokers with insular damage experience less frequent and severe withdrawal symptoms of nicotine (Abdolahi et al., 2015b) and less smoking urges (Abdolahi et al., 2017). Also, damage to the insula was associated with complete abstinence from all nicotine products (Abdolahi et al., 2015a). Furthermore, damage to the basal ganglia was found to significantly increase rates of smoking cessation compared to damage elsewhere (Gaznick et al., 2014). However, when the damage included both the basal ganglia and the insula, it resulted in even higher rates of smoking cessation (Gaznick et al., 2014). Thereby supporting the notion of the insula being a key player in addiction. Nonetheless, one study found no relation between insula damage and smoking status (Bienkowski et al., 2010). It was later suggested that this disparity could be due to the fact that the study took place in Poland, where the harm of smoking is not widely perceived (Naqvi et al., 2014).

Although the vast majority of the evidence pertains to nicotine, other addictions have been shown to be affected by insular damage. For instance, in a comparison between ischemic stroke patients who used opium prior to their stroke, patients with insular damage were significantly more likely to quit using opium; this effect was more significant among younger patients (Yousefzadeh-Fard et al., 2013). Insular lesions were also correlated with the abolishment of cognitive distortions during gambling simulations compared to healthy controls and patients with lesions to other brain regions. This is of importance as problem gamblers are at greater risk of having the examined cognitive distortions such as near misses—a loss that falls close to a jackpot and gambler's fallacy—distorted psychological processing of random sequences (Clark et al., 2014).

Altogether lesion studies show that insular damage improves nicotine and opium cessation outcomes in patients suffering from strokes. Future research should explore if that is also the case in other SUDs.

Neuroimaging Studies

Structural Changes

There is a considerable amount of evidence from structural imaging studies of the insula in addicted individuals. In smokers, researchers have found that cortical thickness and gray matter density of the insula is significantly decreased compared to non-smokers (Fritz et al., 2014; Li et al., 2015; Hanlon et al., 2016; Stoeckel et al., 2016). Furthermore, a meta-analysis of 15 papers (761 smokers and 1,182 non-smokers) found that smoking was associated with decreased gray matter in the insula, specifically the left insular cortex (Sutherland et al., 2016). Although the majority seem to suggest a decrease in cortical thickness and gray matter density, one study found the opposite effect, such that smokers had increased gray matter densities (Zhang et al., 2011). Also, it appears that the changes in insular cortex density are more pronounced in older, more established, smokers as opposed to younger smokers (Hanlon et al., 2016). Young smokers (aged 16–21) did not differ in insula thickness compared to non-smokers (Morales et al., 2014). This suggests that the structural changes could be due to prolonged exposure to smoking. In terms of correlations with smoking behaviors and markers, there is evidence showing that gray matter density of the insula is negatively correlated with daily cigarettes smoked (Stoeckel et al., 2016), Fagerström Test for Nicotine Dependence (FTND) scores (Wang et al., 2019), and pack year smoking (Morales et al., 2014). Smoking cessation outcomes in relation to structural changes of the insula have also been evaluated, but showed no significant difference between smokers who quit, smokers who relapsed and non-smokers (Wang et al., 2019).

Nicotine is not the only drug that has been shown to cause structural changes to the insula; changes have been reported in cocaine, heroin, methamphetamine, cannabis, and alcohol use. For instance, cocaine dependence and duration of dependence has been shown to be correlated with decreased gray matter volume of the insula, which in turn was associated with greater impulsivity (Ersche et al., 2011). Lower cortical thickness of the insula was also found in cocaine users compared to healthy controls (Geng et al., 2017). In addition, cocaine- and heroin-dependent individuals had lower gray matter values in the right pIC compared to healthy controls (Gardini and Venneri, 2011). A meta-analysis of structural changes among stimulant-dependent individuals revealed significant decreases in gray matter in the left insula (Ersche et al., 2013). Similarly, another meta-analysis found cocaine and methamphetamine users had gray matter reductions in the insula. The right insula was more affected in cocaine users, whereas for methamphetamine users it was the left insula. Also, longer methamphetamine abstinence was correlated with an increase in gray matter of the left insula. Interestingly, the duration of methamphetamine use was associated with increased gray matter in the right insula (Hall et al., 2015). With regard to cannabis, regular smokers compared with occasional smokers were found to have a reduction in gray matter volume of the left insula, and this was correlated with the frequency of cannabis use in the 3 months prior to study entry (Battistella et al., 2014). Alcohol use has been subject to both white and gray matter changes. Adolescents with alcohol use disorder had greater white matter volume in the left insula, which was correlated with enhancement motives (i.e., the feeling of "being high") for drinking and with the frequency of binge drinking at baseline and 1-year follow-up. Furthermore, greater volume of white matter in the right insula was correlated with alcohol obsession/craving (Chung and Clark, 2014). In terms of gray matter, adolescents who drank alcohol excessively, but did not meet the criteria for alcohol use disorder, had lower volumes in the right insula compared to light drinkers (Heikkinen et al., 2017).

Behavioral addictions have also been studied. Individuals with the inability to control Internet use even when accompanied by negative consequences to their life showed significantly lower gray matter density in the left insula and lower white matter density in the right insula (Lin et al., 2015). Individuals with online gaming addiction showed gray matter atrophy in the insula, which was correlated with the severity of the subjects' addiction (Weng et al., 2013). A study among subjects who use social media excessively found a correlation between the severity of addiction-like symptoms and a reduction of gray matter volumes in the bilateral pIC, as well as impulsivity (Turel et al., 2018).

Altogether the evidence suggests that structural changes to the insula occur in addicted individuals, thus further demonstrating its involvement in addiction. Although there is not complete consensus on what the changes are, the majority of the findings point toward a decrease in gray matter volumes and density of the insula, rather than an increase.

Functional Changes

Resting State Functional Connectivity

Resting state functional connectivity (rsFC) is a method used to measure brain activity between regions while in a resting state (i.e., task-negative state) (Biswal et al., 1995). It has been widely used in addiction studies to investigate the neurocircuitry, such as large-scale brain networks discussed above, that underlie addiction. For instance, decreased rsFC between the right aIC (component of the SN) and right superior frontal gyrus (component of the ECN) has been reported in smokers (Fedota et al., 2016). Furthermore, smokers were found to have lower rsFC between the insula, executive functions regions, such as the OFC, and superior frontal gyrus, whereas the rsFC between the insula and anterior ACC seems to be negatively correlated with FTND scores (Zhou et al., 2017). Abstaining from smoking for just 12 h resulted in increased rsFC between the right aIC and executive functions regions (i.e., right OFC, and vmPFC) as well as the interconnectivity in the SN (Bi et al., 2017). Acutely abstinent smokers also demonstrate increased rsFC of the insula-DMN when compared to both non-smokers (Huang et al., 2014) and satiated smokers, though satiated smokers still have higher insula-DMN rsFC than non-smokers. Furthermore, a study comparing BOLD data of smokers before and after 48 h of abstinence found that the overall dynamics rsFC was decreased during abstinence and that dorsal and posterior insular connections to the DMN and SN were enhanced, whereas the ventral insular connection to the ECN was reduced. Also, static rsFC in the ventral and posterior insular-seeded circuits were correlated with subjective ratings of aversive affect and withdrawal symptoms (Fedota et al., 2018). However, one study found that increased risky decision making in smokers, which is associated with stronger nicotine dependence, resulted in increased rsFC between the aIC and dorsal ACC (dACC) and the right and left aIC (Wei et al., 2016). A meta-analysis of pharmacological neuroimaging studies found that among smokers, both administration of nicotinic acetylcholine receptor agonists and cigarette smoking were associated with decreased activity in the regions associated with the DMN and SN, such as the insula, vmPFC, PCC, and increased activity in the regions associated with the ECN, such as the lateral PFC and dACC (Sutherland et al., 2015). Interestingly, smokers with higher alexithymia appear to have lower levels of increased rsFC between the right aIC and the vmPFC, a core node of the DMN, and that this mediates craving following overnight withdrawal, though this mediation is disrupted by varenicline or nicotine replacement therapy (Sutherland et al., 2013b). A group of researchers have investigated the functional connectivity of smokers and non-smokers with regard to *CYP2A6* genetic variation. *CYP2A6* variation affects the rate of nicotine metabolism and is associated with smoking outcomes. In smokers, it was found that slow metabolizers of *CYP2A6* had reduced functional connectivity strength in the dACC and ventral striatum, which was driven by the bilateral insula (Li et al., 2017a).

In terms of other SUDs, individuals with cocaine use disorder had greater connectivity within the SN and weaker connectivity between the SN and the striatum. The reduced connectivity was correlated with impulsivity in cocaine users, and can be conceptualize as reduced inhibition of the SN on the striatum. Interestingly, the aberrant connectivity was not correlated to current craving (Wisner et al., 2013). Other researchers have found cocaine users to have decreased connectivity between the right and the left insula, as well as to the dACC, thus affecting the SN (Geng et al., 2017). Similarly, alcohol users had lower SN connectivity than controls and an attenuated blood flow to the insula (Sullivan et al., 2013), whereas individuals with heroin use disorder had an increased SN connectivity (Wang et al., 2010). Reduced connectivity between the aINS and the dACC in regular binge drinkers was found when given alcohol compared to placebo. In addition, the more the connection was reduced, the calmer the participants reported feeling, thus suggesting that the decreased connectivity between these two regions of the SN may be linked to the rewarding effects of alcohol (Gorka et al., 2018). For behavioral addictions, internet gaming disorder subjects exhibited enhanced rsFC between the aIC and a network of regions including the ACC, putamen, angular gyrus, and precuneus; and between the pIC and postcentral gyrus, precentral gyrus, supplemental motor area, and superior temporal gyrus (STG). The addiction severity was positively associated with connectivity between the aIC and angular gyrus, and STG, and with connectivity between the pIC and STG (Hanlon et al., 2018a). Another study found that internet gaming disorder individuals showed decreased functional connectivity between the left pIC, bilateral supplementary motor area and middle cingulated cortex, and between the right pIC and right superior frontal gyrus, and decreased functional integration between insular subregions. This finding can be conceptualized as a reduction in the ability to inhibit motor responses to internet games (Zhang et al., 2016).

In summary, the involvement of the insula in addiction was demonstrated in many rsFC studies. Alterations in the SN function and in the connectivity of the insula to executive functions regions were seen. This may be interpreted as the SN impaired ability to switch from cognitive states of interoceptive cravings to cognitive control. However, more studies are needed to gain a better understanding of brain networks in addictions.

Cue Reactivity

Non-resting state studies have also demonstrated altered connectivity in smokers. Smokers who participated in a memory retrieval task involving smoking and neutral cues were found to have the left insula significantly more active during the retrieval of smoking cues compared to neutral cues. Smokers also reported more cravings when viewing smoking cue images (Janes et al., 2015). Smoking cues resulted in greater left insula functional connectivity with the right insula, OFC, and striatum with that greater connectivity being positively correlated with nicotine dependence, as judged by scores on the FTND (Claus et al., 2013). There was also increased activation in the right aIC and striatal regions in response to cues relating to rewards or losses when nicotine was administered compared to placebo (Moran et al., 2018). Similarly, craving in smokers when viewing smoking cues was associated with increased connectivity, but between the right aIC and the precuneus, which are two regions known to play a role in interoception and self-awareness (Moran-Santa Maria et al., 2015). A meta-analysis of fMRI studies on smoking cue reactivity also concluded that smoking cues, as compared to neutral cues, reliably evoke larger fMRI responses in the insula (Engelmann et al., 2012). The effect of smoking initiation-related cues (e.g., lighter) vs. smoking conclusion-related cues (e.g., cigarette butt in ashtray) on two groups of smokers who were either content or discontent with their behavior further examined temporal relations of smoking cues (Stippekohl et al., 2012), with discontent smokers showed greater insular activation in response to initiation-related cues than content smokers, and aIC activation is observed during intrinsic, but not extrinsic, motivation (Lee and Reeve, 2013).

A study that was done on substance-dependent individuals who used cocaine, alcohol, or nicotine demonstrated an increased BOLD signal to substance cues relative to neutral cues in three distinct clusters: the medial PFC/ACC, the left inferior frontal gyrus/insula, and the right premotor cortex (Hanlon et al., 2018a). This finding may suggest different brain involvement among different individuals with SUD. Interestingly, the three distinct clusters were seen in cocaine, alcohol, or nicotine abuser and, therefore, are not related to the drug of choice. Abstained cannabis users demonstrated greater activation in response to the cannabis cues as compared with the neutral cues in several structures in the reward pathway, including the insula, VTA, thalamus, ACC, and amygdala (Filbey et al., 2009). Surprisingly, a 2011 meta-analysis did not support the role of the insula in drug cue activity- or craving-related activity. However, this might be due to the meta-analysis rigid exclusion criteria (Chase et al., 2011).

In summary, there is evidence suggesting the involvement of the insula in reactivity to drug cues. However, further investigation, such as a meta-analysis, might be of great value. It is important to note that there is debate in the literature about the way drug cues reactivity and craving influence relapse risk, thus additional research should also investigate this question (for further reading on this subject see review by Garavan, 2010).

A Tool for Prognosis and Relapse Prediction

A better understanding of rcFC and cue reactivity led the way to try to find a tool that will enable better prognosis assessment and relapse prediction. In smokers, researchers found a decreased functional connectivity between the insula and the primary sensorimotor cortices (Addicott et al., 2015), as well as the insula, dACC, and dlPFC (Janes et al., 2010), in those who relapsed. Also, abstinent smokers had greater activation in the aIC during an inhibitory control task. Therefore decreased insula activation leads to decreased inhibitory control, which could be an indicator of relapse (Gilman et al., 2018). However, individuals who relapsed had greater brain reactivity to smoking cues in the right insula and dorsal putamen (Janes et al., 2017). Sutherland and Stein suggested that neurocircuits centered in the insula may represent a biomarker for acute withdrawal (Sutherland and Stein, 2018). This was demonstrated by rsFC alterations where abstinent smokers had greater connectivity between the insula and the amygdala (a connectivity which underlines negative affect) (Koob and Le Moal, 2005; Koob and Volkow, 2010), but was down-regulated with nicotine or varenicline administration (Sutherland et al., 2013a).

Additionally, abstinent methamphetamine-dependent individuals who relapsed demonstrated attenuated bilateral insula, bilateral striatum, left inferior frontal gyrus, and left ACC activation in response to outcomes of winning, tying, and losing feedback in a reinforcement learning task, compared to those who remained abstinent (Stewart et al., 2014). Methamphetamine users who remained abstinent showed increased activation of the left aIC and right striatum for large/risky relative to small/safe rewards, whereas individuals who relapsed did not show differential activation between reward types (Gowin et al., 2015). Regarding relapsed cocaine-addicted individuals, they displayed reduced connectivity between the bilateral putamen and pIC, which partially mediates higher impulsivity (Battistella et al., 2014). Researchers have found that occasional stimulant users (amphetamine and cocaine) that developed stimulant use disorders had lower activation of the insula and ACC at baseline during a decision making task compared to individuals who stopped using stimulants (Stewart et al., 2017). Heavy alcohol drinkers had an increased BOLD fMRI signal in response to alcohol cues in the insula (it was significant in the left insula and a trend in the right) and the ventral striatum compared to light drinkers. This links the insula and dorsal striatum to relapse vulnerability. In addition, heavy drinkers had reduced responses in frontal areas to pictures related to higher-order life goals and in the cingulate cortex to appetitive food stimuli, suggesting that they have difficulty finding alternative goals. By using this activation pattern it was possible to differentiate between heavy and light drinkers to a high degree of precision (Ihssen et al., 2011).

In summary, it has been suggested in several studies that insula-related activation patterns can be used as a prognostic tool, as well as the link between the insula and striatum, which might suggest that an adequate striatal inhibition by the insula might be a good prognostic factor. The use of the insula as a biomarker is worth further investigation.

Brain Stimulation Studies

Brain stimulation studies for addiction have mainly targeted the PFC, specifically the dlPFC (Salling and Martinez, 2016). Studies targeting the insula are lacking as there is currently only one study completed thus far (Dinur-Klein et al., 2014). Smokers (n = 115) were randomized to either receive 13 sessions of high frequency, low frequency or sham stimulation to the lateral PFC and insula bilaterally. This stimulation was done using an H-coil for deep TMS. High-frequency deep TMS (10 Hz) was found to significantly reduce cigarette consumption, as well as nicotine dependence. Those who also had smoking cues presented during high-frequency stimulation had the best results (44% abstinence at end of treatment and 33% at 6 months follow-up). It should be noted that they did not exclusively target the insula, thus it is not possible to know if the clinical effect were mediated by the insula or the PFC or both. Nonetheless, given the strong evidence of the insula's role in addiction, as well as the promising results presented by Dinur-Klein et al. (2014), further studies targeting the insula are needed. Currently, there are two smoking cessation trials being conducted using deep rTMS; however, both are targeting the insula along with the PFC (NCT02126124, NCT03264313). On the other hand, our laboratory is working on a clinical trial investigating a combined treatment for smokers using varenicline and deep rTMS targeting the insula. It should be noted that one study found that in healthy volunteers, one session of low-frequency rTMS (1 Hz) to the right aIC using an H-coil was unable to affect the activity of the insula, as measured by behavioral markers (i.e., a blink suppression task and a forced-choice risk-taking task) (Spagnolo et al., 2019).

Secondary Activation

It is evident that the target brain region being stimulated is a very important factor that needs careful consideration. However, the primary stimulation may lead to secondary activations. These activations can occur due to neurotransmitter release or from back propagation of action potentials from the primary site of activation (Diana et al., 2017). Furthermore, these activations are not necessarily confined to the networks associated with the primary site, but can be widespread (Gratton et al., 2013). Secondary activations have been demonstrated by studies combining brain stimulation and brain imaging. For instance, one session of high frequency (10 Hz) of rTMS over the left dlPFC in smokers resulted in inhibition of activity in the right insula and thalamus as measured by fractional amplitude of low-frequency fluctuation (fALFF) (Li et al., 2017b). Also, a single session of bilateral tDCS applied over the dlPFC of abstinent methamphetamine users led to a decrease in subjective craving. The subjective feeling was correlated with a modulation of resting state networks; DMN connectivity decreased, whereas ECN and SN intranetwork functional connectivity increased (Shahbabaie et al., 2018). In alcohol users, a single day of 6 trains of continuous TBS to the left frontal pole decreased evoked BOLD signal in left OFC, insula, and lateral sensorimotor cortex without a significant effect on subjective craving (Hanlon et al., 2018a). Interestingly, a publication about one patient with alcohol dependence, reported that a single rTMS to the dACC led to a temporary abolishment of alcohol craving correlated with a decrease in beta EEG activity in the right insula (De Ridder et al., 2011). There has been one study investigating the changes in dopamine levels following bilateral insula rTMS, but it was done on healthy participants. Low-frequency rTMS (1 Hz) was found to significantly decrease dopamine levels in the substantia nigra, sensorimotor striatum, and associative striatum (Malik et al., 2018).

Altogether, these studies suggest that the effect of brain stimulation is not restricted to the area being targeted, but rather can affect a wide variety of areas, which should be considered when deciding on the parameters used for stimulation. In instances where one session of brain stimulation did not yield behavioral change, further investigation should seek to see whether longer courses of stimulation may lead to a behavioral change.

DISCUSSION

Although there is a vast literature about the use of brain stimulation to treat addictions, there is an ongoing debate about the most effective protocol. Most studies in this field targeted the dlPFC (for recent reviews see Coles et al., 2018; Hanlon et al., 2018b). In this review, we suggested the insula as a novel target to treat addictions. We reviewed brain stimulation techniques and principles that enable stimulation of the insula. In addition, we reviewed relevant preclinical studies which demonstrated the insula's involvement in all stages of addictions: binge/intoxication, withdrawal/negative affect, and preoccupation/anticipation, as well as the clinical studies which demonstrate the major role of the insula in addictions.

At first glance, the evidence presented may seem to be somewhat contradictory. Structural studies showed that addiction resulted in a loss of gray matter in the insula, thus suggesting a loss of function. On the contrary, neuroimaging studies showed increased activation of the insula, thereby suggesting a gain of function. However, it has been previously suggested that the decrease in gray matter actually means an overactive insula (Droutman et al., 2015; Turel et al., 2018). Naqvi et al. (2014) described that with addiction the insula may undergo both a loss and gain of function depending on the specific function investigated. After drug taking, the insula later plays a role in establishing the internal state feeling of the effects of the drug. This role in interoception is what is believed to lead to continuous drug-seeking behavior, as individuals need to reach homeostatic levels. Therefore, this can be thought of as a gain of function of the insula in individuals with addiction. On the other hand, addiction may cause a loss of function in the insula with regard to risky decision making. There is a decreased capability when it comes to weighing out the negative consequences that can occur from decisions involving drug-seeking, leading to the inability to stop this behavior. This dual effect of addiction on the insula further increases the complexity of this area. However, we can learn from lesion studies that a loss of function improves cessation probability, therefore it might be that the gain of function is the key factor in addictions. However, understanding of the reciprocal relationship of the insula and other brain regions will lead to a better understand in its role in addiction, as the insula should not be thought of in isolation but rather as part of a network.

Although the evidence of the involvement of the insula in addiction is convincing, there is a lack of research translating this into treatment for addicted individuals. No studies have yet to investigate brain stimulation of the insula in addiction, with the exception of one clinical trial in smokers that targeted the insula and PFC together (Dinur-Klein et al., 2014). Since the results of the trial were positive and the increasing evidence of the functional role of the insula, the next course of action should be to see whether stimulating the insula exclusively or with other brain regions posits any benefit in the treatment of addiction. Studies will be needed to investigate various addictions, as we have discussed in this review that the insula plays a role in a variety of drug and behavioral addictions. Also, there are currently no established parameters or treatment plans for brain stimulation for addiction, and these factors have been shown to play a major role in the outcomes of stimulation. For instance, although TMS is approved for use for major depression disorder, there is a considerable amount of variance in its effectiveness. Many studies demonstrate that it is efficacious (George et al., 1997; Klein et al., 1999; Berman et al., 2000; George et al., 2000; O'Reardon et al., 2007; George et al., 2010; Harel et al., 2014), including data from meta-analyses (Berlim et al., 2014; Mutz et al., 2018). However, there is also a large number of studies that found no beneficial effect of TMS for depression (Boutros et al., 2002; Loo et al., 2003; Carpenter et al., 2017; Yesavage et al., 2018), as well as meta-analyses (Martin et al., 2002; Couturier, 2005). Others have found that only certain variations of TMS are effective (Li et al., 2014; Blumberger et al., 2016; Brunoni et al., 2017). Given the heterogeneous outcomes in brain stimulation studies for depression, researchers will need to carefully consider the stimulation intensity, frequency, duration, and other parameters. We also described that brain stimulation has been shown to activate secondary sites (i.e., not the primary stimulation site), it is not known what other areas will be activated through this when stimulating the insula. For that reason, studies involving both brain stimulation of the insula and imaging and/or EEG are much needed and could provide a considerable amount of information. Furthermore, electric-field modeling is another tool that may be useful to estimate the insular induced electric field by TMS, thus allowing for better planning and optimization of the stimulation parameters. It is also important to consider the concept of personalized medicine. As we described under the section "A Tool for Prognosis and Relapse Prediction," insular activation patterns and the link between the insula and striatum can be used to predict outcome. We strongly encourage future research to pursue personalized treatment plans, based on a better understanding of the individual brain activation patterns.

Individuals with mental illnesses might also benefit from insular stimulation. The role of the insula and the dACC (which compose the SN) as a common neurological substrate for mental illness was demonstrated in recent meta-analyses studies (Goodkind et al., 2015; Downar et al., 2016), and it is well known that SUDs are more prevalent in this population (Whiteford et al., 2013). Future studies should consider investigating insular stimulation as a dual treatment for symptoms of both mental illnesses and SUDs. In this context, it will also be interesting to see if stimulation of the insula improves the negative affect that is related to withdrawal.

Another factor to consider for future studies should be that of motivation to quit. A person diagnosed with a smoking-related disease is scientifically more likely to cease smoking (Twardella et al., 2006), which could be attributed to an increased motivation to quit. In addition, patients with insular lesions who live in a country with little awareness to smoking-related harm, were not more likely to quit smoking (Bienkowski et al., 2010), this finding suggests that cultural norms may influence individual motivation for quitting. Therefore, it seems that the motivation to quit and the insular damage co-influence the likelihood to cease smoking. Future studies should investigate whether insular stimulation will be more beneficial to individuals who suffer from substance abuse-related diseases. We suggest that it can be of great importance to investigate the role of motivation in patients undergoing insular stimulation, which may further increase the effectiveness of the treatment. This can be done by trying to elevate motivation to quit using patient education programs or cognitive behavioral therapy.

Furthermore, future research could explore the effect of targeting the insula using brain stimulation, as well as with pharmacotherapies. There is evidence that modafinil (Cera et al., 2014), ketamine (Carlson et al., 2013; Höflich et al., 2017; Evans et al., 2018), baclofen (Franklin et al., 2011; Franklin et al., 2012), oxytocin (Riem et al., 2011) and varenicline (Sutherland et al., 2013a) have an effect on the insula. Thus, the effect of dual targeting of the insula could be of interest. As previously mentioned, our laboratory is working on a clinical trial combining varenicline treatment with deep rTMS to the insula for smoking cessation. This will aid in expanding some of the knowledge that is lacking in this field.

An interesting question that arises from this review is to what extent are the described alterations predisposition to addiction and to what extent are they acquired during repeated drug use. Interestingly, a significant reduction in gray matter in the aIC was unique to stimulant-dependent individuals when compared with their siblings (Ersche et al., 2012). On the other hand, individuals with a family history of alcohol dependence showed alternations in insular function compared to controls (Cservenka, 2016). Although this question warrants further investigation, this discussion is not in the scope of this review.

Lastly, there are several limitations concerning the current evidence that should be noted. With regard to the clinical data, the absolute number of participants in these studies is small, and most are males. In addition, studies approached different phases of addiction (i.e., abstinent vs non-abstinent users). The methods of the studies also vary (i.e., different rsFC protocols), which could lead to variability in findings. Also, the imaging studies presented are correlational and not causative, thus making conclusions from these studies should be done with caution. It is important to note that even though there are limitations to the studies and although the majority have found other brain regions to be involved in addiction, the insula is a common area found in all of these findings, thereby further justifying it prominent role in addiction and its potential use as a target for brain stimulation in addicted individuals.

CONCLUSION

In conclusion, the insula has many critical functions pertaining to addiction. Individuals with SUDs have been shown to have structural and functional changes to the insula. Also, preclinical work and human lesion studies have demonstrated that addiction is altered when there is damage to the insula. The convincing evidence leads to the idea of the insula being a promising brain region to target for addiction. Brain stimulation techniques, specifically deep TMS, are advancing and allow the targeting of the insula. This may provide promising treatment outcomes in addicted individuals. Nonetheless, there is a need for further research to determine if that is the case.

AUTHOR CONTRIBUTIONS

CI, DR-K, AP, and MM drafted the manuscript. DB, ZD, AZ, and BF reviewed and edited the manuscript. All authors contributed to the conception of the manuscript.

REFERENCES

Abdolahi, A., Acosta, G., Breslin, F. J., Hemby, S. E., and Lynch, W. J. (2010). Incubation of nicotine seeking is associated with enhanced protein kinase A-regulated signaling of dopamine- and cAMP-regulated phosphoprotein of 32 kDa in the insular cortex. *Eur. J. Neurosci.* 31 (4), 733–741. doi: 10.1111/j.1460-9568.2010.07114.x

Abdolahi, A., Williams, G. C., Benesch, C. G., Wang, H. Z., Spitzer, E. M., Scott, B. E., et al. (2015a). Smoking cessation behaviors three months following acute insular damage from stroke. *Addict. Behav.* 51, 24–30. doi: 10.1016/j.addbeh.2015.07.001

Abdolahi, A., Williams, G. C., Benesch, C. G., Wang, H. Z., Spitzer, E. M., Scott, B. E., et al. (2017). Immediate and sustained decrease in smoking urges after acute insular cortex damage. *Nicotine Tob. Res.* 19 (6), 756–762. doi: 10.1093/ntr/ntx046

Abdolahi, A., Williams, G. C., Benesch, C. G., Wang, H. Z., Spitzer, E. M., Scott, B. E., et al. (2015b). Damage to the insula leads to decreased nicotine withdrawal during abstinence. *Addiction* 110 (12), 1994–2003. doi: 10.1111/add.13061

Addicott, M. A., Sweitzer, M. M., Froeliger, B., Rose, J. E., and McClernon, F. J. (2015). Increased functional connectivity in an insula-based network is associated with improved smoking cessation outcomes. *Neuropsychopharmacology* 40 (11), 2648–2656. doi: 10.1038/npp.2015.114

Allen, G. V., Saper, C. B., Hurley, K. M., and Cechetto, D. F. (1991). Organization of visceral and limbic connections in the insular cortex of the rat. *J. Comp. Neurol.* 311 (1), 1–16. doi: 10.1002/cne.903110102

Alvarez, R. P., Kirlic, N., Misaki, M., Bodurka, J., Rhudy, J. L., Paulus, M. P., et al. (2015). Increased anterior insula activity in anxious individuals is linked to diminished perceived control. *Transl. Psychiatry* 5, e591. doi: 10.1038/tp.2015.84

American Psychiatric Association. (2013). *Diagnostic and Statistical Manual of Mental Disorders.* Arlington, VA: American Psychiatric Association. doi: 10.1176/appi.books.9780890425596

Arguello, A. A., Wang, R., Lyons, C. M., Higginbotham, J. A., Hodges, M. A., and Fuchs, R. A. (2017). Role of the agranular insular cortex in contextual control over cocaine-seeking behavior in rats. *Psychopharmacology* 234 (16), 2431–2441. doi: 10.1007/s00213-017-4632-7

Barker, A. T., Jalinous, R., and Freeston, I. L. (1985). Non-invasive magnetic stimulation of human motor cortex. *Lancet* 325 (8437), 1106–1107. doi: 10.1016/S0140-6736(85)92413-4

Batsikadze, G., Moliadze, V., Paulus, W., Kuo, M.-F., and Nitsche, M. A. (2013). Partially non-linear stimulation intensity-dependent effects of direct current stimulation on motor cortex excitability in humans. *J. Physiol.* 591 (7), 1987–2000. doi: 10.1113/jphysiol.2012.249730

Battistella, G., Fornari, E., Annoni, J.-M., Chtioui, H., Dao, K., Fabritius, M., et al. (2014). Long-term effects of cannabis on brain structure. *Neuropsychopharmacology* 39 (9), 2041–2048. doi: 10.1038/npp.2014.67

Baumgartner, U., Buchholz, H. G., Bellosevich, A., Magerl, W., Siessmeier, T., Rolke, R., et al. (2006). High opiate receptor binding potential in the human lateral pain system. *Neuroimage* 30 (3), 692–699. doi: 10.1016/j.neuroimage.2005.10.033

Bechara, A., and Damasio, A. R. (2005). The somatic marker hypothesis: a neural theory of economic decision. *Games Econ. Behav.* 52 (2), 336–372. doi: 10.1016/j.geb.2004.06.010

Berlim, M. T., Van Den Eynde, F., Tovar-Perdomo, S., and Daskalakis, Z. J. (2014). Response, remission and drop-out rates following high-frequency repetitive transcranial magnetic stimulation (rTMS) for treating major depression: a systematic review and meta-analysis of randomized, double-blind and sham-controlled trials. *Psychol. Med.* 44 (2), 225–239. doi: 10.1017/S0033291713000512

Berman, R. M., Narasimhan, M., Sanacora, G., Miano, A. P., Hoffman, R. E., Hu, X. S., et al. (2000). A randomized clinical trial of repetitive transcranial magnetic stimulation in the treatment of major depression. *Biol. Psychiatry* 47 (4), 332–337. doi: 10.1016/S0006-3223(99)00243-7

Bi, Y., Zhang, Y., Li, Y., Yu, D., Yuan, K., and Tian, J. (2017). 12h abstinence-induced right anterior insula network pattern changes in young smokers. *Drug Alcohol Depend.* 176, 162–168. doi: 10.1016/j.drugalcdep.2017.02.019

Bienkowski, P., Zatorski, P., Baranowska, A., Ryglewicz, D., and Sienkiewicz-Jarosz, H. (2010). Insular lesions and smoking cessation after first-ever ischemic stroke: a 3-month follow-up. *Neurosci. Lett.* 478 (3), 161–164. doi: 10.1016/j.neulet.2010.05.008

Biswal, B., Yetkin, F. Z., Haughton, V. M., and Hyde, J. S. (1995). Functional connectivity in the motor cortex of resting human brain using echo-planar MRI. *Magn. Reson. Med.* 34 (4), 537–541. doi: 10.1002/mrm.1910340409

Blumberger, D. M., Maller, J. J., Thomson, L., Mulsant, B. H., Rajji, T. K., Maher, M., et al. (2016). Unilateral and bilateral MRI-targeted repetitive transcranial magnetic stimulation for treatment-resistant depression: a randomized controlled study. *J. Psychiatry Neurosci.* 41 (4), E58–E66. doi: 10.1503/jpn.150265

Boutros, N. N., Gueorguieva, R., Hoffman, R. E., Oren, D. A., Feingold, A., and Berman, R. M. (2002). Lack of a therapeutic effect of a 2-week sub-threshold transcranial magnetic stimulation course for treatment-resistant depression. *Psychiatry Res.* 113 (3), 245–254. doi: 10.1016/S0165-1781(02)00267-6

Brass, M., and Haggard, P. (2010). The hidden side of intentional action: the role of the anterior insular cortex. *Brain Struct. Funct.* 214 (5–6), 603–610. doi: 10.1007/s00429-010-0269-6

Breit, S., Schulz, J. B., and Benabid, A.-L. (2004). Deep brain stimulation. *Cell Tissue Res.* 318 (1), 275–288. doi: 10.1007/s00441-004-0936-0

Brunoni, A. R., Chaimani, A., Moffa, A. H., Razza, L. B., Gattaz, W. F., Daskalakis, Z. J., et al. (2017). Repetitive transcranial magnetic stimulation for the acute treatment of major depressive episodes: a systematic review with network meta-analysis repetitive transcranial magnetic stimulation for treatment of major depressive episodes repetitive transcranial magnetic stimulation for treatment of major depressive episodes. *JAMA Psychiatry* 74 (2), 143–152. doi: 10.1001/jamapsychiatry.2016.3644

Carlson, P. J., Diazgranados, N., Nugent, A. C., Ibrahim, L., Luckenbaugh, D. A., Brutsche, N., et al. (2013). Neural Correlates of rapid antidepressant response to ketamine in treatment-resistant unipolar depression: a preliminary positron emission tomography study. *Biol. Psychiatry* 73 (12), 1213–1221. doi: 10.1016/j.biopsych.2013.02.008

Carpenter, L. L., Aaronson, S. T., Clarke, G. N., Holtzheimer, P. E., Johnson, C. W., McDonald, W. M., et al. (2017). rTMS with a two-coil array: safety and efficacy for treatment resistant major depressive disorder. *Brain Stimul.* 10 (5), 926–933. doi: 10.1016/j.brs.2017.06.003

Cechetto, D. F., and Saper, C. B. (1987). Evidence for a viscerotopic sensory representation in the cortex and thalamus in the rat. *J. Comp. Neurol.* 262 (1), 27–45. doi: 10.1002/cne.902620104

Cera, N., Tartaro, A., and Sensi, S. L. (2014). Modafinil alters intrinsic functional connectivity of the right posterior insula: a pharmacological resting state fMRI study. *PLoS ONE* 9 (9), e107145. doi: 10.1371/journal.pone.0107145

Chase, H. W., Eickhoff, S. B., Laird, A. R., and Hogarth, L. (2011). The neural basis of drug stimulus processing and craving: an activation likelihood estimation meta-analysis. *Biol. Psychiatry* 70 (8), 785–793. doi: 10.1016/j.biopsych.2011.05.025

Chawla, M., and Garrison, K. A. (2018). Neurobiological considerations for tobacco use disorder. *Curr. Behav. Neurosci. Rep.* 5 (4), 238–248. doi: 10.1007/s40473-018-0168-3

Chiamulera, C., Padovani, L., and Corsi, M. (2017). Drug discovery for the treatment of substance use disorders: novel targets, repurposing, and the need for new paradigms. *Curr. Opin. Pharmacol.* 35, 120–124. doi: 10.1016/j.coph.2017.08.009

Chung, T., and Clark, D. B. (2014). Insula white matter volume linked to binge drinking frequency through enhancement motives in treated adolescents. *Alcohol Clin. Exp. Res.* 38 (7), 1932–1940. doi: 10.1111/acer.12461

Clark, L., Studer, B., Bruss, J., Tranel, D., and Bechara, A. (2014). Damage to insula abolishes cognitive distortions during simulated gambling. *Proc. Natl. Acad. Sci. U. S. A.* 111 (16), 6098–6103. doi: 10.1073/pnas.1322295111

Claus, E. D., Blaine, S. K., Filbey, F. M., Mayer, A. R., and Hutchison, K. E. (2013). Association between nicotine dependence severity, BOLD response to smoking cues, and functional connectivity. *Neuropsychopharmacology* 38 (12), 2363–2372. doi: 10.1038/npp.2013.134

Coles, A. S., Kozak, K., and George, T. P. (2018). A review of brain stimulation methods to treat substance use disorders. *Am. J. Addict.* 27 (2), 71–91. doi: 10.1111/ajad.12674

Contoreggi, C., Herning, R. I., Na, P., Gold, P. W., Chrousos, G., Negro, P. J., et al. (2003). Stress hormone responses to corticotropin-releasing hormone in substance abusers without severe comorbid psychiatric disease. *Biol. Psychiatry* 54 (9), 873–878. doi: 10.1016/S0006-3223(03)00167-7

Contreras, M., Billeke, P., Vicencio, S., Madrid, C., Perdomo, G., González, M. et al., (2012). A role for the insular cortex in long-term memory for context-evoked drug craving in rats. *Neuropsychopharmacology* 37 (9), 2101–2108. doi: 10.1038/npp.2012.59

Contreras, M., Ceric, F., and Torrealba, F. (2007). Inactivation of the interoceptive insula disrupts drug craving and malaise induced by lithium. *Science* 318 (5850), 655–658. doi: 10.1126/science.1145590

Cosme, C. V., Gutman, A. L., and LaLumiere, R. T. (2015). The Dorsal Agranular Insular Cortex Regulates the Cued Reinstatement of Cocaine-Seeking, but not Food-Seeking, Behavior in Rats. *Neuropsychopharmacology* 40 (10), 2425–2433. doi: 10.1038/npp.2015.92

Couturier, J. L. (2005). Efficacy of rapid-rate repetitive transcranial magnetic stimulation in the treatment of depression: a systematic review and meta-analysis. *J. Psychiatry Neurosci.* 30 (2), 83–90.

Craig, A. D. (2002). How do you feel? Interoception: the sense of the physiological condition of the body. *Nat. Rev. Neurosci.* 3 (8), 655–666. doi: 10.1038/nrn894

Craig, A. D. (2003). Interoception: the sense of the physiological condition of the body. *Curr. Opin. Neurobiol.* 13 (4), 500–505. doi: 10.1016/S0959-4388(03)00090-4

Craig, A. D. (2004). Human feelings: why are some more aware than others? *Trends Cogn. Sci.* 8 (6), 239–241. doi: 10.1016/j.tics.2004.04.004

Craig, A. D. (2009). How do you feel–now? The anterior insula and human awareness. *Nat. Rev. Neurosci.* 10 (1), 59–70. doi: 10.1038/nrn2555

Cservenka, A. (2016). Neurobiological phenotypes associated with a family history of alcoholism. *Drug Alcohol Depend.* 158, 8–21. doi: 10.1016/j.drugalcdep.2015.10.021

Daskalakis, Z. J., Christensen, B. K., Fitzgerald, P. B., and Chen, R. (2002). Transcranial magnetic stimulation: a new investigational and treatment tool in psychiatry. *J. Neuropsychiatry Clin. Neurosci.* 14 (4), 406–415. doi: 10.1176/jnp.14.4.406

de Jesus, D. R., Favalli, G.P.d.S., Hoppenbrouwers, S. S., Barr, M. S., Chen, R., Fitzgerald, P. B., et al. (2014). Determining optimal rTMS parameters through changes in cortical inhibition. *Clin. Neurophysiol.* 125 (4), 755–762. doi: 10.1016/j.clinph.2013.09.011

De Ridder, D., Vanneste, S., Kovacs, S., Sunaert, S., and Dom, G. (2011). Transient alcohol craving suppression by rTMS of dorsal anterior cingulate: an fMRI and LORETA EEG study. *Neurosci. Lett.* 496 (1), 5–10. doi: 10.1016/j.neulet.2011.03.074

DeCoteau, W. E., Kesner, R. P., and Williams, J. M. (1997). Short-term memory for food reward magnitude: the role of the prefrontal cortex. *Behav. Brain Res.* 88 (2), 239–249. doi: 10.1016/S0166-4328(97)00044-2

Deen, B., Pitskel, N. B., and Pelphrey, K. A. (2011). Three systems of insular functional connectivity identified with cluster analysis. *Cereb. Cortex* 21 (7), 1498–1506. doi: 10.1093/cercor/bhq186

Dehkordi, O., Rose, J. E., Asadi, S., Manaye, K. F., Millis, R. M., and Jayam-Trouth, A. (2015). Neuroanatomical circuitry mediating the sensory impact of nicotine in the central nervous system. *J. Neurosci. Res.* 93 (2), 230–243. doi: 10.1002/jnr.23477

Deng, Z.-D., Lisanby, S. H., and Peterchev, A. V. (2013). Electric field depth-focality tradeoff in transcranial magnetic stimulation: simulation comparison of 50 coil designs. *Brain Stimul.* 6 (1), 1–13. doi: 10.1016/j.brs.2012.02.005

Di Pietro, N. C., Mashhoon, Y., Heaney, C., Yager, L. M., and Kantak, K. M. (2008). Role of dopamine D1 receptors in the prefrontal dorsal agranular insular cortex in mediating cocaine self-administration in rats. *Psychopharmacology (Berl)* 200 (1), 81–91. doi: 10.1007/s00213-008-1149-0

Diana, M., Raij, T., Melis, M., Nummenmaa, A., Leggio, L., and Bonci, A. (2017). Rehabilitating the addicted brain with transcranial magnetic stimulation. *Nat. Rev. Neurosci.* 18 (11), 685–693. doi: 10.1038/nrn.2017.113

Dinur-Klein, L., Dannon, P., Hadar, A., Rosenberg, O., Roth, Y., Kotler, M., et al. (2014). Smoking cessation induced by deep repetitive transcranial magnetic stimulation of the prefrontal and insular cortices: a prospective, randomized controlled trial. *Biol. Psychiatry* 76 (9), 742–749. doi: 10.1016/j.biopsych.2014.05.020

Downar, J., Blumberger, D. M., and Daskalakis, Z. J. (2016). The neural crossroads of psychiatric illness: an emerging target for brain stimulation. *Trends Cogn. Sci.* 20 (2), 107–120. doi: 10.1016/j.tics.2015.10.007

Droutman, V., Bechara, A., and Read, S. J. (2015). Roles of the different sub-regions of the insular cortex in various phases of the decision-making process. *Front. Behav. Neurosci.* 9, 309. doi: 10.3389/fnbeh.2015.00309

Ehlinger, D. G., Bergstrom, H. C., McDonald, C. G., and Smith, R. F. (2012). Nicotine-induced dendritic remodeling in the insular cortex. *Neurosci. Lett.* 516 (1), 89–93. doi: 10.1016/j.neulet.2012.03.064

Engelmann, J. M., Versace, F., Robinson, J. D., Minnix, J. A., Lam, C. Y., Cui, Y., et al. (2012). Neural substrates of smoking cue reactivity: a meta-analysis of fMRI studies. *Neuroimage* 60 (1), 252–262. doi: 10.1016/j.neuroimage.2011.12.024

Ersche, K. D., Barnes, A., Jones, P. S., Morein-Zamir, S., Robbins, T. W., and Bullmore, E. T. (2011). Abnormal structure of frontostriatal brain systems is associated with aspects of impulsivity and compulsivity in cocaine dependence. *Brain* 134 (Pt 7), 2013–2024. doi: 10.1093/brain/awr138

Ersche, K. D., Jones, P. S., Williams, G. B., Turton, A. J., Robbins, T. W., and Bullmore, E. T. (2012). Abnormal brain structure implicated in stimulant drug addiction. *Science* 335 (6068), 601–604. doi: 10.1126/science.1214463

Ersche, K. D., Williams, G. B., Robbins, T. W., and Bullmore, E. T. (2013). Meta-analysis of structural brain abnormalities associated with stimulant drug dependence and neuroimaging of addiction vulnerability and resilience. *Curr. Opin. Neurobiol.* 23 (4), 615–624. doi: 10.1016/j.conb.2013.02.017

Evans, J. W., Szczepanik, J., Brutsché, N., Park, L. T., Nugent, A. C., and Zarate, C. A. (2018). Default mode connectivity in major depressive disorder measured up to 10 days after ketamine administration. *Biol. Psychiatry* 84 (8), 582–590. doi: 10.1016/j.biopsych.2018.01.027

Fedota, J. R., Ding, X., Matous, A. L., Salmeron, B. J., McKenna, M. R., Gu, H., et al. (2018). Nicotine abstinence influences the calculation of salience in discrete insular circuits. *Biol. Psychiatry Cogn. Neurosci. Neuroimaging* 3 (2), 150–159. doi: 10.1016/j.bpsc.2017.09.010

Fedota, J. R., Matous, A. L., Salmeron, B. J., Gu, H., Ross, T. J., and Stein, E. A. (2016). Insula demonstrates a non-linear response to varying demand for cognitive control and weaker resting connectivity with the executive control network in smokers. *Neuropsychopharmacology* 41 (10), 2557–2565. doi: 10.1038/npp.2016.62

Feil, J., and Zangen, A. (2010). Brain stimulation in the study and treatment of addiction. *Neurosci. Biobehav. Rev.* 34 (4), 559–574. doi: 10.1016/j.neubiorev.2009.11.006

Filbey, F. M., Schacht, J. P., Myers, U. S., Chavez, R. S., and Hutchison, K. E. (2009). Marijuana craving in the brain. *Proc. Natl. Acad. Sci. U S A* 106 (31), 13016–13021. doi: 10.1073/pnas.0903863106

Forget, B., Pushparaj, A., and Le Foll, B. (2010). Granular insular cortex inactivation as a novel therapeutic strategy for nicotine addiction. *Biol. Psychiatry* 68 (3), 265–271. doi: 10.1016/j.biopsych.2010.01.029

Franklin, T. R., Shin, J., Jagannathan, K., Suh, J. J., Detre, J. A., O'Brien, C. P., et al. (2012). Acute baclofen diminishes resting baseline blood flow to limbic structures: a perfusion fMRI study. *Drug Alcohol Depend.* 125 (1-2), 60–66. doi: 10.1016/j.drugalcdep.2012.03.016

Franklin, T. R., Wang, Z., Sciortino, N., Harper, D., Li, Y., Hakun, J., et al. (2011). Modulation of resting brain cerebral blood flow by the GABA B agonist, baclofen: a longitudinal perfusion fMRI study. *Drug Alcohol Depend.* 117 (2-3), 176–183. doi: 10.1016/j.drugalcdep.2011.01.015

Fresquet, N., Angst, M. J., and Sandner, G. (2004). Insular cortex lesions alter conditioned taste avoidance in rats differentially when using two methods of sucrose delivery. *Behav. Brain Res.* 153 (2), 357–365. doi: 10.1016/j.bbr.2003.12.011

Fritz, H.-C., Fritz, H.-C., Wittfeld, K., Wittfeld, K., Schmidt, C. O., Schmidt, C. O., et al. (2014). Current smoking and reduced gray matter volume - a voxel-based morphometry study. *Neuropsychopharmacology* 39 (11), 2594–2600. doi: 10.1038/npp.2014.112

Garavan, H. (2010). Insula and drug cravings. *Brain Struct. Funct.* 214 (5–6), 593–601. doi: 10.1007/s00429-010-0259-8

Gardini, S., and Venneri, A. (2011). Reduced grey matter in the posterior insula as a structural vulnerability or diathesis to addiction. *Brain Res. Bull.* 87 (2), 205–211. doi: 10.1016/j.brainresbull.2011.11.021

Gaspar, P., Berger, B., Febvret, A., Vigny, A., and Henry, J. P. (1989). Catecholamine innervation of the human cerebral cortex as revealed by comparative immunohistochemistry of tyrosine hydroxylase and dopamine-beta-hydroxylase. *J. Comp. Neurol.* 279 (2), 249–271. doi: 10.1002/cne.902790208

Gasquoine, P. G. (2014). Contributions of the insula to cognition and emotion. *Neuropsychol. Rev.* 24 (2), 77–87. doi: 10.1007/s11065-014-9246-9

Gauriau, C., and Bernard, J. F. (2004). Posterior triangular thalamic neurons convey nociceptive messages to the secondary somatosensory and insular cortices in the rat. *J. Neurosci.* 24 (3), 752–761. doi: 10.1523/JNEUROSCI.3272-03.2004

Gaznick, N., Tranel, D., McNutt, A., and Bechara, A. (2014). Basal ganglia plus insula damage yields stronger disruption of smoking addiction than basal ganglia damage alone. *Nicotine Tob. Res.* 16 (4), 445–453. doi: 10.1093/ntr/ntt172

Geng, X., Hu, Y., Gu, H., Salmeron, B. J., Adinoff, B., Stein, E. A., et al. (2017). Salience and default mode network dysregulation in chronic cocaine users predict treatment outcome. *Brain* 140 (5), 1513–1524. doi: 10.1093/brain/awx036

George, M. S., Lisanby, S. H., Avery, D., McDonald, W. M., Durkalski, V., Pavlicova, M., et al. (2010). Daily left prefrontal transcranial magnetic stimulation therapy for major depressive disorder: a sham-controlled randomized trial. *Arch. Gen. Psychiatry* 67 (5), 507–516. doi: 10.1001/archgenpsychiatry.2010.46

George, M. S., Nahas, Z., Molloy, M., Speer, A. M., Oliver, N. C., Li, X.-B., et al. (2000). A controlled trial of daily left prefrontal cortex TMS for treating depression. *Biol. Psychiatry* 48 (10), 962–970. doi: 10.1016/S0006-3223(00)01048-9

George, M. S., Wassermann, E. M., Kimbrell, T. A., Little, J. T., Williams, W. E., Danielson, A. L., et al. (1997). Mood improvement following daily left prefrontal repetitive transcranial magnetic stimulation in patients with depression: a placebo-controlled crossover trial. *Am. J. Psychiatry* 154 (12), 1752–1756. doi: 10.1176/ajp.154.12.1752

Gerfen, C. R., and Clavier, R. M. (1979). Neural inputs to the prefrontal agranular insular cortex in the rat: horseradish peroxidase study. *Brain Res. Bull.* 4 (3), 347–353. doi: 10.1016/S0361-9230(79)80012-X

Gilman, J. M., Radoman, M., Schuster, R. M., Pachas, G., Azzouz, N., Fava, M., et al. (2018). Anterior insula activation during inhibition to smoking cues is associated with ability to maintain tobacco abstinence. *Addict. Behav. Rep.* 7, 40. doi: 10.1016/j.abrep.2018.01.002

Goodkind, M., Eickhoff, S. B., Oathes, D. J., Jiang, Y., Chang, A., Jones-Hagata, L. B., et al. (2015). Identification of a common neurobiological substrate for mental illness. *JAMA Psychiatry* 72 (4), 305–315. doi: 10.1001/jamapsychiatry.2014.2206

Gorelick, D. A., Zangen, A., and George, M. S. (2014). Transcranial magnetic stimulation in the treatment of substance addiction. *Ann. N. Y. Acad. Sci.* 1327 (1), 79–93. doi: 10.1111/nyas.12479

Gorka, S. M., Phan, K. L., and Childs, E. (2018). Acute calming effects of alcohol are associated with disruption of the salience network. *Addict. Biol.* 23 (3), 921–930. doi: 10.1111/adb.12537

Gowin, J. L., Ball, T. M., Wittmann, M., Tapert, S. F., and Paulus, M. P. (2015). Individualized relapse prediction: personality measures and striatal and insular activity during reward-processing robustly predict relapse. *Drug Alcohol Depend.* 152, 93–101. doi: 10.1016/j.drugalcdep.2015.04.018

Grabus, S. D., Martin, B. R., Brown, S. E., and Damaj, M. I. (2006). Nicotine place preference in the mouse: influences of prior handling, dose and strain and attenuation by nicotinic receptor antagonists. *Psychopharmacology (Berl)* 184 (3-4), 456–463. doi: 10.1007/s00213-006-0305-7

Gratton, C., Lee, T., Nomura, E., and D'Esposito, M. (2013). The effect of theta-burst TMS on cognitive control networks measured with resting state fMRI. *Front. Syst. Neurosci.* 7, 1–14. doi: 10.3389/fnsys.2013.00124

Greenberg, B. D., and Rezai, A. R. (2014). Mechanisms and the current state of deep brain stimulation in neuropsychiatry. *CNS Spectrums* 8 (7), 522–526. doi: 10.1017/S109285290001899X

Hall, M. G., Alhassoon, O. M., Stern, M. J., Wollman, S. C., Kimmel, C. L., Perez-Figueroa, A., et al. (2015). Gray matter abnormalities in cocaine versus methamphetamine-dependent patients: a neuroimaging meta-analysis. *Am. J. Drug Alcohol Abuse* 41 (4), 290–299. doi: 10.3109/00952990.2015.1044607

Hanlon, C. A., Dowdle, L. T., Gibson, N. B., Li, X. B., Hamilton, S., Canterberry, M., et al. (2018a). Cortical substrates of cue-reactivity in multiple substance dependent populations: transdiagnostic relevance of the medial prefrontal cortex. *Transl. Psychiatry* 8 (1), 1–8. doi: 10.1038/s41398-018-0220-9

Hanlon, C. A., Dowdle, L. T., and Henderson, J. S. (2018b). Modulating neural circuits with transcranial magnetic stimulation: implications for addiction treatment development. *Pharmacol. Rev.* 70 (3), 661–683. doi: 10.1124/pr.116.013649

Hanlon, C. A., Owens, M. M., Joseph, J. E., Zhu, X., George, M. S., Brady, K. T., et al. (2016). Lower subcortical gray matter volume in both younger smokers and established smokers relative to non-smokers. *Addict. Biol.* 21 (1), 185–195. doi: 10.1111/adb.12171

Hardy, S. G. (1985). Analgesia elicited by prefrontal stimulation. *Brain Res.* 339 (2), 281–284. doi: 10.1016/0006-8993(85)90093-9

Harel, E. V., Rabany, L., Deutsch, L., Bloch, Y., Zangen, A., and Levkovitz, Y. (2014). H-coil repetitive transcranial magnetic stimulation for treatment resistant major depressive disorder: an 18-week continuation safety and feasibility study. *World J. Biol. Psychiatry* 15 (4), 298–306. doi: 10.3109/15622975.2011.639802

Heikkinen, N., Niskanen, E., Kononen, M., Tolmunen, T., Kekkonen, V., Kivimaki, P., et al. (2017). Alcohol consumption during adolescence is associated with reduced grey matter volumes. *Addiction* 112 (4), 604–613. doi: 10.1111/add.13697

Herrington, T. M., Cheng, J. J., and Eskandar, E. N. (2016). Mechanisms of deep brain stimulation. *J. Neurophysiol.* 115 (1), 19–38. doi: 10.1152/jn.00281.2015

Höflich, A., Hahn, A., Küblböck, M., Kranz, G. S., Vanicek, T., Ganger, S., et al. (2017). Ketamine-dependent neuronal activation in healthy volunteers. *Brain Struct. Funct.* 222 (3), 1533–1542. doi: 10.1007/s00429-016-1291-0

Hollander, J. A., Lu, Q., Cameron, M. D., Kamenecka, T. M., and Kenny, P. J. (2008). Insular hypocretin transmission regulates nicotine reward. *Proc. Natl. Acad. Sci.* 105 (49), 19480–19485. doi: 10.1073/pnas.0808023105

Huang, W., King, J. A., Ursprung, W. W., Zheng, S., Zhang, N., Kennedy, D. N., et al. (2014). The development and expression of physical nicotine dependence corresponds to structural and functional alterations in the anterior cingulate-precuneus pathway. *Brain Behav.* 4 (3), 408–417. doi: 10.1002/brb3.227

Huang, Y.-Z., Edwards, M. J., Rounis, E., Bhatia, K. P., and Rothwell, J. C. (2005). Theta burst stimulation of the human motor cortex. *Neuron* 45 (2), 201–206. doi: 10.1016/j.neuron.2004.12.033

Ihssen, N., Cox, W. M., Wiggett, A., Fadardi, J. S., and Linden, D. E. J. (2011). Differentiating heavy from light drinkers by neural responses to visual alcohol cues and other motivational stimuli. *Cereb. Cortex* 21 (6), 1408–1415. doi: 10.1093/cercor/bhq220

Isnard, J., Guenot, M., Sindou, M., and Mauguiere, F. (2004). Clinical manifestations of insular lobe seizures: a stereo-electroencephalographic study. *Epilepsia* 45 (9), 1079–1090. doi: 10.1111/j.0013-9580.2004.68903.x

Janes, A. C., Gilman, J. M., Radoman, M., Pachas, G., Fava, M., and Evins, A. E. (2017). Revisiting the role of the insula and smoking cue-reactivity in relapse: a replication and extension of neuroimaging findings. *Drug Alcohol Depend.* 179, 8–12. doi: 10.1016/j.drugalcdep.2017.06.012

Janes, A. C., Pizzagalli, D. A., Richardt, S., Frederick, B.d., Chuzi, S., Pachas, G., et al. (2010). Brain reactivity to smoking cues prior to smoking cessation predicts ability to maintain tobacco abstinence. *Biol. Psychiatry* 67 (8), 722–729. doi: 10.1016/j.biopsych.2009.12.034

Janes, A. C., Ross, R. S., Farmer, S., Frederick, B. B., Nickerson, L. D., Lukas, S. E., et al. (2015). Memory retrieval of smoking-related images induce greater insula activation as revealed by an fMRI-based delayed matching to sample task. *Addict. Biol.* 20 (2), 349–356. doi: 10.1111/adb.12112

Jaramillo, A. A., Agan, V. E., Makhijani, V. H., Pedroza, S., McElligott, Z. A., and Besheer, J. (2017). Functional role for suppression of the insular - striatal circuit in modulating interoceptive effects of alcohol. *Addict. Biol.* 1020–1031. doi: 10.1111/adb.12551

Jaramillo, A. A., Randall, P. A., Frisbee, S., and Besheer, J. (2016). Modulation of sensitivity to alcohol by cortical and thalamic brain regions. *Eur. J. Neurosci.* 44, 2569–2580. doi: 10.1111/ejn.13374

Jaramillo, A. A., Randall, P. A., Stewart, S., Fortino, B., Van Voorhies, K., and Besheer, J. (2018a). Functional role for cortical-striatal circuitry in modulating alcohol self-administration. *Neuropharmacology.* 130, 42–53. doi: 10.1016/j.neuropharm.2017.11.035

Jaramillo, A. A., Voorhies, K. V., Randall, P. A., and Besheer, J. (2018b). Silencing the insular-striatal circuit decreases alcohol self-administration and increases sensitivity to alcohol. *Behav. Brain Res.* 348 (March), 74–81. doi: 10.1016/j.bbr.2018.04.007

Kalivas, P. W., and Volkow, N. D. (2005). The neural basis of addiction: a pathology of motivation and choice. *Am. J. Psychiatry* 162 (8), 1403–1413. doi: 10.1176/appi.ajp.162.8.1403

Kantak, K. M., Udo, T., Ugalde, F., Luzzo, C., Di Pietro, N., and Eichenbaum, H. B. (2005). Influence of cocaine self-administration on learning related to prefrontal cortex or hippocampus functioning in rats. *Psychopharmacology.* 181 (2), 227–236. doi: 10.1007/s00213-005-2243-1

Kelly, C., Toro, R., Di Martino, A., Cox, C. L., Bellec, P., Castellanos, F. X., et al. (2012). A convergent functional architecture of the insula emerges across imaging modalities. *Neuroimage* 61 (4), 1129–1142. doi: 10.1016/j.neuroimage.2012.03.021

Kim, J.-H., Kim, D.-W., Chang, W. H., Kim, Y.-H., Kim, K., and Im, C.-H. (2014). Inconsistent outcomes of transcranial direct current stimulation may originate from anatomical differences among individuals: electric field simulation using individual MRI data. *Neurosci. Lett.* 564 (2), 6–10. doi: 10.1016/j.neulet.2014.01.054

Kim, Y. T., Song, H. J., Seo, J. H., Lee, J. J., Lee, J., Kwon, D. H., et al. (2011). The differences in neural network activity between methamphetamine abusers and healthy subjects performing an emotion-matching task: functional MRI study. *NMR Biomed.* 24 (10), 1392–1400. doi: 10.1002/nbm.1702

Klein, E., Kreinin, I., Chistyakov, A., Koren, D., Mecz, L., Marmur, S., et al. (1999). Therapeutic efficacy of right prefrontal slow repetitive transcranial magnetic stimulation in major depression: a double-blind controlled study. *Arch. Gen. Psychiatry* 56 (4), 315–320. doi: 10.1001/archpsyc.56.4.315

Koob, G. F., and Le Moal, M. (2005). Plasticity of reward neurocircuitry and the 'dark side' of drug addiction. *Nat. Neurosci.* 8 (11), 1442–1444. doi: 10.1038/nn1105-1442

Koob, G. F., and Volkow, N. D. (2010). Neurocircuitry of addiction [published correction appears in Neuropsychopharmacology. 2010 Mar;35(4):1051]. *Neuropsychopharmacology* 35 (1), 217–238. doi: 10.1038/npp.2009.110

Koob, G. F., and Volkow, N. D. (2016). Neurobiology of addiction: a neurocircuitry analysis. *Lancet Psychiatry* 3 (8), 760–773. doi: 10.1016/S2215-0366(16)00104-8

Krettek, J. E., and Price, J. L. (1977). The cortical projections of the mediodorsal nucleus and adjacent thalamic nuclei in the rat. *J. Comp. Neurol.* 171 (2), 157–191. doi: 10.1002/cne.901710204

Kringelbach, M. L., Jenkinson, N., Owen, S. L. F., and Aziz, T. Z. (2007). Translational principles of deep brain stimulation. *Nat. Rev. Neurosci.* 8, 623+. doi: 10.1038/nrn2196

Kutlu, M. G., Burke, D., Slade, S., Hall, B. J., Rose, J. E., and Levin, E. D. (2013). Role of insular cortex D1 and D2 dopamine receptors in nicotine self-administration in rats. *Behav. Brain Res.* 256, 273–278. doi: 10.1016/j.bbr.2013.08.005

Lee, W., and Reeve, J. (2013). Self-determined, but not non-self-determined, motivation predicts activations in the anterior insular cortex: an fMRI study of personal agency. *Soc. Cogn. Affect. Neurosci.* 8 (5), 538–545. doi: 10.1093/scan/nss029

Lefaucheur, J.-P., André-Obadia, N., Antal, A., Ayache, S. S., Baeken, C., Benninger, D. H., et al. (2014). Evidence-based guidelines on the therapeutic use of repetitive transcranial magnetic stimulation (rTMS). *Clin. Neurophysiol.* 125 (11), 2150–2206. doi: 10.1016/j.clinph.2014.05.021

Lerman, C., Gu, H., Loughead, J., Ruparel, K., Yang, Y., and Stein, E. A. (2014). Large-scale brain network coupling predicts acute nicotine abstinence effects on craving and cognitive function. *JAMA Psychiatry* 71 (5), 523–530. doi: 10.1001/jamapsychiatry.2013.4091

Li, C.-T., Juan, C.-H., Huang, H.-H., Hsieh, J.-C., Chen, L.-F., Chen, M.-H., et al. (2014). Efficacy of prefrontal theta-burst stimulation in refractory depression: a randomized sham-controlled study. *Brain* 137 (7), 2088–2098. doi: 10.1093/brain/awu109

Li, C. L., Zhu, N., Meng, X. L., Li, Y. H., and Sui, N. (2013). Effects of inactivating the agranular or granular insular cortex on the acquisition of the morphine-induced conditioned place preference and naloxone-precipitated conditioned place aversion in rats. *J. Psychopharmacol.* 27 (9), 837–844. doi: 10.1177/0269881113492028

Li, S., Yang, Y., Hoffmann, E., Tyndale, R. F., and Stein, E. A. (2017a). CYP2A6 genetic variation alters striatal-cingulate circuits, network hubs, and executive processing in smokers. *Biol. Psychiatry* 81 (7), 554–563. doi: 10.1016/j.biopsych.2016.09.013

Li, X., Du, L., Sahlem, G. L., Badran, B. W., Henderson, S., and George, M. S. (2017b). Repetitive transcranial magnetic stimulation (rTMS) of the dorsolateral prefrontal cortex reduces resting-state insula activity and modulates functional connectivity of the orbitofrontal cortex in cigarette smokers. *Drug Alcohol Depend.* 174, 98–105. doi: 10.1016/j.drugalcdep.2017.02.002

Li, Y., Yuan, K., Cai, C., Feng, D., Yin, J., Bi, Y., et al. (2015). Reduced frontal cortical thickness and increased caudate volume within fronto-striatal circuits in young adult smokers. *Drug Alcohol Depend.* 151, 211–219. doi: 10.1016/j.drugalcdep.2015.03.023

Lin, X., Dong, G., Wang, Q., and Du, X. (2015). Abnormal gray matter and white matter volume in 'Internet gaming addicts'. *Addict. Behav.* 40, 137–143. doi: 10.1016/j.addbeh.2014.09.010

Loo, C. K., Mitchell, P. B., Croker, V. M., Malhi, G. S., Wen, W., Gandevia, S. C., et al. (2003). Double-blind controlled investigation of bilateral prefrontal transcranial magnetic stimulation for the treatment of resistant major depression. *Psychol. Med.* 33 (1), 33–40. doi: 10.1017/S0033291702006839

Lu, H., and Stein, E. A. (2014). Resting state functional connectivity: its physiological basis and application in neuropharmacology. *Neuropharmacology* 84, 79–89. doi: 10.1016/j.neuropharm.2013.08.023

Ma, H., Wang, N., Wang, X., Jia, M., Li, Y., and Cui, C. (2018). Wnt7a in mouse insular cortex contributes to anxiety-like behavior during protracted abstinence from morphine. *Neuroscience.* 394, 164–176. doi: 10.1016/j.neuroscience.2018.10.032

Ma, P., Liu, H., Li, H., Huang, X., Chen, L., and Zhai, H. (2014). Involvement of the insular nitric oxide signaling pathway in the expression of morphine-induced conditioned place preference in rats. *NeuroReport* 25 (9), 641–646. doi: 10.1097/WNR.0000000000000146

Mackey, W. B., Keller, J., and Van der Kooy, D. (1986). Visceral cortex lesions block conditioned taste aversions induced by morphine. *Pharmacol. Biochem. Behav.* 24 (1), 71–78. doi: 10.1016/0091-3057(86)90047-X

Malik, S., Jacobs, M., Cho, S.-S., Boileau, I., Blumberger, D., Heilig, M., et al. (2018). Deep TMS of the insula using the H-coil modulates dopamine release: a crossover [11C] PHNO-PET pilot trial in healthy humans. *Brain Imaging Behav.* 12 (5), 1306–1317. doi: 10.1007/s11682-017-9800-1

Margeta-Mitrovic, M., Mitrovic, I., Riley, R. C., Jan, L. Y., and Basbaum, A. I. (1999). Immunohistochemical localization of GABA(B) receptors in the rat central nervous system. *J. Comp. Neurol.* 405 (3), 299–321. doi: 10.1002/(SICI)1096-9861(19990315)405:3<299::AID-CNE2>3.0.CO;2-6

Martin, J. L., Barbanoj, M. J., Schlaepfer, T. E., Clos, S., Perez, V., Kulisevsky, J., et al. (2002). Transcranial magnetic stimulation for treating depression. *Cochrane Database Syst. Rev.* (2), Cd003493. doi: 10.1002/14651858.CD003493

Maskos, U., Molles, B. E., Pons, S., Besson, M., Guiard, B. P., Guilloux, J. P., et al. (2005). Nicotine reinforcement and cognition restored by targeted expression of nicotinic receptors. *Nature* 436 (7047), 103–107. doi: 10.1038/nature03694

Matsumoto, H., and Ugawa, Y. (2016). Adverse events of tDCS and tACS: a review. *Clin. Neurophysiol. Pract.* 2, 19–25. doi: 10.1016/j.cnp.2016.12.003

McDonald, A. J., Shammah-Lagnado, S. J., Shi, C., and Davis, M. (1999). Cortical afferents to the extended amygdala. *Ann. N. Y. Acad. Sci.* 877, 309–338. doi: 10.1111/j.1749-6632.1999.tb09275.x

McGeorge, A. J., and Faull, R. L. (1989). The organization of the projection from the cerebral cortex to the striatum in the rat. *Neuroscience* 29 (3), 503–537. doi: 10.1016/0306-4522(89)90128-0

Menon, V. (2011). Large-scale brain networks and psychopathology: a unifying triple network model. *Trends Cogn. Sci.* 15 (10), 483–506. doi: 10.1016/j.tics.2011.08.003

Menon, V., and Uddin, L. Q. (2010). Saliency, switching, attention and control: a network model of insula function. *Brain Struct. Funct.* 214 (5-6), 655–667. doi: 10.1007/s00429-010-0262-0

Mesulam, M. M., and Mufson, E. J. (1982). Insula of the old world monkey. I. Architectonics in the insulo-orbito-temporal component of the paralimbic brain. *J. Comp. Neurol.* 212 (1), 1–22. doi: 10.1002/cne.902120102

Mizoguchi, H., Katahira, K., Inutsuka, A., Fukumoto, K., Nakamura, A., Wang, T., et al. (2015). Insular neural system controls decision-making in healthy and methamphetamine-treated rats. *Proc. Natl. Acad. Sci.* 112 (29), E3930–E3939. doi: 10.1073/pnas.1418014112

Morales, A. M., Ghahremani, D., Kohno, M., Hellemann, G. S., and London, E. D. (2014). Cigarette exposure, dependence, and craving are related to insula thickness in young adult smokers. *Neuropsychopharmacology* 39 (8), 1816–1822. doi: 10.1038/npp.2014.48

Moran-Santa Maria, M. M., Hartwell, K. J., Hanlon, C. A., Canterbery, M., Lematty, T., Owens, M., et al. (2015). Right anterior insula connectivity is important for cue-induced craving in nicotine-dependent smokers. *Addict. Biol.* 20 (2), 407–414. doi: 10.1111/adb.12124

Moran, L. V., Stoeckel, L. E., Wang, K., Caine, C. E., Villafuerte, R., Calderon, V., et al. (2018). Nicotine increases activation to anticipatory valence cues in anterior insula and striatum. *Nicotine Tob. Res.* 20 (7), 851–858. doi: 10.1093/ntr/ntx217

Mueller, V. A., Brass, M., Waszak, F., and Prinz, W. (2007). The role of the preSMA and the rostral cingulate zone in internally selected actions. *Neuroimage* 37 (4), 1354–1361. doi: 10.1016/j.neuroimage.2007.06.018

Muñoz, B., Fritz, B. M., Yin, F., and Atwood, B. K. (2018). Alcohol exposure disrupts mu opioid receptor-mediated long-term depression at insular cortex inputs to dorsolateral striatum. *Nat. Commun.* 9 (1), 1318. doi: 10.1038/s41467-018-03683-1

Mutz, J., Edgcumbe, D. R., Brunoni, A. R., and Fu, C. H. Y. (2018). Efficacy and acceptability of non-invasive brain stimulation for the treatment of adult unipolar and bipolar depression: a systematic review and meta-analysis of randomised sham-controlled trials. *Neurosci. Biobehav. Rev.* 92, 291–303. doi: 10.1016/j.neubiorev.2018.05.015

Naqvi, N. H., and Bechara, A. (2010). The insula and drug addiction: an interoceptive view of pleasure, urges, and decision-making. *Brain Struct. Funct.* 214 (5-6), 435–450. doi: 10.1007/s00429-010-0268-7

Naqvi, N. H., Gaznick, N., Tranel, D., and Bechara, A. (2014). The insula: a critical neural substrate for craving and drug seeking under conflict and risk. *Ann. N. Y. Acad. Sci.* 1316 (1), 53–70. doi: 10.1111/nyas.12415

Naqvi, N. H., Rudrauf, D., Damasio, H., and Bechara, A. (2007). Damage to the insula disrupts addiction to cigarette smoking. *Science* 315 (5811), 531–534. doi: 10.1126/science.1135926

Nitsche, M. A., Doemkes, S., Karaköse, T., Antal, A., Liebetanz, D., Lang, N., et al. (2007). Shaping the Effects of Transcranial Direct Current Stimulation of the Human Motor Cortex. *J. Neurophysiol.* 97 (4), 3109–3117. doi: 10.1152/jn.01312.2006

Nitsche, M. A., and Paulus, W. (2000). Excitability changes induced in the human motor cortex by weak transcranial direct current stimulation. *J. Physiol.* 527 (3), 633–639. doi: 10.1111/j.1469-7793.2000.t01-1-00633.x

Nitsche, M. A., and Paulus, W. (2001). Sustained excitability elevations induced by transcranial DC motor cortex stimulation in humans. *Neurology* 57 (10), 1899–1901. doi: 10.1212/WNL.57.10.1899

Nitsche, M. A. M. D., Cohen, L. G. M. D., Wassermann, E. M. M. D., Priori, A. M. D. P., Lang, N. M. D., Antal, A. P., et al. (2008). Transcranial direct current stimulation: state of the art 2008. *Brain Stimul.* 1 (3), 206–223. doi: 10.1016/j.brs.2008.06.004

O'Brien, C. P. (2008). Review. Evidence-based treatments of addiction. *Philos. Trans. R. Soc. Lond., B, Biol. Sci.* 363 (1507), 3277–3286. doi: 10.1098/rstb.2008.0105

O'Reardon, J. P., Solvason, H. B., Janicak, P. G., Sampson, S., Isenberg, K. E., Nahas, Z., et al. (2007). Efficacy and safety of transcranial magnetic stimulation in the acute treatment of major depression: a multisite randomized controlled trial. *Biol. Psychiatry* 62 (11), 1208–1216. doi: 10.1016/j.biopsych.2007.01.018

Ohara, P. T., Granato, A., Moallem, T. M., Wang, B. R., Tillet, Y., and Jasmin, L. (2003). Dopaminergic input to GABAergic neurons in the rostral agranular insular cortex of the rat. *J. Neurocytol.* 32 (2), 131–141. doi: 10.1023/B:NEUR.0000005598.09647.7f

Paulus, M. P., and Stein, M. B. (2006). An insular view of anxiety. *Biol. Psychiatry* 60 (4), 383–387. doi: 10.1016/j.biopsych.2006.03.042

Paxinos, G., and Watson, C. (1986). *The rat brain in stereotaxic coordinates.* New York: Academic Press.

Pelloux, Y., Murray, J. E., and Everitt, B. J. (2013). Differential roles of the prefrontal cortical subregions and basolateral amygdala in compulsive cocaine seeking and relapse after voluntary abstinence in rats. *Eur. J. Neurosci.* 38, 3018–3026. doi: 10.1111/ejn.12289

Penfield, W., and Faulk, M. E., Jr. (1955). The insula; further observations on its function. *Brain* 78 (4), 445–470. doi: 10.1093/brain/78.4.445

Pietro, N. C. D., Black, Y. D., and Kantak, K. M. (2006). Context-dependent prefrontal cortex regulation of cocaine self-administration and reinstatement behaviors in rats. *Eur. J. Neurosci.* 24, 3285–3298. doi: 10.1111/j.1460-9568.2006.05193.x

Porrino, L. J., Lyons, D., Miller, M. D., Smith, H. R., Friedman, D. P., Daunais, J. B., et al. (2002). Metabolic mapping of the effects of cocaine during the initial phases of self-administration in the nonhuman primate. *J. Neurosci.* 22 (17) 7687–7694. doi: 10.1523/JNEUROSCI.22-17-07687.2002

Priori, A., Berardelli, A., Rona, S., Accornero, N., and Manfredi, M. (1998). Polarization of the human motor cortex through the scalp. *NeuroReport* 9 (10), 2257–2260. doi: 10.1097/00001756-199807130-00020

Pritchard, T. C., Macaluso, D. A., and Eslinger, P. J. (1999). Taste perception in patients with insular cortex lesions. *Behav. Neurosci.* 113 (4), 663–671. doi: 10.1037/0735-7044.113.4.663

Purpura, D. P., and McMurtry, J. G. (1965). Intracellular activities and evoked potential changes during polarization of motor cortex. *J. Neurophysiol.* 28 (1), 166–185. doi: 10.1152/jn.1965.28.1.166

Pushparaj, A., Hamani, C., Yu, W., Shin, D. S., Kang, B., Nobrega, J. N., et al. (2013). Electrical stimulation of the insular region attenuates nicotine-taking and nicotine-seeking behaviors. *Neuropsychopharmacology* 38 (4), 690–698. doi: 10.1038/npp.2012.235

Pushparaj, A., Kim, A. S., Musiol, M., Trigo, J. M., and Le Foll, B. (2015). Involvement of the rostral agranular insular cortex in nicotine self-administration in rats. *Behav. Brain Res.* 290, 77–83. doi: 10.1016/j.bbr.2015.04.039

Pushparaj, A., and Le Foll, B. (2015). Involvement of the caudal granular insular cortex in alcohol self-administration in rats. *Behav. Brain Res.* 293, 203–207. doi: 10.1016/j.bbr.2015.07.044

Ragozzino, M. E., and Kesner, R. P. (1999). The role of the agranular insular cortex in working memory for food reward value and allocentric space in rats. *Behav. Brain Res.* 98 (1), 103–112. doi: 10.1016/S0166-4328(98)00058-8

Riem, M. M., Bakermans-Kranenburg, M. J., Pieper, S., Tops, M., Boksem, M. A., Vermeiren, R. R., et al. (2011). Oxytocin modulates amygdala, insula, and inferior frontal gyrus responses to infant crying: a randomized controlled trial. *Biol. Psychiatry* 70 (3), 291–297. doi: 10.1016/j.biopsych.2011.02.006

Rossi, S., Hallett, M., Rossini, P. M., and Pascual-Leone, A. (2009). Safety, ethical considerations, and application guidelines for the use of transcranial magnetic stimulation in clinical practice and research. *Clin. Neurophysiol.* 120 (12), 2008–2039. doi: 10.1016/j.clinph.2009.08.016

Rotge, J.-y., Cocker, P. J., Daniel, M.-l., Belin-rauscent, A., Everitt, B. J., and Belin, D. (2017). Bidirectional regulation over the development and expression of loss of control over cocaine intake by the anterior insula. *Psychopharmacology (Berl)* 1623–1631. doi: 10.1007/s00213-017-4593-x

Rubboli, F., Court, J. A., Sala, C., Morris, C., Perry, E., and Clementi, F. (1994). Distribution of neuronal nicotinic receptor subunits in human brain. *Neurochem. Int.* 25 (1), 69–71. doi: 10.1016/0197-0186(94)90055-8

Salling, M. C., and Martinez, D. (2016). Brain Stimulation in Addiction. *Neuropsychopharmacology* 41 (12), 2798–2809. doi: 10.1038/npp.2016.80

Sánchez, M. M., Young, L. J., Plotsky, P. M., and Insel, T. R. (1999). Autoradiographic and in situ hybridization localization of corticotropin-releasing factor 1 and 2 receptors in nonhuman primate brain. *J. Comp. Neurol.* 408 (3), 365–377. doi: 10.1002/(SICI)1096-9861(19990607)408:3<365::AID-CNE5>3.3.CO;2-E

Saper, C. B. (1982). Convergence of autonomic and limbic connections in the insular cortex of the rat. *J. Comp. Neurol.* 210 (2), 163–173. doi: 10.1002/cne.902100207

Scott, D., and Hiroi, N. (2011). Deconstructing craving: dissociable cortical control of Cue reactivity in nicotine addiction. *Biol. Psychiatry* 69 (11), 1052–1059. doi: 10.1016/j.biopsych.2011.01.023

Seif, T., Chang, S.-j., Simms, J. A., Gibb, S. L., Dadgar, J., Chen, B. T., et al. (2013). Cortical activation of accumbens hyperpolarization- active NMDARs mediates aversion-resistant alcohol intake. *Nat. Publ. Group* 16 (8), 1094–1100. doi: 10.1038/nn.3445

Shahbabaie, A., Ebrahimpoor, M., Hariri, A., Nitsche, M. A., Hatami, J., Fatemizadeh, E., et al. (2018). Transcranial DC stimulation modifies functional connectivity of large-scale brain networks in abstinent methamphetamine users. *Brain Behav.* 8 (3), e00922–n/a. doi: 10.1002/brb3.922

Shi, C. J., and Cassell, M. D. (1998a). Cascade projections from somatosensory cortex to the rat basolateral amygdala *via* the parietal insular cortex. *J. Comp. Neurol.* 399 (4), 469–491. doi: 10.1002/(SICI)1096-9861(19981005)399:4<469::AID-CNE3>3.0.CO;2-#

Shi, C. J., and Cassell, M. D. (1998b). Cortical, thalamic, and amygdaloid connections of the anterior and posterior insular cortices. *J. Comp. Neurol.* 399 (4), 440–468. doi: 10.1002/(SICI)1096-9861(19981005)399:4<440::AID-CNE2>3.0.CO;2-1

Shillinglaw, J. E., Morrisett, R. A., and Mangieri, R. A. (2018). Ethanol modulates glutamatergic transmission and NMDAR-mediated synaptic plasticity in the agranular insular cortex 9. *Front Pharmacol.* 9, 1–14. doi: 10.3389/fphar.2018.01458

Silvanto, J., and Pascual-Leone, A. (2008). State-dependency of transcranial magnetic stimulation. *Brain Topogr.* 21 (1), 1–10. doi: 10.1007/s10548-008-0067-0

Spagnolo, P. A., Wang, H., Srivanitchapoom, P., Schwandt, M., Heilig, M., and Hallett, M. (2019). Lack of target engagement following low-frequency deep transcranial magnetic stimulation of the anterior insula. *Neuromodulation: Technology at the Neural Interface.* doi: 10.1111/ner.12875

Stewart, J. L., Butt, M., May, A. C., Tapert, S. F., and Paulus, M. P. (2017). Insular and cingulate attenuation during decision making is associated with future transition to stimulant use disorder. *Addiction* 112 (9), 1567–1577. doi: 10.1111/add.13839

Stewart, J. L., Connolly, C. G., May, A. C., Tapert, S. F., Wittmann, M., and Paulus, M. P. (2014). Striatum and insula dysfunction during reinforcement learning differentiates abstinent and relapsed methamphetamine-dependent individuals. *Addiction* 109 (3), 460–471. doi: 10.1111/add.12403

Stippekohl, B., Winkler, M. H., Walter, B., Kagerer, S., Mucha, R. F., Pauli, P., et al. (2012). Neural responses to smoking stimuli are influenced by smokers' attitudes towards their own smoking behaviour. *PLoS ONE* 7 (11), e46782. doi: 10.1371/journal.pone.0046782

Stoeckel, L. E., Chai, X. J., Zhang, J., Whitfield-Gabrieli, S., and Evins, A. E. (2016). Lower gray matter density and functional connectivity in the anterior insula in smokers compared with never smokers. *Addict. Biol.* 21 (4), 972–981. doi: 10.1111/adb.12262

Suhara, T., Nakayama, K., Inoue, O., Fukuda, H., Shimizu, M., Mori, A., et al. (1992). D1 dopamine receptor binding in mood disorders measured by positron emission tomography. *Psychopharmacology (Berl)* 106 (1), 14–18. doi: 10.1007/BF02253582

Sullivan, E. V., Muller-Oehring, E., Pitel, A. L., Chanraud, S., Shankaranarayanan, A., Alsop, D. C., et al. (2013). A selective insular perfusion deficit contributes to compromised salience network connectivity in recovering alcoholic men. *Biol. Psychiatry* 74 (7), 547–555. doi: 10.1016/j.biopsych.2013.02.026

Sun, Y. M., Chen, R. X., Li, Z. F., Spijker, S., Zhai, R. W., and Yang, S. C. (2018). The caudal part of the posterior insula of rats participates in the maintenance but not the acquisition of morphine conditioned place preference. *CNS. Neurosci. Ther.* 24 (5), 420–428. doi: 10.1111/cns.12799

Suñer-Soler, R., Grau, A., Gras, M. E., Font-Mayolas, S., Silva, Y., Dávalos, A., et al. (2012). Smoking cessation 1 year poststroke and damage to the insular cortex. *Stroke* 43 (1), 131–136. doi: 10.1161/STROKEAHA.111.630004

Sutherland, M. T., Carroll, A. J., Salmeron, B. J., Ross, T. J., Hong, L. E., and Stein, E. A. (2013a). Down-regulation of amygdala and insula functional circuits by varenicline and nicotine in abstinent cigarette smokers. *Biol. Psychiatry* 74 (7), 538–546. doi: 10.1016/j.biopsych.2013.01.035

Sutherland, M. T., Carroll, A. J., Salmeron, B. J., Ross, T. J., and Stein, E. A. (2013b). Insula's functional connectivity with ventromedial prefrontal cortex mediates the impact of trait alexithymia on state tobacco craving. *Psychopharmacology* 228 (1), 143–155. doi: 10.1007/s00213-013-3018-8

Sutherland, M. T., McHugh, M. J., Pariyadath, V., and Stein, E. A. (2012). Resting state functional connectivity in addiction: lessons learned and a road ahead. *Neuroimage* 62 (4), 2281–2295. doi: 10.1016/j.neuroimage.2012.01.117

Sutherland, M. T., Ray, K. L., Riedel, M. C., Yanes, J. A., Stein, E. A., and Laird, A. R. (2015). Neurobiological impact of nicotinic acetylcholine receptor agonists: an activation likelihood estimation meta-analysis of pharmacologic neuroimaging studies. *Biol. Psychiatry* 78 (10), 711–720. doi: 10.1016/j.biopsych.2014.12.021

Sutherland, M. T., Riedel, M. C., Flannery, J. S., Yanes, J. A., Fox, P. T., Stein, E. A., et al. (2016). Chronic cigarette smoking is linked with structural alterations in brain regions showing acute nicotinic drug-induced functional modulations. *Behav. Brain Funct.* 12 (1), 16. doi: 10.1186/s12993-016-0100-5

Sutherland, M. T., and Stein, E. A. (2018). Functional neurocircuits and neuroimaging biomarkers of tobacco use disorder. *Trends. Mol. Med.* 24 (2), 129–143. doi: 10.1016/j.molmed.2017.12.002

Turel, O., He, Q., Brevers, D., and Bechara, A. (2018). Delay discounting mediates the association between posterior insular cortex volume and social media addiction symptoms. *Cogn. Affect. Behav. Neurosci.* 18 (4), 694–704. doi: 10.3758/s13415-018-0597-1

Twardella, D., Loew, M., Rothenbacher, D., Stegmaier, C., Ziegler, H., and Brenner, H. (2006). The diagnosis of a smoking-related disease is a prominent trigger for smoking cessation in a retrospective cohort study. *J. Clin. Epidemiol.* 59 (1), 82–89. doi: 10.1016/j.jclinepi.2005.05.003

Ueno, S., Tashiro, T., and Harada, K. (1988). Localized stimulation of neural tissues in the brain by means of a paired configuration of time-varying magnetic fields. *J. Appl. Phys.* 64 (10), 5862–5864. doi: 10.1063/1.342181

Van der Werf, Y. D., Witter, M. P., and Groenewegen, H. J. (2002). The intralaminar and midline nuclei of the thalamus. Anatomical and functional evidence for participation in processes of arousal and awareness. *Brain Res. Brain Res. Rev.* 39 (2–3), 107–140. doi: 10.1016/S0165-0173(02)00181-9

Venniro, M., Caprioli, D., Zhang, M., Whitaker, L. R., Zhang, S., Warren, B. L., et al. (2017). The anterior insular cortex→central amygdala glutamatergic pathway is critical to relapse after contingency management. *Neuron.* 96 (2), 414–427. doi: 10.1016/j.neuron.2017.09.024

Verdejo-Garcia, A., Benbrook, A., Funderburk, F., David, P., Cadet, J. L., and Bolla, K. I. (2007). The differential relationship between cocaine use and marijuana use on decision-making performance over repeat testing with the Iowa Gambling Task. *Drug Alcohol Depend.* 90 (1), 2–11. doi: 10.1016/j.drugalcdep.2007.02.004

Verhagen, J. V., Kadohisa, M., and Rolls, E. T. (2004). Primate insular/opercular taste cortex: neuronal representations of the viscosity, fat texture, grittiness, temperature, and taste of foods. *J. Neurophysiol.* 92 (3), 1685–1699. doi: 10.1152/jn.00321.2004

Vertes, R. P. (2004). Differential projections of the infralimbic and prelimbic cortex in the rat. *Synapse* 51 (1), 32–58. doi: 10.1002/syn.10279

Wang, C., Huang, P., Shen, Z., Qian, W., Li, K., Luo, X., et al. (2019). Gray matter volumes of insular subregions are not correlated with smoking cessation outcomes but negatively correlated with nicotine dependence severity in chronic smokers. *Neurosci. Lett.* 696, 7–12. doi: 10.1016/j.neulet.2018.12.013

Wang, F., Jing, X., Yang, J., Wang, H., Xiang, R., Han, W., et al. (2016). The role of the insular cortex in naloxone-induced conditioned place aversion in morphine-dependent mice. *Physiol. Res./Academia Scientiarum Bohemoslovaca.* 65 (4), 701–709.

Wang, W., Wang, Y. R., Qin, W., Yuan, K., Tian, J., Li, Q., et al. (2010). Changes in functional connectivity of ventral anterior cingulate cortex in heroin abusers. *Chin. Med. J. (Engl)* 123 (12), 1582–1588. doi: 10.3760/cma.j.issn.0366-6999.2010.12.019

Wei, Z., Yang, N., Liu, Y., Yang, L., Wang, Y., Han, L., et al. (2016). Resting-state functional connectivity between the dorsal anterior cingulate cortex and thalamus is associated with risky decision-making in nicotine addicts. *Sci. Rep.* 6 (1), 21778. doi: 10.1038/srep21778

Weng, C. B., Qian, R. B., Fu, X. M., Lin, B., Han, X. P., Niu, C. S., et al. (2013). Gray matter and white matter abnormalities in online game addiction. *Eur. J. Radiol.* 82 (8), 1308–1312. doi: 10.1016/j.ejrad.2013.01.031

Whiteford, H. A., Degenhardt, L., Rehm, J., Baxter, A. J., Ferrari, A. J., Erskine, H. E., et al. (2013). Global burden of disease attributable to mental and substance use disorders: findings from the Global Burden of Disease Study 2010. *Lancet* 382 (9904), 1575–1586. doi: 10.1016/S0140-6736(13)61611-6

Wiese, H., Stude, P., Nebel, K., Forsting, M., and de Greiff, A. (2005). Prefrontal cortex activity in self-initiated movements is condition-specific, but not movement-related. *Neuroimage* 28 (3), 691–697. doi: 10.1016/j.neuroimage.2005.06.044

Wiethoff, S., Hamada, M., and Rothwell, J. C. (2014). Variability in response to transcranial direct current stimulation of the motor cortex. *Brain Stimul.* 7 (3), 468–475. doi: 10.1016/j.brs.2014.02.003

Wills, K. L., Petrie, G. N., Millett, G., Limebeer, C. L., Rock, E. M., Niphakis, M. J. et al., (2016). Double dissociation of monoacylglycerol lipase inhibition and cb 1 antagonism in the central amygdala, basolateral amygdala, and the interoceptive insular cortex on the affective properties of acute naloxone-precipitated morphine withdrawal in rats. *Neuropsychopharmacology* 41, 7, 1865–1873. doi: 10.1038/npp.2015.356

Wisner, K. M., Patzelt, E. H., Lim, K. O., and MacDonald, A. W. (2013). An intrinsic connectivity network approach to insula-derived dysfunctions among cocaine users. *Am. J. Drug Alcohol Abuse* 39 (6), 403–413. doi: 10.3109/00952990.2013.848211

Woolley, J. D., Strobl, E. V., Sturm, V. E., Shany-Ur, T., Poorzand, P., Grossman, S., et al. (2015). Impaired recognition and regulation of disgust is associated with distinct but partially overlapping patterns of decreased gray matter volume in the ventroanterior insula. *Biol. Psychiatry* 78 (7), 505–514. doi: 10.1016/j.biopsych.2014.12.031

Wright, C. I., and Groenewegen, H. J. (1996). Patterns of overlap and segregation between insular cortical, intermediodorsal thalamic and basal amygdaloid afferents in the nucleus accumbens of the rat. *Neuroscience* 73 (2), 359–373. doi: 10.1016/0306-4522(95)00592-7

Yesavage, J. A., Fairchild, J. K., Mi, Z., Biswas, K., Davis-Karim, A., Phibbs, C. S., et al. (2018). Effect of repetitive transcranial magnetic stimulation on treatment-resistant major depression in US veterans: a randomized clinical trial. *JAMA Psychiatry* 75 (9), 884–893. doi: 10.1001/jamapsychiatry.2018.1483

Yousefzadeh-Fard, Y., Gharedaghi, M. H., Esmaeili, S., Pourbakhtyaran, E., Sadaghiani, M. S., Ghorbani, A., et al. (2013). Stroke modifies drug consumption in opium addicts: role of the insula. *Basic Clin. Neurosci.* 4 (4), 307–314.

Zangen, A., Roth, Y., Voller, B., and Hallett, M. (2005). Transcranial magnetic stimulation of deep brain regions: evidence for efficacy of the H-Coil. *Clin. Neurophysiol.* 116 (4), 775–779. doi: 10.1016/j.clinph.2004.11.008

Zhang, X., Salmeron, B. J., Ross, T. J., Geng, X., Yang, Y., and Stein, E. A. (2011). Factors underlying prefrontal and insula structural alterations in smokers. *Neuroimage* 54 (1), 42–48. doi: 10.1016/j.neuroimage.2010.08.008

Zhang, Y., Mei, W., Zhang, J., Wu, Q., and Zhang, W. (2016). Decreased functional connectivity of insula-based network in young adults with internet gaming disorder. *Exp. Brain Res.* 234 (9), 2553–2560. doi: 10.1007/s00221-016-4659-8

Zhou, S., Xiao, D., Peng, P., Wang, S. K., Liu, Z., Qin, H. Y., et al. (2017). Effect of smoking on resting-state functional connectivity in smokers: an fMRI study. *Respirology* 22 (6), 1118–1124. doi: 10.1111/resp.13048

Zito, K. A., Bechara, A., Greenwood, C., and van der Kooy, D. (1988). The dopamine innervation of the visceral cortex mediates the aversive effects of opiates. *Pharmacol. Biochem. Behav.* 30 (3), 693–699. doi: 10.1016/0091-3057(88)90086-X

6

Compensatory Relearning Following Stroke: Cellular and Plasticity Mechanisms in Rodents

Gustavo Balbinot[1] and Clarissa Pedrini Schuch[2]*

[1] Brain Institute, Universidade Federal do Rio Grande do Norte, Natal, Brazil, [2] Graduate Program in Rehabilitation Sciences, Universidade Federal de Ciências da Saúde de Porto Alegre (UFCSPA), Porto Alegre, Brazil

Correspondence:
Gustavo Balbinot
gustavo.balbinot@hotmail.com

von Monakow's theory of diaschisis states the functional 'standstill' of intact brain regions that are remote from a damaged area, often implied in recovery of function. Accordingly, neural plasticity and activity patterns related to recovery are also occurring at the same regions. Recovery relies on plasticity in the periinfarct and homotopic contralesional regions and involves relearning to perform movements. Seeking evidence for a relearning mechanism following stroke, we found that rodents display many features that resemble classical learning and memory mechanisms. Compensatory relearning is likely to be accompanied by gradual shaping of these regions and pathways, with participating neurons progressively adapting cortico-striato-thalamic activity and synaptic strengths at different cortico-thalamic loops – adapting function relayed by the striatum. Motor cortex functional maps are progressively reinforced and shaped by these loops as the striatum searches for different functional actions. Several cortical and striatal cellular mechanisms that influence motor learning may also influence post-stroke compensatory relearning. Future research should focus on *how* different neuromodulatory systems could act before, during or after rehabilitation to improve stroke recovery.

Keywords: stroke, rehabilitation, motor learning, pharmacotherapy, plasticity

INTRODUCTION

Recovery following stroke requires locating reorganization processes in the brain where the necessary motor and sensory signals converge. Once located, descriptions of mechanisms for optimization can provide neural substrates for recovery. In the cortex and striatum, waves of growth inhibiting and promoting factors related to cellular and plastic changes are triggered by the lesion. Cellular death leads to homeostatic destabilization and to a subsequent process of repair leading to partial recovery of cellular function (Carmichael, 2003). Cellular reorganization processes take place in brain regions adjacent or previously connected to the affected cells, such as: periinfarct tissue, cortico-cortical pathways, cortico-striatal pathways and cortico-thalamic pathways. Rehabilitation and pharmacological therapies are used to optimize and guide these cellular and plasticity changes. This complex recovery process following stroke involves several factors, here we suggest that cellular and plasticity mechanisms related to motor learning are likely active.

Stroke induces a permissive environment for axonal sprouting through growth-promoting proteins in the boundary zone to the ischemic core (Li et al., 1998; Carmichael et al., 2005). The permissive environment after stroke leads to cortical and corticospinal tract rewiring (Winship and Murphy, 2008; Wahl and Schwab, 2014) and other forms of long-term plasticity associated with learning (Hess and Donoghue, 1994; Hess et al., 1996). These changes associated with compensatory relearning are expected to produce both increases and decreases in synaptic strength distributed throughout the complex neural networks (bidirectional changes; Cohen and Castro-Alamancos, 2005). The precise homeostatic changes in order to refine synaptic connectivity and to adjust synaptic strengths to promote the stability needed for motor recovery following stroke are still poorly understood (Turrigiano and Nelson, 2004; Murphy and Corbett, 2009).

To enhance stroke recovery, the interaction of fundamental interconnected areas of research - such as motor learning and endogenous plasticity mechanisms, urgently requires new and innovative approaches (Krakauer, 2006; Krakauer et al., 2012). It has been 12 years since Krakauer suggested the relevance of motor learning for stroke recovery and rehabilitation (Krakauer, 2006). A brief review of recent clinical studies on stroke recovery highlights the positive effects of virtual reality for motor learning retention (Carregosa et al., 2018) and also in combination with transcranial stimulation (Fuentes et al., 2018) or exoskeletons (Grimm et al., 2016); and the prominent effects of constraint-induced movement therapy (CIMT) (reviewed elsewhere; Hatem et al., 2016). Motor skill relearning using CIMT is considered a promising and efficient method to improve clinical prognosis in stroke motor rehabilitation. Nevertheless, the authors highlight the need of more information about the integration of other motor skill learning techniques other than CIMT (Hatem et al., 2016). We suggest that using a reverse translation approach, preclinical stroke research may unveil the mechanisms involved in compensatory relearning to gauge the dose and timing of rehabilitation, drug therapy or the combination of both. For example, the use of pharmacotherapy in combination with physical rehabilitation before, during or after the rehabilitation section to maximize relearning effects. In this review, we merge principles and mechanisms of motor learning and stroke recovery and present a new perspective based on *where* and *how* compensatory relearning occurs.

New treatments for post-stroke impairments may depend on a better understanding of the neural mechanisms and influences of compensatory behavior (Jones, 2017). One of the challenges of understanding *how* compensatory relearning occurs is the fluid nature of memories, with participating brain regions dynamically shifting over time (Makino et al., 2016). To test if stroke recovery is mediated by relearning mechanisms, more studies with high temporal and spatial precision are needed (Makino et al., 2016). Recent findings suggest that the 'stroke recovery circuit' may parallel memory formation during learning tasks (Caracciolo et al., 2018); and that thalamo-cortical plasticity promotes stroke recovery (Tennant et al., 2017). These two examples highlight how temporal and spatial information needs to be integrated to unveil the mechanisms of compensatory relearning. The purpose of this review is to condense experimental findings of the large literature on motor skill learning and post-stroke recovery. We refer the reader to other recently published reviews for additional perspectives of cellular and plastic mechanisms of motor skill learning and stroke recovery. We also offer our perspectives on *how* to improve stroke recovery focused on compensatory relearning.

THE CORTICAL CIRCUIT

The cellular and synaptic organization of the somatosensory cortex supports the primary motor neurons and the storage capability needed to encode movements (Penfield and Rasmussen, 1950; Jankowska et al., 1975; Nudo et al., 1996a; Hosp and Luft, 2011). Movements are represented in the motor cortex in regions related to forelimb or hindlimb responses (rostral forelimb area and caudal forelimb area; Neafsey and Sievert, 1982). At each region distinct cortical layers function to receive, integrate and transmit the motor output. The cortical circuit is shaped by redundancy that provides the flexibility needed to network changes, such as during post-stroke recovery (Sanes and Donoghue, 2000). For example, the rostral forelimb area is considered the putative premotor area in the rodent and is involved in post-stroke reorganization of motor representations (Neafsey and Sievert, 1982; Dancause, 2006; Dancause et al., 2015; Touvykine et al., 2016). This reorganization is tailored by thalamo-cortical loops, which are the building blocks of a homeostatic and functional movement network.

Input Stage: Thalamo-Cortico-Thalamic and Thalamo-Cortico-Striatal Loops

At the input stage cortical principal cells receive, but also send information to the thalamus, integrating a redundant system that integrates sensory and motor signals (Haber and Calzavara, 2009; Leyva-Díaz and López-Bendito, 2013). Thalamo-cortical pathways receive higher-order information – already processed by other cortical or extra-cortical regions (Castro-Alamancos and Connors, 1997). For example, thalamo-cortical projections from the basal ganglia terminate in cortical layers I/II, III/IV, and V (McFarland and Haber, 2002); but also from the sensory periphery that projects sparsely to layers V and I (Castro-Alamancos and Connors, 1997). Cortico-thalamic axons are formed by corticofugal pyramidal neurons located in the cortical layer VI, and to a smaller extent layer V (Donoghue and Kitai, 1981; Leyva-Díaz and López-Bendito, 2013) (except where noted, corticofugal, hereafter refers to cortical projections to descending pathways). Interestingly, cortico-thalamic neurons send information that, after relayed by the thalamus, are redirected to a different cortical region integrating different cortical areas into a global network (Leyva-Díaz and López-Bendito, 2013).

As described above, deep layer cortical neurons send projections to thalamus, and thalamus projects back to the striatum and to the superficial, the middle, and the deep cortical layers (layers I/II, III/IV, and V) (Paré and Smith, 1996; McFarland and Haber, 2000, 2002). Thus, projections that terminate in deep cortical layers, e.g., layer V, are likely to form thalamo-cortico-thalamic and thalamo-cortico-striatal loops (Haber and Calzavara, 2009). In other words, deep layer projections may interact with neurons that project back to both the thalamus and striatum. As a result, this interaction can reinforce cortico-thalamic and cortico-striatal inputs to specific cortico-basal ganglia circuits and may be involved in the development of specific learned behaviors (McFarland and Haber, 2002).

Superficial cortical layers I/II also receive thalamo-cortical inputs and can control the activity of any neuron with apical dendrite ascending to layer I (Haber and Calzavara, 2009). Interestingly, due to the more widespread thalamo-cortical terminals in layer I, this input can affect adjacent cortical populations and cortico-cortical connections. Thereby, potentially modulating a different loop at a different cortical region (Haber and Calzavara, 2009). This type of plasticity can be of particular interest during stroke recovery and for compensatory relearning mechanisms. Given that after a cortical ischemia the infarct core is surrounded by functional tissue, it is likely that the surviving tissue can share some of the specific striatal-thalamo-cortical projections with the lesioned tissue. Thus, superficial cortical layers would participate of thalamo-cortico-thalamic and thalamo-cortico-striatal loops that would reinforce new connections during stroke recovery and compensatory relearning of motor tasks (Haber and Calzavara, 2009; Shmuelof and Krakauer, 2011).

In other words, in the rodent agranular motor cortex, asymmetrical thalamic projections target layers I, II/III and V (from basal-ganglia) and layers II/III and V (from cerebellum) (reviewed in Peters et al., 2017). Stroke disrupts these thalamic targets but, the above-mentioned (1) widespread of thalamo-cortical inputs to superficial layers may affect adjacent spared cortical tissue. (2) Superficial layers may act as a preamplifier-like network, which captures these thalamic signals and drives output neurons in lower layers (Weiler et al., 2008). (3) Abundant cortico-cortical communication may affect adjacent and relevant cortical functional columns and integrate the process of augmented responses in deep layers supplemented by (4, 5) compensatory cortical, thalamic and striatal regions. These afferents projecting to layer V may initiate a sequence of synaptic and intrinsic membrane-dependent events, which prime the cortical network and lead to an augmented response due to heightened neuronal excitability in layer V and may favor compensatory relearning of movements (further explored in section "Endogenous Plasticity Mechanisms: Use-Dependent Plasticity, Augmented Responses and Neuromodulation"; Castro-Alamancos and Connors, 1996a) (**Figure 1**).

It is important to consider a few drawbacks of the layer specificity described here. First, that the existence of a layer IV in the rodent motor cortex is still under discussion and can be referred as the deep layer III or the superficial layer Va (Kaneko, 2013; Yamawaki et al., 2014). Second, it has been recently suggested that future studies should focus on specific circuits defined by functional cell type composition rather than the common oversimplification of laminar distribution (Guy and Staiger, 2017). Nevertheless, at the input level an abundant literature supports the importance of lamina-specific activity changes for motor learning (reviewed in Peters et al., 2017). Future studies should take advantage of the recent methods to reveal cell types and their changed post-stroke connectivity, with impact to novel stroke recovery mechanisms focused on compensatory relearning (similarly to striatal microcircuitry; Silberberg and Bolam, 2015).

Output Stage: Redundancy and Intra-Circuit Connectivity

The output cells of the cerebral cortex are the pyramidal cells (70–80% of cortical neurons; Feldman, 1984). Their processing of sensorimotor inputs is beyond a simple output signal to descending motor neurons. The descending corticofugal pathway is complex with several intra- and extra-cortical collaterals and distinct terminations (Donoghue and Kitai, 1981). Primary projections are directed to the spinal cord, with secondary collaterals to the striatum, red nucleus, caudal pons and medulla (Donoghue and Kitai, 1981; Reiner et al., 2003; Leyva-Díaz and López-Bendito, 2013).

Pyramidal cells also show remarkable intra-circuit connectivity – intra-cortical synapses account for ≈70% of total synapses onto pyramidal cells (Amitai and Connors, 1995), both intra-layer (layer V; Markram et al., 1997) and inter-layers (layers II–V or VI–IV; Lund et al., 1993). Cortico-cortical connections are either within the same hemisphere (ipsilateral cortico-cortical connections) or from the opposite hemisphere (callosal connections) (Leyva-Díaz and López-Bendito, 2013). In rodents callosal pyramidal neurons are mainly at cortical layers II/III/IV (≈80%), layer V (≈20%) and, to a lesser extent, layer VI (Leyva-Díaz and López-Bendito, 2013). In addition, a population of layer V medium-sized pyramidal neurons is of cortico-striatal neurons that cross to the contralateral hemisphere (crossed cortico-striatal neurons; Wilson, 1987; Lévesque et al., 1996; Anderson et al., 2010).

The interconnection between hemispheres can lead to short- and long-term motor plasticity. The activation of motor neurons in the contralesional hemisphere can induce activation of cortico-cortical callosal projections to the ipsilesional hemisphere - in the same functional cortical column. For example, neurons from the contralesional caudal forelimb area can prime neurons in the spared ipsilesional caudal forelimb area (e.g., periinfarct region) (Castro-Alamancos and Connors, 1996a). Indeed, callosal cortico-cortical neurons extend axons to mirror-image locations in the same functional area at the contralateral hemisphere (bilateral integration of information; Greig et al., 2013). Ipsilesional neurons would also undergo plastic changes modulated by the newly formed cortico-striatal connections (crossed cortico-striatal neurons; Cheng et al., 1998) during rehabilitation.

In brief, at the output stage pyramidal cells integrate a complex cortical network to produce movement. Including abundant connections with the contralateral hemisphere. Plastic changes of callosal connections is thought as a mechanism underlying the physiological reorganization in the contralesional hemisphere following stroke (Dancause, 2006). In many ways the cortical

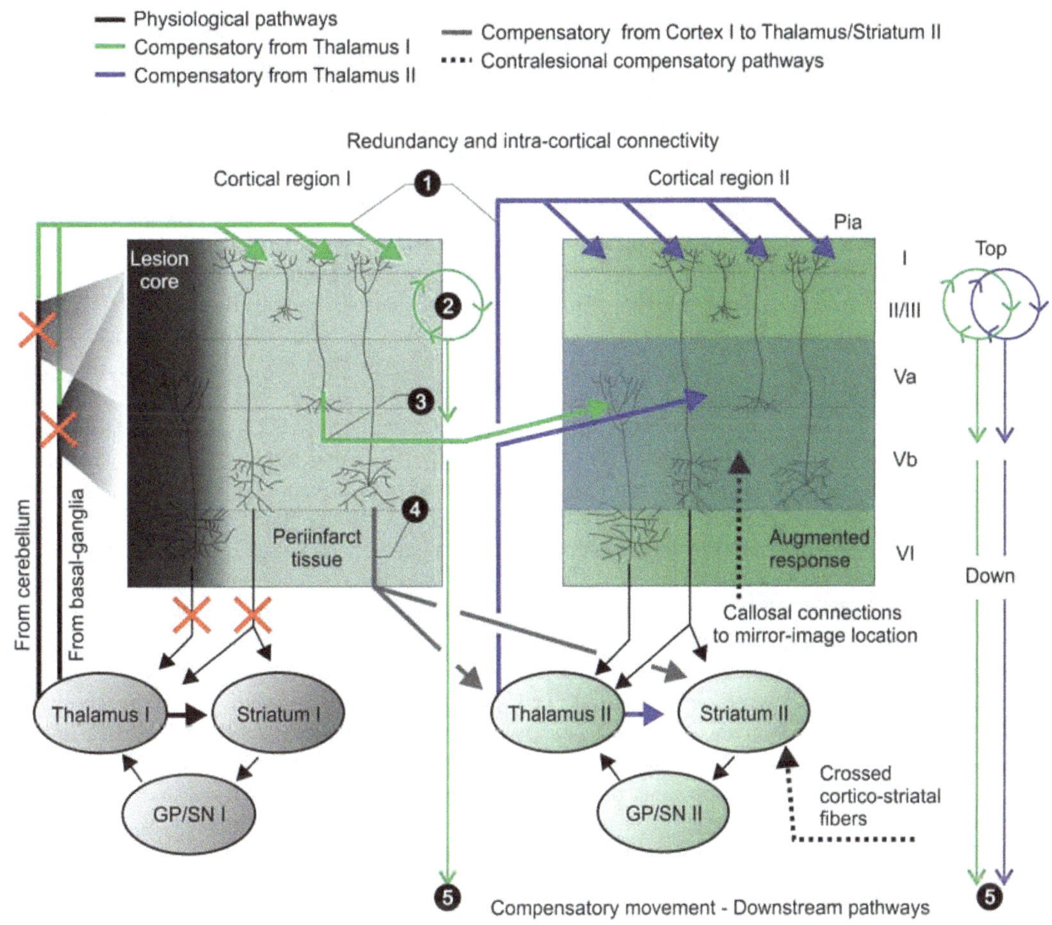

FIGURE 1 | Pronounced intra-cortical connectivity and redundancy are remarkable features of the motor cortex. Motor cortex caudal (e.g., cortical region I) and rostral (e.g., cortical region II) forelimb areas contain the primary motor neurons that encode motor map representations of forelimb skilled movements. Pyramidal neurons project to brainstem and spinal cord (not shown) and send collaterals to striatum and thalamus – integrating thalamo-cortico-thalamic and thalamo-cortico striatal loops. (1) widespread thalamo-cortical connections common to both cortical regions (I and II) target superficial layers and reach damaged, periinfarct and spared areas (upper green and blue solid lines); (2) the preamplifier-like network (green circular loop) captures thalamic I signals and drives output neurons in lower layers (Weiler et al., 2008); (3) horizontal cortico-cortical connections of neurons receive and retransmit this indirect thalamic information (previously shared with the infarct core area) (green solid lines); (4) cortico-thalamic and cortico-striatal projections (from cortical region I to II; gray solid line) integrate another striatal-thalamo-cortical loop (cortical region II). The putative participation of crossed cortico-striatal and cortico-cortical fibers is shown (hashed black lines, bottom right). (5) Cells from adjacent/spared tissue (cortical region II) share thalamo-cortical inputs with interconnected/intertwined thalamo-cortical circuits of the stroke-disrupted network to control compensatory relearning of movements. GP, globus pallidus; SN, substantia nigra.

circuitry is built with redundancy, this allows compensation by spared regions when a lesion occurs.

Endogenous Plasticity Mechanisms: Use-Dependent Plasticity, Augmented Responses and Neuromodulation

Use-dependent plasticity plays a pivotal role on post-stroke functional recovery and on motor learning (Nudo et al., 1996b; Nudo et al., 1996a). For example, potentiation of thalamo- and cortico-cortical afferents by high frequency stimulation of the corpus callosum induces cortical LTP (Chapman et al., 1998) and increases forelimb motor representations, branch complexity, dendritic length and spine density in layer V (Monfils et al., 2004). In the motor cortex the induction of LTP is only possible with partial blockage of cortical $GABA_A$Rs (Castro-Alamancos and Borrell, 1995). Suggesting that a fine tuning between excitation and inhibition is paramount to motor cortex use-dependent plasticity.

Under physiological conditions a strong glutamatergic afferent input from the motor thalamus innervates cortical pyramidal neurons (mainly layer V) (Amitai, 2001; Haber and Calzavara, 2009; Kuramoto et al., 2009). As aforementioned, these projections initiate a sequence of synaptic and intrinsic membrane-dependent events that prime the cortical network and induce an augmented response, i.e., heightened neuronal excitability (Castro-Alamancos and Connors, 1996a,c) (see **Figure 1** – layer V augmented response). Interestingly, this augmented response of layer V is blocked by active exploration or skilled behavioral performance and induced by inactive behavioral states (Castro-Alamancos and Connors, 1996b). Suggesting a dynamic modulation of short-term thalamo-cortical plasticity, which can occur during and after motor skill relearning (Biane et al., 2016). Given that the spread of the augmenting response to upper cortical layers depends of synaptic interconnections and active dendritic conductance (Castro-Alamancos and Connors, 1996a), it is likely that after stroke the more permissive environment (Carmichael et al., 2005; Murphy and Corbett, 2009) could favor this short-term plasticity through horizontal pathways of layers II/III in M1 (Hess et al., 1996), reaching adjacent cortical tissue (e.g., cortical region II – **Figure 1**).

In brief, stroke recovery depends on cortical plasticity and this neuroplasticity is likely to require exploration of spared movements by the striatum (Shmuelof and Krakauer, 2011). We suggest that to unveil *how* these cortico-thalamo-cortical loops act on neuroplasticity mechanisms, a better understanding of the *in vivo* interactions during compensatory relearning is necessary. Previous evidence of *where* these changes occur are abundant, for example skilled training increase: dendritic length and arborization in layer II/III and V motor neurons (Greenough et al., 1985; Withers and Greenough, 1989; Kolb et al., 2008); number of synapses per neuron in layer V (hemisphere contralateral to the trained paw) (Kleim et al., 2004); dendritic arborization of cortical layer V in the contralesional motor cortex (Biernaskie and Corbett, 2001). The bulk of these findings suggests that callosal cortico-cortical, crossed cortico-striatal, and ipsilateral (uncrossed corticospinal projections; Vahlsing and Feringa, 1980) projections undergo neuroplasticity changes related to compensatory relearning of motor tasks.

Neuromodulation

Different types of metabotropic glutamate receptors (mGluRs) are expressed throughout the cortex ($mGlu_{1,2,3,5,7a/b,8a/b}$), where $mGlu_5R$ has the strongest expression (Shigemoto and Mizuno, 2000; Ferraguti and Shigemoto, 2006) (**Figure 2A**); intense expression of $mGlu_5R$ was also detected in cortical GABAergic interneurons (Kerner et al., 1997). mGluRs provide a mechanism by which adjustments of fine-tune activity occurs at the same synapses of fast glutamatergic synaptic responses (Conn and Pin, 1997). Activation of $mGlu_5Rs$ can increase NMDA-evoked responses in the cortical tissue and, for example, $mGlu_5Rs$ antagonism can enhance MK-801 impairments of instrumental learning (Homayoun et al., 2004).

Cortical neurons also express several serotonin (5-HT) receptor subtypes ($5\text{-}HT_{1A/B,2A/C,3,4,6,7}$; Celada et al., 2013), for example, cortical $5\text{-}HT_{1A}Rs$ have high mRNA expression in cortical layers V and VI (Pompeiano et al., 1992; Puig et al., 2005; Singh and Staines, 2015) (**Figure 2B**). It is suggested that 5-HT modulation of motor cortex excitability leans toward facilitation (Singh and Staines, 2015). Interestingly, cortical $5\text{-}HT_{1A}Rs$ activation has an overall excitatory effect on the neural networks that give rise to movement representations (Scullion et al., 2013). Selective serotonin reuptake inhibition improves learning and motor outcomes in animal models of ischemic stroke at different tasks, e.g., rotarod, staircase reaching, cylinder test, adhesive label test (McCann et al., 2014).

Another important cortical neuromodulator is acetylcholine (ACh), which can exert multiple effects on cortical neurons depending on type of target cell, pre- or post-synaptic receptor localization and receptor subtype (Wada et al., 1989, 1990; McGehee et al., 1995; Porter et al., 1999); resulting in a very complex modulation (Lucas-Meunier et al., 2003). Due to its diffuse cortical innervation some authors suggest a modulating rather than direct/synaptic role of ACh on the activity of the cortical circuitry (Lucas-Meunier et al., 2003 for references). Two major classes of ACh receptors are present in the rat cortex: muscarinic receptors (MRs) and nicotinic receptors. In the adult rat brain, cortical MRs subtypes are: m_1 (26.4%), m_2 (21.4%), m_3 (7.7%), m_4 (44.2%), and m_5 (<1%) (Tice et al., 1996); in addition, ACh MRs are located at all cortical layers (Cortés and Palacios, 1986; Frey and Howland, 1992) and are metabotropic (Lucas-Meunier et al., 2003) (**Figure 2C**). Although there is a dense presence of cortical cholinergic receptors, the role of ACh on motor learning is still relatively underexplored. Conner's group pioneer research showed that the basal forebrain cholinergic system is essential for cortical plasticity associated with motor learning (Conner et al., 2003). Later, they showed that cholinergic mechanisms are essential for cortical map plasticity after a skilled motor training (Ramanathan et al., 2009); and that cholinergic activation within the motor cortex modulates cortical map plasticity and motor learning (Conner et al., 2010). Interestingly, the basal forebrain cholinergic system is required for successful post-stroke rehabilitation, with direct impact on cell morphology (Wang et al., 2016).

Dopamine (DA) receptors are selectively expressed in different cortical layers. Motor cortex D_1 receptors are expressed at superficial (low expression; layers II–III) and deep (high expression; layers V–VI) layers (Savasta et al., 1986) (**Figure 2D**). D_2-receptors are expressed in cortical pyramidal layer V but at a lower extent when compared to D_1 expression (Ariano et al., 1993; Awenowicz and Porter, 2002) (**Figure 2E**). D_1 mRNA is present in cortico-cortical, cortico-thalamic and cortico-striatal neurons and D_2 mRNA is restricted to layer V of cortico-striatal and cortico-cortical neurons (Gaspar et al., 1995). The overall effect of DA on cortical pyramidal cell excitability may depend on phasic changes in DA concentration and GABAergic inhibition tone (Gulledge and Jaffe, 2001). D_1/D_2 dopamine receptors activation is necessary for successful motor skill learning (Hosp et al., 2011). And the integrity of the dopaminergic mesencephalic-M1 pathway is also fundamental for motor learning in rats (Hosp and Luft, 2013). Suggesting that the M1 dopaminergic system is paramount to motor skill learning. DA system is also involved on cortical motor map representations (Brown et al., 2009, 2011), movement generation (Parr-Brownlie and Hyland, 2005) and LTP-like plasticity (Korchounov and Ziemann, 2011). Thus, DA has an important role on the modulation of intra-cortical excitability to enhance plasticity and to promote motor skill learning and execution.

Finally, adrenoceptors (ARs) are most present in cortical layers IV and V and the subtypes $\alpha_{1A/B/D,2A/B/C/D}$ and $\beta_{1,2,3}$ are found in the cortical tissue (Wang and McCormick, 1993)

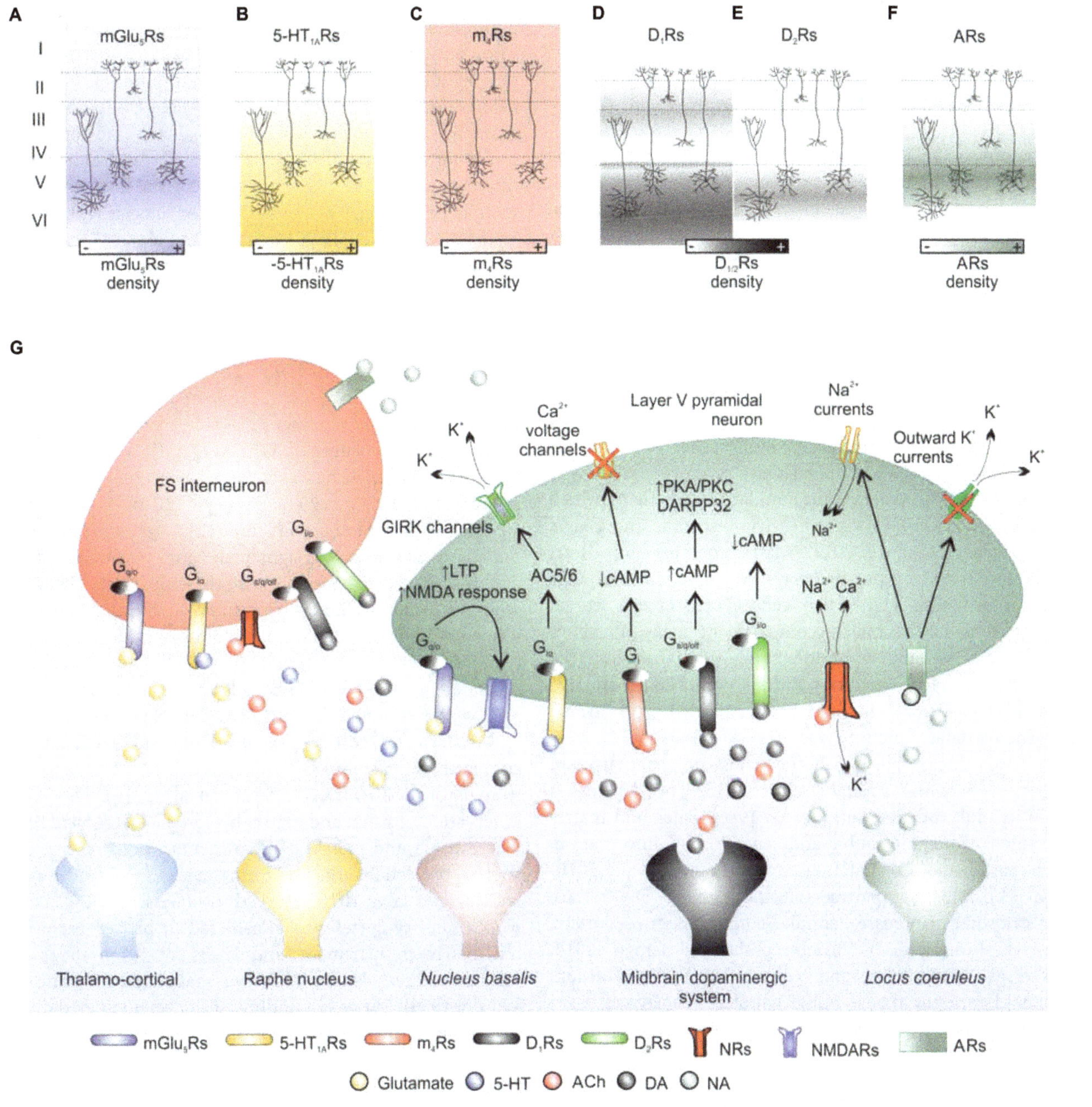

FIGURE 2 | Neuromodulation: main cortical neurotransmitter systems involved in motor learning. **(A)** Glutamate release from cortical or thalamic afferents can modulate cellular excitability and short/long-term plasticity in cortical pyramidal neurons. Metabotropic glutamate receptors ($mGlu_5Rs$) are mainly expressed in cortical layer V and act via $G_{q/O}$ protein on downstream targets. This interaction can enhance NMDARs activity and induce LTP in pyramidal neurons. **(B)** Raphe nucleus serotonin (5-HT) can bind to $5\text{-}HT_{1A}Rs$ (high mRNA expression in cortical layers V and VI) and via a $G_{i\alpha}$ protein-AC5/6 pathway induce K^+ efflux leading to cell hyperpolarization, both in pyramidal cells and FS interneurons. **(C)** *Nucleus basalis* acetylcholine (ACh) binds to muscarinic receptors (MRs; e.g., m_4Rs) or nicotinic receptors (NRs). m_4Rs are expressed in all cortical layers and are coupled to G_i proteins that can reduce cellular activity through cAMP signaling. NMDARs are permeable to Na^+, K^+, and Ca^{2+} ions and are modulated by intra- and extra-Ca^{2+} concentrations (not shown). **(D,E)** Dopamine (DA) released by the midbrain dopaminergic system can bind to D_1Rs (low expression in layers II–III and high expression in layers V–VI) or D_2Rs (expressed in layer V but at a lower extent when compared to D_1 expression) and increase or decrease cellular excitability, respectively, via cAMP acting on downstream targets (e.g., DARPP32). **(F)** *Locus coeruleus* noradrenaline (NA) released to the cerebral cortex binds to adrenoceptors (ARs) highly expressed in cortical layers IV and V. NA may increase cortical excitability via a reduction of outward K^+ currents and increase of Na^+ currents. **(G)** Simplified model of cortical neurotransmitter systems involved in motor learning.

(**Figure 2F**). Overall, noradrenaline (NA) increases the excitability of cortical pyramidal cells, but also the activity of cortical GABAergic non-pyramidal cells (Kawaguchi and Shindou, 1998). In the motor cortex, blockade of NA receptors suppresses the induction of LTP-like plasticity (Korchounov and Ziemann, 2011). **Figure 2G** shows a simplified model of cortical neurotransmitter systems involved in motor learning.

THE STRIATAL CIRCUIT

The striatum is the main input nucleus of the basal ganglia and is a single structure in rodents. In rodents, striatal dorsolateral and medial portions are equivalent to putamen and caudate in primates, respectively (Heilbronner et al., 2016). The striatum can be divided in two compartments based on neurochemical characteristics and connections: patch (μ opiate receptor, substance P and enkephalin) and matrix (ACh esterase and calcium binding protein) (for references see Johnston et al., 1990; Gerfen, 1992; Lopez-Huerta et al., 2016). Anatomically, patch is a structure of interconnected tubes with finger-like branches and matrix is composed of well demarcated "dots" or "islands" of moderate to strong DA fluorescence (Olson et al., 1972; Johnston et al., 1990; Lopez-Huerta et al., 2016). Another recently added compartment is the annular compartment, which surrounds the striosome (or patch) (Brimblecombe and Cragg, 2015; Perrin and Venance, 2019). Matrix contains both direct and indirect striatal output pathways and does not exchange synaptic information with patch cells (Lopez-Huerta et al., 2016). Neurons of the matrix compartment make up about 85% of striatal volume (Johnston et al., 1990), contain the main outputs to globus pallidus and substantia nigra and are suggested to participate in behaviors associated with striatal and cortico-striatal function, such as skill learning (Lopez-Huerta et al., 2016). The patch (or striosome) compartment comprises a maximal striatal area of ≈15% of the rostral striatum in adult rodents (Lança et al., 1986). Patch and matrix compartments integrate limbic and sensorimotor information, through patch and exo-patch neurons (Smith et al., 2016) (**Figure 3A**). This compartmentalization affects DA release among striosomes (increase), annular compartment (decrease), and matrix (unmodified) (Brimblecombe and Cragg, 2015; Salinas et al., 2016; Perrin and Venance, 2019). In addition, cannabinoid receptor type 1 (CB_1R) protein displays elevated expression in striosomes relative to the surrounding matrix (Davis et al., 2018). This complex striatal system is involved in motor skill learning in a medial (early skill learning) to lateral (late skill learning) gradient (Yin et al., 2009) (**Figure 3A**).

Input Stage

The striatum is the input structure of the basal ganglia network. Cortical and thalamic glutamatergic signals converge into the striatum and are modulated by dopaminergic signals from mesolimbic nuclei (for references see Calabresi et al., 1996; Cerovic et al., 2013). In rodents, while cortico-striatal afferents are from several cortical regions, thalamo-striatal afferents are mainly from the parafascicular thalamic nucleus (Calabresi et al., 1996; Smith et al., 2014). Thalamo-striatal afferents have been implicated in controlling presynaptic suppression of cortico-striatal inputs through cholinergic interneurons, with implications on attentional shifts and cessation of ongoing motor programs (Ding et al., 2010). Recently, GABAergic inputs from the motor cortex to the dorsal striatum were described and implicated in motor control (Melzer et al., 2017). Optogenetic stimulation of these GABAergic long-range projections, such as M1 parvalbumin $(PV)^+$ and M2 somatostatin $(SOM)^+$, reduced locomotion (Melzer et al., 2017). These above-mentioned examples challenge the view of how thalamo- and cortico-striatal projections can modulate motor behavior and motor learning. Interestingly, post-stroke changes of cortical inhibitory markers, such as periinfarct PV^+ and SOM^+ have been reported (Zeiler et al., 2013; Alia et al., 2016; Spalletti et al., 2017), suggesting a role of this novel pathway for stroke recovery.

The majority of striatal cellular content is of GABAergic projection neurons, medium spiny neurons (MSNs), which are ≈95% of all neurons in the rat striatum (Kemp and Powell, 1971; Gerfen, 1992; Tepper et al., 2007; Kreitzer, 2009). The remaining glutamatergic afferents target intrastriatal interneurons: large cholinergic aspiny neurons (or cholinergic tonically active neurons), GABAergic PV^+ or neuropeptide Y^+/SOM^+ interneurons (Tepper et al., 2004; for reviews and references see Kreitzer, 2009; Lovinger, 2010).

Cholinergic interneurons are only ≈1% of striatal cells, but their influence is significant due to large cell bodies and widespread axonal connections with MSNs. They receive scattered excitatory innervation mainly from thalamus and to a lesser extent from cortex, and inhibitory synapses from MSNs (Kreitzer, 2009 for references). Striatal cholinergic neurons may regulate functions of motor behavior and can release ACh, or can also co-release glutamate with ACh (Lim et al., 2014).

Motor cortex cortico-striatal afferents to patch and matrix compartments are mostly from layer V and to a lesser extent from layers II/III and VI (Smith et al., 2016). Differences in innervation of patch and matrix by cortical layers were reported, where patch and matrix compartments would receive cortico-striatal projections mostly from layers V/VI and superficial layer V and layer II/III, respectively (Gerfen, 1989). Later, the somatosensory cortex was considered to project exclusively to the matrix compartment, and layers Vb–VI preferentially to patches whereas layers III–Va to matrix axons (Kincaid and Wilson, 1996). But recent findings using genetic-based dissection suggest that cortico-striatal connections target patch and matrix compartments equally, regardless of region. Specifically, in M1, striatal patch/matrix inputs originate at layer V (≈75%), at layers II/III (≈10%) and at layer VI (≈15%). Either striosomes (or pathes) and matrix contain MSNs from direct and indirect pathways (Cerovic et al., 2013).

Output Stage: Direct and Indirect Pathways

Activation of MSNs results in GABA release to the principal MSNs projections: external/internal globus pallidus and substantia nigra (Gerfen, 1992) (**Figure 3B**). The striatal cellular mechanisms provide a continuous balance between direct and indirect pathways. The direct pathway releases movements by disinhibiting thalamic activity and the indirect pathway restrains movements by inhibiting thalamic activity (Gerfen, 1992; Graybiel, 1995).

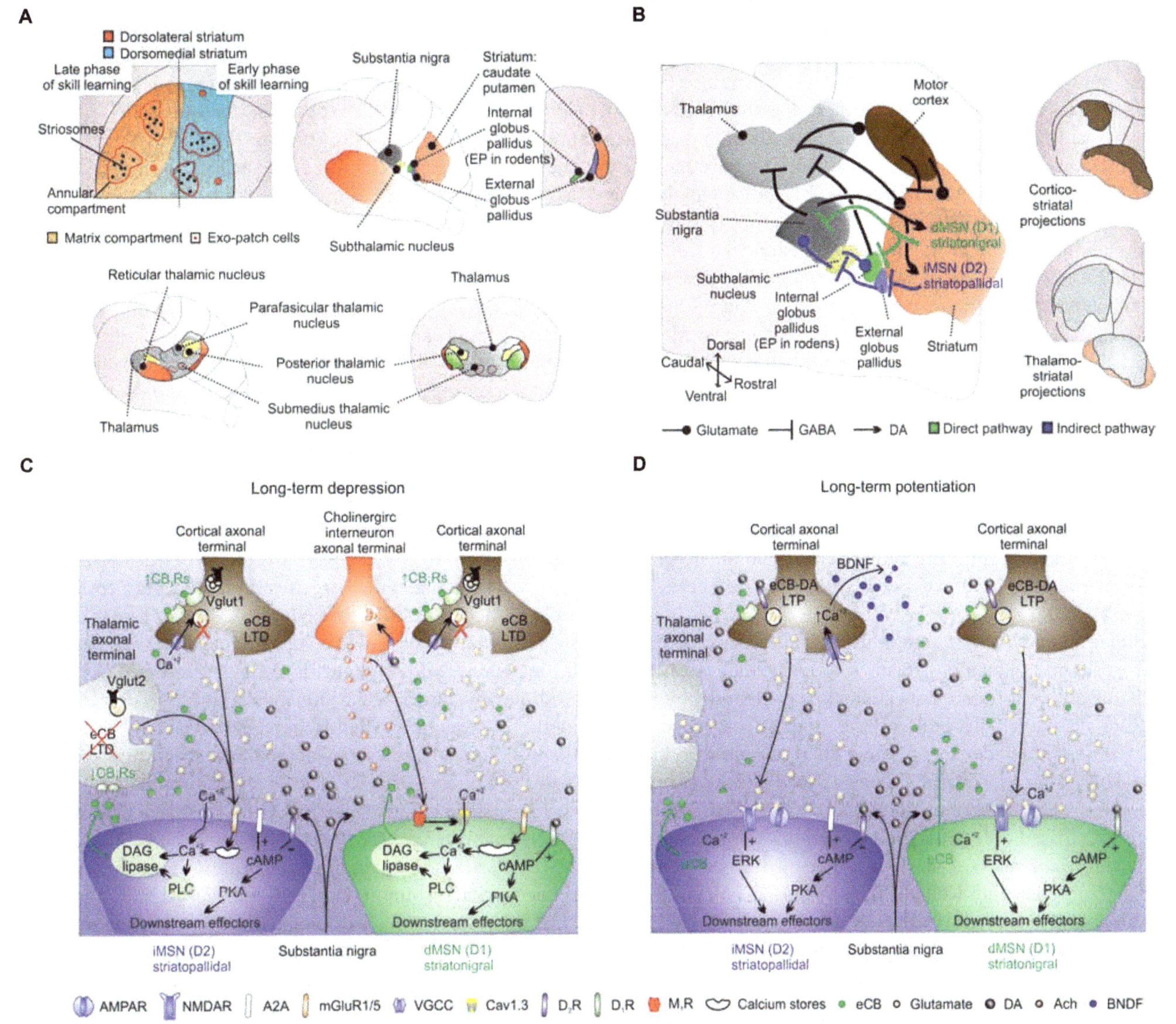

FIGURE 3 | Striatal cellular and synaptic organization. **(A)** Striatum is a single structure in rodents: see striatal theoretical compartmentalization into dorsolateral (red; putamen) and medial (blue; caudate) striatum (Hjornevik, 2007; Heilbronner et al., 2016). Early and late skill learning are suggested to occur in a mediolateral fashion, respectively. (**A**, lower panels) In rodents the main thalamo-striatal afferents originate from the parafascicular nucleus. **(B)** The striatal circuit is composed of several intertwined structures involved in inhibition (indirect-pathway) or disinhibition (direct-pathway) of movement. The indirect-pathway (blue arrows) is formed by striatopallidal MSNs (iMSNs) that project to GABAergic pallidal neurons (external globus pallidus), which exert a powerful inhibitory control into proximal dendrites of glutamatergic neurons in the subthalamic nucleus. Subthalamic nucleus neurons send excitatory afferents to inhibitory output neurons of substantia nigra, and also to internal globus pallidus neurons. The net effect of indirect-pathway activation is inhibition of thalamo-cortical projection neurons, which can reduce cortical premotor drive and inhibit movement. The direct-pathway circuit (green arrows) is formed by striatonigral medium spiny neurons (dMSNs) that provides mainly inhibitory inputs to both GABAergic and dopaminergic cells in substantia nigra, which in turn sends axons to motor nuclei of the thalamus. Direct-pathway activation results in disinhibition of excitatory thalamo-cortical projections, resulting in activation of cortical premotor circuits and the selection/facilitation of movement. Glutamatergic striatal inputs from all cortical areas massively converge into the striatum. Also note the long-range GABAergic projections from the motor cortex to the dorsal striatum. Cortico-striatal and thalamo-striatal glutamatergic inputs target MSNs, large cholinergic interneurons and fast spiking interneurons. Cortico-striatal projections receive several inputs and integrate this information into striatal target neurons. Cholinergic interneurons receive scattered excitatory innervation mainly from thalamus and inhibitory synapses from MSNs. 'Up-states' are modulated by intrastriatal acetylcholine (ACh) and to strong intra-striatal DA release, D_1Rs activation and striatal LTP. Midbrain dopaminergic terminals release dopamine (DA), which exerts a massive effect on all striatal cells. "Down-states" are associated to reduced intra-striatal DA, D_1Rs/D_2Rs activation and striatal LTD. Striatal LTP/LTD is also dependent on NMDARs activation and Ca^{2+} influx in MSNs. (**B**, right panels) Also note the distribution of cortico-striatal and thalamo-striatal afferents (Hunnicutt et al., 2016). **(C)** Long-term depression is dependent on mGLU$_{1/5}$Rs, D_2Rs, M_1Rs, and C_1BRs. For example, in iMSNs, prolonged stimulation of excitatory afferents paired with post-synaptic depolarization triggers the production and release of eCBs (e.g., 2AG) from the precursor diacylglycerol (DAG) through the activation of mGlu$_{1/5}$Rs and phospholipase C (PLC; this process is dependent on Ca^{2+}). **(D)** Long-term potentiation is dependent on NMDARs, D_1Rs, A2ARs and CB_1Rs. LTP is NMDARs dependent and is likely to involve the exocytosis of AMPA receptors. For example, LTP in the indirect pathway is negatively regulated by D_2Rs (dependent on extracellular regulated kinase; ERK) and positively regulated by adenosine A2ARs.

The direct-pathway circuit is formed by striatonigral MSNs (dMSNs) that provides mainly inhibitory inputs to both GABAergic and dopaminergic cells in substantia nigra, which in turn send axons to motor nuclei of the thalamus (Gerfen, 1992; Kreitzer and Malenka, 2008). Direct-pathway activation results in disinhibition of excitatory thalamo-cortical projections and activation of cortical premotor circuits to select/facilitate movement (Kreitzer and Malenka, 2008). The indirect-pathway is formed by striatopallidal MSNs (iMSNs) that projects to external globus pallidus GABAergic neurons (entopeduncular nucleus in rodents; EP); which exert a powerful inhibitory control into proximal dendrites of glutamatergic neurons in the subthalamic nucleus (Smith et al., 1990; Gerfen, 1992; Kreitzer and Malenka, 2008). Subthalamic nucleus neurons send excitatory afferents to inhibitory output neurons (i.e., substantia nigra) and the net effect of indirect-pathway activation is inhibition of thalamo-cortical projection neurons, which can reduce cortical premotor drive and inhibit movement (Kreitzer and Malenka, 2008) (**Figure 3C**). An intertwined function of both striatal pathways was recently proposed and postulated that the striatum would "filter" movement output integrating cortical glutamatergic and nigral dopaminergic inputs (Cui et al., 2013; Calabresi et al., 2014; Wang et al., 2015).

Cellular and synaptic organization is drastically changed in the striatum following stroke. It is likely that the striatal 'search' for different functional actions is accompanied by many structural changes. The bulk of the findings reviewed here supply abundant evidence of *where* these structural changes occur. For example, cortical lesions induce axonal sprouting in the denervated striatum (Uryu et al., 2001), dense network changes of crossed cortico-striatal projections (contralesional to ipsilesional; Napieralski et al., 1996), increased MSNs dendritic lengths (Gonzalez and Kolb, 2003), increased cortico-striatal projections and enkephalin mRNA levels (Napieralski et al., 1996; Uryu et al., 2001). Nevertheless, the post-stroke striatal 'search' task for functional actions is still poorly understood, such as *how* the striatal network would "filter" movement output integrating these novel and compensatory striatal plasticity, e.g., crossed cortico-striatal projections. Crossed cortico-striatal projections are only ≈20% of the total afferents to the contralateral striatum (Smith et al., 2016), but massive collateral sprouting from this minor projection would still be representative (Uryu et al., 2001). Interestingly, crossed cortico-striatal neurons preferentially make synapses with dMSNs, while cortico-striatal neurons with iMSNs (Cowan and Wilson, 1994; Florio et al., 2018). This suggests that the increased post-stroke crossed cortico-striatal inputs would favor movement disinhibition in the ipsilesional motor system. This can modulate excitatory outputs to thalamic neurons in the ipsilesional hemisphere that are the final pathway from the striatal system at the output level.

Endogenous Plasticity Mechanisms: "Up-" and "Down-States"

The striatum exhibits anatomo-functional complexity and intrinsic diversity, such as synaptic transmission may depend on bidirectional plasticity and spike-timing dependent plasticity (STDP). This implies that the precise relative timing and interval between presynaptic and postsynaptic action potentials determine the strength of striatal synaptic potentiation or depression (Cerovic et al., 2013; Perrin and Venance, 2019). Albeit, the role of such type of plasticity for LTP/LTD is still under debate (Lisman and Spruston, 2010). This is a very complex subject, plasticity mechanisms are variable and depend on many factors, such as: stimulation protocol, slice preparation, interplay between receptors, among others. Here, we show a simplified view of striatal plasticity mechanisms, focused on the most recent findings that relate to motor skill learning. The striatum acts as a relay nucleus, which integrates strong cortical and thalamic inputs and retransmit information via indirect thalamic projections. As aforementioned, motor skill learning modifies striatal responses during this relay process, and these changes are suggested to occur in a medial to lateral fashion (Tepper et al., 2007; Kreitzer, 2009; Yin et al., 2009). Hence, these changes in transmission affect the activity of thalamo-cortical projections and, as a consequence, motor behavior (Fisone et al., 2007). Long-lasting changes of cortico-striatal and thalamo-striatal synapses are considered to be a cellular basis of motor learning.

Striatal and thalamic reorganization following a cortical lesion are well documented. For example, Gonzalez and Kolb (2003) showed that small middle cerebral artery occlusion results in increased MSNs dendritic lengths in both hemispheres. Additionally, larger occlusions increased MSNs dendritic length in the contralesional hemisphere, but dendritic branching in the ipsilesional hemisphere (dorsolateral striatum; Gonzalez and Kolb, 2003). Interestingly, in the striatum a single EPSP from cortico-striatal glutamatergic fibers is not sufficient to depolarize MSNs to overcome the voltage-dependent Mg^{2+} blockade of NMDARs. But, in pathological conditions, such as stroke, a single excitatory input can lead to the activation of striatal NMDARs due to the "pathological" removal of the magnesium block (Calabresi et al., 2000 for references). Cortical ischemia also results in reduction of neurons, $GABA_A$ receptors and increase in NMDARs in the ipsilesional thalamus projecting to cortical damaged areas (Qu et al., 1998).

Thus, stroke disrupts cortico-striatal glutamatergic inputs in the damaged site, but also induces MSNs plasticity in both hemispheres. Glutamate has an important role on regulating striatal excitability, such as in response to glutamatergic synaptic input MSNs can transition to a depolarized "up state" near spike threshold. Short-term changes on "up-state" potentials involve KCNQ channels modulated by intrastriatal cholinergic interneurons. ACh binds to m_1Rs in MSNs and activate KCNQ channels through PLCβ/PKC pathway resulting in increased MSNs excitability (Shen et al., 2005). "Up-states" are also suggested to be linked to strong intra-striatal DA release, D_1Rs activation and striatal LTP.

Conversely, "down-states" are associated to low intra-striatal DA, D_1Rs/D_2Rs activation and striatal LTD (Calabresi et al., 1997, 2007; Shen et al., 2008). Striatal LTD reduces the activity of projecting GABAergic MSNs, and influences the output signals from the striatum to other structures that control motor activity (Calabresi et al., 1992). Skill learning and cortico-striatal LTD in the dorsolateral striatum are dependent on AC5 and cAMP signaling (Kheirbek et al., 2009). In addition, the generation of striatal LTD requires Ca^{2+} influx through voltage dependent Ca^{2+} channels, Ca^{2+}-dependent protein kinases (Calabresi et al., 1994) and synthesis of endocannabinoids (eCBs) (Cerovic et al., 2013). eCB signaling integrates signals from different neurotransmitters, such as glutamate and dopamine, with voltage gated Ca^{2+} signals (Cerovic et al., 2013). eCB-LTD is modulated by D_2Rs and dependent on postsynaptic mGluRs activation and L-type calcium channels (Kreitzer and Malenka, 2005). Similarly glutamate-LTD is also modulated by D_2Rs. For example, after high-frequency stimulation of cortico-striatal fibers, mice lacking D_2Rs shift from the expected LTD to a NMDARs-mediated LTP (Calabresi et al., 1997). Another interesting feature of striatal eCB modulation is the differential role on cortico-striatal (high [CB_1Rs]) and thalamo-striatal (low [CB_1Rs]) afferents (Wu et al., 2015). The existence of two forms of striatal LTD induced at up- and down-states (Mathur et al., 2013) and bidirectional DA modulation of eCB-LTD expression (Cui et al., 2015, 2016; Wu et al., 2015; Xu et al., 2018), reflects the complex interactions involved in striatal action control.

Skill learning activates the cortico-striatal pathway, the glutamatergic system and complex cellular mechanisms related to NMDARs activation. In rotarod trained animals, the striatal NMDARs subunit NR1 is up-regulated (D'Amours et al., 2011) and NMDARs or NR2A blockade impairs motor learning in this task in a dose-dependent manner (Lemay-Clermont et al., 2011). Additionally, Yin et al. (2009) demonstrated the medial to lateral gradient of early and late skill learning, respectively, where LTP is observed in iMSNs at the dorsolateral striatum (late skill learning), but not at dMSNs; also that early skill learning plasticity is likely non-NMDARs dependent in the dorsomedial striatum (Yin et al., 2009). Recently, this view has been challenged by a parallel (associative: medial pre-frontal cortex and dorsomedial striatum; sensorimotor: M1 and dorsolateral striatum), but dissociable, processing in cortico-striatal inputs during skill learning (Kupferschmidt et al., 2017). Kupferschmidt et al. (2017) show parallel activity in these associative and sensorimotor circuits while mice refined rotarod performance. Additionally, thalamo-striatal NMDARs-LTD plasticity is also observed in iMSNs and dMSNs (Ding et al., 2008; Ellender et al., 2013; Wu et al., 2015), further that blocking serotonergic signaling favor spike-timing-dependent LTD in dMSNs (Cavaccini et al., 2018). Finally, that presynaptic NMDARs are also involved in cortico-striatal LTP plasticity through BDNF release (Park et al., 2014), but the role of this presynaptic plasticity to stroke relearning is still underexplored. Briefly, abundant findings support the idea that skill learning experience produces changes in cortico-striatal transmission efficacy and induce the formation of sensorimotor links (see suggested reviews at the end of this section). For example, specific context-dependent patterns of cortical activity can engage selected motor programs (Mahon et al., 2004), and such changes partially depend on striatal LTP/LTD mechanisms.

State changes are also involved in striatal plasticity, such as repetitive cortico-striatal transmission during the "up-state" can overcome the threshold for NMDARs activation and, if associated with a strong release of DA, lead to LTP induction. Conversely, repetitive transmission during the "down-state," in association with low DA levels should lead to LTD (Calabresi et al., 1997, 2007; Charpier and Deniau, 1997). The circuitry of relevant motor programs would undergo plastic changes through induction of striatal LTD and LTP (Reynolds et al., 2001). Excitation of dMSNs results in the disinhibition of premotor networks, thus LTP at excitatory striatal inputs would be favorable to the initiation of movements and critical for motor learning (Charpier and Deniau, 1997; Yin et al., 2009; O'Hare et al., 2016).

Striatal cellular mechanisms involved in synaptic modulation are mainly related to presynaptic inhibition of neurotransmitter release through GPCRs (via $G_{i/o}$) and eCBs (Lovinger, 2010; Cerovic et al., 2013). Cortico-striatal terminals are controlled by presynaptic receptors, when activated can result in negative feedback on the striatal release of glutamate (Calabresi et al., 1996). As aforementioned, activation of presynaptic CB_1Rs may have distinct effects on cortico-striatal and thalamo-striatal axonal terminals, due to differential presynaptic CB_1R expression of these inputs (Wu et al., 2015) (**Figures 3C,D**). Finally, it is important to mention the role of striatal fast-spiking interneurons for experience-dependent behavior (O'Hare et al., 2018) and striatum-dependent sequence learning (via feedforward inhibition that restricts MSN bursting and calcium-dependent synaptic plasticity) (Owen et al., 2018).

Here, we highlight the main and most up-to date striatal plasticity mechanisms. This is currently a hot topic in neuroscience and several recent reviews explore this subject in depth. For example, on how (1) dopamine neurotransmission acts in concert with several neurotransmitters to regulate cortical, thalamic and limbic excitatory inputs (Surmeier et al., 2009; Bamford et al., 2018); (2) are the complex interactions between striatal plasticity and learning (Perrin and Venance, 2019); (3) are the complex computations performed by the basal ganglia circuits (Yin, 2017); (4) to clarify the relationship between neuronal plasticity in the basal ganglia and habitual behavior (with focus in kinematics of movement; O'Hare et al., 2018); (5) eCB-DA interaction affects striatal synaptic plasticity (Mathur and Lovinger, 2012); (6) genetic tools enabled new experimental protocols to reveal striatal cell types and connectivity (Silberberg and Bolam, 2015); (7) the thalamo-striatal system changes in diseased states (Smith et al., 2014). Perrin and Venance (2019) suggest that a new period of abundant and constructive debates is opened in the field of striatal plasticity. We suggest that the post-stroke recovery field should take advantage of this fruitful period to establish new mechanisms and therapies for stroke recovery.

TWO PHASES OF STROKE RECOVERY – 'FAST' AND 'SLOW' MOTOR RELEARNING

Cortical and striatal circuits work together during the development of motor skills characterized in two phases. A 'fast' improvement of motor performance with rapid behavioral outcomes, which can be observed both within a single training session and across the first few sessions. And a 'slow' improvement that develops across sessions, with more moderate gains in performance that progress across multiple training sessions (Karni et al., 1998; Kleim et al., 2004). During 'fast' motor learning cortical and striatal circuits undergo rapid and extensive recruitment with parallel activity; conversely, during 'slow' learning the activity patterns differs between structures (Costa et al., 2004). This suggests that both structures work to rapidly adapt the motor system to the new task. During 'slow' learning parallel recruitment is less often and cortical or striatal recruitment are likely associated to distinct movement features (Costa et al., 2004).

In the same line of thoughts, cortical motor representation changes do not contribute to the initial acquisition of motor skills – but represent the consolidation of motor skills that occur during the later 'slow' phase of learning (Kleim et al., 1998; Kleim et al., 2004; Krakauer and Shadmehr, 2006). This suggests that 'fast' skill improvement is related to an ongoing process, not yet consolidated intra-cortically, thus dependent on parallel striatal activity. For example, post-stroke relearning could activate a large number of cortical cells during initial stages, but with practice increase the number of cells active that correlate with the motor task (as for motor learning; Peters et al., 2014; Makino et al., 2016). This would translate in a functional motor map/engram if sufficient reinforcement of motor action render behavior habitual (Hosp and Luft, 2011).

In other words, if during this striatal 'search' task the rewiring does not elicit functional movements, the reward-related reinforcement is poor. Hence, this dysfunctional motor map should not consolidate and the striatal 'search' should continue. Recovery would rely on this parallel cortico-striatal processing until permanent and relevant changes are reinforced and stored intra-cortically. In search for spared/functional movements the striatal network attempts to integrate the remaining pieces of cortico-thalamic network. Callosal cortico-cortical connections from the contralesional homotopic motor cortex and crossed cortico-striatal connections help to direct and guide this changing network - in search for functional movements. In addition, thalamo-cortical loops relayed by the striatum have the flexibility needed for adaptation to imposed behavioral demands following motor skill training (Biane et al., 2016). Striatal 'up' and 'down' states modulated by changed glutamatergic inputs – in some regions reduced (lesion) and in others increased (compensatory connections), redirects information flow throughout the circuits. Hebbian plasticity in the associated population of cells may change synaptic strengths to favor plasticity of pathways coincidently active and eventually results in a refined ensemble and stereotyped functional behavior (Makino et al., 2016). Thus, remainings of previous loops that are disrupted by the lesion can join this novel network assisted by intense cortico-striatal parallel processing – a novel cortical representation is later formed. This idea is supported by recent findings on how optogenetic rewiring of thalamo-cortical circuits can restore function in the stroke injured brain (Tennant et al., 2017). Rehabilitation would offer the repeated opportunity to explore, select and refine impaired movements (Makino et al., 2016).

Interestingly, post-stroke, a relatively 'fast' behavioral motor recovery is followed by a plateau of 'slow' or absent recovery (62–70% proportional to the initial impairment; Jeffers et al., 2018). Rehabilitation is thought to help guidance and pruning of new connections, which due widespread activation of growth and plasticity mechanisms following the lesion may form unbalanced, non-functional connections (Murphy and Corbett, 2009). This would fit perfectly with the striatal 'search task' during relearning, adding specificity and homeostatic balance to novel functional connections. Indeed, early onset of rehabilitation during this 'fast' period consistently results in better functional outcomes (Biernaskie et al., 2004; Murphy and Corbett, 2009).

At chronic phases of 'slow' motor recovery the motor circuits would constantly modify to select and refine novel skills. How this process occurs is still unclear, it is likely that the 'fast' attempt to recover function involves the old cortical/striatal circuits, or what is left of it. It is reasonable to think that this is a less demanding homeostatic adaptation, compared to novel long-distance connections and changes of regions remote from the lesion – previously minimally involved in the motor skill.

Indeed, facilitation of LTP (1 week; Hagemann et al., 1998) and use-dependent neuronal activation (10 days; Clarke et al., 2014) in the dysfunctional perilesional cortex occur early after stroke and may indicate 'fast' changes of function in this region. Such changes are absent in homotopic contralateral areas at this early time point (Hagemann et al., 1998; Clarke et al., 2014). In chronic post-stroke, reorganization of functional circuits of parallel projecting cortical areas in the ipsilesional and contralesional hemispheres suggests that long-term or 'slow' reorganizational changes involve undamaged regions adjacent and distant to the lesion core (3–4 weeks; squirrel monkeys; Nudo et al., 1996b, 2001). Examples of such 'slow' changes include: damaged ipsilesional cortico-striatal connections that are functionally 'replaced' by increased crossed cortico-striatal projections to the denervated striatum (Cheng et al., 1998); axonal sprouting in the contralesional striatum (Uryu et al., 2001) that may be linked to increased crossed cortico-striatal projections (ipsilateral to contralateral; Napieralski et al., 1996; Uryu et al., 2001). These processes would slowly evolve during relearning of movements through striatal exploration, selection and refinement of functional movements. We suggest that these features would be part of a 'slow' compensatory relearning mechanism by which the motor function would be restored (**Figure 4**).

Are Cortical Motor Maps a Reflection of Consolidation?

Here we discuss how the motor map may reflect consolidation–reconsolidation processes. If the motor map is a reflection of consolidation of motor memories it should stabilize and persist over time. Evidence, both in humans (Ward et al., 2003; Tombari et al., 2004) and rodents (Molina-Luna et al., 2008; Reed et al., 2011), indicates that this is indeed not the case. According to the expansion-renormalization theory, learning-related neural processes often follow the sequence of

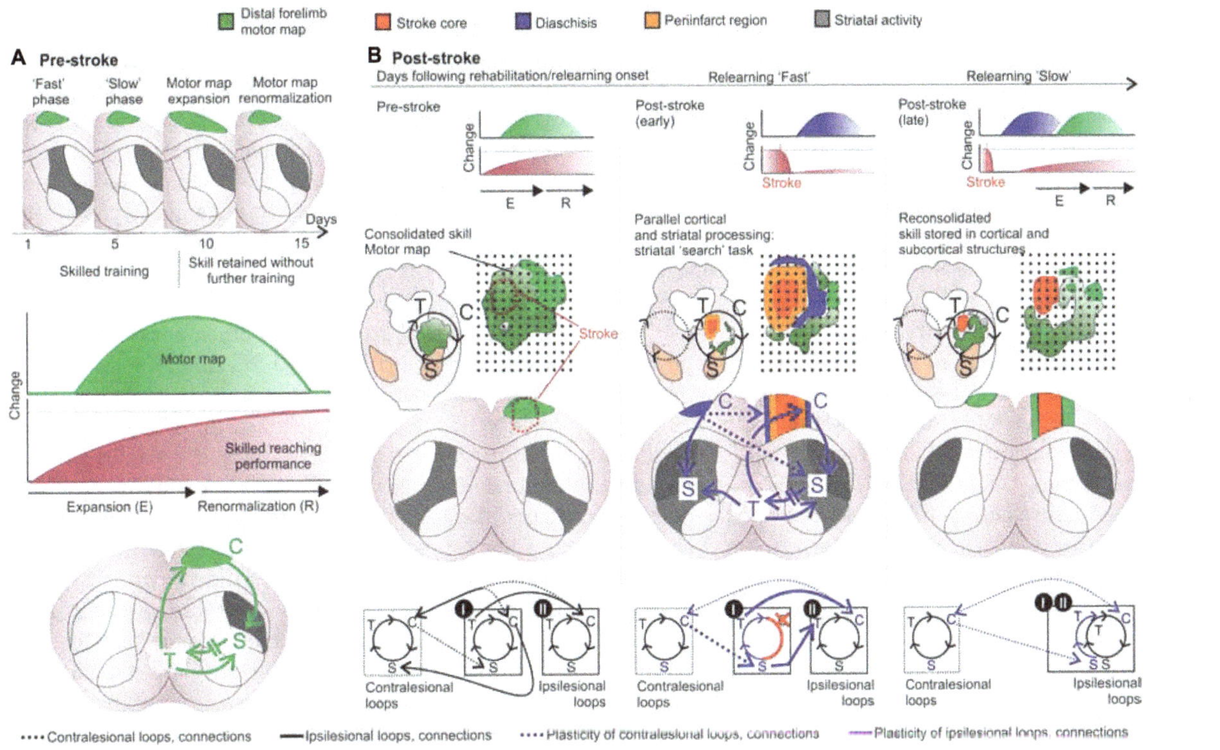

FIGURE 4 | Motor learning and post-stroke relearning. (**A**, upper and middle panels) Motor learning is divided into a fast phase, with rapid improvement in performance, and a slow phase related to a "cortical learning mode" likely involved in the consolidation of motor skills. After 8–10 days of training the motor skill is acquired and transient changes imply in motor map expansion-renormalization according to the trained skill (Kleim et al., 2003; Molina-Luna et al., 2008; Wenger et al., 2017). (**A**, lower panel) The motor map/engram is composed by the motor map of the acquired skill and by specific cortico-striatal-thalamo-cortical loops (green). (**B**, left panels) From top to bottom, the respective motor map (green) is sustained by specific cortico-striatal-thalamo-cortical loops following motor map expansion-renormalization related to the acquired skill. The loop diagram describes the ipsilesional (black lines) and crossed (black hashed lines) connections from specific cortical, striatal and thalamic regions I and II (bottom). (**B**, middle and right panels) From top to bottom, post-stroke, diaschisis may affect motor representations with, respectively, impaired skilled function. The lesion core is surrounded by dysfunctional tissue, such as periinfarct tissue (orange) and regions of focal and non-focal diaschisis (blue). Connectivity is changed and the putative participation of adjacent cortico-striatal-thalamo-cortical loops in the ipsi- and contralesional hemispheres is shown. Cortical stroke (red cross and connections) induces cellular and plastic changes (blue arrows and letters). Post-stroke cellular and plastic changes during relearning of the skilled movements may also occur in a medial to lateral fashion, similarly to motor learning and may include: increased activity in the medial portion of the ipsilesional striatum (gray); increased activity of uncrossed corticospinal fibers and of mirror-image neurons in the contralesional hemisphere (blue lines); increased activation of crossed corticostriatal fibers (blue hashed lines); short- and long-term striatal plasticity that results in increased dendritic branching and spines in the ipsi and contralesional hemispheres; the putative participation of the contralesional medial striatum during later phases of slow relearning; motor maps are reorganized and potentiated corticospinal projections to the affected muscles are available, both in the ipsi and contralesional hemispheres (i.e., crossed and uncrossed corticospinal fibers) (Pruitt et al., 2016). Connections and loops are rearranged and the newly formed motor configurations are encoded into the lateral portions of bilateral striatum. C, cortex; S, striatum; T, thalamus.

expansion, selection and renormalization (reviewed in Wenger et al., 2017). Motor map expansion may be thought as a transitory "cortical learning mode", which according to the expansion-renormalization model should subsequently refine and compact, maintaining the readiness of the learned skill (Molina-Luna et al., 2008; Wenger et al., 2017). It is reasonable to think that following motor skill learning prolonged map expansion may reduce the flexibility needed to acquire subsequent novel motor skills.

Nevertheless, several studies indicate that the motor map may encompass some features of consolidated motor memories, such as synaptogenesis (Kleim et al., 2004), susceptibility to protein synthesis inhibition (anisomycin, ANI; Kleim et al., 2003), dependence of DA (following intrastriatal 6-hydroxydopamine injections; Brown et al., 2009 – also see Hosp and Luft, 2013) and influence of cholinergic (Conner et al., 2005; Ramanathan et al., 2009) and serotonergic (Scullion et al., 2013) mechanisms. It is also the case of post-stroke motor maps, rehabilitative training may drive the reemergence and reorganization of motor maps (Nudo et al., 1996b; Conner et al., 2005; Ramanathan et al., 2006) and infusion of ANI can decrease the reorganized motor map, synaptic density and post-stroke performance improvement (Kim et al., 2018).

Similarly, studies support the role of the motor cortex for skilled behavior (Guo et al., 2015; Miri et al., 2017; Galiñanes et al., 2018), for motor learning (Peters et al., 2014) and of the somatosensory cortex for motor memory update and motor adaptation (Mathis et al., 2017). Conversely, evidence also indicates that non-dexterous motor performance is not dependent on the motor cortex (Kawai et al., 2015; Miri et al., 2017; also see Papale and Hooks, 2018). According to systems consolidation theory, at remote points the memory trace should depend more on cortical areas rather than subcortical regions (Hardt and Nadel, 2018). It is plausible to think the motor map expansion as the learning mode that further consolidate the motor memory in the complex cortico-striatal-thalamo-cortical loops. Further studies should demonstrate the role of striatal and thalamic lesions on motor maps following learned skilled behavior and in non-dexterous motor controls. In non-trained animals, motor maps are not affected by either medial or lateral striatal lesions, suggesting that motor impairments after such lesions are not simply related to motor map alterations (Karl et al., 2008). It is still to be answered if this is the case for skilled trained animals, and also for post-stroke reemergence and reorganization of motor maps. In a recent study, it was shown that striatal lesions are important for spontaneous recovery of non-skilled tasks (i.e., cylinder task) but not for dexterous reaching behavior (i.e., staircase task) (Karthikeyan et al., 2018). This is in accordance with the emerging consensus on the concept of cortical control over skilled motor behavior (Papale and Hooks, 2018).

Does motor map size really matter for consolidated motor skills? We suggest that future studies should focus more on the complexity and quality of the motor output, not strictly the size, given the above-mentioned dynamic nature of motor map size on short time scales (Molina-Luna et al., 2008; Reed et al., 2011). One suggested possibility is that M1 outputs captured by motor mapping may be necessary for driving plasticity in downstream structures or for initiating consolidation processes (Papale and Hooks, 2018). This consolidation would take place somewhere along the cortico-striatal-thalamo-cortical loops. The reflection of such consolidation should not always relate to increased size of motor representations, but to its efficiency in driving functional combinations of movements. For example, motor maps can be categorized in complex multiplanar movements such as abduction and adduction (Harrison et al., 2012; Bonazzi et al., 2013). Additionally, post-stroke emergence of abnormal movements or synergies in rats suggests that relearning may involve motor map reorganization to generate functional control of such complex movements (Balbinot et al., 2018). In our opinion this may not always be reflected by a greater size of motor representation, but to its content, such as the combination of different cortical modules for efficient post-stroke compensation.

DIASCHISIS AS A CONSOLIDATION-RECONSOLIDATION PROCESS

von Monakow's theory of diaschisis describes neurophysiological changes distant to a focal brain lesion (von Monakow, 1914; Carrera and Tononi, 2014). Accordingly, this concept posits that functional changes in brain structures remote from the site of a focal brain damage can underlie functional recovery following stroke (Witte, 1998; Seitz et al., 1999). Diaschisis can be subdivided into two types: (1 – focal diaschisis) reduction of energy metabolism at rest or during activation in anatomically intact brain regions distant from the lesion; (2 – non-focal diaschisis) change in coupling between two regions of a defined network or connectome involving areas distant from the lesion (Carrera and Tononi, 2014). For example, ipsilesional thalamic diaschisis is characterized by thalamic hypoperfusion in the acute phase of stroke patients (Reidler et al., 2018). Ginsberg et al. (1989) showed evidence of functional thalamic diaschisis following small thrombotic infarct in rats-in the form of impaired thalamo-cortical activation, in other words, thalamic activation was normal at rest but failed to exhibit the expected increment in response when stimulated. Similarly, Carmichael et al. (2004) described acute hypometabolism in a broad region of cortex adjacent to the stroke, striatum and thalamus – not related to cerebral blood flow reduction or reperfusion injury. At chronic stages, the ipsilesional cortical diaschisis still encompassed an area ≈13 times larger than the infarct (Carmichael et al., 2004). The authors suggest that the overlap of axonal sprouting and cortical hypometabolism are likely related to a process of neuronal reorganization and reconnection following stroke (Carmichael et al., 2004). Interestingly, functional diaschisis may involve reduced activation of some areas, but increased responsiveness of others (Carrera and Tononi, 2014). Suggesting that diaschisis is more than simple loss of function, but changed function of areas distant to the lesion.

Is diaschisis a cause or consequence of this process of neuronal reorganization and reconnection? It is interestingly how diaschisis occurs early following stroke and that rehabilitation optimally affect behavioral outcome also at this early time point. It is likely that diaschisis is a gross, brain wide process of reorganization, much less subtle than a reconsolidation process, for example. Albeit different, this neuronal reorganization and reconnection must involve the classical and well described mechanisms of consolidation and reconsolidation of motor memories. Motor map/engram integrity requires continuous expression of specific proteins, such as local injections of protein synthesis inhibitors (e.g., ANI, cycloheximide) results in loss of movement representations (Kleim et al., 2003). A possibility is that motor maps are constitutively plastic, its existence relies upon constant presence of specific neural signals (Monfils et al., 2005). Once stroke disrupts these specific neural signals to distant regions, the related regions change functionality. Thus, it is reasonable to think that diaschisis would not be a cause, but a consequence of neuronal reorganization and reconnection processes.

Given the aforementioned positive role of rehabilitation during this early period of changed function, it is possible that learning mechanisms can tailor this neuronal reorganization and reconnection process. In the light of the motor learning school, this process of neuronal reorganization and reconnection could be described as a process of 'rebuilding' the motor engram/map to regain function - such as during consolidation/reconsolidation of motor memories.

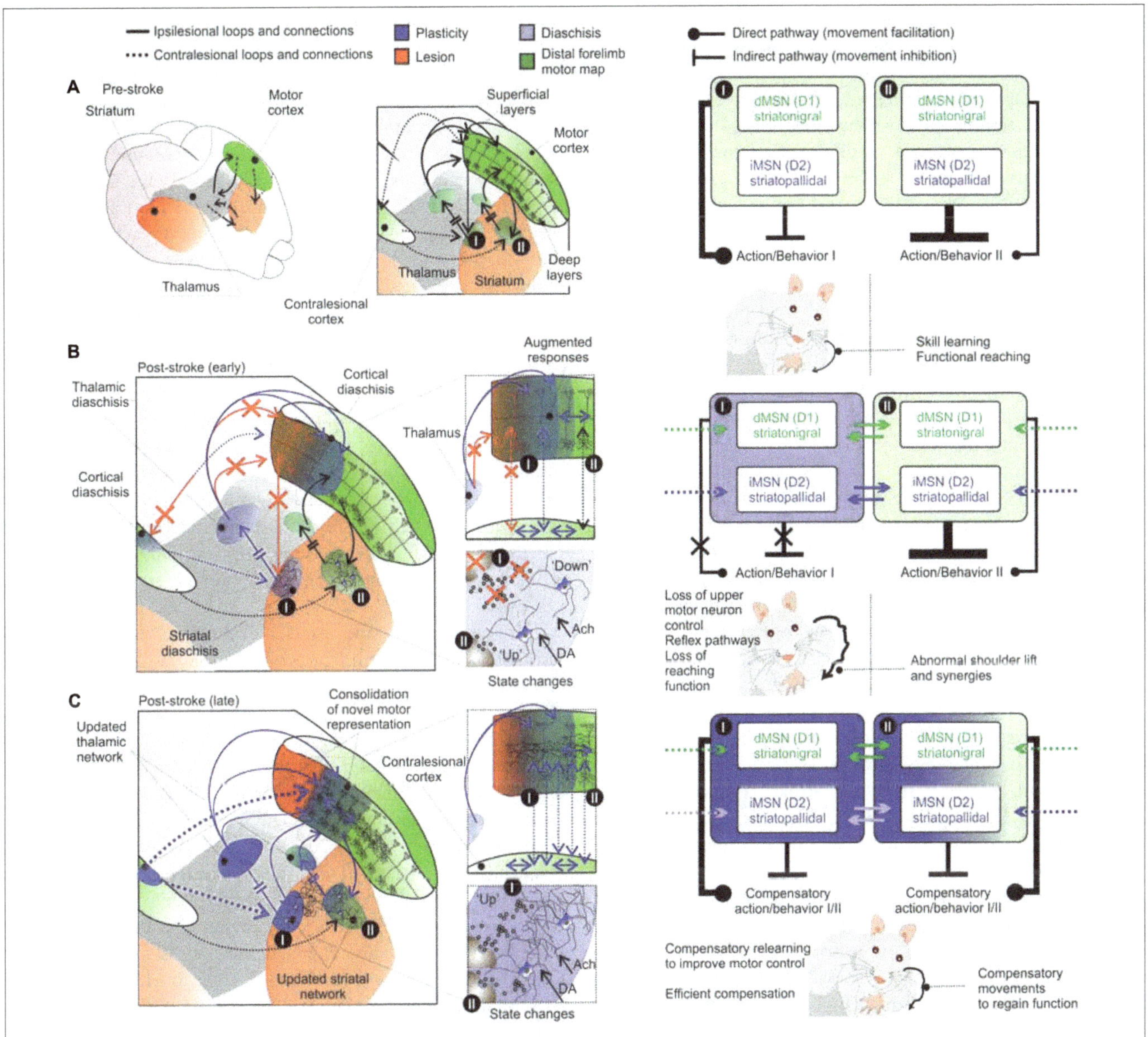

FIGURE 5 | Diaschisis as a consolidation-reconsolidation process. (**A**, left) Movement before stroke involves the selection of the appropriate motor program for the specific action (cortico-striatal-thalamo-cortical loops). (**A**, right) Specific actions are linked to specific cortico-striatal-thalamo-cortical loops. This specific functional region may control a voluntary movement, using the appropriate motor sequence for a coordinated muscular action. (**B**, left panels) Following stroke, diaschisis of regions close or distant to the infarct core (light blue) affects the functionality of the motor network and disrupts or change the specific action (red arrows: lost connections; blue and black arrows: remaining connections). (**B**, right panels) This results in loss of upper motor neuron control over voluntary movements and the emergence of abnormal movements (Balbinot et al., 2018). Compensatory relearning is unlikely to fully restitute movements of the paretic limb, which should retain some of the abnormalities and deficits in the specific action. Functional compensatory movements may be reinforced by lateral inhibition between ipsilesional MSNs (solid lines; the striatal region I influence striatal region II) and/or contralesional cortico-striatal connections (hashed lines). This reinforcement is shaped by striatal state changes and cortical plasticity. **(C)** Rehabilitation provides the recollection of visual, tactile and motor cues: the motor output is a changed action tailored over many rehabilitation sections during the "striatal search task" and the "cortical learning mode". It is likely that consolidation–reconsolidation mechanisms are slowly acting to shape these circuits during rehabilitation. Compensatory brain regions may supplement function of damaged areas and a novel motor engram is formed (dark blue) (e.g., Kim et al., 2018). The system is shaped toward the specific actions used over rehabilitation sections. Hence, the generation of a novel motor engram is supported by a series of adjustments in connections of the redundant motor system network. Right panels in **(A–C)** are inspired by a new perspective for striatal local circuitry plasticity (Burke et al., 2017). The authors explore how lateral inhibition (between MSNs) can contribute to the formation of functional units to process, integrate and filter inputs to generate motor patterns and learned behaviors (Burke et al., 2017).

Indeed, previously consolidated motor memories can undergo a labile state upon reactivation. The reactivated motor memory can be modified through reconsolidation (Walker et al., 2003; Censor et al., 2010; de Beukelaar et al., 2014, 2016). If this is the case, rehabilitation would promote such recollection of visual, tactile and spatial cues to provide cortical and striatal systems with relevant information to rebuild the motor engram. Relearning should involve the reconsolidation of previous motor loops that were not completely destroyed by the lesion, they are updated. For example, in remote regions that undewent diaschisis following stroke. Additionally, consolidation of novel compensatory motor engrams – novel connections to compensate for the loss of tissue and motor network function (**Figure 5**).

Abundant evidence of learning-like plasticity at both, close and remote regions, have been reported following stroke. For example, axonal sprouting within local projections, intra-cortical projections, long distance interhemispheric projections and cortico-striatal projections (Wilson, 1987; Lévesque et al., 1996; Carmichael and Chesselet, 2002; Carmichael, 2003). These cortical plastic changes are supported by the induction of growth-promoting genes (Brown and Murphy, 2007), also induced by motor learning (Cheung et al., 2013; Hertler et al., 2016). Striatal gene expression also occurs after a new complex motor task is memorized and most of the upregulated genes are associated with synaptic plasticity (D'Amours et al., 2011). Overall, the permissive environment following stroke leads to cortical rewiring (Winship and Murphy, 2008) and this phenomenon may be experience- and time-dependent. This suggests that plasticity, experience- and time-dependence are common attributes of both stroke recovery and consolidation-reconsolidation processes. In addition, recent evidence shows that the classic molecule CREB, involved in many learning processes, controls cortical circuit plasticity and functional recovery following stroke (Caracciolo et al., 2018). These learning-like plastic changes may relate to consolidation-reconsolidation of 'novel' or 'updated' motor engrams/maps.

Rehabilitative experience may slowly shape these new connections in a constant process of consolidation-reconsolidation of motor memories. Given the complex and continuous nature of the rehabilitation stimulus, these processes would evolve and change continuously. In other words, the consolidation-reconsolidation process of motor memories would change throughout multiple trials. This is more challenging to understand compared to declarative or fear memories that often are treated as a single trial event. Despite these differences, the understanding that recovery/relearning of movements may share the same classic mechanisms involved in learning and memory opens a new venue of timed and focused interventions during rehabilitation. For example, the timed use of learning enhancing drugs before, during or after rehabilitation sections. Or, use of protein synthesis inhibitors upon reactivation of maladaptive motor programs, such as dysfunctional compensation or learned bad-use.

CONCLUSION

Optimization of stroke recovery focused on learning mechanisms should follow the same logic of previous learning and memory studies. The fact that the motor skill redevelops slower, across multiple trials, presents a challenge for preclinical studies on the mechanisms of post-stroke compensatory relearning (Schubring-Giese et al., 2007). Recovery following stroke is related to rewiring at many corticospinal tract regions and requires *upstream* cortical commands (Lindau et al., 2014; Wahl and Schwab, 2014; Wahl et al., 2014). The deep cortico-striatal network plays a pivotal role on the selection of actions (Arber and Costa, 2018) and a putative role on selection of compensatory actions following stroke. Cortico-thalamo-cortical loops are relayed by the striatal network that is drastically changed following stroke. The denervated striatum receives increased crossed cortico-striatal connections and undergo plastic changes. In search for functional action, the striatal network participates on the reorganization of the motor system and uses spared and compensatory motor networks. As the system reorganizes, rehabilitation should induce functional compensatory movements (large lesions) or full restitution of functional movements (smaller lesions) (Murphy and Corbett, 2009; Jones, 2017). Rehabilitation therapies should focus on *how* to improve relearning.

Several cortical and striatal cellular mechanisms that influence motor learning may also influence post-stroke compensatory relearning, such as: $mGlu_5Rs$ agonists (Homayoun et al., 2004), 5-HT reuptake inhibition (McCann et al., 2014), cholinergic system manipulation to induce plasticity (Ramanathan et al., 2009; Conner et al., 2010) and improve post-stroke rehabilitation/relearning (Wang et al., 2016), dopaminergic manipulation (Ogura et al., 2005; Akita et al., 2006; Brown et al., 2009, 2011; Hosp et al., 2011; Kawashima et al., 2012; Hosp and Luft, 2013), selective manipulation of dorsolateral striatum matrix compartment (Lopez-Huerta et al., 2016), NMDARs manipulation in the dorsolateral striatum (Dang et al., 2006; Beutler et al., 2011; Lemay-Clermont et al., 2011) and modulation of FS interneurons in the dorsolateral striatum (Kao et al., 2015; Xu et al., 2016).

If the motor recovery process is directly shaped by cortical-striatal-thalamic interactions, whatever changes *downstream* must be secondary to this relearning process. For example, the importance of spinal cord (Lindau et al., 2014; Wahl et al., 2014) and red nucleus (Mosberger et al., 2018) plasticity for stroke recovery. Thus, optimizing relearning focusing on cortical-striatal-thalamic interactions is likely acting directly on the mechanism that induce learning-related plasticity both, *in site* and *downstream* to the lesion. Despite the importance of the striatum to learning, evidence of striatal participation on stroke recovery is lacking. In addition, the majority of basic stroke research studies does not fully address the role of striatal lesions and mechanisms (Edwardson et al., 2017).

In vivo recordings have changed the way we think about motor learning (Costa et al., 2004), motor recovery (Ramanathan et al., 2018) and sensorimotor representation plasticity following stroke (Harrison et al., 2013). The most pressing question facing researchers have evolved from *where* recovery occurs, to *how* it occurs. We suggest that unveiling *how* the recovery/relearning process occurs is like to take a walk on a well know path of motor learning. This path should remind us that neural activity and synaptic plasticity are constantly interacting, both at individual synapses and within neural circuits. Our challenge is to understand *how* they operate in a behaving brain to support post-stroke compensatory relearning.

AUTHOR CONTRIBUTIONS

GB wrote the manuscript and drawn the figures. CS reviewed the manuscript.

FUNDING

This work was supported by a grant from the Canadian Government - Emerging Leaders in the Americas Program (ELAP; CIC #509/2016) and by Coordenação de Aperfeiçoamento de Pessoal de Nível Superior (CAPES/Brazil).

ACKNOWLEDGMENTS

We thank Ph.D. Numa Dancause for insightful comments and directions in a previous version of this manuscript. We also thank Ph.D. Martín Cammarota and Ph.D. Adriano B.L. Tort for supervision and support, respectively.

REFERENCES

Akita, H., Ogata, M., Jitsuki, S., Ogura, T., Oh-Nishi, A., Hoka, S., et al. (2006). Nigral injection of antisense oligonucleotides to synaptotagmin I using HVJ-liposome vectors causes disruption of dopamine release in the striatum and impaired skill learning. *Brain Res.* 1095, 178–189. doi: 10.1016/j.brainres.2006.04.039

Alia, C., Spalletti, C., Lai, S., Panarese, A., Micera, S., and Caleo, M. (2016). Reducing GABAA-mediated inhibition improves forelimb motor function after focal cortical stroke in mice. *Sci. Rep.* 6:37823. doi: 10.1038/srep37823

Amitai, Y. (2001). Thalamocortical synaptic connections: efficacy, modulation, inhibition and plasticity. *Rev. Neurosci.* 12, 159–173. doi: 10.1515/REVNEURO.2001.12.2.159

Amitai, Y., and Connors, B. W. (1995). "Intrinsic physiology and morphology of single neurons in neocortex," in *The Barrel Cortex of Rodents*, eds E. G. Jones and I. Diamond (New York, NY: Plenum Press), 299–331.

Anderson, C. T., Sheets, P. L., Kir-itani, T., and Shepherd, G. M. (2010). Sublayer-specific microcircuits of corticospinal and corticostriatal neurons in motor cortex. *Nat. Neurosci.* 13, 739–744. doi: 10.1038/nn.2538

Arber, S., and Costa, R. M. (2018). Connecting neuronal circuits for movement. *Science* 360, 1403–1404. doi: 10.1126/science.aat5994

Ariano, M. A., Fisher, R. S., Smyk-Randall, E., Sibley, D. R., and Levine, M. S. (1993). D2 dopamine receptor distribution in the rodent CNS using anti-peptide antisera. *Brain Res.* 609, 71–80. doi: 10.1016/0006-8993(93)90857-J

Awenowicz, P. W., and Porter, L. L. (2002). Local application of dopamine inhibits pyramidal tract neuron activity in the rodent motor cortex. *J. Neurophysiol.* 88, 3439–3451. doi: 10.1152/jn.00078.2002

Balbinot, G., Schuch, C. P., Jeffers, M. S., McDonald, M. W., Livingston-Thomas, J. M., and Corbett, D. (2018). Post-stroke kinematic analysis in rats reveals similar reaching abnormalities as humans. *Sci. Rep.* 8:8738. doi: 10.1038/s41598-018-27101-0

Bamford, N. S., Wightman, R. M., and Sulzer, D. (2018). Dopamine's effects on corticostriatal synapses during reward-based behaviors. *Neuron* 97, 494–510. doi: 10.1016/j.neuron.2018.01.006

Beutler, L. R., Eldred, K. C., Quintana, A., Keene, C. D., Rose, S. E., Postupna, N., et al. (2011). Severely impaired learning and altered neuronal morphology in mice lacking NMDA receptors in medium spiny neurons. *PLoS One* 6:11. doi: 10.1371/journal.pone.0028168

Biane, J. S., Takashima, Y., Scanziani, M., Conner, J. M., and Tuszynski, M. H. (2016). Thalamocortical projections onto behaviorally relevant neurons exhibit plasticity during adult motor learning. *Neuron* 89, 1173–1179. doi: 10.1016/j.neuron.2016.02.001

Biernaskie, J., Chernenko, G., and Corbett, D. (2004). Efficacy of rehabilitative experience declines with time after focal ischemic brain injury. *J. Neurosci.* 24, 1245–1254. doi: 10.1523/JNEUROSCI.3834-03.2004

Biernaskie, J., and Corbett, D. (2001). Enriched rehabilitative training promotes improved forelimb motor function and enhanced dendritic growth after focal ischemic injury. *J. Neurosci.* 21, 5272–5280. doi: 10.1523/JNEUROSCI.21-14-05272.2001

Bonazzi, L., Viaro, R., Lodi, E., Canto, R., Bonifazzi, C., and Franchi, G. (2013). Complex movement topography and extrinsic space representation in the rat forelimb motor cortex as defined by long-duration intracortical microstimulation. *J. Neurosci.* 33, 2097–2107. doi: 10.1523/JNEUROSCI.3454-12.2013

Brimblecombe, K. R., and Cragg, S. J. (2015). Substance P weights striatal dopamine transmission differently within the striosome-matrix axis. *J. Neurosci.* 35, 9017–9023. doi: 10.1523/JNEUROSCI.0870-15.2015

Brown, A. R., Antle, M. C., Hu, B., and Teskey, G. C. (2011). High frequency stimulation of the subthalamic nucleus acutely rescues motor deficits and neocortical movement representations following 6-hydroxydopamine administration in rats. *Exp. Neurol.* 231, 82–90. doi: 10.1016/j.expneurol.2011.05.017

Brown, C. E., Aminoltejari, K., Erb, H., Winship, I. R., and Murphy, T. H. (2009). In vivo voltage-sensitive dye imaging in adult mice reveals that somatosensory maps lost to stroke are replaced over weeks by new structural and functional circuits with prolonged modes of activation within both the peri-infarct zone and distant sites. *J. Neurosci.* 29, 1719–1734. doi: 10.1523/JNEUROSCI.4249-08.2009

Brown, C. E., and Murphy, T. H. (2007). Livin' on the edge: imaging dendritic spine turnover in the peri-infarct zone during ischemic stroke and recovery. *Neuroscientist* 14, 139–146. doi: 10.1177/1073858407309854

Burke, D. A., Rotstein, H. G., and Alvarez, V. A. (2017). Striatal local circuitry: a new framework for lateral inhibition. *Neuron* 96, 267–284. doi: 10.1016/j.neuron.2017.09.019

Calabresi, P., Centonze, D., Gubellini, P., Marfia, G. A., Pisani, A., Sancesario, G., et al. (2000). Synaptic transmission in the striatum: from plasticity to neurodegeneration. *Prog. Neurobiol.* 61, 231–265. doi: 10.1016/S0301-0082(99)00030-1

Calabresi, P., Picconi, B., Tozzi, A., and Di Filippo, M. (2007). Dopamine-mediated regulation of corticostriatal synaptic plasticity. *Trends Neurosci.* 30, 211–219. doi: 10.1016/j.tins.2007.03.001

Calabresi, P., Picconi, B., Tozzi, A., Ghiglieri, V., and Di Filippo, M. (2014). Direct and indirect pathways of basal ganglia: a critical reappraisal. *Nat. Neurosci.* 17, 1022–1030. doi: 10.1038/nn.3743

Calabresi, P., Pisani, A., Mercuri, N. B., and Bernardi, G. (1992). Long-term potentiation in the striatum is unmasked by removing the voltage-dependent magnesium block of NMDA receptor channels. *Eur. J. Neurosci.* 4, 929–935. doi: 10.1111/j.1460-9568.1992.tb00119.x

Calabresi, P., Pisani, A., Mercuri, N. B., and Bernardi, G. (1994). Post-receptor mechanisms underlying striatal long-term depression. *J. Neurosci.* 14, 4871–4881. doi: 10.1523/JNEUROSCI.14-08-04871.1994

Calabresi, P., Pisani, A., Mercuri, N. B., and Bernardi, G. (1996). The corticostriatal projection: from synaptic plasticity to dysfunctions of the basal ganglia. *Trends Neurosci.* 19, 19–24. doi: 10.1016/0166-2236(96)81862-5

Calabresi, P., Saiardi, A., Pisani, A., Baik, J. H., Centonze, D., Mercuri, N. B., et al. (1997). Abnormal synaptic plasticity in the striatum of mice lacking dopamine

D2 receptors. *J. Neurosci.* 17, 4536–4544. doi: 10.1523/JNEUROSCI.17-12-04536.1997

Caracciolo, L., Marosi, M., Mazzitelli, J., Latifi, S., Sano, Y., Galvan, L., et al. (2018). CREB controls cortical circuit plasticity and functional recovery after stroke. *Nat. Commun.* 9:2250. doi: 10.1038/s41467-018-04445-9

Carmichael, S. T. (2003). Plasticity of cortical projections after stroke. *Neuroscientist* 9, 64–75. doi: 10.1177/1073858402239592

Carmichael, S. T., Archibeque, I., Luke, L., Nolan, T., Momiy, J., and Li, S. (2005). Growth-associated gene expression after stroke: evidence for a growth-promoting region in peri-infarct cortex. *Exp. Neurol.* 193, 291–311. doi: 10.1016/j.expneurol.2005.01.004

Carmichael, S. T., and Chesselet, M. F. (2002). Synchronous neuronal activity is a signal for axonal sprouting after cortical lesions in the adult. *J. Neurosci.* 22, 6062–6070. doi: 10.1523/JNEUROSCI.22-14-06062.2002

Carmichael, S. T., Tatsukawa, K., Katsman, D., Tsuyuguchi, N., and Kornblum, H. I. (2004). Evolution of diaschisis in a focal stroke model. *Stroke* 35, 758–763. doi: 10.1161/01.STR.0000117235.11156.55

Carregosa, A. A., Aguiar Dos Santos, L. R., Masruha, M. R., Coêlho, M. L. D. S., Machado, T. C., Souza, D. C. B., et al. (2018). Virtual rehabilitation through Nintendo Wii in poststroke patients: follow-up. *J. Stroke Cerebrovasc. Dis.* 27, 494–498. doi: 10.1016/j.jstrokecerebrovasdis.2017.09.029

Carrera, E., and Tononi, G. (2014). Diaschisis: past, present, future. *Brain* 137(Pt 9), 2408–2422. doi: 10.1093/brain/awu101

Castro-Alamancos, M. A., and Borrell, J. (1995). Contribution of NMDA and nonNMDA glutamate receptors to synchronized excitation and cortical output in the primary motor cortex of the rat. *Brain Res. Bull.* 37, 539–543. doi: 10.1016/0361-9230(95)00059-N

Castro-Alamancos, M. A., and Connors, B. W. (1996a). Cellular mechanisms of the augmenting response: short-term plasticity in a thalamocortical pathway. *J. Neurosci.* 16, 7742–7756.

Castro-Alamancos, M. A., and Connors, B. W. (1996b). Short-term plasticity of a thalamocortical pathway dynamically modulated by behavioral state. *Science* 272, 274–277.

Castro-Alamancos, M. A., and Connors, B. W. (1996c). Spatiotemporal properties of short-term plasticity sensorimotor thalamocortical pathways of the rat. *J. Neurosci.* 16, 2767–2779.

Castro-Alamancos, M. A., and Connors, B. W. (1997). Thalamocortical synapses. *Prog. Neurobiol.* 6, 581–606. doi: 10.1016/S0301-0082(97)00002-6

Cavaccini, A., Gritti, M., Giorgi, A., Locarno, A., Heck, N., Migliarini, S., et al. (2018). Serotonergic signaling controls input-specific synaptic plasticity at striatal circuits. *Neuron* 98, 801.e7–816.e7. doi: 10.1016/j.neuron.2018.04.008

Celada, P., Puig, M. V., and Artigas, F. (2013). Serotonin modulation of cortical neurons and networks. *Front. Integr. Neurosci.* 7:25. doi: 10.3389/fnint.2013.00025

Censor, N., Dimyan, M. A., and Cohen, L. G. (2010). Modification of existing human motor memories is enabled by primary cortical processing during memory reactivation. *Curr. Biol.* 20, 1545–1549. doi: 10.1016/j.cub.2010.07.047

Cerovic, M., D'Isa, R., Tonini, R., and Brambilla, R. (2013). Molecular and cellular mechanisms of dopamine-mediated behavioral plasticity in the striatum. *Neurobiol. Learn. Mem.* 105, 63–80. doi: 10.1016/j.nlm.2013.06.013

Chapman, C. A., Trepel, C., Ivanco, T. L., Froc, D. J., Wilson, K., and Racine, R. J. (1998). Changes in field potentials and membrane currents in rat sensorimotor cortex following repeated tetanization of the corpus callosum in vivo. *Cereb. Cortex* 8, 730–742. doi: 10.1093/cercor/8.8.730

Charpier, S., and Deniau, J. M. (1997). In vivo activity-dependent plasticity at cortico-striatal connections: evidence for physiological long-term potentiation. *Proc. Natl. Acad. Sci. U.S.A.* 94, 7036–7040. doi: 10.1073/pnas.94.13.7036

Cheng, H. W., Tong, J., and McNeill, T. H. (1998). Ultrastructural evidence for cortical axon sprouting in the deafferented striatum of adult rat. *Neurosci. Lett.* 241, 1–4.

Cheung, V. C., Deboer, C., Hanson, E., Tunesi, M., D'Onofrio, M., Arisi, I., et al. (2013). Gene expression changes in the motor cortex mediating motor skill learning. *PLoS One* 8:e61496. doi: 10.1371/journal.pone.0061496

Clarke, J., Langdon, K. D., and Corbett, D. (2014). Early poststroke experience differentially alters periinfarct layer II and III cortex. *J. Cereb. Blood Flow Metab.* 34, 630–637. doi: 10.1038/jcbfm.2013.237

Cohen, J. D., and Castro-Alamancos, M. A. (2005). Skilled motor learning does not enhance long-term depression in the motor cortex in vivo. *J. Neurophysiol.* 93, 1486–1497. doi: 10.1152/jn.00958.2004

Conn, J. P., and Pin, J. P. (1997). Pharmacology and functions of metabotropic glutamate receptors. *Ann. Rev. Pharmacol. Toxicol.* 37, 205–237. doi: 10.1146/annurev.pharmtox.37.1.205

Conner, J. M., Chiba, A. A., and Tuszynski, M. H. (2005). The basal forebrain cholinergic system is essential for cortical plasticity and functional recovery following brain injury. *Neuron* 46, 173–179. doi: 10.1016/j.neuron.2005.03.003

Conner, J. M., Culberson, A., Packowski, C., Chiba, A. A., and Tuszynski, M. H. (2003). Lesions of the basal forebrain cholinergic system impair task acquisition and abolish cortical plasticity associated with motor skill learning. *Neuron* 38, 819–829. doi: 10.1016/S0896-6273(03)00288-5

Conner, J. M., Kulczycki, M., and Tuszynski, M. H. (2010). Unique contributions of distinct cholinergic projections to motor cortical plasticity and learning. *Cereb. Cortex* 20, 2739–2748. doi: 10.1093/cercor/bhq022

Cortés, R., and Palacios, J. M. (1986). Muscarinic cholinergic receptor subtypes in the rat brain. I. Quantitative autoradiographic studies. *Brain Res.* 362, 227–238. doi: 10.1016/0006-8993(86)90448-8

Costa, R. M., Cohen, D., and Nicolelis, M. A. (2004). Differential corticostriatal plasticity during fast and slow motor skill learning in mice. *Curr. Biol.* 14, 1124–1134. doi: 10.1016/j.cub.2004.06.053

Cowan, R. L., and Wilson, C. J. (1994). Spontaneous firing patterns and axonal projections of single corticostriatal neurons in the rat medial agranular cortex. *J. Neurophysiol.* 71, 17–32. doi: 10.1152/jn.1994.71.1.17

Cui, G., Jun, S. B., Jin, X., Pham, M. D., Vogel, S. S., Lovinger, D. M., et al. (2013). Concurrent activation of striatal direct and indirect pathways during action initiation. *Nature* 494, 238–242. doi: 10.1038/nature11846

Cui, Y., Paillé, V., Xu, H., Genet, S., Delord, B., Fino, E., et al. (2015). Endocannabinoids mediate bidirectional striatal spike-timing-dependent plasticity. *J. Physiol.* 593, 2833–2849. doi: 10.1113/JP270324

Cui, Y., Prokin, I., Xu, H., Delord, B., Genet, S., Venance, L., et al. (2016). Endocannabinoid dynamics gate spike- timing dependent depression and potentiation. *eLife* 5:e13185. doi: 10.7554/eLife.13185

D'Amours, G., Bureau, G., Boily, M. J., and Cyr, M. (2011). Differential gene expression profiling in the mouse brain during motor skill learning: focus on the striatum structure. *Behav. Brain Res.* 221, 108–117. doi: 10.1016/j.bbr.2011.02.030

Dancause, N. (2006). Vicarious function of remote cortex following stroke: recent evidence from human and animal studies. *Neuroscientist* 12, 489–499. doi: 10.1177/1073858406292782

Dancause, N., Touvykine, B., and Mansoori, B. (2015). Inhibition of the contralesional hemisphere after stroke: reviewing a few of the building blocks with a focus on animal models. *Prog. Brain Res.* 218, 361–387. doi: 10.1016/bs.pbr.2015.01.002

Dang, M. T., Yokoi, F., Yin, H. H., Lovinger, D. M., Wang, Y., and Li, Y. (2006). Disrupted motor learning and long-term synaptic plasticity in mice lacking NMDAR1 in the striatum. *Proc. Natl. Acad. Sci. U.S.A.* 103, 15254–15259. doi: 10.1073/pnas.0601758103

Davis, M. I., Crittenden, J. R., Feng, A. Y., Kupferschmidt, D. A., Naydenov, A., Stella, N., et al. (2018). The cannabinoid-1 receptor is abundantly expressed in striatal striosomes and striosome-dendron bouquets of the substantia nigra. *PLoS One* 13:e0191436. doi: 10.1371/journal.pone.0191436

de Beukelaar, T. T., Woolley, D. G., Alaerts, K., Swinnen, S. P., and Wenderoth, N. (2016). Reconsolidation of motor memories is a time-dependent process. *Front. Hum. Neurosci.* 10:408. doi: 10.3389/fnhum.2016.00408

de Beukelaar, T. T., Woolley, D. G., and Wenderoth, N. (2014). Gone for 60 seconds: reactivation length determines motor memory degradation during reconsolidation. *Cortex* 59, 138–145. doi: 10.1016/j.cortex.2014.07.008

Ding, J., Peterson, J. D., and Surmeier, D. J. (2008). Corticostriatal and thalamostriatal synapses have distinctive properties. *J. Neurosci.* 28, 6483–6492. doi: 10.1523/JNEUROSCI.0435-08.2008

Ding, J. B., Guzman, J. N., Peterson, J. D., Goldberg, J. A., and Surmeier, D. J. (2010). Thalamic gating of corticostriatal signaling by cholinergic interneurons. *Neuron* 67, 294–307. doi: 10.1016/j.neuron.2010.06.017

Donoghue, J. P., and Kitai, S. T. (1981). A collateral pathway to the neostriatum from corticofugal neurons of the rat sensorimotor cortex: an intracellular study. *J. Comp. Neurol.* 201, 1–13. doi: 10.1002/cne.902010102

Edwardson, M. A., Wang, X., Liu, B., Ding, L., Lane, C. J., Park, C., et al. (2017). Stroke lesions in a large upper limb rehabilitation trial cohort rarely match lesions in common preclinical models. *Neurorehabil. Neural Repair* 31, 509–520. doi: 10.1177/1545968316688799

Ellender, T. J., Harwood, J., Kosillo, P., Capogna, M., and Bolam, J. P. (2013). Heterogeneous properties of central lateral and parafascicular thalamic synapses in the striatum. *J. Physiol.* 591, 257–272. doi: 10.1113/jphysiol.2012.245233

Feldman, M. L. (1984). "Morphology of the neocortical pyramidal neuron," in *Cellular Components of the Cerebral Cortex*, eds A. Peters and E. G. Jones (New York, NY: Plenum Press), 123–200.

Ferraguti, F., and Shigemoto, R. (2006). Metabotropic glutamate receptors. *Cell Tissue Res.* 326, 483–504. doi: 10.1007/s00441-006-0266-5

Fisone, G., Hakansson, K., Borgkvist, A., and Santini, E. (2007). Signaling in the basal ganglia: postsynaptic and presynaptic mechanisms. *Physiol. Behav.* 92, 8–14. doi: 10.1016/j.physbeh.2007.05.028

Florio, T. M., Scarnati, E., Rosa, I., Di Censo, D., Ranieri, B., Cimini, A., et al. (2018). The basal ganglia: more than just a switching device. *CNS Neurosci. Ther.* 24, 677–684. doi: 10.1111/cns.12987

Frey, K. A., and Howland, M. M. (1992). Quantitative autoradiography of muscarinic cholinergic receptor binding in the rat brain: distinction of receptor subtypes in antagonist competition assays. *J. Pharmacol. Exp. Ther.* 263, 1391–1400.

Fuentes, M. A., Borrego, A., Latorre, J., Colomer, C., Alcañiz, M., Sánchez-Ledesma, M. J., et al. (2018). Combined transcranial direct current stimulation and virtual reality-based paradigm for upper limb rehabilitation in individuals with restricted movements. A feasibility study with a chronic stroke survivor with severe hemiparesis. *J. Med. Syst.* 42:87. doi: 10.1007/s10916-018-0949-y

Galiñanes, G. L., Bonardi, C., and Huber, D. (2018). Directional reaching for water as a cortex-dependent behavioral framework for mice. *Cell Rep.* 22, 2601–2614. doi: 10.1016/j.celrep.2018.02.042

Gaspar, P., Bloch, B., and Le Moine, C. (1995). D1 and D2 receptor gene expression in the rat frontal cortex: cellular localization in different classes of efferent neurons. *Eur. J. Neurosci.* 7, 1050–1063. doi: 10.1111/j.1460-9568.1995.tb01092.x

Gerfen, C. R. (1989). The neostriatal mosaic: striatal patch-matrix organization is related to cortical lamination. *Science* 246, 385–388. doi: 10.1126/science.2799392

Gerfen, C. R. (1992). The neostriatal mosaic: multiple levels of compartmental organization in the basal ganglia. *Annu. Rev. Neurosci.* 15, 285–320. doi: 10.1146/annurev.ne.15.030192.001441

Ginsberg, M. D., Castella, Y., Dietrich, W. D., Watson, B. D., and Busto, R. (1989). Acute thrombotic infarction suppresses metabolic activation of ipsilateral somatosensory cortex: evidence for functional diaschisis. *J. Cereb. Blood Flow Metab.* 9, 329–341. doi: 10.1038/jcbfm.1989.51

Gonzalez, C. L., and Kolb, B. (2003). A comparison of different models of stroke on behaviour and brain morphology. *Eur. J. Neurosci.* 18, 1950–1962. doi: 10.1046/j.1460-9568.2003.02928.x

Graybiel, A. M. (1995). Building action repertoires: memory and learning functions of the basal ganglia. *Curr. Opin. Neurobiol.* 5, 733–741. doi: 10.1016/0959-4388(95)80100-6

Greenough, W. T., Larson, J. R., and Withers, G. S. (1985). Effects of unilateral and bilateral training in a reaching task on dendritic branching of neurons in the rat motor-sensory forelimb cortex. *Behav. Neural Biol.* 44, 301–314. doi: 10.1016/S0163-1047(85)90310-3

Greig, L. F. C., Woodworth, M. B., Galazo, M. J., Padmanabhan, H., and Macklis, J. D. (2013). Molecular logic of neocortical projection neuron specification, development and diversity. *Nat. Rev. Neurosci.* 14, 755–769. doi: 10.1038/nrn3586

Grimm, F., Naros, G., and Gharabaghi, A. (2016). Closed-loop task difficulty adaptation during virtual reality reach-to-grasp training assisted with an exoskeleton for stroke rehabilitation. *Front. Neurosci.* 10:518. doi: 10.3389/fnins.2016.00518

Gulledge, A. T., and Jaffe, D. B. (2001). Multiple effects of dopamine on layer V pyramidal cell excitability in rat prefrontal cortex. *J. Neurophysiol.* 86, 586–595. doi: 10.1152/jn.2001.86.2.586

Guo, J. Z., Graves, A. R., Guo, W. W., Zheng, J., Lee, A., Rodríguez-Gonzá, J., et al. (2015). Cortex commands the performance of skilled movement. *eLife* 4:e10774. doi: 10.7554/eLife.10774

Guy, J., and Staiger, J. F. (2017). The functioning of a cortex without layers. *Front. Neuroanat.* 11:54. doi: 10.3389/fnana.2017.00054

Haber, S. N., and Calzavara, R. (2009). The cortico-basal ganglia integrative network: the role of the thalamus. *Brain Res. Bull.* 78, 69–74. doi: 10.1016/j.brainresbull.2008.09.013

Hagemann, G., Redecker, C., Neumann-Haefelin, T., Freund, H. J., and Witte, O. W. (1998). Increased long-term potentiation in the surround of experimentally induced focal cortical infarction. *Ann. Neurol.* 44, 255–258. doi: 10.1002/ana.410440217

Hardt, O., and Nadel, L. (2018). Systems consolidation revisited, but not revised: the promise and limits of optogenetics in the study of memory. *Neurosci. Lett.* 680, 54–59. doi: 10.1016/j.neulet.2017.11.062

Harrison, T. C., Ayling, O. G. S., and Murphy, T. H. (2012). Distinct cortical circuit mechanisms for complex forelimb movement and motor map topography. *Neuron* 74, 397–409. doi: 10.1016/j.neuron.2012.02.028

Harrison, T. C., Silasi, G., Boyd, J. D., and Murphy, T. H. (2013). Displacement of sensory maps and disorganization of motor cortex after targeted stroke in mice. *Stroke* 44, 2300–2306. doi: 10.1161/STROKEAHA.113.001272

Hatem, S. M., Saussez, G., della Faille, M., Prist, V., Zhang, X., Dispa, D., et al. (2016). Rehabilitation of motor function after stroke: a multiple systematic review focused on techniques to stimulate upper extremity recovery. *Front. Hum. Neurosci.* 10:442. doi: 10.3389/fnhum.2016.0044

Heilbronner, S. R., Rodriguez-Romaguera, J., Quirk, G. J., Groenewegen, H. J., and Haber, S. N. (2016). Circuit based cortico-striatal homologies between rat and primate. *Biol. Psychiatry* 80, 509–521. doi: 10.1016/j.biopsych.2016.05.012

Hertler, B., Buitrago, M. M., Luft, A. R., and Hosp, J. A. (2016). Temporal course of gene expression during motor memory formation in primary motor cortex of rats. *Neurobiol. Learn. Mem.* 136, 105–115. doi: 10.1016/j.nlm.2016.09.018

Hess, G., Aizenman, C. D., and Donoghue, J. P. (1996). Conditions for the induction of long-term potentiation in layer II/III horizontal connections of the rat motor cortex. *J. Neurophysiol.* 75, 1765–1778. doi: 10.1152/jn.1996.75.5.1765

Hess, G., and Donoghue, J. P. (1994). Long-term potentiation of horizontal connections provides a mechanism to reorganize cortical motor maps. *J. Neurophysiol.* 71, 2543–2547. doi: 10.1152/jn.1994.71.6.2543

Hjornevik, T. (2007). Three-dimensional atlas system for mouse and rat brain imaging data. *Front. Neuroinform.* 1:4. doi: 10.3389/neuro.11.004.2007

Homayoun, H., Stefani, M. R., Adams, B. W., Tamagan, G. D., and Moghaddam, B. (2004). Functional interaction between NMDA and mGlu5 receptors: effects on working memory, instrumental learning, motor behaviors, and dopamine release. *Neuropsychopharmacology* 29, 1259–1269. doi: 10.1038/sj.npp.1300417

Hosp, J., and Luft, A. R. (2013). Dopaminergic meso-cortical projections to M1: role in motor learning and motor cortex plasticity. *Front. Neurol.* 4:145. doi: 10.3389/fneur.2013.00145

Hosp, J. A., and Luft, A. R. (2011). Cortical plasticity during motor learning and recovery after ischemic stroke. *Neural Plast.* 2011:871296. doi: 10.1155/2011/871296

Hosp, J. A., Pekanovic, A., Rioult-Pedotti, M. S., and Luft, A. R. (2011). Dopaminergic projections from midbrain to primary motor cortex mediate motor skill learning. *J. Neurosci.* 31, 2481–2487. doi: 10.1523/JNEUROSCI.5411-10.2011

Hunnicutt, B. J., Jongbloets, B. C., Birdsong, W. T., Gertz, K. J., Zhong, H., and Mao, T. (2016). A comprehensive excitatory input map of the striatum reveals novel functional organization. *eLife* 5:e19103. doi: 10.7554/eLife.19103

Jankowska, E., Padel, Y., and Tanaka, R. (1975). Projections of pyramidal tract cells to alpha motoneurons innervating hindlimb muscles in the monkey. *J. Physiol.* 249, 637–667. doi: 10.1113/jphysiol.1975.sp011035

Jeffers, M., Karthikeyan, S., and Corbett, D. (2018). Does stroke rehabilitation really matter? Part A: proportional stroke recovery in the rat. *Neurorehabil. Neural Repair* 32, 3–6. doi: 10.1177/1545968317751210

Johnston, J. G., Gerfen, C. R., Haber, S. N., and van der Kooy, D. (1990). Mechanisms of striatal pattern formation: conservation of mammalian compartmentalization. *Brain Res. Dev. Brain Res.* 57, 93–102. doi: 10.1016/0165-3806(90)90189-6

Jones, T. A. (2017). Motor compensation and its effects on neural reorganization after stroke. *Nat. Rev. Neurosci.* 8, 267–280. doi: 10.1038/nrn.2017.26

Kaneko, T. (2013). Local connections of excitatory neurons in motor-associated cortical areas of the rat. *Front. Neural Circuits* 7:75. doi: 10.3389/fncir.2013.00075

Kao, F. C., Su, S. H., Carlson, G. C., and Liao, W. (2015). MeCP2-mediated alterations of striatal features accompany psychomotor deficits in a mouse model of Rett syndrome. *Brain Struct. Funct.* 220, 419–434. doi: 10.1007/s00429-013-0664-x

Karl, J. M., Sacrey, L. A. R., McDonald, R. J., and Whishaw, I. Q. (2008). Intact intracortical microstimulation (ICMS) representations of rostral and caudal forelimb areas in rats with quinolinic acid lesions of the medial or lateral caudate-putamen in an animal model of Huntington's disease. *Brain Res. Bull.* 77, 42–48. doi: 10.1016/j.brainresbull.2008.04.012

Karni, A., Meyer, G., Rey-Hipolito, C., Jezzard, P., Adams, M. M., Turner, R., et al. (1998). The acquisition of skilled motor performance: fast and slow experience-driven changes in primary motor cortex. *Proc. Natl. Acad. Sci. U.S.A.* 95, 861–868. doi: 10.1073/pnas.95.3.861

Karthikeyan, S., Jeffers, M. S., Carter, A., and Corbett, D. (2018). Characterizing spontaneous motor recovery following cortical and subcortical stroke in the rat. *Neurorehabil. Neural Repair* doi: 10.1177/1545968318817823 [Epub ahead of print].

Kawaguchi, Y., and Shindou, T. (1998). Noradrenergic excitation and inhibition of GABAergic cell types in rat frontal cortex. *J. Neurosci.* 18, 6963–6976. doi: 10.1523/JNEUROSCI.18-17-06963.1998

Kawai, R., Markman, T., Poddar, R., Ko, R., Fantana, A. L., Dhawale, A. K., et al. (2015). Motor cortex is required for learning but not for executing a motor skill. *Neuron* 86, 800–812. doi: 10.1016/j.neuron.2015.03.024

Kawashima, S., Ueki, Y., Kato, T., Matsukawa, N., Mima, T., Hallett, M., et al. (2012). Changes in striatal dopamine release associated with human motor-skill acquisition. *PLoS One* 7:e31728. doi: 10.1371/journal.pone.0031728

Kemp, J. M., and Powell, T. P. (1971). The termination of fibres from the cerebral cortex and thalamus upon dendritic spines in the caudate nucleus: a study with the Golgi method. *Philos. Trans. R. Soc. Lond. B Biol. Sci.* 262, 429–439. doi: 10.1098/rstb.1971.0105

Kerner, J. A., Standaert, D. G., Penney, J. B., Young, A. B., and Landwehrmeyer, G. B. (1997). Expression of group one metabotropic glutamate receptor subunit mRNAs in neurochemically identified neurons in the rat neostriatum, neocortex, and hippocampus. *Brain Res. Mol. Brain Res.* 48, 259–269. doi: 10.1016/S0169-328X(97)00102-2

Kheirbek, M. A., Britt, J. P., Beeler, J. A., Ishikawa, Y., McGehee, D. S., and Zhuang, X. (2009). Adenylyl cyclase type 5 contributes to corticostriatal plasticity and striatum-dependent learning. *J. Neurosci.* 29, 12115–12124. doi: 10.1523/JNEUROSCI.3343-09.2009

Kim, S. Y., Hsu, J. E., Husbands, L. C., Kleim, J. A., and Jones, T. A. (2018). Coordinated plasticity of synapses and astrocytes underlies practice-driven functional vicariation in peri-infarct motor cortex. *J. Neurosci.* 38, 93–107. doi: 10.1523/JNEUROSCI.1295-17.2017

Kincaid, A. E., and Wilson, C. J. (1996). Corticostriatal innervation of the patch and matrix in the rat neostriatum. *J. Comp. Neurol.* 374, 578–592. doi: 10.1002/(SICI)1096-9861(19961028)374:4<578::AID-CNE7>3.0.CO;2-Z

Kleim, J. A., Barbay, S., and Nudo, R. J. (1998). Functional reorganization of the rat motor cortex following motor skill learning. *J. Neurophysiol.* 80, 3321–3325. doi: 10.1152/jn.1998.80.6.3321

Kleim, J. A., Bruneau, R., Calder, K., Pocock, D., VandenBerg, P. M., MacDonald, E., et al. (2003). Functional organization of adult motor cortex is dependent upon continued protein synthesis. *Neuron* 40, 167–176. doi: 10.1016/S0896-6273(03)00592-0

Kleim, J. A., Hogg, T. M., VandenBerg, P. M., Cooper, N. R., Bruneau, R., and Remple, M. (2004). Cortical synaptogenesis and motor map reorganization occur during late, but not early, phase of motor skill learning. *J. Neurosci.* 24, 628–633. doi: 10.1523/JNEUROSCI.3440-03.2004

Kolb, B., Cioe, J., and Comeau W. (2008). Contrasting effects of motor and visual spatial learning tasks on dendritic arborization and spine density in rats. *Neurobiol. Learn. Mem.* 90, 295–300. doi: 10.1016/j.nlm.2008.04.012

Korchounov, A., and Ziemann, U. (2011). Neuromodulatory neurotransmitters influence LTP-like plasticity in human cortex: a pharmaco-TMS study. *Neuropsychopharmacology* 36, 1894–1902. doi: 10.1038/npp.2011.75

Krakauer, J. W. (2006). Motor learning: its relevance to stroke recovery and neurorehabilitation. *Curr. Opin. Neurol.* 19, 84–90. doi: 10.1097/01.wco.0000200544.29915.cc

Krakauer, J. W., Carmichael, S. T., Corbett, D., and Wittenberg, G. F. (2012). Getting neurorehabilitation right: what can be learned from animal models? *Neurorehabil. Neural Repair* 26, 923–931. doi: 10.1177/1545968312440745

Krakauer, J. W., and Shadmehr, R. (2006). Consolidation of motor memory. *Trends Neurosci.* 29, 58–64. doi: 10.1016/j.tins.2005.10.003

Kreitzer, A. C. (2009). Physiology and pharmacology of striatal neurons. *Annu. Rev. Neurosci.* 32, 127–147. doi: 10.1146/annurev.neuro.051508.135422

Kreitzer, A. C., and Malenka, R. C. (2005). Dopamine modulation of state-dependent endocannabinoid release and long-term depression in the striatum. *J. Neurosci.* 25, 10537–10545. doi: 10.1523/JNEUROSCI.2959-05.2005

Kreitzer, A. C., and Malenka, R. C. (2008). Striatal plasticity and basal ganglia circuit function. *Neuron* 60, 543–554. doi: 10.1016/j.neuron.2008.11.005

Kupferschmidt, D. A., Juczewski, K., Cui, G., Johnson, K. A., and Lovinger, D. M. (2017). Parallel, but dissociable, processing in discrete corticostriatal inputs encodes skill learning. *Neuron* 96, 476.e5–489.e5. doi: 10.1016/j.neuron.2017.09.040

Kuramoto, E., Furuta, T., Nakamura, K. C., Unzai, T., Hioki, H., and Kaneko, T. (2009). Two types of thalamocortical projections from themotor thalamic nuclei of the rat: a single neuron-tracing study using viral vectors. *Cereb. Cortex* 19, 2065–2077. doi: 10.1093/cercor/bhn231

Lança, A. J., Boyd, S., Kolb, B. E., and van der Kooy, D. (1986). The development of a patchy organization of the rat striatum. *Dev. Brain Res.* 27, 1–10. doi: 10.1016/0165-3806(86)90226-9

Lemay-Clermont, J., Robitaille, C., Auberson, Y. P., Bureau, G., and Cyr, M. (2011). Blockade of NMDA receptors 2A subunit in the dorsal striatum impairs the learning of a complex motor skill. *Behav. Neurosci.* 125, 714–723. doi: 10.1037/a0025213

Lévesque, M., Charara, A., Gagnon, S., Parent, A., and Deschênes, M. (1996). Corticostriatal projections from layer V cells in rat are collaterals of long-range corticofugal axons. *Brain Res.* 709, 311–315. doi: 10.1016/0006-8993(95)01333-4

Leyva-Díaz, E., and López-Bendito, G. (2013). In and out from the cortex: development of major forebrain connections. *Neuroscience* 254, 26–44. doi: 10.1016/j.neuroscience.2013.08.070

Li, Y., Jiang, N., Powers, C., and Chopp, M. (1998). Neuronal damage and plasticity identified by microtubule-associated protein 2, growth-associated protein 43, and cyclin D1 immunoreactivity after focal cerebral ischemia in rats. *Stroke* 29, 1972–1998. doi: 10.1161/01.STR.29.9.1972

Lim, S. A., Kang, U. J., and McGehee, D. S. (2014). Striatal cholinergic interneuron regulation and circuit effects. *Front. Synaptic Neurosci.* 6:22. doi: 10.3389/fnsyn.2014.00022

Lindau, N. T., Bänninger, B. J., Gullo, M., Good, N. A., Bachmann, L. C., Starkey, M. L., et al. (2014). Rewiring of the corticospinal tract in the adult rat after unilateral stroke and anti-Nogo-A therapy. *Brain* 137(Pt 3), 739–756. doi: 10.1093/brain/awt336

Lisman, J., and Spruston, N. (2010). Questions about STDP as a general model of synaptic plasticity. *Front. Synaptic Neurosci.* 2:140. doi: 10.3389/fnsyn.2010.00140

Lopez-Huerta, V. G., Nakano, Y., Bausenwein, J., Jaidar, O., Lazarus, M., Cherassse, Y., et al. (2016). The neostriatum: two entities, one structure? *Brain Struct. Funct.* 221, 1737–1749. doi: 10.1007/s00429-015-1000-4

Lovinger, D. M. (2010). Neurotransmitter roles in synaptic modulation, plasticity and learning in the dorsal striatum. *Neuropharmacology* 58, 951–961. doi: 10.1016/j.neuropharm.2010.01.008

Lucas-Meunier, E., Fossier, P., Baux, G., and Amar, M. (2003). Cholinergic modulation of the cortical neuronal network. *Pflugers Arch.* 446, 17–29. doi: 10.1007/s00424-002-0999-2

Lund, J. S., Yoshioka, T., and Levitt, J. B. (1993). Comparison of intrinsic connectivity in different areas of macaque monkey cerebral cortex. *Cereb. Cortex* 3, 148–162. doi: 10.1093/cercor/3.2.148

Mahon, S., Deniau, J. M., and Charpier, S. (2004). Corticostriatal plasticity: life after the depression. *Trends Neurosci.* 27, 460–467. doi: 10.1016/j.tins.2004.06.010

Makino, H., Hwang, E. J., Hedrick, N. G., and Komiyama, T. (2016). Circuit mechanisms of sensorimotor learning. *Neuron* 92, 705–721. doi: 10.1016/j.neuron.2016.10.029

Markram, H., Lübke, J., Frotscher, M., Roth, A., and Sakmann, B. (1997). Physiology and anatomy of synaptic connections between thick tufted pyramidal neurones in the developing rat neocortex. *J. Physiol.* 500(Pt 2), 409–440. doi: 10.1113/jphysiol.1997.sp022031

Mathis, M. W., Mathis, A., and Uchida, N. (2017). Somatosensory cortex plays an essential role in forelimb motor adaptation in mice. *Neuron* 93, 1493.e6–1503.e6. doi: 10.1016/j.neuron.2017.02.049

Mathur, B. N., and Lovinger, D. M. (2012). Endocannabinoid-dopamine interactions in striatal synaptic plasticity. *Front. Pharmacol.* 3:66. doi: 10.1017/S0040298217000092

Mathur, B. N., Tanahira, C., Tamamaki, N., and Lovinger, D. M. (2013). Voltage drives diverse endocannabinoid signals to mediate striatal microcircuit-specific plasticity. *Nat. Neurosci.* 16, 1275–1283. doi: 10.1038/nn.3478

McCann, S. K., Irvine, C., Mead, G. E., Sena, E. S., Currie, G. L., Egan, K. E., et al. (2014). Efficacy of antidepressants in animal models of ischemic stroke: a systematic review and meta-analysis. *Stroke* 45, 3055–3063. doi: 10.1161/STROKEAHA.114.006304

McFarland, N. R., and Haber, S. N. (2000). Convergent inputs from thalamic motor nuclei and frontal cortical areas to the dorsal striatum in the primate. *J. Neurosci.* 20, 3798–3813. doi: 10.1523/JNEUROSCI.20-10-03798.2000

McFarland, N. R., and Haber, S. N. (2002). Thalamic relay nuclei of the basal ganglia form both reciprocal and nonreciprocal cortical connections, linking multiple frontal cortical areas. *J. Neurosci.* 22, 8117–8132. doi: 10.1523/JNEUROSCI.22-18-08117.2002

McGehee, D. S., Heath, M. J., Gelber, S., Devay, P., and Role, L. W. (1995). Nicotine enhancement of fast excitatory synaptic transmission in CNS by pre-synaptic receptors. *Science* 269, 1692–1696. doi: 10.1126/science.7569895

Melzer, S., Gil, M., Koser, D. E., Michael, M., and Huang, K. W. (2017). Distinct corticostriatal GABAergic neurons modulate striatal output neurons and motor activity article distinct corticostriatal GABAergic neurons modulate striatal output neurons and motor activity. *Cell Rep.* 19, 1045–1055. doi: 10.1016/j.celrep.2017.04.024

Miri, A., Warriner, C. L., Seely, J. S., Elsayed, G. F., Cunningham, J. P., Churchland, M. M., et al. (2017). Behaviorally selective engagement of short-latency effector pathways by motor cortex. *Neuron* 95, 683.e11–696.e11. doi: 10.1016/j.neuron.2017.06.042

Molina-Luna, K., Hertler, B., Buitrago, M. M., and Luft, A. R. (2008). Motor learning transiently changes cortical somatotopy. *Neuroimage* 40, 1748–1754. doi: 10.1016/j.neuroimage.2007.11.018

Monfils, M. H., Plautz, E. J., and Kleim, J. A. (2005). In search of the motor engram: motor map plasticity as a mechanism for encoding motor experience. *Neuroscientist* 11, 471–483. doi: 10.1177/1073858405278015

Monfils, M. H., VandenBerg, P. M., Kleim, J. A., and Teskey, G. C. (2004). Long-term potentiation induces expanded movement representations and dendritic hypertrophy in layer V of rat sensorimotor cortex. *Cereb. Cortex* 14, 586–593. doi: 10.1093/cercor/bhh020

Mosberger, A. C., Miehlbradt, J. C., Bjelopoljak, N., Schneider, M. P., Wahl, A. S., Ineichen, B. V., et al. (2018). Axotomized corticospinal neurons increase supra-lesional innervation and remain crucial for skilled reaching after bilateral pyramidotomy. *Cereb. Cortex* 28, 625–643. doi: 10.1093/cercor/bhw405

Murphy, T. H., and Corbett, D. (2009). Plasticity during stroke recovery: from synapse to behaviour. *Nat. Rev. Neurosci.* 10, 861–872. doi: 10.1038/nrn2735

Napieralski, J. A., Butler, A. K., and Chesselet, M. F. (1996). Anatomical and functional evidence for lesion-specific sprouting of corticostriatal input in the adult rat. *J. Comp. Neurol.* 373, 484–497. doi: 10.1002/(SICI)1096-9861(19960930)373:4<484::AID-CNE2>3.0.CO;2-Y

Neafsey, E. J., and Sievert, C. (1982). A second forelimb motor area exists in rat frontal cortex. *Brain Res.* 232, 151–156. doi: 10.1016/0006-8993(82)90617-5

Nudo, R. J., Milliken, G. W., Jenkins, W. M., and Merzenich, M. M. (1996a). Use dependent alterations of movement representations in primary motor cortex of adult squirrel monkeys. *J. Neurosci.* 16, 785–807.

Nudo, R. J., Wise, B. M., SiFuentes, F., and Milliken, G. W. (1996b). Neural substrates for the effects of rehabilitative training on motor recovery after ischemic infarct. *Science* 272, 1791–1794.

Nudo, R. J., Plautz, E. J., and Frost, S. B. (2001). Role of adaptive plasticity in recovery of function after damage to motor cortex. *Muscle Nerve* 24, 1000–1019. doi: 10.1002/mus.1104

Ogura, T., Ogata, M., Akita, H., Jitsuki, S., Akiba, L., Noda, K., et al. (2005). Impaired acquisition of skilled behavior in rotarod task by moderate depletion of striatal dopamine in a pre-symptomatic stage model of Parkinson's disease. *Neurosci. Res.* 51, 299–308. doi: 10.1016/j.neures.2004.12.006

O'Hare, J., Calakos, N., and Yin, H. H. (2018). Recent insights into corticostriatal circuit mechanisms underlying habits. *Curr. Opin. Behav. Sci.* 20, 40–46. doi: 10.1016/j.cobeha.2017.10.001

O'Hare, J. K., Ade, K. K., Sukharnikova, T., Van Hooser, S. D., Palmeri, M. L., Yin, H. H., et al. (2016). Pathway-specific striatal substrates for habitual behavior. *Neuron* 89, 472–479. doi: 10.1016/j.neuron.2015.12.032

Olson, L., Seiger, A., and Fuxe, K. (1972). Heterogeneity of striatal and limbic dopamine innervation: highly fluorescent islands in developing and adult rats. *Brain Res.* 44, 283–288. doi: 10.1016/0006-8993(72)90385-X

Owen, S. F., Berke, J. D., and Kreitzer, A. C. (2018). Fast-spiking interneurons supply feedforward control of bursting, calcium, and plasticity for efficient learning. *Cell* 172, 683.e15–695.e15. doi: 10.1016/j.cell.2018.01.005

Papale, A. E., and Hooks, B. M. (2018). Circuit changes in motor cortex during motor skill learning. *Neuroscience* 368, 283–297. doi: 10.1016/j.neuroscience.2017.09.010

Paré, D., and Smith, Y. (1996). Thalamic collaterals of corticostriatal axons: their termination field and synaptic targets in cats. *J. Comp. Neurol.* 372, 551–567. doi: 10.1002/(SICI)1096-9861(19960902)372:4<551::AID-CNE5>3.0.CO;2-3

Park, H., Popescu, A., and Poo, M. M. (2014). Essential role of presynaptic NMDA receptors in activity-dependent BDNF secretion and corticostriatal LTP. *Neuron* 84, 1009–1022. doi: 10.1016/j.neuron.2014.10.045

Parr-Brownlie, L. C., and Hyland, B. I. (2005). Bradykinesia induced by dopamine D2 receptor blockade is associated with reduced motor cortex activity in the rat. *J. Neurosci.* 25, 5700–5709. doi: 10.1523/JNEUROSCI.0523-05.2005

Penfield, W., and Rasmussen, T. (1950). *The Cerebral Cortex of Man.* New York, NY: MacMillan Press.

Perrin, E., and Venance, L. (2019). Bridging the gap between striatal plasticity and learning. *Curr. Opin. Neurobiol.* 54, 104–112. doi: 10.1016/j.conb.2018.09.007

Peters, A. J., Chen, S. X., and Komiyama, T. (2014). Emergence of reproducible spatiotemporal activity during motor learning. *Nature* 510, 263–267. doi: 10.1038/nature13235

Peters, A. J., Liu, H., and Komiyama, T. (2017). Learning in the rodent motor cortex. *Annu. Rev. Neurosci.* 40, 77–97. doi: 10.1146/annurev-neuro-072116-031407

Pompeiano, M., Palacios, J. M., and Mengod, G. (1992). Distribution and cellular localization of mRNA coding for 5-HT1A receptor in rat brain: correlation with receptor binding. *J. Neurosci.* 12, 440–453. doi: 10.1523/JNEUROSCI.12-02-00440.1992

Porter, J. T., Cauli, B., Tsuzuki, K., Lambolez, B., Rossier, J., and Audinat, E. (1999). Selective excitation of subtypes of neocortical interneurons by nicotinic receptors. *J. Neurosci.* 19, 5228–5235. doi: 10.1523/JNEUROSCI.19-13-05228.1999

Pruitt, D. T., Schmid, A. N., Danaphongse, T. T., Flanagan, K. E., Morrison, R. A., Kilgard, M. P., et al. (2016). Forelimb training drives transient map reorganization in ipsilateral motor cortex. *Behav. Brain Res.* 313, 10–16. doi: 10.1016/j.bbr.2016.07.005

Puig, M. V., Artigas, F., and Celada, P. (2005). Modulation of the activity of pyramidal neurons in rat prefrontal cortex by raphe stimulation in vivo: involvement of serotonin and GABA. *Cereb. Cortex* 15, 1–14. doi: 10.1093/cercor/bhh104

Qu, M., Mittmann, T., Luhmann, H. J., Schleicher, A., and Zilles, K. (1998). Long-term changes of ionotropic glutamate and GABA receptors after unilateral permanent focal cerebral ischemia in the mouse brain. *Neuroscience* 85, 29–43. doi: 10.1016/S0306-4522(97)00656-8

Ramanathan, D., Conner, J. M., and Tuszynski, M. H. (2006). A form of motor cortical plasticity that correlates with recovery of function after brain injury. *Proc. Natl. Acad. Sci. U.S.A.* 103, 11370–11375. doi: 10.1073/pnas.0601065103

Ramanathan, D., Tuszynski, M. H., and Conner, J. M. (2009). The basal forebrain cholinergic system is required specifically for behaviorally mediated cortical map plasticity. *J. Neurosci.* 29, 5992–6000. doi: 10.1523/JNEUROSCI.0230-09.2009

Ramanathan, D. S., Guo, L., Gulati, T., Davidson, G., Hishinuma, A. K., Won, S. J., et al. (2018). Low-frequency cortical activity is a neuromodulatory target that tracks recovery after stroke. *Nat. Med.* 24, 1257–1267. doi: 10.1038/s41591-018-0058-y

Reed, A., Riley, J., Carraway, R., Carrasco, A., Perez, C., Jakkamsetti, V., et al. (2011). Cortical map plasticity improves learning but is not necessary for improved performance. *Neuron* 70, 121–131. doi: 10.1016/j.neuron.2011.02.038

Reidler, P., Thierfelder, K. M., Fabritius, M. P., Sommer, W. H., Meinel, F. G., Dorn, F., et al. (2018). Thalamic diaschisis in acute ischemic stroke: occurrence, perfusion characteristics, and impact on outcome. *Stroke* 49, 931–937. doi: 10.1161/STROKEAHA.118.020698

Reiner, A., Jiao, Y., Del Mar, N., Laverghetta, A. V., and Lei, W. L. (2003). Differential morphology of pyramidal tract-type and intratelencephalically projecting-type corticostriatal neurons and their intrastriatal terminals in rats. *J. Comp. Neurol.* 457, 420–440. doi: 10.1002/cne.10541

Reynolds, J. N., Hyland, B. I., and Wickens, J. R. (2001). A cellular mechanism of reward-related learning. *Nature* 413, 67–70. doi: 10.1038/35092560

Salinas, A. G., Davis, M. I., Lovinger, D. M., and Mateo, Y. (2016). Dopamine dynamics and cocaine sensitivity differ between striosome and matrix compartments of the striatum. *Neuropharmacology* 108, 275–283. doi: 10.1016/j.neuropharm.2016.03.049

Sanes, J. N., and Donoghue, J. P. (2000). Plasticity and primary motor cortex. *Annu. Rev. Neurosci.* 23, 393–415. doi: 10.1146/annurev.neuro.23.1.393

Savasta, M., Dubois, A., and Scatton, B. (1986). Autoradiographic localization of D1 dopamine receptors in the rat brain with [3H]SCH 23390. *Brain Res.* 375, 291–301. doi: 10.1016/0006-8993(86)90749-3

Schubring-Giese, M., Molina-Luna, K., Hertler, B., Buitrago, M. M., Hanley, D. F., and Luft, A. R. (2007). Speed of motor re-learning after experimental stroke depends on prior skill. *Exp. Brain Res.* 181, 359–365. doi: 10.1007/s00221-007-0930-3

Scullion, K., Boychuk, J. A., Yamakawa, G. R., Rodych, J. T., Nakanishi, S. T., Seto, A., et al. (2013). Serotonin 1A receptors alter expression of movement representations. *J. Neurosci.* 33, 4988–4999. doi: 10.1523/JNEUROSCI.4241-12.2013

Seitz, R. J., Azari, N. P., Knorr, U., Binkofski, F., Herzog, H., and Freund, H. J. (1999). The role of diaschisis in stroke recovery. *Stroke* 30, 1844–1850. doi: 10.1161/01.STR.30.9.1844

Shen, W., Flajolet, M., Greengard, P., and Surmeier, D. J. (2008). Dichotomous dopaminergic control of striatal synaptic plasticity. *Science* 321, 848–851. doi: 10.1126/science.1160575

Shen, W., Hamilton, S. E., Nathanson, N. M., and Surmeier, D. J. (2005). Cholinergic suppression of KCNQ channel currents enhances excitability of striatal medium spiny neurons. *J. Neurosci.* 25, 7449–7458. doi: 10.1523/JNEUROSCI.1381-05.2005

Shigemoto, R., and Mizuno, N. (2000). "Metabotropic glutamate receptors-immunocytochemical and in situ hybridization analyses," in *Handbook of Chemical Neuroanatomy: Glutamate*, Vol. 18, eds O. P. Ottersen and J. Storm-Mathisen (New York, NY: Elsevier Press), 63–98.

Shmuelof, L., and Krakauer, J. W. (2011). Are we ready for a natural history of motor learning? *Neuron* 72, 469–476. doi: 10.1016/j.neuron.2011.10.017

Silberberg, G., and Bolam, J. P. (2015). Local and afferent synaptic pathways in the striatal microcircuitry. *Curr. Opin. Neurobiol.* 33, 182–187. doi: 10.1016/j.conb.2015.05.002

Singh, A. M., and Staines, W. R. (2015). The effects of acute aerobic exercise on the primary motor cortex. *J. Mot. Behav.* 47, 328–339. doi: 10.1080/00222895.2014.983450

Smith, J. B., Klug, J. R., Ross, D. L., Howard, C. D., Hollon, N. G., Ko, V. I., et al. (2016). Genetic-based dissection unveils the inputs and outputs of striatal patch and matrix compartments. *Neuron* 91, 1069–1084. doi: 10.1016/j.neuron.2016.07.046

Smith, Y., Bolam, J. P., and Krosigk, M. V. (1990). Topographical and synaptic organization of the GABA-containing pallido subthalamic projection in the rat. *Eur. J. Neurosci.* 2, 500–511. doi: 10.1111/j.1460-9568.1990.tb00441.x

Smith, Y., Galvan, A., Ellender, T. J., Doig, N., Villalba, R. M., Huerta-Ocampo, I., et al. (2014). The thalamostriatal system in normal and diseased states. *Front. Syst. Neurosci.* 8:5. doi: 10.3389/fnsys.2014.00005

Spalletti, C., Alia, C., Lai, S., Panarese, A., Conti, S., Micera, S., et al. (2017). Combining robotic training and inactivation of the healthy hemisphere restores pre-stroke motor patterns in mice. *eLife* 6:e28662. doi: 10.7554/eLife.28662

Surmeier, D. J., Plotkin, J., and Shen, W. (2009). Dopamine and synaptic plasticity in dorsal striatal circuits controlling action selection. *Curr. Opin. Neurobiol.* 19, 621–628. doi: 10.1016/j.conb.2009.10.003

Tennant, K. A., Taylor, S. L., White, E. R., and Brown, C. E. (2017). Optogenetic rewiring of thalamocortical circuits to restore function in the stroke injured brain. *Nat. Commun.* 23:15879. doi: 10.1038/ncomms15879

Tepper, J. M., Abercrombie, E. D., and Bolam, J. P. (2007). Basal ganglia macrocircuits. *Prog. Brain Res.* 160, 3–7. doi: 10.1016/S0079-6123(06)60001-0

Tepper, J. M., Koós, T., and Wilson, C. J. (2004). GABAergic microcircuits in the neostriatum. *Trends Neurosci.* 27, 662–669. doi: 10.1016/j.tins.2004.08.007

Tice, M. A., Hashemi, T., Taylor, L. A., and McQuade, R. D. (1996). Distribution of muscarinic receptor subtypes in rat brain from postnatal to old age. *Dev. Brain. Res.* 92, 70–76. doi: 10.1016/0165-3806(95)01515-9

Tombari, D., Loubinoux, I., Pariente, J., Gerdelat, A., Albucher, J. F., Tardy, J., et al. (2004). A longitudinal fMRI study: in recovering and then in clinically stable sub-cortical stroke patients. *Neuroimage* 23, 827–839. doi: 10.1016/j.neuroimage.2004.07.058

Touvykine, B., Mansoori, B. K., Jean-Charles, L., Deffeyes, J., Quessy, S., and Dancause, N. (2016). The effect of lesion size on the organization of the ipsilesional and contralesional motor cortex. *Neurorehabil. Neural Repair* 30, 280–292. doi: 10.1177/1545968315585356

Turrigiano, G. G., and Nelson, S. B. (2004). Homeostatic plasticity in the developing nervous system. *Nat. Rev. Neurosci.* 5, 97–107. doi: 10.1038/nrn1327

Uryu, K., MacKenzie, L., and Chesselet, M. F. (2001). Ultrastructural evidence for differential axonal sprouting in the striatum after thermocoagulatory and aspiration lesions of the cerebral cortex in adult rats. *Neuroscience* 105, 307–316. doi: 10.1016/S0306-4522(01)00203-2

Vahlsing, H. L., and Feringa, E. R. (1980). A ventral uncrossed corticospinal tract in the rat. *Exp. Neurol.* 70, 282–287. doi: 10.1016/0014-4886(80)90027-8

von Monakow, C. (1914). *Lokalisation im Gehirn und Funktionelle Sta'rungen Induziert Durch Kortikale Läsionen.* Wiesbaden: Bergmann JF.

Wada, E., McKinnon, D., Heinemann, S., Patrick, J., and Swanson, L. W. (1990). The distribution of mRNA encoded by a new member of the neuronal nicotinic acetylcholine receptor gene family (a5) in the rat central nervous system. *Brain Res.* 526, 45–53. doi: 10.1016/0006-8993(90)90248-A

Wada, E., Wada, K., Boulter, J., Deneris, E., Heinemann, S., Patrick, J., et al. (1989). Distribution of a2, a3, a4, and b2 neuronal nicotinic receptor subunit mRNAs in the central nervous system: a hybridization histochemical study in the rat. *J. Comp. Neurol.* 284, 314–335. doi: 10.1002/cne.902840212

Wahl, A. S., Omlor, W., Rubio, J. C., Chen, J. L., Zheng, H., Schröter, A., et al. (2014). Neuronal repair. asynchronous therapy restores motor control by rewiring of the rat corticospinal tract after stroke. *Science* 344, 1250–1255. doi: 10.1126/science.1253050

Wahl, A. S., and Schwab, M. E. (2014). Finding an optimal rehabilitation paradigm after stroke: enhancing fiber growth and training of the brain at the right moment. *Front. Hum. Neurosci.* 8:381. doi: 10.3389/fnhum.2014.00381

Walker, M. P., Brakefield, T., Hobson, J. A., and Stickgold, R. (2003). Dissociable stages of human memory consolidation and reconsolidation. *Nature* 425, 616–620. doi: 10.1038/nature01930

Wang, K. S., McClure, J. P., Alselehdar, S. K., and Kanta, V. (2015). Direct and indirect pathways of the basal ganglia: opponents or collaborators? *Front. Neuroanat.* 9:20. doi: 10.3389/fnana.2015.00020

Wang, L., Conner, J. M., Nagahara, A. H., and Tuszynski, M. H. (2016). Rehabilitation drives enhancement of neuronal structure in functionally relevant neuronal subsets. *Proc. Natl. Acad. Sci. U.S.A.* 113, 2750–2755. doi: 10.1073/pnas.1514682113

Wang, Z., and McCormick, D. A. (1993). Control of firing mode of corticotectal and corticopontine layer V burst-generating neurons by norepinephrine, acetylcholine, and 1S,3R-ACPD. *J. Neurosci.* 13, 2199–2216. doi: 10.1523/JNEUROSCI.13-05-02199.1993

Ward, N. S., Brown, M. M., Thompson, A. J., and Frackowiak, R. S. J. (2003). Neural correlates of motor recovery after stroke: a longitudinal fMRI study. *Brain* 126, 2476–2496. doi: 10.1093/brain/awg245

Weiler, N., Wood, L., Yu, J., Solla, S. A., and Shepherd, G. M. G. (2008). Top-down laminar organization of the excitatory network in motor cortex. *Nat. Neurosci.* 11, 360–366. doi: 10.1038/nn2049

Wenger, E., Brozzoli, C., Lindenberger, U., and Lövdén, M. (2017). Expansion and renormalization of human brain structure during skill acquisition. *Trends Cogn. Sci.* 21, 930–939. doi: 10.1016/j.tics.2017.09.008

Wilson, C. J. (1987). Morphology and synaptic connections of crossed corticostriatal neurons in the rat. *J. Comp. Neurol.* 263, 567–580. doi: 10.1002/cne.902630408

Winship, I. R., and Murphy, T. H. (2008). In vivo calcium imaging reveals functional rewiring of single somatosensory neurons after stroke. *J. Neurosci.* 28, 6592–6606. doi: 10.1523/JNEUROSCI.0622-08.2008

Withers, G. S., and Greenough, W. T. (1989). Reach training selectively alters dendritic branching in subpopulations of layer II-III pyramids in rat motor-somatosensory forelimb cortex. *Neuropsychologia* 27, 61–69. doi: 10.1016/0028-3932(89)90090-0

Witte, O. W. (1998). Lesion-induced plasticity as a potential mechanism for recovery and rehabilitative training. *Curr. Opin. Neurol.* 11, 655–662. doi: 10.1097/00019052-199812000-00008

Wu, Y. W., Kim, J. I., Tawfik, V. L., Lalchandani, R. R., Scherrer, G., and Ding, J. B. (2015). Input- and cell-type-specific endocannabinoid-dependent LTD in the striatum. *Cell Rep.* 10, 75–87. doi: 10.1016/j.celrep.2014.12.005

Xu, H., Perez, S., Cornil, A., Detraux, B., Prokin, I., Cui, Y., et al. (2018). Dopamine–endocannabinoid interactions mediate spike-timing-dependent potentiation in the striatum. *Nat. Commun.* 9:4118. doi: 10.1038/s41467-018-06409-5

Xu, M., Li, L., and Pittenger, C. (2016). Ablation of fast-spiking interneurons in the dorsal striatum, recapitulating abnormalities seen post-mortem in Tourette syndrome, produces anxiety and elevated grooming. *Neuroscience* 324, 321–329. doi: 10.1016/j.neuroscience.2016.02.074

Yamawaki, N., Borges, K., Suter, B. A., Harris, K. D., and Shepherd, G. M. G. (2014). A genuine layer 4 in motor cortex with prototypical synaptic circuit connectivity. *eLife* 3:e05422. doi: 10.7554/eLife.05422

Yin, H. H. (2017). The basal ganglia in action. *Neuroscientist* 23, 299–313. doi: 10.1177/1073858416654115

Yin, H. H., Prasad-Mulcare, S., Hilário, M. R. F., Clouse, E., Davis, M. I., Hansson, A. C., et al. (2009). Dynamic reorganization of striatal circuits during the acquisition and consolidation of a skill. *Nat. Neurosci.* 12, 333–341. doi: 10.1038/nn.2261

Zeiler, S. R., Gibson, E. M., Hoesch, R. E., Li, M. Y., Worley, P. F., O'Brien, R. J., et al. (2013). Medial premotor cortex shows a reduction in inhibitory markers and mediates recovery in a mouse model of focal stroke. *Stroke* 44, 483–489. doi: 10.1161/STROKEAHA.112.676940

7

Off-Label Use of Bumetanide for Brain Disorders

*Shivani C. Kharod[1], Seok Kyu Kang[1] and Shilpa D. Kadam[1,2]**

[1] *Neuroscience Laboratory, Hugo W. Moser Research Institute at Kennedy Krieger, Baltimore, MD, United States,*

[2] *Department of Neurology and Neurosurgery, Johns Hopkins University School of Medicine, Baltimore, MD, United States*

Correspondence:
Shilpa D. Kadam
skadam1@jhmi.edu;
kadam@kennedykrieger.org

Bumetanide (BTN or BUM) is a FDA-approved potent loop diuretic (LD) that acts by antagonizing sodium-potassium-chloride (Na-K-Cl) cotransporters, NKCC1 (SLc12a2) and NKCC2. While NKCC1 is expressed both in the CNS and in systemic organs, NKCC2 is kidney-specific. The off-label use of BTN to modulate neuronal transmembrane Cl^- gradients by blocking NKCC1 in the CNS has now been tested as an anti-seizure agent and as an intervention for neurological disorders in pre-clinical studies with varying results. BTN safety and efficacy for its off-label use has also been tested in several clinical trials for neonates, children, adolescents, and adults. It failed to meet efficacy criteria for hypoxic-ischemic encephalopathy (HIE) neonatal seizures. In contrast, positive outcomes in temporal lobe epilepsy (TLE), autism, and schizophrenia trials have been attributed to BTN in studies evaluating its off-label use. NKCC1 is an electroneutral neuronal Cl^- importer and the dominance of NKCC1 function has been proposed as the common pathology for HIE seizures, TLE, autism, and schizophrenia. Therefore, the use of BTN to antagonize neuronal NKCC1 with the goal to lower internal Cl^- levels and promote GABAergic mediated hyperpolarization has been proposed. In this review, we summarize the data and results for pre-clinical and clinical studies that have tested off-label BTN interventions and report variable outcomes. We also compare the data underlying the developmental expression profile of NKCC1 and KCC2, highlight the limitations of BTN's brain-availability and consider its actions on non-neuronal cells.

Keywords: bumetanide (BTN), Na-K-Cl cotransporter 1 (NKCC1), neonatal seizures, autism, schizophrenia, temporal lobe epilepsy (TLE)

INTRODUCTION

Bumetanide is a fast-acting LD, acting on the widely distributed NKCC1 (Slc12a2), and renal-specific NKCC2. LDs act on the loop of Henle and are often used clinically for palliative treatment of renal insufficiency, heart failure, nephrotic syndrome, and hypertension (Wittner et al., 1991; Brater, 2000). Patients that were prone to seizures but administered LDs to induce diuresis for these previously mentioned indications, reported notable anti-seizure effects (Hesdorffer et al., 1996; Hesdorffer et al., 2001; Kanner, 2002; Maa et al., 2011). While various mechanisms for

---

Abbreviations: BBB, blood–brain barrier; BTN, bumetanide; Cl^-, chloride; CNS, central nervous system; DLPFC, dorsolateral prefrontal cortex; FCD, focal cortical dysplasia; GABA, gamma-aminobutyric acid; HIE, hypoxic-ischemic encephalopathy; IP, intraperitoneal; IV, intravenous; KCC2, K-Cl cotransporter 2; LD, loop diuretic; NKCC, Na-K-Cl cotransporter; OAT, organic anion transporter; PB, phenobarbital; PD, pharmacodynamics; PK, pharmacokinetic; TLE, temporal lobe epilepsy.

the seizure alleviation were proposed, the use of loop-diuretics as anti-seizure drugs remains under investigation.

In the brain, the Cl^- importer NKCC1 is balanced by the function of Cl^- extruder, potassium-chloride-cotransporter 2 (KCC2). Increased expression of NKCC1, not balanced with the efflux action of KCC2, has been the rationale behind administration of BTN as an antiseizure agent. BTN has been administered for HIE neonatal seizures (NCT01434225, 2015; NCT00830531, 2017), but was reported inefficacious (Pressler et al., 2015). BTN administered to patients with autism (Lemonnier and Ben-Ari, 2010; Lemonnier et al., 2012, 2017), schizophrenia (Rahmanzadeh et al., 2017) and TLE (Eftekhari et al., 2013), however, reported beneficial effects.

The developmental expression profile of BTN's primary target, NKCC1 (Morita et al., 2014; Sedmak et al., 2016), has recently been elucidated. Studies conducted to analyze BTN's BBB penetration (Puskarjov et al., 2014), interaction with efflux transporters (Donovan et al., 2014, 2016; Römermann et al., 2017), blood plasma-binding properties (Donovan et al., 2016), diuresis (Asbury et al., 1972; Maa et al., 2011) and pharmacokinetic (PK) properties (Puskarjov et al., 2014) all have addressed questions about BTN's brain availability. Of interest are BTN's possible interactions with NKCC1 in non-neuronal cells (Zhang et al., 2014).

MAINTAINING THE TRANSMEMBRANE Cl^- GRADIENT

Cl^- cotransporters, NKCC1 and KCC2, are the primary mediators that maintain neuronal transmembrane Cl^- gradient (Rivera et al., 1999; Ben-Ari et al., 2012; Côme et al., 2019). NKCC1 is expressed in multiple cell types in the CNS, including neurons, contributing to Cl^- intracellular accumulation (Dzhala et al., 2005; Nicholls et al., 2012). KCC2 expression, while thought to be neuronal specific (Song et al., 2002; Zhang et al., 2014), has been found outside the CNS as well (Antrobus et al., 2012), and extrudes Cl^- to maintain lower $[Cl^-]_i$. These two co-transporters mediate the GABA "switch," and their functions contribute to inhibitory actions of $GABA_A$ receptor ($GABA_AR$) agonists (Owens and Kriegstein, 2002; Lee et al., 2005). Excitation/inhibition imbalance has been attributed to the developmental profiles of NKCC1 and KCC2 protein expression (Ben-Ari et al., 2012). In the immature brain and in certain pathological states, activation of GABA channels leads to the efflux of Cl^- ions due to high $[Cl^-]_i$, resulting in membrane depolarization. Achieving a balance between NKCC1 (Cl^- influx) and KCC2 (Cl^- efflux), by curbing excessive NKCC1 function has been the reasoning behind the off-label use of BTN, both in pre-clinical models and clinical studies (see **Table 1** for details). Despite being a potent NKCC1 antagonist, BTN can also antagonize KCC2 at higher concentrations (Delpire et al., 2009). The developmental upregulation of KCC2 has been elucidated and confirmed with a wide span of experimental techniques (Uvarov et al., 2013; Sedmak et al., 2016). The expression profile of KCC2 correlates with maturation of different brain regions (Watanabe and Fukuda, 2015; Côme et al., 2019). The KCC2b isoform is developmentally upregulated, but KCC2a expression remains steady over brain maturation (Uvarov et al., 2007, 2009; Côme et al., 2019). Until recently, however, the developmental profile of NKCC1 isoforms has remained uncertain, mainly due to experimental limitations (Morita et al., 2014; **Figure 1**).

DEVELOPMENTAL PROFILE OF NKCC1 ISOFORM EXPRESSION IN THE BRAIN

The developmental expression profile of NKCC1 mRNA has been examined in postmortem human brains with RT-PCR and was found to be stable postnatally (Morita et al., 2014). This contrasts with the age-dependent reduction of NKCC1 protein expression levels reported with rodent and human western blotting data (Dzhala et al., 2005; Kang et al., 2015) (**Figure 1A**). NKCC1 mRNA has been shown to have predominant expression in ventricular and periventricular cell populations at embryonic and early neonatal ages in the brain (Li et al., 2002). Toward P0, there was no more significant increase in expression of mRNA but distribution within cortical layers changed from ventricular zones to cortical layers (Li et al., 2002). After mRNA splicing, NKCC1 results in two main isoforms, NKCC1a and NKCC1b, that span across many tissue types in humans, including the brain (Vibat et al., 2001). Commercially available, NKCC1 western blotting antibodies, used in many of the earlier pre-clinical and human studies, failed to detect NKCC1b, one of the two main isoforms of NKCC1 in the brain (Dzhala et al., 2005; Morita et al., 2014; Kang et al., 2015). The western blotting probes and antibodies targeted exon 21, found in NKCC1a, but not NKCC1b (Clayton et al., 1998; Vibat et al., 2001; Kaila et al., 2014; Morita et al., 2014; Puskarjov et al., 2014; Kang et al., 2015). Since NKCC1b is the predominant isoform expressed in the brain, (Vibat et al., 2001), the apparent downregulation of NKCC1 total protein in maturing brains could be attributed to this experimental artifact. Additionally, (Morita et al., 2014) identified multiple isoforms with different developmental profiles in the human brain. Along with NKCC1a and b, the mRNA expression of recently discovered NKCC1 transcripts, 1-27 (21a), 1-4a and 1-2a were identified and verified in the DLPFC (Morita et al., 2014). The mRNA expressions of NKCC1a, NKCC1b, and 1-4a were low during fetal development, increased after birth through adolescence and reached stable levels in adulthood. This is further supported in a study that evaluated NKCC1 mRNA in P5-P90 rats. While high at P5, there was a significant drop at P10 that then remained stable with advancing age. Since P7 in rodents is close to term birth in humans, this would indicate stable NKCC1 mRNA expression in neurons after birth (Lee et al., 2010). Transcript 1-2a decreased after birth but was stable throughout postnatal life (Morita et al., 2014). Additionally, qRT-PCR was utilized in another study to determine developmental expression of NKCC1 (Hyde et al., 2011). An upregulation was seen after birth before leveling off at 20 and 23 years of age in the DLPFC and hippocampus, respectfully. Isoform specific quantification was not conducted in this study, however, and probes utilized spanned exons 4-5.

TABLE 1 | BTN off-label studies.

	Study	Model	Strain	Age	Sex as a biological variable	BTN dose	Number of BTN doses	Dose delivery	Experimental paradigm	Reported effect
Pre-clinical rodent studies (*in vivo*)										
Neonatal seizures	Dzhala et al., 2005	KA	Long–Evans rats, Wistar rats and C57 mice	(P9–12), (P5–23), and (P7–9), respectively	EEG: M (Wistar), sex not specified for Long-Evans or C57	0.1–0.2 mg/kg (*in vivo*); 10 μM *in vitro*	1 *in vivo* and bath-applied *in vitro*	IP, *in vivo* and bath-applied *in vitro*	Bath applied post-elevated K+ (*in vitro*) and Injected 15 min post-KA (*in vivo*)	Epileptiform activity in hippocampal slices *in vitro*↓; KA-induced seizure's *in vivo* ↓ EEG power
Neonatal seizures	Mares, 2009	PTZ	Wistar rats	P7, P12, P18	M	0.2, 0.5, 1, and 2.5 mg/kg	1	*In vivo*, IP	Pretreatment 20 min before PTZ (*in vivo*)	Dose-dependent effect in P12 (anticonvulsant at 1 mg/kg, and proconvulsant at 2.5 mg/kg); No effect in P7/P18.
Neonatal seizures	Mazarati et al., 2009	Rapid kindling	Wistar rats	P11, P14, P21	M	0.2, 0.5, or 2.5 mg/kg	1.5	*In vivo*, IP	Once upon detection of ADT (+ 1/2 dose during kindling procedure	Anticonvulsant at P11, no effect at P14/P21
Neonatal Sseizures	Liu et al., 2012	Right carotid ligation	Sprague–Dawley rats	P7	M/F	2.5 and 10 mg/kg	1	*In vivo*, IP	10 min after PB injection, which was administered 15 min post-hypoxia	Anticonvulsant effect together with PB (BTN: 10 mg/kg), no effect with 2.5 mg/kg BTN
Febrile seizures	Koyama et al., 2012	Hyperthermia	Sprague–Dawley rats	P11	M	0.1 mg/kg *in vivo*	6	IP, *in vivo* and bath-applied *in vitro*	Once daily from P11–P17 *in vivo* post-hyperthermia on P11	Rescue of granule cell ectopia, limbic seizure susceptibility and development of epilepsy
Neonatal seizures	Cleary et al., 2013	Hypoxia	Long–Evans rats	P10	M	0.15 or 0.3 mg/kg	1	*In vivo*, IP	15 min prior to seizure induction by hypoxia	Reversal of seizure-induced changes in E_{GABA} when compared to PB and/or BTN applied alone
Neonatal seizures	Kang et al., 2015	Right carotid ligation	CD-1 mice	P7, P10	M/F	0.1–0.2 mg/kg	1	*In vivo*, IP	1 h post-PB, 2 h post- unilateral carotid ligation	No effect/seizure aggravation at P10

(Continued)

TABLE 1 | Continued

	Study	Model	Strain	Age	Sex as a biological variable	BTN dose	Number of BTN doses	Dose delivery	Experimental paradigm	Reported effect
Neonatal seizures	Wang et al., 2015	Hypoxia	Wistar rats	P10	Not indicated	0.5 mg/kg/day	21	*In vivo*, IP	Daily for 3 weeks post-hypoxia	Alteration of newborn DG cell structure and ↓ spontaneous EEG seizure's after HI
Neonatal seizures	Holmes et al., 2015	Flurothyl	Sprague–Dawley rats	Induced seizure's P5–14, tested for developmental alterations from P18–25	M	0.5 mg/kg	10	*In vivo*, IP	Twice daily, once before first flurothyl-induced seizure and again after the last seizure each day	Normalization of voltage correlation, sociability and seizure threshold
Neonatal seizures	Hu et al., 2017	PTZ after HI (Rice-Vanucci method)	Sprague–Dawley rats	P7	Unsexed	0.5 mg/kg	6	*In vivo*, IP	Twice daily for 3 days after surgery	PTZ-induced seizure susceptibility ↓, restoration of hippocampal neurogenesis, improved cognitive function
Neonatal seizures	Kharod et al., 2018	PTZ	CD-1 mice	P7	M/F	0.1–0.2 mg/kg	1	*In vivo*, IP	1 h post-PB, 2 h post-PTZ	No effect/seizure aggravation post-PB suppression in P7 females
TLE	Brandt et al., 2010	Pilocarpine	Sprague–Dawley rats	Adult	F	Three dosing protocols: (1) 0.2 mg/kg, (2) 10 mg/kg, (3) 0.8 mg/kg/h	(1) Multiple doses first 24 h, then 14, (2) multiple doses first 24 h, then 14, (3) continuous	(1) *In vivo*, IP (2) *in vivo*, IP (3) *in vivo*, IV	(1) First 24 h all 3–7 h, then twice daily for 2 weeks, (2) first 24 h all 3–7 h, then twice daily for 2 weeks, (3) continuous infusion after bolus of 2 mg/kg/ for 5 days	Combined PB/BTN treatment altered behavior consequences of epileptic rats
TLE	Sivakumaran and Maguire, 2016	KA	C57BL/6 mice	Adult	M	0.2 mg/kg or 2.0 mg/kg, i.p. (*in vivo*), and 54.8 μM (*in vitro*)	1 *in vivo* and bath applied *in vitro*	IP, *in vivo* and intrahippocampal administration *in vitro*	BTN 30, 60, 90, and 120 min prior KA administration (*in vivo*) and direct hippocampal injection of BTN 30 min prior to KA injection (*in vitro*)	↓ KA-induced ictal activity *in vivo* and SLEs *in vitro*, restoration of diazepam efficacy *in vitro* and *in vivo*

(Continued)

TABLE 1 | Continued

	Study	Model	Strain	Age	Sex as a biological variable	BTN dose	Number of BTN doses	Dose delivery	Experimental paradigm	Reported effect
TLE	Kourdougli et al., 2017	Pilocarpine	Wistar rats	Adult	M	86 ng/day	Continuous	*In vivo,* Osmotic minipumps	Continuous infusion for 3 days	Restored post-SE NKCC1/KCC2, normalized Cl^- homeostasis, ↓ of glutamatergic recurrent mf sprouting in DG
Autism	Tyzio et al., 2014	Rats exposed *in utero* to valproate (VPA rats) and mice carrying the Fragile X mutation (FRX mice)	Wistar rats, mice strain not specified	E18, P0, P2, P4, P7, P8, P15 and P30 (mice); E20, P0, P2, P4, P7, P15, and P30 (rats)	M/F	2–2.5 mg/kg *(in vivo)*, 10 μM *(in vitro)*	1	In drinking water (*in vivo*) + *in vitro*	BTN pretreatment – given to dams in drinking water (*in vivo*) and bath-applied *in vitro*	Maternal pretreatment restored electrophysiological and behavioral phenotypes in pups
Stroke	Xu et al., 2017	Endothelin stroke model	Wistar rats	Adult	M	0.2 mg/kg/day	Continuous	*In vivo*, IV; mini-osmotic pumps	21 days - continuous infusion	Enhancement of neurogenesis and behavioral recovery, no effects on inflammation
Periventricular leukomalacia	Jantzie et al., 2015	Unilateral carotid artery ligation followed by hypoxia	Long–Evans rats, protein-enhanced green fluorescent protein transgenic mouse pups (B6/CBA background)	P6	M	0.3 mg/kg	6	*In vivo*, IP	Every 12 h for 60 h post-HI	Attenuation of myelin base protein loss and neuronal degeneration 7 days post-HI
TBI	Lu et al., 2006	Weight drop device	Wistar rats	Adult	M	15 mg/kg	1	*In vivo*, IV	20 min before TBI	↓ Brain contusion volume
TBI	Lu et al., 2007	Weight drop device	Wistar rats	Adult	M	15 mg/kg	1	*In vivo*, IV	20 min before TBI	Attenuation of inflammatory response and neuronal loss
Neuropathic pain	Mòdol et al., 2014	Sciatic nerve injury	Sprague–Dawley rats	Adult	F	30 mg/kg	16	*In vivo*, IP	Days 1–16 - post injury	Prevented spinothalamic tract projecting area changes and hyperalgesia

(Continued)

TABLE 1 | Continued

	Study	Model	Strain	Age	Sex as a biological variable	BTN dose	Number of BTN doses	Dose delivery	Experimental paradigm	Reported effect
Intracerebral hemorrhage	Wilkinson et al., 2019	Collagenase	Sprague–Dawley rats	Adult	M	10 and 40 mg/kg	Multiple doses and treatment groups	*In vivo*, oral and IP	2 h or 7 days post-ICH, either 6 or 12 h interval orally or IP for 3 days	Minor ↓ in edema after early dosing, no effect on behavior or injury volume, no normalization of ion concentration after late dosing
Pre-clinical rodent studies (*in vitro* only)										
Neonatal seizures	Dzhala et al., 2008	Low Mg^{2+}	Sprague–Dawley rats	P4–P7	M	10 μM	Bath-applied	*In vitro*	Bath-applied after 5–8 recurrent ictal-like episodes	Efficacious adjunct to PB, ↓ recurrent tonic-clonic epileptiform activity
Febrile seizures	Reid et al., 2013	Lipopoly-saccharide/ KA + behavioral febrile seizure	Long–Evans rats	P14	M	10 μM	Bath-applied	*In vitro*	Bath-applied 30 min after application of 4-AP	↓ *In vitro* 4-AP-induced inter-ictal activity in the inflammation and inflammation + FS groups
TLE	Bragin et al., 2009	Pilocarpine	Wistar rats	Adult	M	10 μM	Bath-applied	*In vitro*	Bath-applied; 20 min superfusion 3 weeks post-SE	Restoration of IPSP reversal potential and ↓ polysynaptic burst discharge
Schizophrenia and autism	Amin et al., 2017	22q11.2 DS hippocampal neurons	C57BL/6 J mice	Neurons from E18	Not indicated	10 μM	Applied to cell culture media	In vitro	Applied to cell culture media at 16 DIV, then after 16 DIVs (+ baseline spiking activity	(hyperexcitable action of $GABA_A$ receptor signaling, restored network homeostatic plasticity in *Lgdel*$^{+/-}$ networks
Off-label clinical studies										
Neonatal seizures	Kahle et al., 2009	Human (case report)	n/a	6 weeks	F	0.1 mg/kg	1	IV	Single dose, post-PB and fosphenytoin	↓ Mean seizure duration and frequency
Neonatal seizures	NCT01434225, 2015	Human	n/a	Gestational age of 37–43 weeks and postnatal age <48 h	M/F	0.05, 0.1, 0.2, or 0.3 mg/kg	4	IV	Up to four times, 12 h intervals	No anticonvulsant effect, ototoxicity

(Continued)

TABLE 1 | Continued

	Study	Model	Strain	Age	Sex as a biological variable	BTN dose	Number of BTN doses	Dose delivery	Experimental paradigm	Reported effect
Neonatal seizures	NCT00830531, 2017	Human	n/a	Post-conceptual age of 33–44 weeks	M/F	0.1, 0.2, or 0.3 mg/kg	1	IV	One dose together with PB after establishing PB-resistance with a first-line PB only dose	Results and summary statement on clinical trials.gov awaited
TLE	Eftekhari et al., 2013	Human	n/a	Adult – 31, 32, and 37 years	M	2 mg/day	Long-term administration	Oral	~3/4 months + pre-existing anti-epileptic drugs	Seizure frequency ↓, epileptiform discharges ↓ on pre-vs. post EEG in 2 out of 3 patients
Autism	Lemonnier and Ben-Ari, 2010	Human	n/a	Age span from 3 years and 8 months to 11 years and 5 months	M/F	1 mg/day	Long-term administration	Oral	0.5 mg twice a day for 3 months	Improvement in IAS with no side effects
Autism	Lemonnier et al., 2012	Human	n/a	6.8 years ± 13.2 months	M/F	1 mg/day	Long-term administration	Oral	0.5 mg twice a day for 3 months, followed by 1 month washout	Improved CARS, CGI and Autism Diagnostic Observation Schedule values
Autism	Du et al., 2015	Human	n/a	2.5–6.5 years	M/F	1 mg/day	Long-term administration	Oral	0.5 mg twice a day for 3 months	ABC and CGI scores improved when ABA training combined with BTN treatment, compared to ABA training alone
Autism	Lemonnier et al., 2017	Human	n/a	2–18 years	M/F	1.0, 2.0, and 4.0 mg/day	Long-term administration	Oral	0.5, 1.0, and 2.0 mg twice daily for 3 months	Improved CARS, SRS and CGI scores
Autism	Hadjikhani et al., 2018	Human	n/a	14.8–28.5 years	M/F	1 mg/day	Long-term administration	Oral	Once daily for 10 months	More eye contact, less amygdala activation
Schizophrenia	Lemonnier et al., 2016	Human (case report)	n/a	14 years	M	2 mg/day	Long-term administration	Oral	Once daily for 11 months	↓ Hallucinations
Schizophrenia	Rahmanzadeh et al., 2016	Human	n/a	55.9 ± 13.9 years	M/F	1 mg	Long-term administration	Oral	Twice daily for 2 months	No effect on PANSS scores/subscores or BPRS score

(Continued)

TABLE 1 | Continued

	Study	Model	Strain	Age	Sex as a biological variable	BTN dose	Number of BTN doses	Dose delivery	Experimental paradigm	Reported effect
Schizophrenia	Rahmanzadeh et al., 2017	Human	n/a	38–67 years	M/F	1 mg	Long-term administration	Oral	Twice daily for 2 months	↓ Hallucinations
Parkinson's disease	Damier et al., 2016	Human	n/a	(> 50 years (n (=4)	M/F	5 mg	Long-term administration	Oral	Once daily for 2 months	Improvement of PD motor symptoms in all four patients, improvement of gait and freezing in 2 of these patients
Human *in vitro* studies										
Neonatal seizures (tuberous sclerosis complex and focal cortical dysplasia)	Talos et al., 2012	Human, TSC cortical slices	n/a	Infancy through adulthood (1.4–57 years)	M/F	10 μM	Bath-applied	*In vitro*	Bath-applied with NBQX and DL-AP5	Suppression of PSC amplitude and frequency
TLE	Palma et al., 2006	Human, surgical resection from hippocampus and temporal neocortex injected into oocytes	n/a	Adult (27, 29, 41, and 43 years)	M/F	12 μM	Bath-applied	*In vitro*	Oocytes treated with BTN (3 h)	Shifted the E_{GABA} to more negative in oocytes injected with membranes from TLE hippocampal subiculum
Brain tumor related epileptogenesis	Conti et al., 2011	Human, membranes from peritumoral cortical tissues of epileptic patients injected into oocytes	n/a	Adult (21–67 years)	M/F	12 μM	Bath-applied	*In vitro*	Oocytes pretreated with BTN (2 h)	Abolished difference of depolarized E_{GABA} in oocytes injected with epileptic peritumoral cerebral cortex
Sturge–Weber Syndrome	Tyzio et al., 2009	Human, neurons from human pediatric SWS cortex *in vitro*	n/a	Infancy (6, 9, 13, and 14 months)	M/F	10 μM	Bath-applied	*In vitro*	Bath-applied	No prominent effects on epileptiform activity

(Continued)

TABLE 1 | Continued

	Study	Model	Strain	Age	Sex as a biological variable	BTN dose	Number of BTN doses	Dose delivery	Experimental paradigm	Reported effect
Focal cortical dysplasia	Blauwblomme et al., 2018	Human, slices from resected tissue from patients with FCD	n/a	2.8–16.9 years; BTN tested in 12 slices from 7 patients	M/F	8 μM	Bath-applied	*In vitro*	Bath-applied	Suppressed IIDs in 9 of 12 slices, IIDs reappeared after washout. No effect in 1 case, and reduced frequency and amplitude in 2 cases of FCD Type 1c

NBQX, 2,3-dihydroxy-6-nitro-7-sulfamoyl-benzo[f]quinoxaline-2,3-dione; ADT, after discharge threshold; ABA, applied behavior analysis; ABC, autism behavior checklist; BPRS, Brief Psychiatric Rating Scale; BTN, bumetanide; CARS, Childhood Autism Rating Scale; CGI, clinical global impressions; DIV, days in vitro; DG, dentate gyrus; DL-AP5, DL-2-Amino-5-phosphonopentanoic acid; EEG, electroencephalogram; F, female; FCD, focal cortical dysplasia; HI, hypoxia-ischemia; IAS, infantile autistic syndromes; ICH, intracerebral hemorrhage; IIDs, interictal discharges; M, male; mf, mossy fiber; IPSP, inhibitory post-synaptic potential; KA, kainic acid; PD, Parkinson's disease; PTZ, pentylenetetrazole; PB, phenobarbital; PANSS, Positive and Negative Syndrome Scale; PSC, post-synaptic current; sz, seizure; SRS, Social Responsive Scale; SE, status epilepticus; SWS, Sturge-Weber Syndrome; TLE, temporal lobe epilepsy; TBI, traumatic brain injury; TSC, tuberous sclerosis complex; yrs, years.

Brain Cloud^{TM} is an open-access online tool[1], containing genetic and epigenetic data from human prefrontal cortex postmortem brains (Colantuoni et al., 2011). Microarray conducted on human postmortem brain tissue showed NKCC1 mRNA expression profiles from post-conceptual ages through adulthood. These data has been quantitated with two Illumina microarray probes (hHA034657 and hHC001510, Brain Cloud Expression data) spanning the length of all introns and exons to quantitate both isoform transcripts. Both microarray probes show an increase in expression of NKCC1 mRNA as the brain matures (UCSC Genome Browser, Brain Cloud Expression Data). The developmental upregulation of NKCC1 mRNA via microarray mRNA expression data has been reported in many brain regions (Sedmak et al., 2016). In contrast, however, NKCC1 mRNA has been shown to be downregulated in rat neocortical neurons with advancing age (P1–21) when assessed with RT-PCR (Yamada et al., 2004). Other studies utilized *in situ* hybridization to demonstrate downregulation in visual cortex from P0 to P28 (Ikeda et al., 2003), cerebral cortex and hippocampus [Plotkin et al., 1997b (P0-adult); Shimizu-Okabe et al., 2002 (P1–P28)]. Different parts of the brain express different levels of NKCC1 at different developmental timepoints. With advancing age, the expressions of certain transcripts are different than of others. With the availability of probes that target different parts of NKCC1 mRNA sequence, it is confounding on how to properly assess isoform-specific developmental NKCC1 profile. To validate their NKCC1 knockout mouse model, one study utilized multiple probes like mouse, rabbit and goat SLC12a2 antibodies against total protein, C-terminus and N-terminus (Antoine et al., 2013). Revalidation of western blot data with NKCC1-isoform-specific antibodies that can help quantify both NKCC1 isoforms accurately in humans and rodents is needed. Monoclonal antibodies targeting both NKCC1 and NKCC2 are currently available (Developmental Studies Hybridoma Bank at the University of Iowa). While these antibodies cannot help clarify the developmental expression profile of multiple NKCC1 isoform proteins in the brain (Morita et al., 2014), their specificity has only been validated using NKCC1-knockout mouse brains (Deidda et al., 2015). Some studies have tried to tackle this issue by reporting NKCC1 mRNA and comparing it to KCC2 total protein to help evaluate simultaneous expression (Reid et al., 2013). No western blotting probe currently allows us to identify and quantitate each isoform of NKCC1 independently. Western blotting samples from different brain regions also contain empty blood vessels lined with ependymal tissue and glial cells, both of which express NKCC1, representing contamination to assertions about neuronal NKCC1 expression profiles. This would be especially true both in embryonic and neonatal developmental brain studies.

ACTION IN NON-NEURONAL CELLS

NKCC1 has a widespread distribution throughout the body (Vibat et al., 2001) and maintains cellular ionic homeostasis

[1]http://braincloud.jhmi.edu/

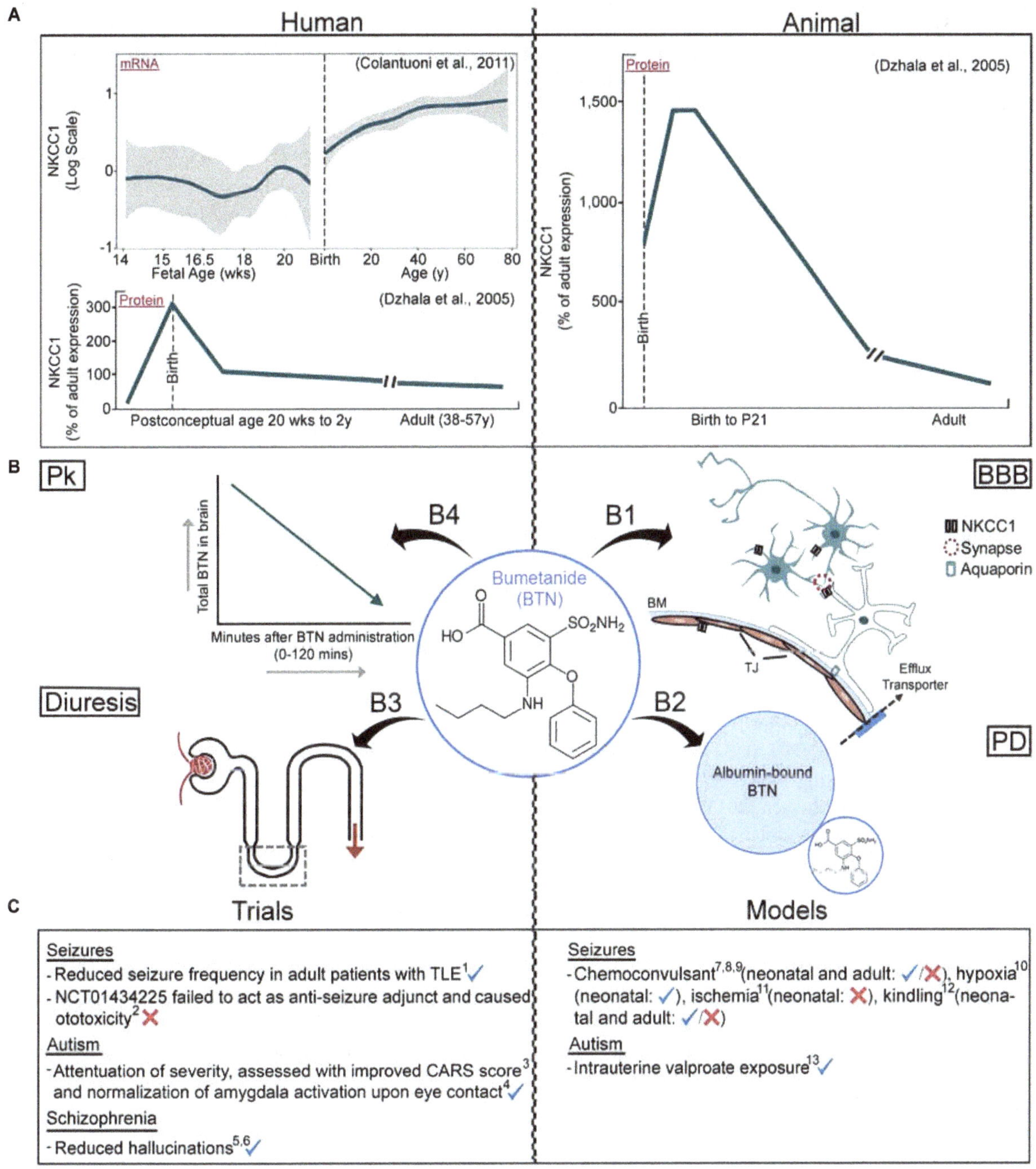

FIGURE 1 | Parsing information about NKCC1 isoforms and BTN **(A)** Human vs. rodent NKCC1 expression profiles. mRNA data from microarray probe (hH034657, Illumina Technologies - probe chosen specifically because it spans most of NKCC1) shows developmental upregulation, followed by NKCC1a protein data using western blotting techniques showing a developmental downregulation. Rodent data of NKCC1a protein shows a developmental downregulation, quantitated with western blotting techniques and consistent with human data analyzed with western blotting using the same probes. **(B)** Pharmacological attributes of BTN affecting its direct neuronal modulation; **(B1)** BBB, neuronal and non-neuronal NKCC1, **(B2)** Albumin's high affinity to BTN, **(B3)** BTN's diuretic effects, **(B4)** BTN's short half-life in serum and brain. **(C)** Clinical trials and pre-clinical models with varying results of BTN efficacy, see **Table 1** for further details. Pk, pharmacokinetics; BBB, Blood–Brain Barrier; PD, pharmacodynamics; BM, basement membrane; TJ, tight junction. Panel A data adapted from Dzhala et al., 2005 with permission and Colantuoni et al., 2011 (graphed brain cloud data replotted with R statistical software).

through electroneutral movement of ions across the membrane (Geck et al., 1980; Markadieu and Delpire, 2014). In the CNS, NKCC1 is also expressed in ependymal and glial cells (Plotkin et al., 1997a; Wu et al., 1998; Hubner et al., 2001; Kanaka et al., 2001; Yan et al., 2001a,b; Mikawa et al., 2002; Su et al., 2002; Wang et al., 2003; Sun, 2010). NKCC1, assessed with RNA-seq, shows higher concentration of transcripts in mature astrocytes (human ages 8–63) than fetal astrocytes (18 gestational weeks) (Zhang et al., 2014). BTN improved ischemic cerebral edema in the post-ischemic brain (Yan et al., 2001b; O'Donnell et al., 2004). This effect is perhaps through BTN's actions on ependymal NKCC1 (Patyal and Alvarez-Leefmans, 2016).

Na-K-Cl co-transport is responsible for regulating K^+ concentration gradient in astrocytes (Hertz, 1965; Walz, 1987). This function is especially crucial in attempts to avoid excessive K^+ accumulation that occurs after astrocyte swelling in pathological conditions, such as ischemia and traumatic brain injury (TBI) (Kimelberg, 1992; Rutledge and Kimelberg, 1996; Walz, 2000). Additionally, NKCC1 is involved in control of extracellular Ca^{2+} ions (Lenart et al., 2004; Annunziato et al., 2013) and astrocytes regulate neuronal Ca^{2+} levels through Ca^{2+}-dependent glutamate release (Parpura et al., 1994). When NKCC1 activity was ablated or pharmaceutically inhibited in astrocytes, filling of Ca^{2+} endoplasmic-reticulum Ca^{2+} stores in astrocytes was absent following oxygen/glucose deprivation and reoxygenation (Lenart et al., 2004). Astrocytes are active modulators of neuronal activity. The vital relationship between neurons and astrocytes that allows for proper brain homeostasis could be indicative of further neuronal regulation via astrocytes (**Figure 1B1**). This concept could underlie one of the multifactorial mechanisms of BTN responsiveness in the CNS due to the role of astrocyte pathologies in the different neurological diseases.

The relationship between aquaporin 4 (AQP4) and NKCC1 has been investigated in the CNS; AQP4 effluxes water in response to NKCC1 transporting water (Østby et al., 2009; Zeuthen, 2010; Nagelhus and Ottersen, 2013), indicating other possible sites for BTN mediated modulation. NKCC1 expressed in the mouse choroid plexus is the main contributor to cerebrospinal fluid production, through its water-translocating properties (Steffensen et al., 2018). While once thought to be a passive process, recent studies show NKCC1 plays an active role in producing nearly half of the brains daily quota of CSF through the choroid plexus (Steffensen et al., 2018). NKCC1 is also robustly expressed in oligodendrocytes and has a pivotal role in GABAergic functions (Plotkin et al., 1997b; Wang et al., 2003; Annunziato et al., 2013). Muscimol-induced activation of $GABA_AR$'s resulted in reduced $[Cl^-]_I$, cell shrinkage and NKCC1 activity (Wang et al., 2003). In fact, NKCC1 is most robustly expressed in newly formed oligodendrocytes when compared to all other neural cell types including astrocytes, neurons, oligodendrocyte progenitor cells, myelinating oligodendrocytes, microglia and epithelia (Zhang et al., 2014). BTN increased neurogenesis and alleviated stroke-induced behavioral impairments in adult rats (Xu et al., 2017). For the following studies, (O'Donnell et al., 2005, 2006), authors utilized T4 hybridoma pan NKCC1 and NKCC2 antibody. Since endothelial cells in the brain solely express NKCC1 and not NKCC2, one can infer that the quantifications reported were of NKCC1 only. Authors, however, reported it as NKCC protein since probe was not NKCC1 specific. NKCC1 function in endothelial cells, lining CNS microvasculature are significantly controlled by endogenous factors like arginine vasopressin and estradiol, (O'Donnell et al., 2005, 2006). It was previously shown that antagonizing NKCC with BTN reduced edema formation in a rat stroke model (O'Donnell et al., 2004). Arginine vasopressin stimulates NKCC activity during ischemia and promotes edema formation (O'Donnell et al., 2005). Estradiol was shown to reduce activity of NKCC and decreased edema formation (O'Donnell et al., 2006). Therefore, NKCC1 antagonist, BTN, could play a significant role over brain activity even before it crosses the BBB.

Outside the CNS, NKCC1 is expressed in the epithelial cells of the inner ear (Delpire et al., 1999). Maintenance of homeostasis of inner ear fluids is crucial for proper functioning of the auditory organs, and the inner ear is known to be sensitive to systemic offsets (Juhn et al., 1991). NKCC1 is expressed in the inner and middle ear (Crouch et al., 1997; Kim et al., 2007; Abbas and Whitfield, 2009). Interestingly, NKCC1-null mice exhibit deafness at birth (Delpire et al., 1999). NKCC1 suppression can cause both reversible and irreversible hearing loss (Watabe et al., 2017). Transgenic mice generated to selectively manipulate cochlear NKCC1 resulted in reversible hearing loss in the postnatal mice (Watabe et al., 2017). Therefore, systemic BTN delivery for CNS disorders during critical developmental periods would also inhibit the cochlear-specific NKCC1 isoform (Delpire et al., 2009). The ototoxicity reported following BTN interventions in the HIE trial (NCT01434225, 2015) have been discussed taking the above findings into consideration (Pressler et al., 2015; Allegaert et al., 2016). Interestingly, a animal model study that utilized mice with mutations of Slc12a2 found that the associated inner ear dysfunction additionally caused motor hyperactivity via increased levels of pCREB and pERK in the nucleus accumbens (Antoine et al., 2013). These brain circuit effects were independent of loss of NKCC1 in the brain. Acute diuretic effects of BTN could also lead to dyshomeostasis and fluid imbalance in the inner ear, further aggravating ototoxicity, but in a reversible way. NKCC1-null mice exhibit decreased blood pressure (Flagella et al., 1999), intestinal bleeding (Flagella et al., 1999), infertility (Pace et al., 2000), and salivary secretion reduction (Evans et al., 2000; Sun, 2010). These findings indicate NKCC1 function plays a significant role in multiple organs other than the kidney and brain.

BTN's BRAIN AVAILABILITY

Prenatal brains have been thought to be more vulnerable to drugs, toxins and pathological conditions due to an immature BBB (Saunders et al., 2012). However, the prevalence of efflux transporters present in the placenta may provide protection *in utero*. This protection is lost after birth and may cause the neonatal period to be more vulnerable than the fetal period (Saunders et al., 2012). However, this understanding has been challenged, especially with regard to neurotoxicology (Ek et al., 2012; Saunders et al., 2012). Trypan blue and other acidic dyes administered systemically have been utilized to investigate the integrity of the BBB (Saunders et al., 2012). Functionally effective tight junctions are present in the embryonic brain (Nitta et al., 2003; Ek et al., 2006; Saunders et al., 2012). Therefore, the neonatal BBB is present and functional during development.

The OAT efflux transporter family is responsible for efficacious drug transport (Kusuhara et al., 1999; Urquhart and Kim, 2009; Nigam et al., 2015). OAT3 mediates the necessary uptake for BTN to reach NKCC in the kidney (Burckhardt, 2012). Probenecid, while an inhibitor of all members of the OAT family, is a more selective inhibitor of OAT3, and was utilized to study the effects of the PKs of BTN in the brain (Donovan et al., 2014, 2016). Probenecid increased the brain levels of BTN (Donovan et al., 2014; Töllner et al., 2015). Therefore, activity of OAT3 may contribute significantly to the poor brain access of BTN after systemic administration (Löscher et al., 2013) (**Figure 1B1**). Both restricted passive diffusion and active efflux transport by OAT3, murine OAT polypeptide (Oatp1a4), and multidrug resistance protein 4 (MRP4) lowered the concentrations of systemically administered BTN to the brain in *in vivo* experiments (Römermann et al., 2017). While initially thought that OAT3 is the only transporter that actively effluxes BTN, later studies confirmed that additional transporters may be involved (Römermann et al., 2017). Excitotoxic insults, however, could result in the failure of the BBB via glutamatergic actions on NMDA receptors expressed on endothelial cells lining the CNS vasculature (Xhima et al., 2016). This could have potential implications on both the influx and efflux kinetics of BTN in conditions where this is known to occur.

Just as low brain concentrations and rapid CNS efflux of BTN leads to low plasma/brain ratios for BTN; only unbound and non-ionized forms of BTN are able to diffuse across membranes to begin with (**Figure 1B2**). Based on the calculated pKa of BTN, >99% is ionized at the plasma pH of 7.4 when assessed with nuclear magnetic resonance (NMR) spectroscopy and ultraviolet visible (UV) spectroscopy (Song et al., 2011), with additional variations if using pooled human blood (Walker et al., 1989) or *in vitro* bovine albumin (Donovan et al., 2016) to test binding. Free and unionized BBB-permeable BTN is much lower after systemic administration, compared to what would be warranted for efficacious brain penetration and NKCC1 antagonization in neurons (Puskarjov et al., 2014). Less than 1% of the IP administered BTN (0.15–0.3mg/kg) reached the brain in hypoxic-ischemic insulted P10 rats, showing a similar penetration to those who didn't receive the insult (Puskarjov et al., 2014) (**Figure 1B4**). These results indicate that even ischemic injury to the P10 BBB did not help BTN penetrate the brain at higher concentrations.

Overall, systemic IP injections of BTN yield lower levels of free BTN than IV infusions or injections (Olsen, 1977; Brandt et al., 2010; Puskarjov et al., 2014; Wang et al., 2015). Once in plasma, only BTN that is not bound by albumin can enter the brain, skewing the ratio of BTN presence in the brain compared to plasma. Since the concentration of BTN detected in the brain after systemic administration was much lower than what would be needed to antagonize neuronal NKCC1, higher doses of BTN would have to be administered. Doing so, however, would also aggravate all the other systemic or non-neuronal effects of BTN (Löscher et al., 2013). A short half-life and the presence of efflux transporters further challenges the maintenance of BTN levels in the brain. All of these factors indicate poor CNS interaction of BTN from a therapeutic efficacy standpoint. However, BTN, while only approved as a diuretic, has been reported to show beneficial effects in some neurological disorders. Systemic effects due to non-neuronal action on NKCC1 expressed inside and outside of the BBB needs consideration.

SYSTEMIC EFFECTS

Low doses of BTN (0.5–2 mg in adults, 0.1–0.3 mg/kg in neonates and children) are sufficient to induce diuresis. With the above concentrations, diuresis is complete in about 4h's (FDA Bumetanide Label, 2009). The elimination of BTN is considerably slower in neonatal patients compared with adults (FDA Bumetanide Label, 2009), with ranges from 8 to 27 h in neonates and 33–100 min in adults (Pacifici, 2012; Puskarjov et al., 2014). BTN is also utilized in the treatment of nephrotic syndrome and massive edema (2–6 mg/day) (Lemieux et al., 1981), heart failure (1–3 mg/day) (Kourouklis et al., 1976), and liver disease (0.5–4 mg/day) (Moult et al., 1974). BTN can be administered orally, intravenously, or intramuscularly and increases urinary output by inhibiting Na^+ and Cl^- in the loop of Henle (**Figure 1B3**) with secondary actions on the proximal tubules (Bourke et al., 1973; Murdoch and Auld, 1975; Ward and Heel, 1984; FDA Bumetanide Label, 2009). Side effects of the induced diuresis include volume depletion, electrolyte depletion, and hypokalemia (FDA Bumetanide Label, 2009). Repeated doses require caution and should not exceed 10 mg a day (FDA Bumetanide Label, 2009).

Off-Label Studies

Neonatal Seizures

The anti-seizure efficacy of BTN by itself or as an adjunct has been evaluated in several pre-clinical models of neonatal seizures (Dzhala et al., 2005, 2008; Cleary et al., 2013; Kang et al., 2015; Kharod et al., 2018). BTN alone hyperpolarized the equilibrium potential of Cl^- in immature neurons, suppressed epileptiform activity in hippocampal slices *in vitro* and reduced kainic acid induced seizures *in vivo* (Dzhala et al., 2005). BTN seizure suppression data reported in this study resulted in the initiation of clinical trials for BTN for HIE seizures. This was attributed to the hypothesized higher expression of NKCC1 in immature human and rodent brains (see **Figure 1A** human and animal WB data). However, the developmentally regulated low expression and function of KCC2 at birth may also play a significant role in determining Cl^- gradients during early postnatal weeks (Rivera et al., 1999; Lee et al., 2005). Additionally, microarray data show that human NKCC1 mRNA increases into adulthood, and therefore contradicts the developmental hypothesis of high NKCC1 transporter function and its association with early life seizure susceptibility.

In vitro, BTN served as an efficacious adjunct to PB to decrease recurrent tonic-clonic epileptiform activity after application of Mg^{2+} free ACSF in the intact immature hippocampus (Dzhala et al., 2008). PB and BTN applied in combination to *ex vivo* hippocampal slices following hypoxia-induced seizures reversed seizure-induced changes in E_{GABA} when compared to PB and/or BTN applied alone (Cleary et al., 2013). In a *in vivo* model of ischemic seizures, BTN failed as an adjunct to PB in P10 CD-1 mice (Kang et al., 2015). The implications in utilizing *in vivo* models boils down to the simplification that many other factors are at play, often times, these attributes are ones that cannot be controlled as in *in vitro* model counterparts. Post-ischemic P7 CD-1 brains were significantly less susceptible to necrotic infarct injury compared to P10 and P12 for the same insult, with no signs of stroke infarcts detected at P7 in the hypoxic-ischemic model (Kang et al., 2015). While P10 and P12 CD-1 pups responded to PB, P7 pups did not respond to the same loading dose (Kang et al., 2015). PB-inefficacy at P7 was not rescued with co-administration of BTN when administered 1 h post-PB and PB efficacy witnessed in the P10 age group was shunted when BTN was administered, meaning there was significant increase in seizure burden after effective seizure suppression with PB (Kang et al., 2015). In a recent model of pentylenetetrazole (PTZ)-induced acute episodic seizures at the same age (P7) and same mouse strain (CD-1), PB effectively suppressed an even higher seizure burden than what was witnessed in the ischemic seizure model where PB was inefficacious (Kang et al., 2015; Kharod et al., 2018). BTN administration 1h post-PB reversed PB efficacy (Kharod et al., 2018), similar to the ischemic model at P10 (Kang et al., 2015). In contrast, BTN significantly reduced PTZ induced seizure susceptibility following hypoxic-ischemic injury at P7 in a rat model (Hu et al., 2017). The 3-day BTN treatment also helped restore hippocampal neurogenesis and improved cognitive function in the treated rats (Hu et al., 2017). These improvements may suggest the long-term benefits of acute BTN intervention unrelated to the acute modulation of neuronal Cl^-.

Cl^- co-transporter expression levels, following seizure induction, not only differ by type of insults used to induce neonatal seizures in models of pre-clinical research but also by temporal changes from time of the insult (Cleary et al., 2013; Puskarjov et al., 2014; Kharod et al., 2018). In the CD-1 mouse ischemia model, there was a downregulation of KCC2 total protein, while a PTZ insult in the same strain at the same age resulted in a upregulation of KCC2 (Kang et al., 2015; Kharod et al., 2018). No significant changes were detected in NKCC1 expression in either model, indicating KCC2 may play a critical role in acute post-insult brain plasticity in acquired models of seizures. In the ischemia model of neonatal seizures, it is possible the reported BTN-induced aggravation of PB-suppressed seizures was due to PB-rebound seizures. If BTN aggravated the seizures independently, the mechanism is not understood at this point. Furthermore, it is of interest that BTN aggravated PB-suppressed seizures both in the ischemic and PTZ induced models in a sex-specific manner (see **Table 1**), highlighting the importance of testing sex as a biological variable in every pre-clinical study. **Table 1** highlights the bias toward using only male rodents for pre-clinical studies. In summary, BTN has been reported to have varying efficacies in animal models of neonatal seizures (Dzhala et al., 2008; Mares, 2009; Mazarati et al., 2009; Khirug et al., 2010; Cleary et al., 2013; Kang et al., 2015; Kharod et al., 2018) (see **Figure 1C** and **Table 1**). These model-specific efficacies of BTN could be explained by multiple factors including but not limited to: (1) post-insult response of Cl^- cotransporter expression (both KCC2 and NKCC1), (2) presence of cell-death, edema, albumin leak through disrupted BBB, (3) maturity of the of the BBB (Kang and Kadam, 2014) and (4) the role of non-neuronal cells like astrocytes at tight junctions. Developmentally high NKCC1 expression proposed to result in high $[Cl-]_i$ and thus depolarizing GABA was the hypothesis that formed the basis for the clinical trial for BTN intervention in HIE neonates, but BTN failed as an anti-seizure adjunct to PB (NCT01434225, 2015; Pressler et al., 2015).

Focal Cortical Dysplasia

Focal cortical dysplasia is a malformation of cortical development (Kabat and Król, 2012). The histological characteristics were first described by Taylor et al. (1971). Three types of cortical dysplasia are recognized (Blümcke et al., 2011), types I, II, and III. Characterization of Type I to Type III FCD is based on the location and extent of histopathological changes associated with cortical dysplasias. In the case of Type III FCD, the dysplasia extends beyond the temporal lobe and is associated with other principal lesions like hippocampal sclerosis or vascular malformations (Blümcke et al., 2011; Kabat and Król, 2012). Dysregulated GABAergic transmissions, either due to disrupted chloride cotransporter function or altered $GABA_AR$ mediation are some of the reported characteristics of FCD (Blauwblomme et al., 2018). The effect of BTN was assessed in slices from tissue resected from FCD patients. Bath-applied BTN suppressed interictal discharges, in slices from resected tissue which resumed after washout in physiological artificial CSF (Blauwblomme et al., 2018). In this study, the effects of BTN were variable. However, it suppressed interictal discharges in 9 of 12 slices (see **Table 1**). The conclusions tied the BTN effects on suppression of the interictal discharges to a hypothesized upregulation of NKCC1, without quantification of NKCC1. The results, however, did report reduced membrane KCC2 expression in ictogenic zones within the resected FCD brain slices.

Temporal Lobe Epilepsy

Spontaneous rhythmic activity has been reported in brain slices derived from patients with TLE, that were suppressed by glutamatergic or GABAergic signaling antagonists (Cohen et al., 2002). Brain tissue resected from TLE patients showed alterations in the relative expression of KCC2 and NKCC1 in neurons, which may contribute to epileptiform activity in the subiculum of patients with hippocampal sclerosis (Munoz et al., 2007). BTN attenuated seizure frequency in two out of three patients with TLE (Eftekhari et al., 2013). Seizure models for TLE, including amygdala-kindled rats, pilocarpine-induced SE, post-traumatic seizures, neuronal hyperactivity, ischemia-induced seizures and febrile seizures have been utilized to study altered chloride cotransporter levels (Hochman and Schwartzkroin, 2000; Okabe et al., 2002; Yamada et al., 2004; Li et al., 2008; Lee et al., 2011; Koyama et al., 2012; Kaila et al., 2014; Sivakumaran and Maguire, 2016). The excitatory GABA caused by NKCC1 upregulation remains the proposed rationale behind testing BTN's efficacy (Ben-Ari, 2017). The contributing role of KCC2 hypofunction in seizure susceptibilities is also being explored (Chen et al., 2017). In a recent study, it was shown that local ablation of KCC2 activity in a subset of hippocampal neurons resulted in compromised GABAergic inhibition and development of spontaneous seizures and hippocampal sclerosis (Kelley et al., 2018).

Autism

Autism and prevalence of seizures go hand-in-hand (Besag, 2017). The seizures in patients with autism are often treatment-resistant (Sansa et al., 2011). High $[Cl^-]_i$ makes GABA excitatory, and was proposed to be the basis of the contradictory actions of PB in autistic patients with seizures (Lemonnier et al., 2012). Based on these hypotheses, reducing the $[Cl^-]_i$ via BTN proved efficacious in an animal model of autism using valproic acid exposure (Tyzio et al., 2014). In a commentary response to this study, however, it was noted that it is premature to consider BTN as a prenatal intervention suitable for ASD due to the lack of proper technical tests and failures to assess the long lasting modifications (Bambini-Junior et al., 2014).

In three separate clinical trials where BTN was administered to patients with autism ranging from infancy to adulthood, BTN significantly improved Childhood Autistic Rating Scale (CARS) scores and attenuated the severity of the disorder overall, with no major side effects other than diuresis (Lemonnier and Ben-Ari, 2010; Ben-Ari, 2017; Lemonnier et al., 2017). In a recent study, BTN given to a subset of the patients with autism showed the normalization of amygdala activation upon eye contact (Hadjikhani et al., 2018) (**Figure 1C**), long-after cessation of the BTN therapy suggesting permanent and corrective alterations to the underlying circuits.

Schizophrenia

Increased NKCC1 mRNA expression in patients with schizophrenia was also the proposed rationale underlying BTN treatment trials in these patients. Many patients with schizophrenia manifest clinical symptoms that suggest prefrontal cortex dysfunction (Weinberger, 1988), and so this region remains of interest to study under pathological conditions. A 7.4-fold upregulation of NKCC1 mRNA was detected in the Brodmann's area 46 in schizophrenia patients (Dean et al., 2007). However, more recent data elucidate DLPFC NKCC1b mRNA was significantly decreased in patients with schizophrenia and NKCC1a mRNA remained unchanged when compared to controls (Morita et al., 2014). This finding indicates that NKCC1 isoform expression underlying different pathological conditions could differ by the neurological disorder. In both a case study (Lemonnier et al., 2016) and a small pilot study (Rahmanzadeh et al., 2017), BTN reduced hallucinations in schizophrenic patients. In additional tests, however, where the brief psychiatric rating scale (BPRS) was assessed, BTN treatment had no significant effect when compared to the placebo group (Rahmanzadeh et al., 2016).

In schizophrenia and autism, and in the cases where increased NKCC1 expression has been determined, either by western blotting or PCR, it would be of interest to investigate whether the developmental profile of NKCC1 expression is impaired. The potential developmental and functional alterations in NKCC1 isoform expression and distribution both in healthy and diseased brains could help understand the role of NKCC1 in CNS disorders.

SHARED MECHANISMS WITH OSMOTIC AGENTS

Osmotic agents have been administered for treatment of seizures and alleviation of brain injury and edema (Cruz et al., 2004; Maa et al., 2011; Walcott et al., 2012). Osmotic agents may share mechanism of action(s) with BTN due to their shared diuretic properties. Mannitol (an osmolyte), much like BTN, has been reported to have varying efficacies. The anti-seizure effects of mannitol have long been studied in animal models and humans. In a kainic acid rat model, mannitol (1.5 g/kg, IV, 10 min, 1.5 and 3 h, respectively, after kainic acid administration) yielded a protective effect at 1.5 h after kainic acid seizure induction (Baran et al., 1987). Along with anti-seizure effects, mannitol prevented the formations of lesions and other potential neurochemical changes. Additionally, rat CA1 hippocampal slices in solutions made 5–30 mosmol/kg hyperosmotic by additions of mannitol, sucrose, raffinose, L-glucose and dextran blocked $[K+]o$-induced spontaneous seizures (Traynelis and Dingledine, 1989). In contrast, a recent study did not find any anticonvulsant effects of NKCC blockers (LD's) in a electroconvulsive adult seizure model, while other diuretics exhibited some activity at high doses (Zaluska et al., 2018). Haglund and Hochman (2005) administered a single dose of either 20 mg furosemide (cation-Cl^- cotransporter antagonist) or 50 g mannitol to epileptic patients during their surgical procedures for the treatment of intractable epilepsy; both drugs significantly suppressed epileptic-spikes and electrical stimulation-evoked epileptiform discharges in all subjects recorded from electrodes directly placed on the cortical surface. In another study, mannitol was given to pediatric patients experiencing status epilepticus (SE) and raised intracranial pressure. While success rates were not provided in detail, authors concluded that all seizures cannot be treated with one drug. Underlying pathologies must be taken into consideration when choosing what anti-seizure drug to employ, especially in regards to the utilization of diuretics, which have preexisting conflicting success rates (Smith et al., 1996). One prominent mechanism shared by diuretics in general, with proposed antiepileptic efficacy is inhibition of carbonic anhydrase. Carbonic anhydrases catalyze reversible hydration/dehydration of CO_2/HCO_3^-, respectively (Aggarwal et al., 2013). These actions suppress seizures through disruption of CO_2 equilibrium with inhibitory action on ion channels (Aggarwal et al., 2013). However, carbonic anhydrase inhibition likely is not one of the mechanisms of action of BTN, since BTN is a weak carbonic anhydrase inhibitor (isoforms I, II, III, and XIII) (Carta and Supuran, 2013). BTN was inhibitory to carbonic anhydrase for tumor-associated isoforms (Carta and Supuran, 2013). Therefore, BTN's mechanism of action via carbonic anhydrase requires further investigations to fully understand its anti-convulsive properties.

BTN PRO-DRUGS AND ANALOGS

To improve BTN accessibility to the brain, pro-drugs with lipophilic and uncharged esters, alcohol and amide analogs have been created. These pro-drugs convert to BTN after gaining access into the brain. There was a significantly higher concentration of ester prodrug, BUM5 (*N,N* – dimethylaminoethyl ester), in mouse brains compared to the parent BTN (10 mg/kg, IV of BTN and equimolar dose of 13 mg/kg, IV of BUM5) (Töllner et al., 2014). BUM5 stopped seizures in adult animal models where BTN failed to work (Töllner et al., 2014; Erker et al., 2016). BUM5 was also less diuretic and showed better brain access when compared to the other prodrugs, BUM1 (ester prodrug), BUM7 (alcohol prodrug) and BUM10 (amide prodrug). BUM5 was reported to be more effective than BTN in altering seizure thresholds in epileptic animals post-SE and post-kindling (Töllner et al., 2014). Furthermore, BUM5 (13 mg/kg, IV) was more efficacious than BTN (10 mg/kg, IV) in promoting the anti-seizure effects of PB, in a maximal electroshock seizure model (Erker et al., 2016). Compared to BUM5 which was an efficacious adjunct to PB in the above mentioned study, BTN was not efficacious when administered as an adjunct (Erker et al., 2016). In addition to seizure thresholds, further studies need to be conducted to assess effects of BUM5 on seizure burdens, ictal events, duration and latencies.

Recently, a benzylamine derivative, bumepamine, has been investigated in pre-clinical models. Since benzylamine derivatives lack the carboxylic group of BTN, it results in lower diuretic activity (Nielsen and Feit, 1978). This prompted Brandt et al. (2018) to explore the proposed lower diuretic activity, higher lipophilicity and lower ionization rate of bumepamine at physiological pH. Since it is known that rodents metabolize BTN quicker than humans, the study used higher doses of 10 mg/kg of bumepamine similar to their previous BTN studies (Olsen, 1977; Brandt et al., 2010; Töllner et al., 2014). Bumepamine, while only being nominally metabolized to BTN, was more effective than BTN to support anticonvulsant effects of PB in rodent models of epilepsy. This GABAergic response, however, was not due to antagonistic actions on NKCC1; suggesting bumepamine may have an off-target effect, which remains unknown. However, the anticonvulsive effects of bumepamine, in spite of its lack of action on NKCC1, are to be noted. Additionally, in another study by the same group, it was shown that azosemide was 4-times more potent an inhibitor of NKCC1 than BTN, opening additional avenues for better BBB penetration and NKCC1-antagonizing compounds for potential neurological drug discovery (Hampel et al., 2018).

CONCLUSION

The beneficial effects of BTN reported in cases of autism, schizophrenia and TLE, given its poor-brain bioavailability are intriguing. The mechanisms underlying the effects of BTN, as a neuromodulator for developmental and neuropsychiatric disorders could be multifactorial due to prominent NKCC1 function at neuronal and non-neuronal sites within the CNS. Investigation of the possible off-target and systemic effects of BTN may help further this understanding with the advent of a new generation of brain-accessible BTN analogs.

AUTHOR CONTRIBUTIONS

SCK, SKK, and SDK contributed to writing of this manuscript. SDK supervised and made final edits.

FUNDING

The work associated with this review was supported by the Eunice Kennedy Shriver National Institute of Child Health & Human Development of the National Institutes of Health under Award Number R01HD090884 (SDK). The content is solely the responsibility of the authors and does not necessarily represent the official views of the National Institutes of Health.

ACKNOWLEDGMENTS

The authors thank Brennan Sullivan for helpful comments and discussions.

REFERENCES

Abbas, L., and Whitfield, T. T. (2009). Nkcc1 (Slc12a2) is required for the regulation of endolymph volume in the otic vesicle and swim bladder volume in the zebrafish larva. *Development* 136, 2837–2848. doi: 10.1242/dev.034215

Aggarwal, M., Kondeti, B., and McKenna, R. (2013). Anticonvulsant/antiepileptic carbonic anhydrase inhibitors: a patent review. *Expert Opin. Ther. Pat.* 23, 717–724. doi: 10.1517/13543776.2013.782394

Allegaert, K., Lahav, A., and Van den Anker, J. N. (2016). A mechanism to explain ototoxicity in neonates exposed to bumetamide: lessons to help improve future product development in neonates. *Pediatr. Drugs* 18, 331–333. doi: 10.1007/s40272-016-0190-4

Amin, H., Marinaro, F., De Pietri Tonelli, D., and Berdondini, L. (2017). Developmental excitatory-to-inhibitory GABA-polarity switch is disrupted in 22q11.2 deletion syndrome: a potential target for clinical therapeutics. *Sci. Rep.* 7:15752. doi: 10.1038/s41598-017-15793-9

Annunziato, L., Boscia, F., and Pignataro, G. (2013). Ionic transporter activity in astrocytes, microglia, and oligodendrocytes during brain ischemia. *J. Cereb. Blood Flow Metab.* 33, 969–982. doi: 10.1038/jcbfm.2013.44

Antoine, M. W., Hübner, C. A., Arezzo, J. C., and Hébert, J. M. (2013). A causative link between inner ear defects and long-term striatal dysfunction. *Science* 341, 1120–1123. doi: 10.1126/science.1240405

Antrobus, S. P., Lytle, C., and Payne, J. A. (2012). K+-Cl- cotransporter-2 KCC2 in chicken cardiomyocytes. *Am. J. Physiol. Cell Physiol.* 303, C1180–C1191. doi: 10.1152/ajpcell.00274.2012

Asbury, M. J., Gatenby, P. B., O'Sullivan, S., and Bourke, E. (1972). Bumetanide: potent new 'Loop' diuretic. *Br. Med. J.* 1, 211–213. doi: 10.1136/bmj.1.5794.211

Bambini-Junior, V., Nunes, G. D., Schneider, T., and Gottfried, C. (2014). Comment on 'oxytocin-mediated gaba inhibition during delivery attenuates autism pathogenesis in rodent offspring.' *Science* 346:176. doi: 10.1126/science.1255679

Baran, H., Lassmann, H., Sperk, G., Seitelberger, F., and Hornykiewicz, O. (1987). Effect of mannitol treatment on brain neurotransmitter markers in kainic acid-induced epilepsy. *Neuroscience* 21, 679–684. doi: 10.1016/0306-4522(87)90029-7

Ben-Ari, Y. (2017). NKCC1 chloride importer antagonists attenuate many neurological and psychiatric disorders. *Trends Neurosci.* 40, 536–554. doi: 10.1016/j.tins.2017.07.001

Ben-Ari, Y., Khalilov, I., Kahle, K. T., and Cherubini, E. (2012). The GABA excitatory/inhibitory shift in brain maturation and neurological disorders. *Neuroscientist* 18, 467–486. doi: 10.1177/1073858412438697

Besag, F. M. (2017). Epilepsy in patients with autism: links, risks and treatment challenges. *Neuropsychiatr. Dis. Treat.* 14, 1–10. doi: 10.2147/NDT.S120509

Blauwblomme, T., Dossi, E., Pellegrino, C., Goubert, E., Iglesias, B. G., Sainte-Rose, C., et al. (2018). Gamma-aminobutyric acidergic transmission underlies interictal epileptogenicity in pediatric focal cortical dysplasia. *Ann. Neurol.* 85, 204–217. doi: 10.1002/ana.25403

Blümcke, I., Thom, M., Aronica, E., Armstrong, D. D., Vinters, H. V., Palmini, A., et al. (2011). The clinicopathologic spectrum of focal cortical dysplasias: a consensus classification proposed by an ad hoc task force of the ILAE diagnostic methods commission. *Epilepsia* 52, 158–174. doi: 10.1111/j.1528-1167.2010.02777.x

Bourke, E., Asbury, M. J., O'Sullivan, S., and Gatenby, P. B. (1973). The sites of action of bumetanide in man. *Eur. J. Pharmacol.* 23, 283–289. doi: 10.1016/0014-2999(73)90096-4

Bragin, D. E., Sanderson, J. L., Peterson, S., Connor, J. A., and Müller, W. S. (2009). Development of epileptiform excitability in the deep entorhinal cortex after status epilepticus. *Eur. J. Neurosci.* 30, 611–624. doi: 10.1111/j.1460-9568.2009.06863.x

Brandt, C., Nozadze, M., Heuchert, N., Rattka, M., and Löscher, W. (2010). Disease-modifying effects of phenobarbital and the NKCC1 inhibitor bumetanide in the pilocarpine model of temporal lobe epilepsy. *J. Neurosci.* 30, 8602–8612. doi: 10.1523/JNEUROSCI.0633-10.2010

Brandt, C., Seja, P., Töllner, K., Römermann, K., Hampel, P., Kalesse, M., et al. (2018). Bumepamine, a brain-permeant benzylamine derivative of bumetanide, does not inhibit NKCC1 but is more potent to enhance phenobarbital's anti-seizure efficacy. *Neuropharmacology* 143, 186–204. doi: 10.1016/j.neuropharm.2018.09.025

Brater, C. D. (2000). Pharmacology of diuretics. *Am. J. Med. Sci.* 319, 38–50. doi: 10.1016/S0002-9629(15)40678-0

Burckhardt, G. (2012). Drug transport by organic anion transporters (OATs). *Pharmacol. Ther.* 136, 106–130. doi: 10.1016/j.pharmthera.2012.07.010

Carta, F., and Supuran, C. T. (2013). Diuretics with carbonic anhydrase inhibitory action: a patent and literature review (2005 – 2013). *Expert Opin. Ther. Pat.* 23, 681–691. doi: 10.1517/13543776.2013.780598

Chen, L., Wan, L., Wu, Z., Ren, W., Huang, Y., Qian, B., et al. (2017). KCC2 downregulation facilitates epileptic seizures. *Sci. Rep.* 7:156. doi: 10.1038/s41598-017-00196-7

Clayton, G. H., Owens, G. C., Wolff, J. S., and Smith, R. L. (1998). Ontogeny of cation-Cl- cotransporter expression in rat neocortex. *Brain Res. Dev. Brain Res.* 109, 281–292. doi: 10.1016/S0165-3806(98)00078-9

Cleary, R. T., Sun, H., Huynh, T., Manning, S. M., Li, Y., Rotenberg, A., et al. (2013). Bumetanide enhances phenobarbital efficacy in a rat model of hypoxic neonatal seizures. *PLoS One* 8:e57148. doi: 10.1371/journal.pone.0057148

Cohen, I., Navarro, V., Clemenceau, S., Baulac, M., and Miles, R. (2002). On the origin of interictal activity in human temporal lobe epilepsy in vitro. *Science* 298, 1418–1421. doi: 10.1126/science.1076510

Colantuoni, C., Lipska, B. K., Ye, T., Hyde, T. M., Tao, R., Leek, J. T., et al. (2011). Temporal dynamics and genetic control of transcription in the human prefrontal cortex. *Nature* 478, 519–523. doi: 10.1038/nature10524. Available at: http://braincloud.jhmi.edu/ for Brain Cloud Expression data information.

Côme, E., Heubl, M., Schwartz, E. J., Poncer, J. C., and Lévi, S. (2019). Reciprocal regulation of KCC2 trafficking and synaptic activity. *Front. Cell. Neurosci.* 13:48. doi: 10.3389/fncel.2019.00048

Conti, L., Palma, E., Roseti, C., Lauro, C., Cipriani, R., de Groot, M., et al. (2011). Anomalous levels of Cl- transporters cause a decrease of GABAergic inhibition in human peritumoral epileptic cortex. *Epilepsia* 52, 1635–1644. doi: 10.1111/j.1528-1167.2011.03111.x

Crouch, J. J., Sakaguchi, N., Lytle, C., and Schulte, B. A. (1997). Immunohistochemical localization of the Na-K-Cl Co-transporter (NKCC1) in the gerbil inner ear. *J. Histochem. Cytochem.* 45, 773–778. doi: 10.1177/002215549704500601

Cruz, J., Minoja, G., Okuchi, K., and Facco, E. (2004). Successful use of the new high-dose mannitol treatment in patients with Glasgow coma scale scores of 3 and bilateral abnormal pupillary widening: a randomized trial. *J. Neurosurg.* 100, 376–383. doi: 10.3171/jns.2004.100.3.0376

Damier, P., Hammond, C., and Ben-Ari, Y. (2016). Bumetanide to treat Parkinson disease: a report of 4 cases. *Clin. Neuropharmacol.* 39, 57–59. doi: 10.1097/WNF.0000000000000114

Dean, B., Keriakous, D., Scarr, E., and Thomas, E. A. (2007). Gene expression profiling in brodmann's area 46 from subjects with schizophrenia. *Aust. N. Z. J. Psychiatry* 41, 308–320. doi: 10.1080/00048670701213245

Deidda, G., Parrini, M., Naskar, S., Bozarth, I. F., Contestabile, A., and Cancedda, L. (2015). Reversing excitatory GABAAR signaling restores synaptic plasticity and memory in a mouse model of down syndrome. *Nat. Med.* 21, 318–326. doi: 10.1038/nm.3827

Delpire, E., Days, E., Lewis, L. M., Mi, D., Kim, K., Lindsley, C. W., et al. (2009). Small-molecule screen identifies inhibitors of the neuronal K-Cl cotransporter KCC2. *Proc. Natl. Acad. Sci. U.S.A.* 106, 5383–5388. doi: 10.1073/pnas.0812756106

Delpire, E., Lu, J., England, R., Dull, C., and Thorne, T. (1999). Deafness and imbalance associated with inactivation of the secretory Na-K-2Cl Co-transporter. *Nat. Genet.* 22, 192–195. doi: 10.1038/9713

Donovan, M. D., O'Brien, F. E., Boylan, G. B., Cryan, J. F., and Griffin, B. T. (2014). The effect of organic anion transporter 3 inhibitor probenecid on bumetanide levels in the brain: an integrated in vivo microdialysis study in the rat. *J. Pharm. Pharmacol.* 67, 501–510. doi: 10.1111/jphp.12341

Donovan, M. D., Schellekens, H., Boylan, G. B., Cryan, J. F., and Griffin, B. T. (2016). In vitro bidirectional permeability studies identify pharmacokinetic limitations of NKCC1 inhibitor bumetanide. *Eur. J. Pharmacol.* 770, 117–125. doi: 10.1016/j.ejphar.2015.12.001

Du, L., Shan, L., Wang, B., Li, H., Xu, Z., Staal, W. G., et al. (2015). A pilot study on the combination of applied behavior analysis and bumetanide treatment for children with autism. *J. Child Adolesc. Psychopharmacol.* 25, 585–588. doi: 10.1089/cap.2015.0045

Dzhala, V. I., Brumback, A. C., and Staley, K. J. (2008). Bumetanide enhances phenobarbital efficacy in a neonatal seizure model. *Ann. Neurol.* 63, 222–235. doi: 10.1002/ana.21229

Dzhala, V. I., Talos, D. M., Sdrulla, D. A., Brumback, A. C., Mathews, G. C., Benke, T. A., et al. (2005). NKCC1 transporter facilitates seizures in the developing brain. *Nat. Med.* 11, 1205–1213. doi: 10.1038/nm1301

Eftekhari, S., Habibabadi, J. M., Ziarani, M. N., Fesharaki, S. S. H., Gharakhani, M., Mostafavi, H., et al. (2013). Bumetanide reduces seizure frequency in patients with temporal lobe epilepsy. *Epilepsia* 54, e9–e12. doi: 10.1111/j.1528-1167.2012.03654.x

Ek, C. J., Dziegielewska, K. M., Habgood, M. D., and Saunders, N. R. (2012). Barriers in the developing brain and neurotoxicology. *Neurotoxicology* 33, 586–604. doi: 10.1016/j.neuro.2011.12.009

Ek, C. J., Dziegielewska, K. M., Stolp, H., and Saunders, N. R. (2006). Functional effectiveness of the blood-brain barrier to small water soluble molecules in developing and adult opossum (*Monodelphis domestica*). *J. Comp. Neurol.* 496, 13–26. doi: 10.1002/cne.20885

Erker, T., Brandt, C., Töllner, K., Schreppel, P., Twele, F., Schidlitzki, A., et al. (2016). The bumetanide prodrug BUM5, but not bumetanide, potentiates the antiseizure effect of phenobarbital in adult epileptic mice. *Epilepsia* 57, 698–705. doi: 10.1111/epi.13346

Evans, R. L., Park, K., Turner, R. J., Watson, G. E., Nguyen, H. V., Dennnett, M. R., et al. (2000). Severe impairment of salivation in Na+/K+/2Cl- cotransporter (NKCC1)-deficient mice. *J. Biol. Chem.* 275, 26720–26726. doi: 10.1074/jbc.M003753200

FDA Bumetanide Label (2009). *FDA Label*. Silver Spring, MD: FDA.

Flagella, M., Clarke, L. L., Miller, M. L., Erway, L. C., Giannella, R. A., Andringa, A., et al. (1999). Mice lacking the basolateral Na-K-2Cl cotransporter have impaired epithelial chloride secretion and are profoundly deaf. *J. Biol. Chem.* 274, 26946–26955. doi: 10.1074/jbc.274.38.26946

Geck, P., Pietrzyk, C., Burckhardt, B. C., Pfeifferl, B., and Heinz, E. (1980). Electrically silent cotransport of Na+, K+ and Cl- in Ehrlich cells. *Biochim. Biophys. Acta* 600, 432–447. doi: 10.1016/0005-2736(80)90446-0

Hadjikhani, N., Asberg Johnels, J., Lassalle, A., Zurcher, N. R., Hippolyte, L., Gillberg, C., et al. (2018). Bumetanide for autism: more eye contact, less amygdala activation. *Sci. Rep.* 8:3602. doi: 10.1038/s41598-018-21958-x

Haglund, M. M., and Hochman, D. W. (2005). Furosemide and mannitol suppression of epileptic activity in the human brain. *J. Neurophysiol.* 94, 907–918. doi: 10.1152/jn.00944.2004

Hampel, P., Römermann, K., MacAulay, N., and Löscher, W. (2018). Azosemide is more potent than bumetanide and various other loop diuretics to inhibit the sodium-potassium-chloride-cotransporter human variants HNKCC1A and HNKCC1B. *Sci. Rep.* 8:9877. doi: 10.1038/s41598-018-27995-w

Hertz, L. (1965). Possible role of neuroglia: a potassium-mediated neuronal – neuroglial – neuronal impulse transmission system. *Nature* 206, 1091–1094. doi: 10.1038/2061091a0

Hesdorffer, D. C., Hauser, W. A., Annegers, J. F., and Rocca, W. A. (1996). Severe, uncontrolled hypertension and adult-onset seizures: a case-control study in Rochester, Minnesota. *Epilepsia* 37, 736–741. doi: 10.1111/j.1528-1157.1996.tb00644.x

Hesdorffer, D. C., Stables, J. P., Hauser, W. A., Annegers, J. F., and Cascino, G. (2001). Are certain diuretics also anticonvulsants? *Ann. Neurol.* 50, 458–462.

Hochman, D. W., and Schwartzkroin, P. A. (2000). Chloride-cotransport blockade desynchronizes neuronal discharge in the 'Epileptic' hippocampal slice. *J. Neurophysiol.* 83, 406–417. doi: 10.1152/jn.2000.83.1.406

Holmes, G. L., Tian, C., Hernan, A. E., Flynn, S., Camp, D., and Barry, J. (2015). Alterations in sociability and functional brain connectivity caused by early-life seizures are prevented by bumetanide. *Neurobiol. Dis.* 77, 204–219. doi: 10.1016/j.nbd.2015.02.015

Hu, J. J., Yang, X. L., Luo, W. D., Han, S., Yin, J., Liu, W. H., et al. (2017). Bumetanide reduce the seizure susceptibility induced by pentylenetetrazol via inhibition of aberrant hippocampal neurogenesis in neonatal rats after hypoxia-ischemia. *Brain Res. Bull.* 130, 188–199. doi: 10.1016/j.brainresbull.2017.01.022

Hubner, C. A., Stein, V., Hermans-Borgmeyer, I., Meyer, T., Ballanyi, K., and Jentsch, T. J. (2001). Disruption of KCC2 reveals an essential role of K-Cl cotransport already in early synaptic inhibition. *Neuron* 30, 515–524. doi: 10.1016/S0896-6273(01)00297-5

Hyde, T. M., Lipska, B. K., Ali, T., Mathew, S. V., Law, A. J., Metitiri, O. E., et al. (2011). Expression of GABA signaling molecules KCC2, NKCC1, and GAD1 in cortical development and schizophrenia. *J. Neurosci.* 31, 11088–11095. doi: 10.1523/JNEUROSCI.1234-11.2011

Ikeda, M., Toyoda, H., Yamada, J., Okabe, A., Sato, K., Hotta, Y., et al. (2003). Differential development of cation-chloride cotransporters and Cl- homeostasis contributes to differential GABAergic actions between developing rat visual cortex and dorsal lateral geniculate nucleus. *Brain Res.* 984, 149–159. doi: 10.1016/S0006-8993(03)03126-3

Jantzie, L. L., Hu, M. Y., Park, H. K., Jackson, M. C., Yu, J., Maxwell, J. R., et al. (2015). Chloride cotransporter NKCC1 inhibitor bumetanide protects against white matter injury in a rodent model of periventricular leukomalacia. *Pediatr. Res.* 77, 554–562. doi: 10.1038/pr.2015.9

Juhn, S. K., Ikeda, K., Morizono, T., and Murphy, M. (1991). Pathophysiology of inner ear fluid imbalance. *Acta Otolaryngol. Suppl.* 485, 9–14. doi: 10.3109/00016489109128038

Kabat, J., and Król, P. (2012). Focal cortical dysplasia - review. *Pol. J. Radiol.* 77, 35–43. doi: 10.12659/PJR.882968

Kahle, K. T., Barnett, S. M., Sassower, K. C., and Staley, K. J. (2009). Decreased seizure activity in a human neonate treated with bumetanide, an inhibitor of the Na+-K+-2Cl- cotransporter NKCC1. *J. Child Neurol.* 24, 572–576. doi: 10.1177/0883073809333526

Kaila, K., Price, T. J., Payne, J. A., Puskarjov, M., and Voipio, J. (2014). Cation-chloride cotransporters in neuronal development, plasticity and disease. *Nat. Rev. Neurosci.* 15, 637–654. doi: 10.1038/nrn3819

Kanaka, C., Ohno, K., Okabe, A., Kuriyama, K., Itoh, T., Fukuda, A., et al. (2001). The differential expression patterns of messenger RNAs encoding K-Cl cotransporters (KCC1,2) and Na-K-2Cl cotransporter (NKCC1) in the rat nervous system. *Neuroscience* 104, 933–946. doi: 10.1016/S0306-4522(01)00149-X

Kang, S. K., and Kadam, S. D. (2014). Pre-clinical models of acquired neonatal seizures: differential effects of injury on function of chloride Co-transporters. *Austin J. Cerebrovasc. Dis. Stroke* 1:1026.

Kang, S. K., Markowitz, G. J., Kim, S. T., Johnston, M. V., and Kadam, S. D. (2015). Age- and sex-dependent susceptibility to phenobarbital-resistant neonatal seizures: role of chloride Co-transporters. *Front. Cell. Neurosci.* 9:173. doi: 10.3389/fncel.2015.00173

Kanner, A. M. (2002). Diuretics as antiepileptic drugs. *Epilepsy Curr.* 2, 39–40. doi: 10.1046/j.1535-7597.2002.00013.x

Kelley, M. R., Cardarelli, R. A., Smalley, J. L., Ollerhead, T. A., Andrew, P. M., Brandon, N. J., et al. (2018). Locally reducing KCC2 activity in the hippocampus is sufficient to induce temporal lobe epilepsy. *EBiomedicine* 32, 62–71. doi: 10.1016/j.ebiom.2018.05.029

Kharod, S. C., Carter, B. M., and Kadam, S. D. (2018). Pharmaco-resistant neonatal seizures: critical mechanistic insights from a chemoconvulsant model. *Dev. Neurobiol.* 78, 1117–1130. doi: 10.1002/dneu.22634

Khirug, S., Ahmad, F., Puskarjov, M., Afzalov, R., Kaila, K., and Blaesse, P. (2010). A single seizure episode leads to rapid functional activation of KCC2 in the neonatal rat hippocampus. *J. Neurosci.* 30, 12028–12035. doi: 10.1523/JNEUROSCI.3154-10.2010

Kim, S. J., Choi, J. Y., Son, E. J., Namkung, W., Lee, M. G., and Yoon, J. H. (2007). Interleukin-1β upregulates Na+-K+-2Cl- cotransporter in human middle ear epithelia. *J. Cell. Biochem.* 101, 576–586. doi: 10.1002/jcb.21216

Kimelberg, H. K. (1992). Astrocytic edema in CNS trauma. *J. Neurotrauma* 9(Suppl. 1), S71–S81.

Kourdougli, N., Pellegrino, C., Renko, J. M., Khirug, S., Chazal, G., Kukko-Lukjanov, T. K., et al. (2017). Depolarizing γ-aminobutyric acid contributes to glutamatergic network rewiring in epilepsy. *Ann. Neurol.* 81, 251–265. doi: 10.1002/ana.24870

Kourouklis, C., Christensen, O., and Augoustakis, D. (1976). Bumetanide in congestive heart failure. *Curr. Med. Res. Opin.* 4, 422–431. doi: 10.1185/03007997609111998

Koyama, R., Tao, K., Sasaki, T., Ichikawa, J., Miyamoto, D., Muramatsu, R., et al. (2012). GABAergic excitation after febrile seizures induces ectopic granule cells and adult epilepsy. *Nat. Med.* 18, 1271–1278. doi: 10.1038/nm.2850

Kusuhara, H., Sekine, T., Utsunomiya-Tate, N., Tsuda, M., Kojima, R., Cha, S. H., et al. (1999). Molecular cloning and characterization of a new multispecific organic anion transporter from rat brain. *J. Biol. Chem.* 274, 13675–13680. doi: 10.1074/jbc.274.19.13675

Lee, H., Chen, C. X., Liu, Y. J., Aizenman, E., and Kandler, K. (2005). KCC2 expression in immature rat cortical neurons is sufficient to switch the polarity of GABA responses. *Eur. J. Neurosci.* 21, 2593–2599. doi: 10.1111/j.1460-9568.2005.04084.x

Lee, H. A., Hong, S. H., Kim, J. W., and Jang, I. S. (2010). Possible involvement of DNA methylation in NKCC1 gene expression during postnatal development and in response to ischemia. *J. Neurochem.* 114, 520–529. doi: 10.1111/j.1471-4159.2010.06772.x

Lee, H. H., Deeb, T. Z., Walker, J. A., Davies, P. A., and Moss, S. J. (2011). NMDA receptor activity downregulates KCC2 resulting in depolarizing GABA(A) receptor mediated currents. *Nat. Neurosci.* 14, 736–743. doi: 10.1038/nn.2806

Lemieux, G., Beauchemin, M., Gougoux, A., and Vinay, P. (1981). Treatment of nephrotic edema with bumetanide. *Can. Med. Assoc. J.* 125, 1111–1112.

Lemonnier, E., and Ben-Ari, Y. (2010). The diuretic bumetanide decreases autistic behaviour in five infants treated during 3 months with no side effects. *Acta Paediatr.* 99, 1885–1888. doi: 10.1111/j.1651-2227.2010.01933.x

Lemonnier, E., Degrez, C., Phelep, M., Tyzio, R., Josse, F., Grandgeorge, M., et al. (2012). A randomised controlled trial of bumetanide in the treatment of autism in children. *Transl. Psychiatry* 2:e202. doi: 10.1038/tp.2012.124

Lemonnier, E., Lazartigues, A., and Ben-Ari, Y. (2016). Treating schizophrenia with the diuretic bumetanide: a case report. *Clin. Neuropharmacol.* 39, 115–117. doi: 10.1097/WNF.0000000000000136

Lemonnier, E., Villeneuve, N., Sonie, S., Serret, S., Rosier, A., Roue, M., et al. (2017). Effects of bumetanide on neurobehavioral function in children and adolescents with autism spectrum disorders. *Transl. Psychiatry* 7:e1056. doi: 10.1038/tp.2017.10

Lenart, B., Kintner, D. B., Shull, G. E., and Sun, D. (2004). Na-K-Cl cotransporter-mediated intracellular Na+ accumulation affects Ca2+ signaling in astrocytes in an in vitro ischemic model. *J. Neurosci.* 24, 9585–9597. doi: 10.1523/JNEUROSCI.2569-04.2004

Li, H., Tornberg, J., Kaila, K., Airaksinen, M. S., and Rivera, C. (2002). Patterns of cation-chloride cotransporter expression during embryonic rodent CNS development. *Eur. J. Neurosci.* 16, 2358–2370. doi: 10.1046/j.1460-9568.2002.02419.x

Li, X., Zhou, J., Chen, Z., Chen, S., Zhu, F., and Zhou, L. (2008). Long-term expressional changes of Na+ - K+ - Cl- Co-transporter 1 (NKCC1) and K+ - Cl- Co-transporter 2 (KCC2) in CA1 region of hippocampus following lithium-pilocarpine induced status epilepticus (PISE). *Brain Res.* 1221, 141–146. doi: 10.1016/j.brainres.2008.04.047

Liu, Y., Shangguan, Y., Barks, J. D., and Silverstein, F. S. (2012). Bumetanide augments the neuroprotective efficacy of phenobarbital plus hypothermia in a neonatal hypoxia-ischemia model. *Pediatr. Res.* 71, 559–565. doi: 10.1038/pr.2012.7

Löscher, W., Puskarjov, M., and Kaila, K. (2013). Cation-chloride cotransporters NKCC1 and KCC2 as potential targets for novel antiepileptic and antiepileptogenic treatments. *Neuropharmacology* 69, 62–74. doi: 10.1016/j.neuropharm.2012.05.045

Lu, K. T., Wu, C. Y., Cheng, N. C., Wo, Y. Y., Yang, J. T., Yen, H. H., et al. (2006). Inhibition of the Na+-K+-2Cl-cotransporter in choroid plexus attenuates traumatic brain injury-induced brain edema and neuronal damage. *Eur. J. Pharmacol.* 548, 99–105. doi: 10.1016/j.ejphar.2006.07.048

Lu, K. T., Wu, C. Y., Yen, H. H., Peng, J. H., Wang, C. L., and Yang, Y. L. (2007). Bumetanide administration attenuated traumatic brain injury through IL-1 overexpression. *Neurol. Res.* 29, 404–409. doi: 10.1179/016164107X204738

Maa, E. H., Kahle, K. T., Walcott, B. P., Spitz, M. C., and Staley, K. J. (2011). Diuretics and epilepsy: will the past and present meet? *Epilepsia* 52, 1559–1569. doi: 10.1111/j.1528-1167.2011.03203.x

Mares, P. (2009). Age- and dose-specific anticonvulsant action of bumetanide in immature rats. *Physiol. Res.* 58, 927–930.

Markadieu, N., and Delpire, E. (2014). Physiology and pathophysiology of SLC12A1/2 transporters. *Pflugers Arch.* 466, 91–105. doi: 10.1007/s00424-013-1370-5

Mazarati, A., Shin, D., and Sankar, R. (2009). Bumetanide inhibits rapid kindling in neonatal rats. *Epilepsia* 50, 2117–2122. doi: 10.1111/j.1528-1167.2009.02048.x

Mikawa, S., Wang, C., Shu, F., Wang, T., Fukuda, A., and Sato, K. (2002). Developmental changes in KCC1, KCC2 and NKCC1 MRNAs in the rat cerebellum. *Dev. Brain Res.* 136, 93–100. doi: 10.1016/S0165-3806(02)00345-0

Mòdol, L., Cobianchi, S., and Navarro, X. (2014). Prevention of NKCC1 phosphorylation avoids downregulation of KCC2 in central sensory pathways and reduces neuropathic pain after peripheral nerve injury. *Pain* 155, 1577–1590. doi: 10.1016/j.pain.2014.05.004

Morita, Y., Callicott, J. H., Testa, L. R., Mighdoll, M. I., Dickinson, D., Chen, Q., et al. (2014). Characteristics of the cation cotransporter NKCC1 in human brain: alternate transcripts, expression in development, and potential relationships to brain function and schizophrenia. *J. Neurosci.* 34, 4929–4940. doi: 10.1523/JNEUROSCI.1423-13.2014

Moult, P. J., Lunzer, M. R., Trash, D. B., and Sherlock, S. (1974). Use of bumetanide in the treatment of ascites due to liver disease. *Gut* 15, 988–992. doi: 10.1136/gut.15.12.988

Munoz, A., Mendez, P., DeFelipe, J., and Alvarez-Leefmans, F. J. (2007). Cation-chloride cotransporters and GABA-ergic innervation in the human epileptic hippocampus. *Epilepsia* 48, 663–673. doi: 10.1111/j.1528-1167.2007.00986.x

Murdoch, W. R., and Auld, W. H. (1975). Bumetanide—acute and long term studies of a new high potency diuretic. *Postgrad. Med. J.* 51, 10–14. doi: 10.1136/pgmj.51.591.10

Nagelhus, E. A., and Ottersen, O. P. (2013). Physiological roles of aquaporin-4 in brain. *Physiol. Rev.* 93, 1543–1562. doi: 10.1152/physrev.00011.2013

NCT00830531 (2017). *Pilot Study of Bumetanide for Newborn Seizures.* Available at: https://clinicaltrials.gov/ct2/show/NCT00830531 (accessed on January 20, 2019).

NCT01434225 (2015). *NEMO1:NEonatal Seizure Using Medication Off-Patent (NEMO1).* Available at: https://clinicaltrials.gov/ct2/show/NCT01434225 (accessed on January 20, 2019).

Nicholls, J. G., Martin, A. R., Fuchs, P. A., Brown, D. A., Diamond, M. E., and Weisblat, D. A. (2012). *From Neuron to Brain*, 5th Edn. Sunderland, MA: Sinauer Associates.

Nielsen, O. B., and Feit, P. W. (1978). Structure-activity relationships of aminobenzoic acid diuretics and related compounds (1). *Diuretic Agents* 83, 12–23. doi: 10.1021/bk-1978-0083.ch002

Nigam, S. K., Bush, K. T., Martovetsky, G., Ahn, S. Y., Liu, H. C., Richard, E., et al. (2015). The organic anion transporter (OAT) family: a systems biology perspective. *Physiol. Rev.* 95, 83–123. doi: 10.1152/physrev.00025.2013

Nitta, T., Hata, M., Gotoh, S., Seo, Y., Sasaki, H., Hashimoto, N., et al. (2003). Size-selective loosening of the blood-brain barrier in claudin-5–deficient mice. *J. Cell Biol.* 161, 653–660. doi: 10.1083/jcb.200302070

O'Donnell, M. E., Duong, V., Suvatne, J., Foroutan, S., and Johnson, D. M. (2005). Arginine vasopressin stimulation of cerebral microvascular endothelial cell Na-K-Cl cotransporter activity is V1 receptor and [Ca] dependent. *Am. J. Physiol. Cell Physiol.* 289, C283–C292. doi: 10.1152/ajpcell.00001.2005

O'Donnell, M. E., Lam, T. I., Tran, L. Q., Foroutan, S., and Anderson, S. E. (2006). Estradiol reduces activity of the blood-brain barrier Na-K-Cl cotransporter and decreases edema formation in permanent middle cerebral artery occlusion. *J. Cereb. Blood Flow Metab.* 26, 1234–1249. doi: 10.1038/sj.jcbfm.9600278

O'Donnell, M. E., Tran, L., Lam, T. I., Liu, X. B., and Anderson, S. E. (2004). Bumetanide inhibition of the blood-brain barrier Na-K-Cl cotransporter reduces edema formation in the rat middle cerebral artery occlusion model of stroke. *J. Cereb. Blood Flow Metab.* 24, 1046–1056. doi: 10.1097/01.WCB.0000130867.32663.90

Okabe, A., Ohno, K., Toyoda, H., Yokokura, M., Sato, K., and Fukuda, A. (2002). Amygdala kindling induces upregulation of MRNA for NKCC1, a Na+, K+-2Cl- cotransporter, in the rat piriform cortex. *Neurosci. Res.* 44, 225–229. doi: 10.1016/S0168-0102(02)00093-7

Olsen, U. B. (1977). The pharmacology of bumetanide. *Acta Pharmacol. Toxicol.* 41, 1–28. doi: 10.1111/j.1600-0773.1977.tb03209.x

Østby, I., Øyehaug, L., Einevoll, G. T., Nagelhus, E. A., Plahte, E., Zeuthen, T., et al. (2009). Astrocytic mechanisms explaining neural-activity-induced shrinkage of extraneuronal space. *PLoS Comput. Biol.* 5:e1000272. doi: 10.1371/journal.pcbi.1000272

Owens, D. F., and Kriegstein, A. R. (2002). Is there more to gaba than synaptic inhibition? *Nat. Rev. Neurosci.* 3, 715–727. doi: 10.1038/nrn919

Pace, A. J., Lee, E., Athirakul, K., Coffman, T. M., O'Brien, D. A., and Koller, B. H. (2000). Failure of spermatogenesis in mouse lines deficient in the Na(+)-K(+)-2Cl(-) cotransporter. *J. Clin. Investig.* 105, 441–450. doi: 10.1172/JCI8553

Pacifici, G. M. (2012). Clinical pharmacology of the loop diuretics furosemide and bumetanide in neonates and infants. *Pediatr. Drugs* 14, 233–246. doi: 10.2165/11596620-000000000-00000

Palma, E., Amici, M., Sobrero, F., Spinelli, G., Di Angelantonio, S., Ragozzino, D., et al. (2006). Anomalous levels of Cl- transporters in the hippocampal subiculum from temporal lobe epilepsy patients make GABA excitatory. *Proc. Natl. Acad. Sci. U.S.A.* 103, 8465–8468. doi: 10.1073/pnas.0602979103

Parpura, V., Basarsky, T. A., Liu, F., Jeftinija, K., Jeftinija, S., and Haydon, P. G. (1994). Glutamate-mediated astrocyte-neuron signalling. *Nature* 369, 744–747. doi: 10.1038/369744a0

Patyal, P., and Alvarez-Leefmans, F. J. (2016). Expression of NKCC1 and aquaporins 4, 7 and 9 in mouse choroid plexus and ependymal cells. *FASEB J.* 30:lb621. doi: 10.1096/fasebj.30.1_supplement.lb621

Plotkin, M. D., Kaplan, M. R., Peterson, L. N., Gullans, S. R., Hebert, S. C., and Delpire, E. (1997a). Expression of the Na(+)-K(+)-2Cl- cotransporter BSC2 in the nervous system. *Am. J. Physiol. Cell Physiol.* 272, C173–C183. doi: 10.1152/ajpcell.1997.272.1.C173

Plotkin, M. D., Snyder, E. Y., Hebert, S. C., and Delpire, E. (1997b). Expression of the Na-K-2Cl cotransporter is developmentally regulated in postnatal rat brains: a possible mechanism underlying GABA's excitatory role in immature brain.

J. Neurobiol. 33, 781–795. doi: 10.1002/(SICI)1097-4695(19971120)33:6<781::AID-NEU6>3.0.CO;2-5

Pressler, R. M., Boylan, G. B., Marlow, N., Blennow, M., Chiron, C., Cross, J. H., et al. (2015). Bumetanide for the treatment of seizures in newborn babies with hypoxic ischaemic encephalopathy (NEMO): an open-label, dose finding, and feasibility phase 1/2 trial. *Lancet Neurol.* 14, 469–477. doi: 10.1016/S1474-4422(14)70303-5

Puskarjov, M., Kahle, K. T., Ruusuvuori, E., and Kaila, K. (2014). Pharmacotherapeutic targeting of cation-chloride cotransporters in neonatal seizures. *Epilepsia* 55, 806–818. doi: 10.1111/epi.12620

Rahmanzadeh, R., Eftekhari, S., Shahbazi, A., Ardakani, M. K., Rahmanzade, R., Mehrabi, S., et al. (2017). Effect of bumetanide, a selective NKCC1 inhibitor, on hallucinations of schizophrenic patients; a double-blind randomized clinical trial. *Schizophr. Res.* 184, 145–146. doi: 10.1016/j.schres.2016.12.002

Rahmanzadeh, R., Shahbazi, A., Ardakani, M. K., Mehrabi, S., Rahmanzade, R., and Joghataei, M. T. (2016). Lack of the effect of bumetanide, a selective NKCC1 inhibitor, in patients with schizophrenia: a double-blind randomized trial. *Psychiatry Clin. Neurosci.* 71, 72–73. doi: 10.1111/pcn.12475

Reid, A. Y., Riazi, K., Campbell Teskey, G., and Pittman, Q. J. (2013). Increased excitability and molecular changes in adult rats after a febrile seizure. *Epilepsia* 54, e45–e48. doi: 10.1111/epi.12061

Rivera, C., Voipio, J., Payne, J. A., Ruusuvuori, E., Lahtinen, H., Lamsa, K., et al. (1999). The K+/Cl- Co-transporter KCC2 renders GABA hyperpolarizing during neuronal maturation. *Nature* 397, 251–255. doi: 10.1038/16697

Römermann, K., Fedrowitz, M., Hampel, P., Kaczmarek, E., Töllner, K., Erker, T., et al. (2017). Multiple blood-brain barrier transport mechanisms limit bumetanide accumulation, and therapeutic potential, in the mammalian brain. *Neuropharmacology* 117, 182–194. doi: 10.1016/j.neuropharm.2017.02.006

Rutledge, E. M., and Kimelberg, H. K. (1996). Release of [3H]-D-aspartate from primary astrocyte cultures in response to raised external potassium. *J. Neurosci.* 16, 7803–7811. doi: 10.1523/JNEUROSCI.16-24-07803.1996

Sansa, G., Carlson, C., Doyle, W., Weiner, H. L., Bluvstein, J., Barr, W., et al. (2011). Medically refractory epilepsy in autism. *Epilepsia* 52, 1071–1075. doi: 10.1111/j.1528-1167.2011.03069.x

Saunders, N. R., Liddelow, S. A., and Dziegielewska, K. M. (2012). Barrier mechanisms in the developing brain. *Front. Pharmacol.* 3:46. doi: 10.3389/fphar.2012.00046

Sedmak, G., Jovanov-Miloševiæ, N., Puskarjov, M., Ulamec, M., Krušlin, B., Kaila, K., et al. (2016). Developmental expression patterns of KCC2 and functionally associated molecules in the human brain. *Cereb. Cortex* 26, 4574–4589. doi: 10.1093/cercor/bhv218

Shimizu-Okabe, C., Yokokura, M., Okabe, A., Ikeda, M., Sato, K., Kilb, W., et al. (2002). Layer-specific expression of Cl- transporters and differential [Cl-]i in newborn rat cortex. *Neuroreport* 13, 2433–2437. doi: 10.1097/00001756-200212200-00012

Sivakumaran, S., and Maguire, J. (2016). Bumetanide reduces seizure progression and the development of pharmacoresistant status epilepticus. *Epilepsia* 57, 222–232. doi: 10.1111/epi.13270

Smith, R. A., Martland, T., and Lowry, M. F. (1996). Children with seizures presenting to accident and emergency. *J. Accid. Emerg. Med.* 13, 54–58. doi: 10.1136/emj.13.1.54

Song, B., Galande, A. K., Kodukula, K., Moos, W. H., and Miller, S. M. (2011). Evaluation of the PKa values and ionization sequence of bumetanide using 1H and 13C NMR and UV spectroscopy. *Drug Dev. Res.* 72, 416–426. doi: 10.1002/ddr.20443

Song, L., Mercado, A., Vázquez, N., Xie, Q., Desai, R., George, A. L. Jr., et al. (2002). Molecular, functional, and genomic characterization of human KCC2, the neuronal K-Cl cotransporter. *Mol. Brain Res.* 103, 91–105. doi: 10.1016/S0169-328X(02)00190-0

Steffensen, A. B., Oernbo, E. K., Stoica, A., Gerkau, N. J., Barbuskaite, D., Tritsaris, K., et al. (2018). Cotransporter-mediated water transport underlying cerebrospinal fluid formation. *Nat. Commun.* 9:2167. doi: 10.1038/s41467-018-04677-9

Su, G., Kintner, D. B., Flagella, M., Shull, G. E., and Sun, D. (2002). Astrocytes from Na+-K+-Cl-cotransporter-null mice exhibit absence of swelling and decrease in EAA release. *Am. J. Physiol. Cell Physiol.* 282, C1147–C1160. doi: 10.1152/ajpcell.00538.2001

Sun, D. (2010). "The 'Loop' diuretic drug bumetanide-sensitive Na+-K+-Cl-cotransporter in cerebral ischemia," in *New Strategies in Stroke Intervention: Ionic Transporters, Pumps, and New Channels*, ed. L. Annunziato (New York, NY: Humana Press).

Talos, D. M., Sun, H., Kosaras, B., Joseph, A., Folkerth, R. D., Poduri, A., et al. (2012). Altered inhibition in tuberous sclerosis and type IIb cortical dysplasia. *Ann. Neurol.* 71, 539–551. doi: 10.1002/ana.22696

Taylor, D. C., Falconer, M. A., Bruton, C. J., and Corsellis, J. A. (1971). Focal dysplasia of the cerebral cortex in epilepsy. *J. Neurol. Neurosurg. Psychiatry* 34, 369–387. doi: 10.1136/jnnp.34.4.369

Töllner, K., Brandt, C., Römermann, K., and Löscher, W. (2015). The organic anion transport inhibitor probenecid increases brain concentrations of the NKCC1 inhibitor bumetanide. *Eur. J. Pharmacol.* 746, 167–173. doi: 10.1016/j.ejphar.2014.11.019

Töllner, K., Brandt, C., Töpfer, M., Brunhofer, G., Erker, T., Gabriel, M., et al. (2014). A novel prodrug-based strategy to increase effects of bumetanide in epilepsy. *Ann. Neurol.* 75, 550–562. doi: 10.1002/ana.24124

Traynelis, S. F., and Dingledine, R. (1989). Role of extracellular space in hyperosmotic suppression of potassium-induced electrographic seizures. *J. Neurophysiol.* 61, 927–938. doi: 10.1152/jn.1989.61.5.927

Tyzio, R., Khalilov, I., Represa, A., Crepel, V., Zilberter, Y., Rheims, S., et al. (2009). Inhibitory actions of the gamma-aminobutyric acid in pediatric sturge-weber syndrome. *Ann. Neurol.* 66, 209–218. doi: 10.1002/ana.21711

Tyzio, R., Nardou, R., Ferrari, D. C., Tsintsadze, T., Shahrokhi, A., Eftekhari, S., et al. (2014). Oxytocin-mediated GABA inhibition during delivery attenuates autism pathogenesis in rodent offspring. *Science* 343, 675–679. doi: 10.1126/science.1247190

Urquhart, B. L., and Kim, R. B. (2009). Blood-brain barrier transporters and response to CNS-active drugs. *Eur. J. Clin. Pharmacol.* 65, 1063–1070. doi: 10.1007/s00228-009-0714-8

Uvarov, P., Llano, O., Ludwig, A., Airaksinen, M., and Rivera, C. (2013). "Multiple roles of KCC2 in the developing brain," in *Cellular Migration and Formation of Neuronal Connections*, eds J. Rubenstein and P. Rakic (Cambridge, MA: Academic Press), 975–998. doi: 10.1016/B978-0-12-397266-8.00190-3

Uvarov, P., Ludwig, A., Markkanen, M., Pruunsild, P., Kaila, K., Delpire, E., et al. (2007). A novel N-terminal isoform of the neuron-specific K-Cl cotransporter KCC2. *J. Biol. Chem.* 282, 30570–30576. doi: 10.1074/jbc.M705095200

Uvarov, P., Ludwig, A., Markkanen, M., Soni, S., Hübner, C. A., Rivera, C., et al. (2009). Coexpression and heteromerization of two neuronal K-Cl cotransporter isoforms in neonatal brain. *J. Biol. Chem.* 284, 13696–13704. doi: 10.1074/jbc.M807366200

Vibat, C. R., Holland, M. J., Kang, J. J., Putney, L. K., and O'Donnell, M. E. (2001). Quantitation of Na+-K+-2Cl- cotransport splice variants in human tissues using kinetic polymerase chain reaction. *Anal. Biochem.* 298, 218–230. doi: 10.1006/abio.2001.5398

Walcott, B. P., Kahle, K. T., and Simard, J. M. (2012). Novel treatment targets for cerebral edema. *Neurotherapeutics* 9, 65–72. doi: 10.1007/s13311-011-0087-4

Walker, P. C., Berry, N. S., and Edwards, D. J. (1989). Protein binding characteristics of bumetanide. *Dev. Pharmacol. Ther.* 12, 13–18. doi: 10.1159/000480977

Walz, W. (1987). Swelling and potassium uptake in cultured astrocytes. *Can. J. Physiol. Pharmacol.* 65, 1051–1057. doi: 10.1139/y87-166

Walz, W. (2000). Role of astrocytes in the clearance of excess extracellular potassium. *Neurochem. Int.* 36, 291–300. doi: 10.1016/S0197-0186(99)00137-0

Wang, H., Yan, Y., Kintner, D. B., Lytle, C., and Sun, D. (2003). GABA-mediated trophic effect on oligodendrocytes requires Na-K-2Cl cotransport activity. *J. Neurophysiol.* 90, 1257–1265. doi: 10.1152/jn.01174.2002

Wang, S., Zhang, X. Q., Song, C. G., Xiao, T., Zhao, M., Zhu, G., et al. (2015). In vivo effects of bumetanide at brain concentrations incompatible with NKCC1 inhibition on newborn DGC structure and spontaneous EEG seizures following hypoxia-induced neonatal seizures. *Neuroscience* 286, 203–215. doi: 10.1016/j.neuroscience.2014.11.031

Ward, A., and Heel, R. C. (1984). Bumetanide. A review of its pharmacodynamic and pharmacokinetic properties and therapeutic use. *Drugs* 28, 426–464. doi: 10.2165/00003495-198428050-00003

Watabe, T., Xu, M., Watanabe, M., Nabekura, J., Higuchi, T., Hori, K., et al. (2017). Time-controllable Nkcc1 knockdown replicates reversible hearing loss in postnatal mice. *Sci. Rep.* 7:13605. doi: 10.1038/s41598-017-13997-7

Watanabe, M., and Fukuda, A. (2015). Development and regulation of chloride homeostasis in the central nervous system. *Front. Cell. Neurosci.* 9:371. doi: 10.3389/fncel.2015.00371

Weinberger, D. R. (1988). Schizophrenia and the frontal lobe. *Trends Neurosci.* 11, 367–370. doi: 10.1016/0166-2236(88)90060-4

Wilkinson, C. M., Fedor, B. A., Aziz, J. R., Nadeau, C. A., Brar, P. S., Clark, J. J. A., et al. (2019). Failure of bumetanide to improve outcome after intracerebral hemorrhage in rat. *PLoS One* 14:e0210660. doi: 10.1371/journal.pone.0210660

Wittner, M., Di Stefano, A., Wangemann, P., and Greger, R. (1991). How do loop diuretics act? *Drugs* 41, 1–13. doi: 10.2165/00003495-199100413-00003

Wu, Q., Delpire, E., Hebert, S. C., and Strange, K. (1998). Functional demonstration of Na+-K+-2Cl-cotransporter activity in isolated, polarized choroid plexus cells. *Am. J. Physiol. Cell Physiol.* 275, C1565–C1572. doi: 10.1152/ajpcell.1998.275.6.C1565

Xhima, K., Weber-Adrian, D., and Silburt, J. (2016). Glutamate induces blood-brain barrier permeability through activation of N-methyl-D-aspartate receptors. *J. Neurosci.* 36, 12296–12298. doi: 10.1523/JNEUROSCI.2962-16.2016

Xu, W., Mu, X., Wang, H., Song, C., Ma, W., Jolkkonen, J., et al. (2017). Chloride co-transporter NKCC1 inhibitor bumetanide enhances neurogenesis and behavioral recovery in rats after experimental stroke. *Mol. Neurobiol.* 54, 2406–2414. doi: 10.1007/s12035-016-9819-0

Yamada, J., Okabe, A., Toyoda, H., Kilb, W., Luhmann, H. J., and Fukuda, A. (2004). Cl(-) uptake promoting depolarizing GABA actions in immature rat neocortical neurones is mediated by NKCC1. *J. Physiol.* 557(Pt 3), 829–841. doi: 10.1113/jphysiol.2004.062471

Yan, Y., Dempsey, R. J., and Sun, D. (2001a). Expression of Na+-K+-Cl- cotransporter in rat brain during development and its localization in mature astrocytes. *Brain Res.* 911, 43–55. doi: 10.1016/S0006-8993(01)02649-X

Yan, Y., Dempsey, R. J., and Sun, D. (2001b). Na+-K+-Cl- cotransporter in rat focal cerebral ischemia. *J. Cereb. Blood Flow Metab.* 21, 711–721. doi: 10.1097/00004647-200106000-00009

Załuska, K., Kondrat-Wróbel, M. W., and Łuszczki, J. J. (2018). Comparison of the anticonvulsant potency of various diuretic drugs in the maximal electroshock-induced seizure threshold test in mice. *Adv. Clin. Exp. Med.* 27, 609–613. doi: 10.17219/acem/68694

Zeuthen, T. (2010). Water transporting proteins. *J. Membr. Biol.* 234, 57–73. doi: 10.1007/s00232-009-9216-y

Zhang, Y., Chen, K., Sloan, S. A., Bennett, M. L., Scholze, A. R., and O'Keefe, S. (2014). An RNA-sequencing transcriptome and splicing database of glia, neurons, and vascular cells of the cerebral cortex. *J. Neurosci.* 34, 11929–11947. doi: 10.1523/JNEUROSCI.1860-14.2014. Available at: http://web.stanford.edu/group/barre_lab/brain_rnaseq.html and http://web.stanford.edu/group/barres_lab/brainseq2/brainseq2.html

8

Immunomodulatory Therapeutic Strategies in Stroke

*Kyle Malone[1], Sylvie Amu[2], Anne C. Moore[3] and Christian Waeber[1]**

[1] Department of Pharmacology and Therapeutics, School of Pharmacy, University College Cork, Cork, Ireland, [2] Cancer Research @UCC, University College Cork, Cork, Ireland, [3] School of Biochemistry and Cell Biology, University College Cork, Cork, Ireland

***Correspondence:**
Christian Waeber
c.waeber@ucc.ie

The role of immunity in all stages of stroke is increasingly being recognized, from the pathogenesis of risk factors to tissue repair, leading to the investigation of a range of immunomodulatory therapies. In the acute phase of stroke, proposed therapies include drugs targeting pro-inflammatory cytokines, matrix metalloproteinases, and leukocyte infiltration, with a key objective to reduce initial brain cell toxicity. Systemically, the early stages of stroke are also characterized by stroke-induced immunosuppression, where downregulation of host defences predisposes patients to infection. Therefore, strategies to modulate innate immunity post-stroke have garnered greater attention. A complementary objective is to reduce longer-term sequelae by focusing on adaptive immunity. Following stroke onset, the integrity of the blood–brain barrier is compromised, exposing central nervous system (CNS) antigens to systemic adaptive immune recognition, potentially inducing autoimmunity. Some pre-clinical efforts have been made to tolerize the immune system to CNS antigens pre-stroke. Separately, immune cell populations that exhibit a regulatory phenotype (T- and B- regulatory cells) have been shown to ameliorate post-stroke inflammation and contribute to tissue repair. Cell-based therapies, established in oncology and transplantation, could become a strategy to treat the acute and chronic stages of stroke. Furthermore, a role for the gut microbiota in ischaemic injury has received attention. Finally, the immune system may play a role in remote ischaemic preconditioning-mediated neuroprotection against stroke. The development of stroke therapies involving organs distant to the infarct site, therefore, should not be overlooked. This review will discuss the immune mechanisms of various therapeutic strategies, surveying published data and discussing more theoretical mechanisms of action that have yet to be exploited.

Keywords: stroke, immunomodulation, ischaemia, immune, therapy, neuroinflammation

INTRODUCTION

Stroke remains a major cause of morbidity and mortality worldwide (Krishnamurthi et al., 2013). Despite the clear impact of acute ischaemic stroke (AIS) on patients, recombinant tissue plasminogen activator (tPA) is the only medication specifically approved for its treatment. Beyond a therapeutic window of 4.5 h, however, the benefits of thrombolysis are outweighed by its risks, with the incidence of haemorrhagic transformation increasing dramatically (Lees et al., 2010). Consequently, only a small percentage of patients receive tPA. Separately, mechanical thrombectomy is indicated for up to 6 h after the onset of ischaemic stroke symptoms, though recent trials have allowed for an extension to 24 h in selected patients (Robinson, 2018).

Additional agents for the treatment of AIS are now required, not only as adjuncts to increase the therapeutic potential of thrombolysis and thrombectomy, but also for patients who, for various reasons, cannot receive standard care. Ideally, such therapies, through curtailing damage to the brain post-stroke or contributing to long-term tissue remodelling, would improve patient survival and functional outcomes.

In the last few decades, hundreds of agents targeting numerous pathophysiological mechanisms have failed clinical trials (O'Collins et al., 2006). Yet from this research, important lessons have been learned. The role of immunity in all stages of stroke, for instance, is becoming better understood. Consequently, a range of immune-targeted therapies are now in development and testing (Malone et al., 2018).

A number of reviews have examined the individual components of the immune response to stroke, or the immunomodulatory agents currently enrolled in stroke clinical trials (Iadecola and Anrather, 2011; Smith et al., 2015; Drieu et al., 2018). However, many aspects of the immune response play multifaceted roles in stroke, and the interaction between the brain and immune system post-stroke is an ever-evolving picture. Future stroke treatment may involve a range of mechanical, immunological, and pharmacological therapies, all working in concert (Neuhaus et al., 2017). If clinically translated, strategies manipulating the immune response could play a crucial part. In this review, we provide an update on immune-targeted strategies in AIS, from the level of pathology to pre-clinical evidence and clinical trials. The aim of this review, therefore, is to discuss immunomodulatory therapeutic strategies in stroke (listed in **Table 1**), surveying published data and highlighting more theoretical mechanisms of action that have yet to be explored.

STROKE AND THE BLOOD–BRAIN BARRIER

The brain was long thought to be hidden from our immune system. This is in large part due to the lack of an obvious lymphatic system and the presence of a blood–brain barrier (BBB). This barrier separates the blood compartment from the central nervous system (CNS) at the level of brain endothelial cells, thus rigorously controlling immune cell trafficking between the CNS and the periphery (Wilson et al., 2010). Correspondingly, breakdown of this barrier may underlie the pathophysiology of immune-based CNS disorders. However, while the BBB is indeed compromised in some CNS disorders and brain injury, the recent discovery of meningeal lymphatics suggests that, even under basal conditions, the "immune privilege" of the brain is not as absolute as was once thought (Louveau et al., 2015).

The BBB is composed of specialized endothelial cells in capillaries and post-capillary venules of the brain and spinal cord, characterized by low pinocytotic activity and by complex tight junctions composed of transmembrane and cytoplasmic adhesion molecules (Serlin et al., 2015). These endothelial cells produce a basement membrane containing embedded pericytes. Another basement membrane, produced by astrocytes, constitutes together with the astrocytic end feet, the glia limitans perivascularis. While these two basement membranes are indistinguishable at the capillary level, they are separate at the level of post-capillary venules, where they form a perivascular space containing cerebrospinal fluid (CSF) and antigen-presenting cells. Under basal conditions, leukocytes rarely penetrate the glia limitans but accumulate in this perivascular space during inflammation (as well as in the leptomeningeal and ventricular spaces) (**Figure 1**). Here, they fulfil an immune-surveillance function by interacting with antigen-presenting bone marrow-derived macrophages and dendritic cells.

The fact that oxidative stress leads to BBB breakdown has been observed in various neurological diseases, including multiple sclerosis (MS) and stroke (Rosenberg, 2012). Oxidative stress is not associated with the ischaemic episode itself but rather with reperfusion, which, although essential to limit brain injury, also causes an initial breakdown of the BBB by activating matrix metalloproteinases (MMPs) and upregulating inflammatory mediators. In experimental studies, BBB opening is biphasic. The initial BBB breakdown occurs within 2–3 h of stroke onset, is associated with activation of MMP-2, and is accompanied by the development of vasogenic oedema (i.e., excess accumulation of fluid in the brain extracellular spaces). Following a partial recovery of BBB function, a second increase in BBB permeability, occurring 24 to 48 h after stroke, is characterized by inflammatory processes with upregulation of inducible MMPs (MMP-3 and MMP-9) and cyclooxygenase (COX)-2, tight junction redistribution, and neutrophil infiltration (Jiang et al., 2018). It is worth mentioning that the biphasic profile of BBB opening has been questioned (as discussed in Merali et al., 2017), and the BBB might in fact be continuously opened for up to a week.

Although neutrophils are the first subset of leukocytes to appear in the ischaemic brain (detected within the first hour), these neutrophils are not found in parenchyma but remain in the cerebral microvessels, which they occlude (contributing to the no-reflow phenomenon) and from where they can damage the BBB by releasing proteolytic enzymes and reactive oxygen species (ROS). Neutrophils penetrate the CNS parenchyma mainly following the more damaging second opening of the BBB, which leads to severe endothelial damage, gross destruction of adjacent blood vessels, and in some cases haemorrhagic transformation (Perez-de-Puig et al., 2015).

Despite the relatively early opening of the BBB, lymphocytes are only detected within the ischaemic territory 24 h after stroke onset, their number increasing over the following days (Schroeter et al., 1994; Brait et al., 2010). Larger infarctions may be associated with earlier appearance of lymphocytes in the brain (Chu et al., 2014). Following stroke, antigen presentation to lymphocytes can rapidly occur in the spleen and lymph nodes, since BBB opening and cell damage following stroke enable CNS antigens to access the blood compartment early after the onset of ischaemia. Indeed, CNS antigens are found in the cervical lymph nodes 24 h after middle cerebral artery occlusion in mice (van Zwam et al., 2009), and the concentration of these antigens seems to correlate with stroke severity (Jauch et al., 2006). Brain-derived

TABLE 1 | Immunomodulatory therapeutic strategies in stroke.

Target	Role in stroke pathology	Proposed therapy
Astrocytes	–Promote neurotoxicity through pro-inflammatory cytokine release (e.g., IL-15) and glial scar formation (Roy-O'Reilly and McCullough, 2017). –Provide neuroprotection *via* reduced excitotoxicity, neurotrophin production, and angiogenic and synaptogenic effects (Wang et al., 2018).	–CDK5-knockdown astrocyte cell therapy (Becerra-Calixto and Cardona-Gómez, 2017)
Macrophage/microglia	–Increase ischaemic injury (M1 type) *via* release of ROS, NO, and pro-inflammatory cytokines (e.g., TNF-α and IL-12) (Chiba and Umegaki, 2013). –Promote tissue repair (M2 type) *via* growth factors, anti-inflammatory cytokines (e.g., IL-4), and phagocytosis of dead cells (Kanazawa et al., 2017).	–Minocycline (macrophage deactivator) (Lampl et al., 2007) –Edaravone (free radical scavenger) (Chen et al., 2014)
Complement pathway	–Contributes to neuronal cell death through C3a and C5a anaphylatoxins (Alawieh et al., 2015a). –Contributes to subacute/chronic neurogenesis and repair (Alawieh and Tomlinson, 2016).	–CR2-Crry (complement inhibitor) (Alawieh et al., 2015b) –B4Crry (complement inhibitor) (Alawieh et al., 2018)
Nitric oxide	–Provides beneficial reductions in platelet aggregation and leukocyte adhesion as well as improved vascular tone and host defence (Kim et al., 2014). –Directly neurotoxic in high levels (Venkataramana et al., 2015).	–Glyceryl trinitrate (nitric oxide donor) (Chen et al., 2017)
IL-1β	–Promotes neurotoxicity through NF-κB-mediated generation of a pro-inflammatory environment (Boutin et al., 2001).	–Anakinra (recombinant IL-1 receptor antagonist) (Smith et al., 2018)
TNF-α	–Promotes BBB breakdown, leukocyte infiltration, and brain oedema (acute stage) (Amantea et al., 2009). –Contributes to neuronal and microvasculature repair (chronic stage) (Amantea et al., 2009).	–Etanercept (TNF-inhibitor) (Tobinick et al., 2014)
COX/LO pathway	–COX: PGE_2 increases ischaemic injury (Iadecola and Gorelick, 2005). PGE_1 contributes to post-stroke neurogenesis and angiogenesis (Ling et al., 2016). –LO: LTC4 promotes BBB dysfunction (Baskaya et al., 1996).	–NS398 (COX-2 inhibitor) (Sugimoto and Iadecola, 2003) –Montelukast (cysteinyl leukotriene receptor-1 antagonist) (Saad et al., 2015)
MMPs	–Increased MMP activity causes neuronal apoptosis, BBB breakdown, leukocyte infiltration, and brain oedema (Rosell and Lo, 2008). –Involved in late-stage neovascularization and neurovascular remodelling (Zhao et al., 2006).	–Minocycline (MMP-9 inhibitor) (Murata et al., 2008)
Chemokines	–Involved in acute ischaemic injury *via* increased leukocyte infiltration, ROS production, and BBB disruption (Chen et al., 2018a). –Possible function in chronic stem cell recruitment to the infarct site (Wang et al., 2002).	–NR58-3.14.3 (pan-chemokine inhibitor) (Mirabelli-Badenier et al., 2011)
Adhesion molecules	–Upregulation of selectins, immunoglobulins, and integrins post-stroke increase leukocyte infiltration with resulting infarct growth (Yilmaz and Granger, 2008).	–Enlimomab (anti-ICAM-1 antibody) (Investigators, 2001) –Hu23F2G (anti-Mac-1 antibody) (Becker, 2002) –Natalizumab (anti-VLA-4 antibody) (Elkins et al., 2017) –Fingolimod (S1P receptor modulator) (Zhu et al., 2015)
Regulatory immune cells	–Regulatory B and T-cells provide neuroprotection and enhance post-stroke repair through dampening excessive immune responses and producing anti-inflammatory cytokines (e.g., IL-10) (Liesz and Kleinschnitz, 2016; Bodhankar et al., 2013)	–IL-2/IL-2 antibody complex (Zhang et al., 2018) –Adoptive cell transfer (Ren et al., 2011)

IL-15, interleukin-15; CDK5, cyclin-dependent kinase 5; ROS, reactive oxygen species; NO, nitric oxide; TNF-α, tumour necrosis factor alpha; IL-12, interleukin-12; IL-4, interleukin 4; NF-κB, COX, cyclooxygenase; LO, lipoxygenase; BBB, blood brain barrier; PGE2, prostaglandin E2; LTC4, leukotriene C4; MMP, matrix metalloproteinase; S1P, sphingosine 1-phosphate; VLA-4, very late antigen-4; ICAM-1, intercellular adhesion molecule-1.

antigens are also found in cervical lymph node cells expressing costimulatory major histocompatibility complex II (MHC-II) receptors in patients with acute stroke (Planas et al., 2012). This suggests that improving BBB function following stroke or at least preventing lymphocytes from entering the brain following their activation with brain antigens might improve functional outcome after stroke. The latter mechanism of action might explain why fingolimod was found to be effective in rodent models of stroke (Wei et al., 2011), reduced the risk of haemorrhagic transformation associated with delayed administration of tPA (Campos et al., 2013), and showed promising results in small clinical trials (Fu et al., 2014a; Fu et al., 2014b).

ACUTE POST-STROKE IMMUNE RESPONSES

In 87% of cases, stroke is due to a drastic reduction in cerebral blood flow (CBF) that results in metabolic and functional deficits. At a pathophysiological level, however, a much more complex web of interactions is seen. Following the onset of cerebral ischaemia, an orderly sequence of events involving the CNS, the lymphoid organs, the blood, and the wider vasculature is triggered (Iadecola and Anrather, 2011). Hypoperfusion causes an immediate deprivation of glucose and oxygen to the brain, leading to a fall in ATP production. Within minutes of the ischaemic insult, the

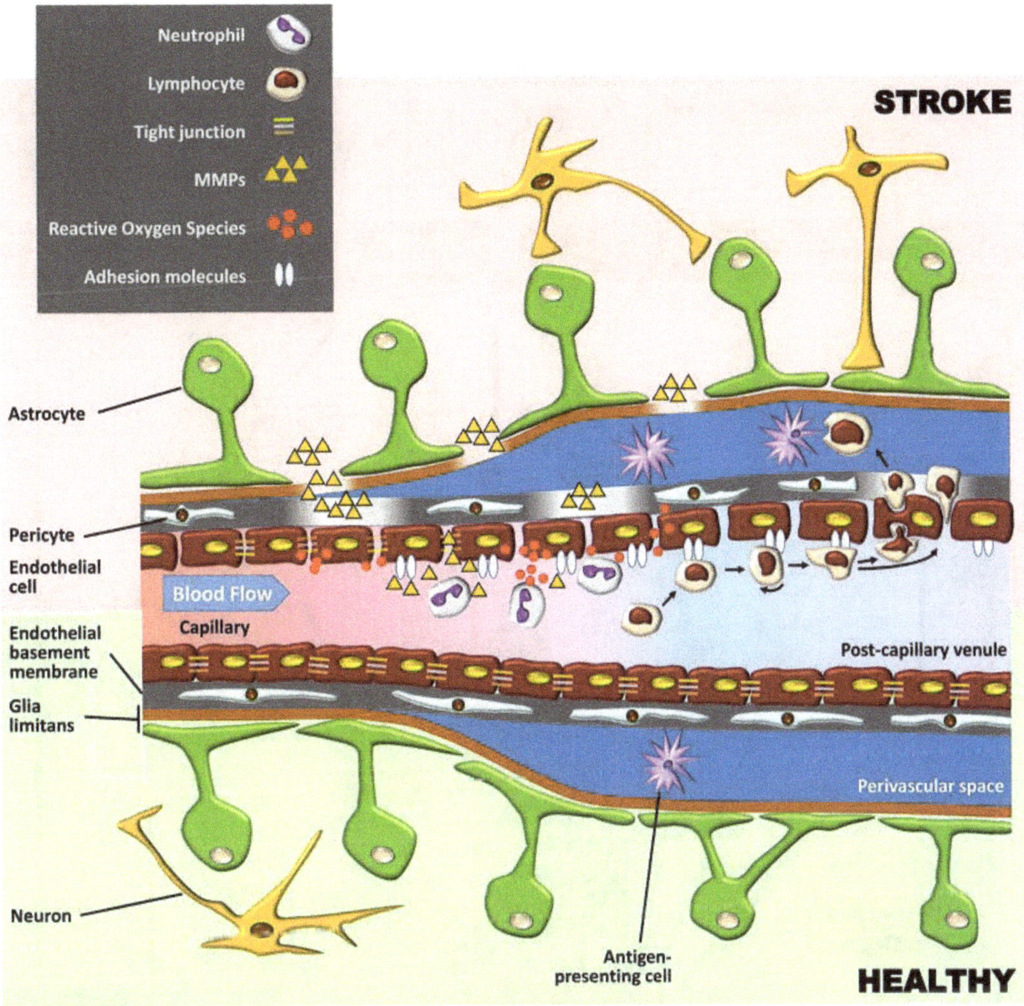

FIGURE 1 | Schematic representation of the blood–brain barrier (BBB) under healthy conditions (bottom part of the figure) and during its early breakdown following stroke (top part). The BBB is composed of a layer of endothelial cells with tight junctions composed of transmembrane and cytoplasmic adhesion molecules. These cells produce a basement membrane containing embedded pericytes. Astrocytes and their end feet constitute the glia limitans perivascularis. At the capillary level (left side of the figure), the endothelial basement membrane and the glia limitans are indistinguishable, but at the level of post-capillary venules (on the right), they are separated by a perivascular space containing cerebrospinal fluid (CSF) and antigen-presenting bone marrow-derived macrophages and dendritic cells. Following reperfusion, reactive oxygen species (ROS) cause an initial breakdown of the BBB by activating matrix metalloproteinases (MMPs) and upregulating inflammatory mediators. Stroke leads to an increased expression of integrin molecules on the leukocyte surface (not shown) and of the corresponding adhesion molecules on the endothelium. Leukocytes tether and roll onto the vascular endothelium before being activated by chemokines (not shown). They then firmly adhere to the endothelium and undergo either transcellular or paracellular diapedesis through the endothelial layer.

downstream processes of acidotoxicity, excitotoxicity, oxidative stress, and inflammation begin, giving rise to widespread neuronal cell death (Fann et al., 2013). The release of danger/damage-associated molecular patterns (DAMPs) from dying neurons induces a new phase of innate inflammatory response (**Figure 2**). Pattern-recognition receptor (PRR) activation on microglia results in the inflammasome-mediated production of interleukin 1-beta (IL-1β) and tumour necrosis factor-α (TNF-α) (Marsh et al., 2009). The subsequent release of cytokines/chemokines from astrocytes and endothelial cells creates an inflammatory environment, containing IL-17, granzyme, ROS, and perforin (Fann et al., 2013). In the vasculature, platelets are activated alongside endothelial cells and proteins of the complement system (Iadecola and Anrather, 2011). Fibrin, the end-product of the coagulation cascade, traps leukocytes and platelets, forming microvascular occlusions (del Zoppo et al., 1991). A fall in the bioavailability of nitric oxide (NO), which normally inhibits platelet aggregation, exacerbates this intravascular plugging (Chen et al., 2017). Capillary occlusions are further promoted by pro-inflammatory signalling, the constriction of pericytes, and the translocation of the adhesion molecule P-selectin to cell membranes. As mentioned above, this combination of oxidative stress, inflammatory cytokines, downregulated endothelial junction proteins, and increased MMP activity increases BBB permeability (Engelhardt and Sorokin, 2009). In the perivascular space, proteins released from macrophages (ROS, IL-1β,

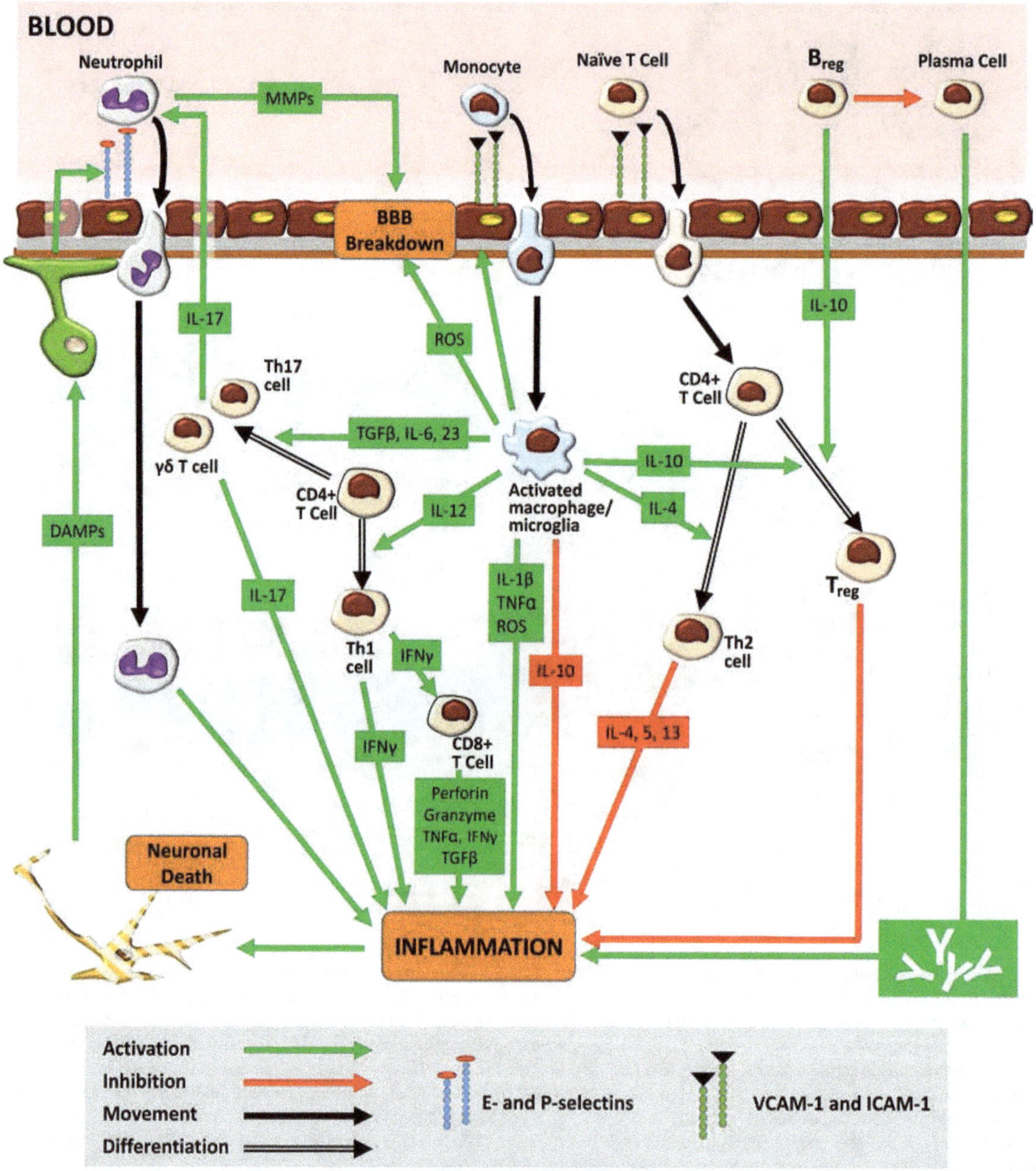

FIGURE 2 | Immune response to stroke. Hypoperfusion causes an immediate deprivation of glucose and oxygen to the brain, leading to widespread neuronal cell death. The release of danger/damage-associated molecular patterns (DAMPs) from dying neurons results in the secondary activation of astrocytes and microglia. The release of chemokines/cytokines from glial cells generates an inflammatory environment featuring ROS, activated leukocytes, and the upregulated expression of adhesion molecules on endothelial cell membranes. Adhesion molecules such as E- and P-selectin mediate the initial tethering of circulating leukocytes to the endothelium. Separate surface molecules such as ICAM-1 and VCAM-1 then facilitate firm adhesion and transmigration. Neutrophils, entering the brain as early as 1 h post-stroke, increase BBB permeability *via* MMPs, further exacerbating ischaemic injury. Monocytes, infiltrating 1–2 days later, function as tissue macrophages. The M1 macrophage/microglia phenotype increases ischaemic injury through the production of ROS and pro-inflammatory cytokines (TNF-α and IL-1β). The M1 subtype also secretes cytokines [IL-12, IL-6, transforming growth factor beta 1 (TGF-β), and IL-23], which encourage the differentiation of infiltrated naïve CD4+ T-cells into pro-inflammatory Th1 and Th17 forms. Th1 cells, through release of interferon gamma (IFNγ), promote the cytotoxic activity of CD8+ T-cells. Th17 cells (as well as their γδ T-cell counterparts) further increase neutrophilic activity and enhance ischaemic through the production of IL-17. Ultimately, the pro-inflammatory milieu seen in the acute stages of ischaemic stroke gives way to a second, subacute anti-inflammatory phase typified by increased M2 microglial/macrophagic activity. The release of IL-10 from both glial cells and circulating Bregs encourages the generation of Tregs, a cell type that promotes neuroprotection and repair. Bregs may also play a role in the chronic immune response to stroke where they serve to reduce the effect of long-term antibody-mediated neurotoxicity.

and TNF-α) and mast cells (histamine and proteases) further degrade BBB structures (Iadecola and Anrather, 2011). Swelling of endothelial cells first causes protein extravasation and interstitial oedema. Detachment of endothelial cells from the basement membrane then results in unimpeded entry of free water and serum into the brain, ultimately leading to haemorrhage (Petrovic-Djergovic et al., 2016). A compromise in BBB integrity also allows leukocyte entry into the infarct site. Endothelial cell-derived prostaglandins and chemoattractant molecules drive the trafficking process (Engblom et al., 2002; Huang et al., 2006). The infiltration of macrophages, neutrophils, and lymphocytes into the brain is mediated by interactions between high-avidity integrin molecules on the leukocyte surface and the corresponding ligands on the endothelium. The expression of such proteins, including vascular cell adhesion molecule-1 (VCAM-1) and intracellular adhesion molecule-1 (ICAM-1), is upregulated post-stroke (Supanc et al., 2011). Activated leukocytes secrete a mix of collagenases, gelatinases, ROS, cytokines, leukotrienes, and platelet-activating factor, promoting vasoconstriction, platelet aggregation, and further neurotoxicity (Kim et al., 2016). As the ischaemic penumbra expands, a combination of fresh excitotoxic responses, oxidative stress, and mitochondrial dysfunction drives the next phase of both the local and systemic immune responses.

THERAPEUTIC STRATEGIES TARGETING ASTROCYTES AND MICROGLIA

Astrocytes undergo numerous changes post-ischaemia, including rapid swelling, increased intracellular calcium signalling, and upregulated expression of glial fibrillary acidic protein (GFAP) (Petrovic-Djergovic et al., 2016). The astroglial response begins in the infarct site as early as 4 h post-stroke, reaching peak activity around day 4 (Kim et al., 2016). Although this "reactive gliosis" contributes to long-term healing, the initial formation of the glial scar is thought to be detrimental. The scar acts as both a physical and chemical barrier to axonal re-growth, preventing reinnervation (Barreto et al., 2011). Several studies have shown that decreased astrogliosis correlates with reduced infarct size (reviewed in Barreto et al., 2011). Separate research has highlighted how astrocytes can play a similarly detrimental role in AIS as traditional leukocytes, increasing interest in immunomodulatory strategies targeting these cells. Astrocytes have been shown to express various pro-inflammatory mediators in the acute phase including cytokines, chemokines, and inducible nitric oxide synthase (iNOS) (Dong and Benveniste, 2001). Astrocyte-derived IL-15, for example, augments cell-mediated immunity post-stroke, promoting ischaemic injury (Roy-O'Reilly and McCullough, 2017). More recent work, however, points to astrocytes as promising therapeutic targets for neuroprotection and neurorestoration (Liu and Chopp, 2016). Fundamentally, the glial scar divides the site of injury from surrounding viable tissue, hindering infarct growth. During the acute phase, astrocytes also limit neuronal cell death by reducing excitotoxicity and releasing neurotrophins (Liu and Chopp, 2016). Finally, astrocytes contribute to the chronic processes of angiogenesis, neurogenesis, and synaptogenesis (Wang et al., 2018). As for many other immune targets in AIS, the manipulation of the astrocytic response may involve a combination of pharmacological [e.g., cyclin-dependent kinase 5 (CDK5) inhibitors] and cell-based therapies (Becerra-Calixto and Cardona-Gómez, 2017).

In the resting state, microglia exhibit a ramified appearance. However, in the event of acute brain injury, they undergo a morphological transformation to an active amoeboid state, making them virtually indistinguishable from circulating macrophages (Kim et al., 2016). Microglia activate within minutes of brain ischaemia, with products detectable as early as 1 h post-stroke (Xu and Jiang, 2014). Peripheral macrophages infiltrate 1–2 days later, reaching peak levels 3–7 days after the onset of ischaemia (Xu and Jiang, 2014). Overall, microglial activity predominates in the early stages of ischaemia, while blood-derived cells contribute more to the subacute and chronic phases of neuroinflammation. The destructive effects of microglia/macrophages in AIS are well documented (Chiba and Umegaki, 2013). Other studies, however, in which the selective ablation of microglial cells leads to worsened stroke outcomes suggest a protective function (Lalancette-Hébert et al., 2007). Indeed, blocking macrophage infiltration abolished long-term behavioural recovery and led to reduced anti-inflammatory signalling in the brain (Wattananit et al., 2016). Importantly, the overall net effect of microglia/macrophages in AIS depends on the M1/M2 polarization status. It has been demonstrated that the anti-inflammatory M2 phenotype gives way to the pro-inflammatory M1 phenotype during disease progression (Xu and Jiang, 2014). The shift between the M1 and M2 subtypes depends on specific cytokine signals from the local inflammatory milieu. Several molecular switches, such as triggering receptor expressed on myeloid cells 2 (TREM2), have been shown to control the functional polarization in the setting of AIS, making them potential immunomodulatory targets (Kawabori et al., 2015). At pre-clinical level, agents that prevent microglial activation, such as minocycline, hyperbaric oxygen, or the free radical scavenger, edaravone, are neuroprotective, possibly as a result of reduced M1 activity (Chen et al., 2014). Minocycline, a semi-synthetic tetracycline compound, progressed to human trials. Two phase II open-label, placebo-controlled trials concluded that the drug was safe and significantly improved clinical outcome (Lampl et al., 2007; Padma Srivastava et al., 2012). In a third study, however, minocycline did not prove efficacious (Kohler et al., 2013). Evidently, a more nuanced understanding of the M1/M2 phenomenon in AIS is needed, alongside a greater appreciation of the differences between resident microglia and circulating macrophages. Some authors contend that microglia/macrophages may yet prove an attractive immunomodulatory target in the context of cell-based therapies (Kanazawa et al., 2017).

THERAPEUTIC STRATEGIES TARGETING INFLAMMATORY MEDIATORS

The Complement Pathway

The proteins and receptors of the complement pathway, once thought to be restricted to immune cells, are now known to be expressed by neurons, microglia, and astrocytes

(Alawieh et al., 2015a). The complement pathway contributes to neuroinflammation in the initial phase of AIS (Iadecola and Anrather, 2011), but other studies indicate a second function for these proteins in the subacute and chronic stages, predominantly in post-stroke neurogenesis and repair (Alawieh and Tomlinson, 2016). As with many facets of the immune response to stroke, the dual role of complement has hindered the development of effective therapies. A number of pre-clinical studies have shown that the anaphylatoxins C3a and C5a promote tissue inflammation and neurotoxicity. Administration of a C3a receptor antagonist in a mouse model of stroke, for example, reduced infarct size and improved neurological outcome, while similar results were seen in $C3a^{-/-}$ mice (Mocco et al., 2006a). C3a receptor antagonism has also been shown to promote neuroblast formation, curb T-cell infiltration, and lead to better overall histologic and functional outcomes (Ducruet et al., 2012). Use of a C5a receptor blocker, meanwhile, significantly reduced infarct volume and improved neurological outcomes 24 h after ischaemia (Kim et al., 2008). Evidence also exists for a pathological role for complement in human stroke. Patients deficient in mannose-binding lectin, for example, display smaller infarct size (Osthoff et al., 2011). The plasma levels of complement proteins are also raised following AIS (Cojocaru et al., 2008). Despite these findings, none of the complement inhibitors tested pre-clinically have progressed to clinical trials. Several concerns remain around these drugs including poor bioavailability, questionable efficacy, increased risk of infection, and potential interference with homeostatic function. As a result, several other complement receptor-based inhibitors [e.g., soluble complement receptor 1 (sCR1) and sialyl Lewis x glycosylated soluble complement receptor 1 ($sCR1sLe^x$)] have been developed. However, while sCR1 reduced ischaemic injury in mice, it failed to provide the same neuroprotection in a non-human primate model of stroke (Huang et al., 1999; Mocco et al., 2006b). Similarly, while $sCR1sLe^x$ decreased cerebral infarct volume and inhibited platelet/neutrophil accumulation in mice, the effect was not replicated in either rats or non-human primates (Huang et al., 1999; Ducruet et al., 2007). No further development of $sCR1sLe^x$ has been reported. More promise has been shown by compounds attached to a recombinant form of complement receptor type 2 (CR2). Both CR2-Crry (an inhibitor of all complement pathways) and CR2-fH (an inhibitor of the alternative pathway) significantly reduced infarct size, apoptotic cell death, and neurological deficits in a mouse model of transient middle cerebral artery occlusion (tMCAO) (Alawieh et al., 2015b). The same research group observed improved long-term motor and cognitive recovery using B4Crry, another site-targeted inhibitor (Alawieh et al., 2018). Separately, recent evidence has shown that tPA upregulates complement cascade activity in ischaemic stroke models through plasmin-mediated cleavage of the C3 protein. The resulting C3a anaphylatoxin promotes post-ischaemic brain haemorrhage and cerebral oedema. Inhibition of the C3a receptor, however, abrogates such adverse effects, indicating a potential role for complement inhibitors as adjuncts to tPA. Currently, the risk of haemorrhagic transformation limits the clinical use of thrombolysis. However, complement inhibition could enhance the therapeutic window of tPA through the mechanism described above (Zhao et al., 2017).

Nitric Oxide

The protective functions of NO in AIS include regulation of vascular tone, inhibition of platelet aggregation, prevention of leukocyte adhesion, and host defence (Kim et al., 2014). High levels of nitric oxide, however, have been shown to be neurotoxic (Venkataramana et al., 2015). NO is generated *in vivo* through nitric oxide synthase (NOS), and though all three isoforms (endothelial NOS, neuronal NOS, and inducible NOS) have been implicated in AIS, iNOS in particular contributes to neuroinflammatory processes (Iadecola et al., 1995). Inhibition/knockdown of the iNOS enzyme has been shown to be neuroprotective, and separate studies in which iNOS generation was indirectly reduced have supported this hypothesis (Zhao et al., 2000; Han et al., 2002; Coughlan et al., 2005; Park et al., 2006). Due to a possible role in both neuroprotection and neurotoxicity, a number of NO-based therapies have been suggested for the treatment of AIS, including NO donors, L-arginine (NO precursor), and iNOS inhibitors (Chen et al., 2017). To date, only glyceryl trinitrate (GTN), an NO donor commonly used in the management of angina, has progressed to clinical trials. A recent systematic review, however, highlighted that despite reductions in blood pressure, there is insufficient evidence to recommend GTN in AIS (Bath et al., 2017). Further pre-clinical evidence is required before other NO-based candidate therapies can progress to the clinical stage.

Pro-Inflammatory Cytokines

The levels of IL-1β in the brain are upregulated over 40-fold within the first 24 h after AIS (Clausen et al., 2005). The pathogenic role of IL-1β in rodent models of stroke is well established; exogenous administration of IL-1β increased brain oedema, while IL-1α/β double-knockout mice showed ameliorated infarct size (Boutin et al., 2001). Separately, deficiency or inhibition of the IL-1 receptor (IL-1R1) improved long-term functional outcomes (Basu et al., 2005). Similarly, overexpression or treatment with IL-1Ra proved neuroprotective (Yang et al., 1997; Mulcahy et al., 2003). A recent systematic review concluded that anakinra, a recombinant IL-1 receptor antagonist (IL-1Ra), reduced infarct volume by 36.2% in experimental models of ischaemic stroke (McCann et al., 2016). In human studies, a phase II trial in 2005 showed anakinra to be safe and well tolerated in AIS patients (Emsley et al., 2005). With the replacement of the intravenous formulation by a subcutaneous injection, the effects of anakinra have since been re-investigated at a twice-daily dose (Sobowale et al., 2016). Although anakinra significantly decreased plasma levels of IL-6 and C-reactive protein, a possible negative interaction between IL-1Ra and tPA was revealed (Smith et al., 2018). Further pre-clinical and clinical studies are therefore required to determine whether anakinra or other IL-1 based therapies could be safely used as an adjunct in AIS treatment. Separately, reports of a potential neuroprotective role of IL-1β post-stroke must be re-examined (Amantea et al., 2010). Suggested mechanisms for this beneficial effect include the IL-1β-mediated release of high-mobility group box 1 (HMGB1) from reactive astrocytes as well as the production of neurotrophic factors (Hayakawa et al., 2010; Hewett et al., 2012).

TNF-α can be found in the CSF and serum of patients within 24 h of the onset of ischaemia (Zaremba and Losy, 2001; Lambertsen et al., 2012). The circulating levels of TNF-α are correlated with infarct size and the severity of neurological impairment. Inhibition of TNF-α also protects the brain against ischaemic injury (Chiba and Umegaki, 2013). Conversely, pre-treatment with recombinant TNF-α proved neuroprotective, while mice lacking TNF-α receptors showed larger infarct size (Bruce et al., 1996; Ginis et al., 2002). Arguably, the action of TNF-α depends on timing. In the early stages of stroke, TNF-α promotes BBB breakdown, leukocyte infiltration, and brain oedema, while further along the timeline, it mediates neuronal and microvasculature repair (Amantea et al., 2009). The location of TNF-α release could also be a factor; increased production in the striatum, for instance, promotes neurodegeneration, whereas release in the hippocampus promotes neuroprotection (Sriram and O'Callaghan, 2007). Separately, receptor subtype, gene polymorphism, or cell signalling pathways could determine what type of response TNF-α causes (Pradillo et al., 2005; Cui et al., 2012). To date, no clinical trials of TNF-α-based therapies in AIS have been published. However, etanercept, a biologic TNF-α inhibitor, has been studied experimentally in the setting of traumatic brain injury and clinically for the treatment of stroke-induced neurological dysfunction (Wang et al., 2013). In both studies, etanercept attenuated motor deficits. In humans, a single perispinal dose also improved psychological outcomes and reduced post-stroke complications (Tobinick et al., 2014). As TNF-α receptor inhibitors, such as etanercept, are already licensed for the treatment of certain autoimmune diseases, clinical trials in AIS could be expedited. The possibility of anti-TNF-α therapies leading to increased infection rates in the setting of stroke, however, would have to be addressed (Zeng et al., 2013).

Cyclooxygenase/Lipoxygenase Pathways

Arachidonic acid metabolites from the COX or lipoxygenase (LO) pathways play a role in stroke injury (Yagami et al., 2016). Increased phospholipase A2 (PLA2) activity has been documented in several experimental models of stroke, while mice lacking PLA2 showed improved disease outcomes (Bonventre et al., 1997; Muralikrishna Adibhatla and Hatcher, 2006). Inhibition of COX-1/COX-2 enhanced survival of neurons in mouse hippocampus, suggesting the enzyme has a neurotoxic activity (Candelario-Jalil et al., 2003). Likewise, the delayed administration of COX-2 inhibitor NS398 reduced infarct volume and neurological deficits in an experimental model of stroke, whereas COX-2 overexpression exacerbated ischaemic injury (Doré et al., 2003; Sugimoto and Iadecola, 2003). Development of COX-2 inhibitors for the treatment of cerebral ischaemia was hindered by the finding that long-term use of COX-2 inhibitors themselves increased the risk of stroke (though strategies to prevent this adverse effect may yet be achieved) (Huang et al., 2016). Separately, leukotriene C4 (LTC4), an end-product of the 5-LO enzyme pathway, may play a more pronounced role in BBB dysfunction than do products of the COX pathway, with a biphasic expression pattern closely correlated to BBB opening (Rao et al., 1999). Use of a 5-LO inhibitor in an experimental model of transient ischaemia led to decreased brain levels of LTC4 and reduced cerebral oedema (Baskaya et al., 1996). Likewise, montelukast, a cysteinyl leukotriene receptor-1 antagonist licensed clinically for use in asthma, ameliorated hippocampal injury (Saad et al., 2015). The protective effect, however, could not be replicated in 5-LO knockout mice, casting doubt on leukotriene involvement in infarct development (Kitagawa et al., 2004). As for the COX pathway, a possible neuroprotective function has been argued. COX-1-deficient mice, for example, showed increased susceptibility to ischaemic injury, possibly as a result of compromised CBF (Iadecola et al., 2001). Several studies have highlighted a neuroprotective effect of prostaglandin E1, while accumulating evidence also demonstrates the beneficial effects of Prostaglandin E2 receptor 2/4 (EP2/EP4) receptor activation (Huang et al., 2016; Ling et al., 2016). The development of pharmacological agents targeting arachidonic acid (AA) metabolites in stroke may therefore yet move away from COX-2 inhibition towards manipulation of downstream EP receptors in the acute post-stroke phase.

Matrix Metalloproteinases

MMPs, a family of zinc-binding endopeptidases, become dysregulated in the setting of AIS. Increased MMP activity leads to neuronal apoptosis, BBB breakdown, leukocyte infiltration, brain oedema, and, under certain circumstances, haemorrhage (Rosell and Lo, 2008). Various MMPs, including MMP-2, MMP-3, MMP-7, and MMP-9, have been implicated in infarct growth. MMP-2, which is constitutively expressed in the brain, contributes to ischaemic damage in the early stages (<24 h) through extracellular matrix disruption, tight junction protein degradation, and oxidative stress injury (Gasche et al., 2001; Yang et al., 2007). Conversely, MMP-9, an inducible enzyme secreted by microglia, macrophages, and infiltrating neutrophils, mediates the more intense and irreversible damage to the BBB associated with haemorrhage (Montaner et al., 2001). MMP-9, upregulated 15–48 h after the onset of ischaemia, has also been intimately linked to stroke pathology, with higher serum levels, a predictor of poor disease outcome (Abdelnaseer et al., 2017). Studies of MMP-9 knockout/inhibition highlighted decreased infarct volume and an overall reduction in ischaemic damage (Asahi et al., 2001; Gu et al., 2005). The same neuroprotective effect, however, was not noted in mice lacking MMP-2, leading to the theory that the enzyme is instead involved in post-stroke repair (Lucivero et al., 2007). Indeed, a wealth of evidence now points to a role for MMPs in processes such as neovascularization and neurovascular remodelling (Lee et al., 2006, Zhao et al., 2006). Treatment with MMP inhibitors at 7 days, for example, increased brain injury, impaired functional outcome, and reduced remodelling of the infarct site (Zhao et al., 2006). As a result, the clinical translation of therapies targeting MMPs may involve administration of modulators in the subacute stages of stroke that promote longer-term recovery. Separately, studies suggest MMP-9 is responsible for haemorrhagic transformation associated with tPA therapy, as levels of the enzyme are elevated in response to thrombolysis (Ning et al., 2006). As a result, MMP-9 inhibitors (e.g., minocycline) may yet find a role in the acute phase of AIS therapy as adjuncts to lengthen the therapeutic window for thrombolysis (Murata et al., 2008).

Chemokines

Chemoattractant molecules are expressed by a range of cell types in AIS, including circulating immune cells, activated microglia, endothelial cells, astrocytes, and neurons (Kim et al., 1995b; Che et al., 2001). Chemokines, the expression of which are upregulated post-stroke, play a detrimental role in the early stages through leukocyte infiltration, ROS production, and BBB disruption (Kawabori and Yenari, 2015; Chen et al., 2018a). Mice lacking CCL5 or the neuronally expressed CX3CL1 (fractalkine), for example, showed reduced infarct size (Soriano et al., 2002; Terao et al., 2008). Similarly, inhibition of CXCL8 provided neuroprotection in transient brain ischaemia (Garau et al., 2005). Likewise, the genetic deletion of both CCR2 and CX3CR1 receptors proved neuroprotective in a ferric chloride model of ischaemia (Cisbani et al., 2018). However, evidence now also points to a second, neuroprotective function for chemokines in AIS, possibly as a result of increased stem cell recruitment to the infarct site (Wang et al., 2002). Several therapeutic strategies targeting chemokines—including small molecule receptor antagonists, neutralizing antibodies, pathogen-derived receptor antagonists, and modified chemokines—have been trialled in AIS, with moderate success (reviewed in Mirabelli-Badenier et al., 2011). Administration of an anti-MIP-3α antibody in rats, for example, reduced infarct size while TAK-779, a nonpeptide CCR5 antagonist, protected mice against focal cerebral ischaemia (Takami et al., 2002; Terao et al., 2009). Similarly, the pan-chemokine specific inhibitor NR58-3.14.3 also improved outcome in experimental stroke, while anti-CCL2 and CXCL8 antibodies decreased brain oedema and BBB permeability, respectively (Mirabelli-Badenier et al., 2011). Furthermore, the viral peptide, macrophage inflammatory protein-1α (MIP-II) (a chemokine analogue of MIP-II encoded by human herpesvirus-8 DNA), proved neuroprotective against focal cerebral ischaemia in mice (Takami et al., 2001). Despite these successes, however, issues preventing the clinical translation of chemokine-targeted therapies remain, including the correct timing of administration and drug concentration. While some research has shown the benefit of broad-spectrum chemokine inhibition, the risks that blanket-blocking the system poses to host defence and neuroprotective immune cell recruitment has also yet to be resolved (Lee et al., 2015). As a result, drugs such as JWH-133, which inhibit CXCL2-mediated neutrophil migration to the CNS without affecting the response in the periphery, may provide the way forward (Mirabelli-Badenier et al., 2011).

THERAPEUTIC STRATEGIES TARGETING LEUKOCYTE INFILTRATION

E-, L-, and P-selectins, a family of transmembrane glycoproteins, have all been implicated in leukocyte trafficking in AIS (Yilmaz and Granger, 2008). In animal models, the selective blockade of E- or P-selectin resulted in improved neurological outcome (Huang et al., 2000; Mocco et al., 2002). Similarly, P-selectin-deficient mice showed decreased BBB breakdown (Jin et al., 2010). However, the use of an anti-L-selectin antibody in a rabbit model of stroke did not reduce ischaemic injury (Yenari et al., 2001).

Among the immunoglobulin superfamily, ICAM-1 and VCAM-1 have been the most studied in the setting of AIS (Stanimirovic et al., 1997). These molecules facilitate the adhesion of leukocytes to the endothelial wall and extravasation into the infarct site. The results of both *in vitro* experiments and human studies confirm increased ICAM-1 expression under conditions of ischaemia (Hess et al., 1994; Bitsch et al., 1998). As ICAM-1 levels peak at 12–48 h post-stroke, they are ideal targets for the acute phase. Studies of ICAM-1 deficiency/inhibition showed reduced ischaemic injury and decreased leukocyte infiltration (Kitagawa et al., 1998; Kanemoto et al., 2002; Vemuganti et al., 2004). ICAM-1 knockout mice also displayed reduced infarct size, as well as improvements in CBF and neurological function (Connolly et al., 1996). A phase III clinical trial of anti-ICAM-1 antibody enlimomab, however, failed to replicate these results, with the antibody-treated group reporting higher mortality (Investigators, 2001). Increased neutrophil activity in enlimomab-treated patients has been attributed to the antigenicity of the murine antibody used. As a result, the benefit of ICAM-1 modulation in AIS awaits confirmation. Likewise, there remains doubt as to the validity of VCAM-1 as an immunomodulatory target. Several groups have shown improved stroke outcomes in association with decreased VCAM-1 expression (Zhang and Wei, 2003; Cervera et al., 2004). A study of VCAM-1 knockdown, for example, led to decreased T lymphocyte infiltration and reduced infarct volume (Liesz et al., 2011). However, use of an anti-VCAM-1 antibody did not prove neuroprotective in either rats or mice, casting further doubt on the viability of this target in AIS (Justicia et al., 2006).

Integrin molecules, such as leukocyte function-associated antigen-1 (LFA-1 or CD11a/CD18), macrophage-1 (Mac-1 or CD11b/CD18), and very late adhesion molecule-4 (VLA-4 or CD49d), facilitate the binding of leukocytes to areas of activated endothelium in AIS (Iadecola and Anrather, 2011). The expression of CD11a/CD18 is upregulated in stroke patients (Kim et al., 1995a). In an experimental model of CD11a/CD18 deficiency, reductions in infarct volume and neurological deficit were noted (Arumugam et al., 2004). Administration of an anti-CD11b antibody produced the same result (Chen et al., 1994). Likewise, in mice lacking CD18 or Mac-1, reduced infarct size, decreased neutrophil infiltration, and decreased mortality were shown (Prestigiacomo et al., 1999; Soriano et al., 1999). The use of Hu23F2G, an anti-Mac-1 antibody, caused a similar amelioration of ischaemic injury (Yenari et al., 1998). In the phase III clinical trial "LeukArrest," however, Hu23F2G did not prove neuroprotective (Becker, 2002). A second human study—Acute Stroke Therapy by Inhibition of Neutrophils (ASTIN)—instead investigated the effect of Mac-1 inhibitor, UK-279,276 (neutrophil inhibitor factor), in AIS patients (Krams et al., 2003). Again, however, despite good pre-clinical evidence, ASTIN failed to meet the predetermined endpoint of a 3-point additional mean recovery on the Scandinavian Stroke Scale, and the study was terminated early (Jiang et al., 1995). Plausible confounding factors in both trials include the timing of drug administration, differences in integrin molecules between humans and rodents, and the variability in reperfusion in human stroke vs. animal models (Jickling et al., 2015). On this last point, it has been noted that anti-integrin therapies provide more benefit in transient compared with permanent models of ischaemia in animals (Zhang et al., 1995). The observation that an anti-Mac-1 antibody extends the therapeutic window of tPA suggests a possible place for these therapies as an adjunct in AIS treatment (Zhang et al., 2003). Another integrin-based therapy, which has progressed to the clinical trial stage is natalizumab—an anti-VLA-4 antibody used to attenuate neuroinflammation in relapsing-remitting MS. The "ACTION" trial (phase II) explored the safety and efficacy of natalizumab in stroke (Elkins et al., 2017). While natalizumab did not affect infarct volume, improvements in functional outcomes at 30 days warranted further investigation. The follow-up phase IIb trial, however, did not meet its primary or secondary endpoints. This likely concludes the investigation into natalizumab in AIS at this time.

Perhaps, as a result of poor clinical translation, research into strategies targeting leukocyte infiltration in AIS has shifted away from global inhibition to specific subsets. Therapies aimed at reducing T-cell extravasation, for example, have received increased interest. Fingolimod, a sphingosine-1-phosphate receptor modulator used in the treatment of relapsing-remitting MS, is one such treatment. A wealth of pre-clinical evidence now supports the benefits of fingolimod on AIS outcome (Liu et al., 2013). The suppression of T-cell infiltration into the CNS plays a role in this efficacy, though other mechanisms such as decreased BBB dysfunction, reduced microglial activation, and direct neuroprotection are also likely to be involved (Kraft et al., 2013; Li et al., 2016). At the clinical level, fingolimod has been investigated in a small number of pilot studies (either alone or in combination with thrombolysis). Both studies confirmed a beneficial effect of fingolimod on infarct size, rates of haemorrhagic transformation, and neurological function (Fu et al., 2014b; Zhu et al., 2015).

STROKE-INDUCED IMMUNODEPRESSION

The early activation of the peripheral immune system post-stroke gives way 2 days after initial ischaemia to a second phenomenon termed stroke-induced immunodepression (SIID). Theoretically, SIID may have evolved as an adaptive response, protecting the CNS from harmful autoimmune responses. The active depression of immune defence mechanisms, however, dramatically increases the susceptibility of the host to infection. Indeed, large studies have estimated approximately 30% of stroke patients contract infections, the most prevalent of which are urinary tract infections (UTIs) and pneumonia (Westendorp et al., 2011). Microorganisms routinely implicated in post-stroke infection include *Staphylococcus aureus*, *Pseudomonas aeruginosa*, *Klebsiella pneumoniae*, and *Escherichia coli*. Anatomical factors seem to be important in post-stroke infection. The extent of lesion size, for example, is associated with occurrence of pneumonia, though whether infarct location influences events remains unclear (Minnerup et al., 2010). The fact that most cases of pneumonia and UTI are diagnosed within the first few days after stroke, however, implies SIID is involved and that infections are not simply a manifestation of poor patient care (Westendorp et al., 2011). Regarding outcome, almost all major studies of post-stroke infection have shown a significant impact of infection on functional outcome and patient mortality (Vermeij et al., 2018). As a result, strategies that aim to prevent or cure such infections are currently receiving greater interest.

SIID is typified by lymphopenia, increased levels of anti-inflammatory cytokines such as IL-10 and transforming growth factor beta 1 (TGF-β), and splenic atrophy (Kamel and Iadecola, 2012). Mechanistically, the CNS causes immunological changes through a variety of humoral and neural pathways, including the sympathetic nervous system (SNS), the parasympathetic nervous system (PNS), and the hypothalamic–pituitary–adrenal (HPA) axis (Brambilla et al., 2013). Glucocorticoids, end-products of HPA axis activation, curb the peripheral immune response post-stroke through promoting lymphopenia, impairing lymphocyte/neutrophil function, and deactivating macrophages (Prass et al., 2003; Mracsko et al., 2014). Glucocorticoid receptor blockade reduced splenocyte apoptosis and corrected lymphopenia in an experimental model of stroke, though this antagonism did not prevent pneumonia (Prass et al., 2003). The beneficial effect of glucocorticoid blockade on lymphocyte counts was confirmed in a further mouse study, though this intervention did increase levels of the SNS mediator, metanephrine (Mracsko et al., 2014). Both of these studies suggest that modulation of the glucocorticoid pathway can reduce the manifestation of SIID, though whether this leads to reduced incidence of infection or deleterious signalling elsewhere still needs to be reconciled.

Increased transmission in the PNS, chiefly through vagal nerve activity, is also capable of altering peripheral immune function. Studies have shown the detrimental effect that acetylcholine (ACh), secreted by both parasympathetic nerves and splenic memory T cells, has on macrophage function (Rosas-Ballina et al., 2011; Trakhtenberg and Goldberg, 2011). Activation of nicotinic acetylcholine receptor α7 (nAChRα7) results in decreased pro-inflammatory cytokine secretion, predisposing the host to infection (Rosas-Ballina et al., 2011; Trakhtenberg and Goldberg, 2011). As of yet, however, therapies targeting the PNS have focused more on reducing innate immune function at the infarct site (Kox and Pickkers, 2015).

One branch of the autonomic nervous system that modulates peripheral immune function post-stroke and has progressed to human studies is the SNS. Increased levels of adrenaline and noradrenaline post-ischaemia skews leukocytes towards an anti-inflammatory phenotype, while also disabling hepatic invariant natural killer T cells (iNKT) in mice (Chamorro et al., 2012). The latter cell type in particular has been shown to be pivotal in host defence against post-stroke infection (Wong et al., 2011). The inhibition of iNKT function, however, can be reversed pharmacologically through administration of the glycolipid, α-galactosylceramide, or beta blockers such as propranolol (Shi et al., 2018). In the clinic, the beneficial effects of beta blockers on infection rates and early mortality have been replicated several times (Dziedzic et al., 2007; Sykora et al., 2015). Controversially, separate studies showed a negative effect of beta blockers, coupled with higher rates of adverse events (Westendorp et al., 2016). In theory, beta blockers could affect CBF or aggravate pro-inflammatory responses in the brain. Evidently, further studies into immunomodulatory therapies of the SNS are required.

In terms of post-stroke infection outcomes, the most recent systematic reviews of prophylactic antibiotic therapy suggest that this approach is not effective (Vermeij et al., 2018). Despite a meta-analysis finding that preventative antibacterial drugs reduced overall infection rates, no effect on functional outcome (modified Rankin scale) or mortality was seen (Zheng et al., 2017). Importantly, however, the pathophysiology of post-stroke infection is still poorly understood, while certain classes of antibiotics (e.g., fluoroquinolones) have known neurotoxic properties. The use of prophylactic antibiotic therapy, therefore, may yet prove effective in certain patient subgroups. Nevertheless, in order to achieve improved functional outcomes, a combination of antibiotics and immunomodulatory drugs could show greater promise.

BRAIN ANTIGEN TOLERIZATION

Increased permeability in the BBB, coupled with significant levels of cell death, results in greater exposure and presentation of brain antigens to the immune system. This can lead to the generation of autoimmune B- and T-cell responses. A likely function of SIID is to reduce the number of auto-reactive IFN-γ-secreting T-cells; this was demonstrated in a 2D2 transgenic mouse model where the T-cell receptor is specific for myelin oligodendrocyte glycoprotein (MOG), a CNS antigen (Römer et al., 2015). Clinical evidence demonstrates a strong correlation between Th1 responses and poorer stroke outcome up to 3 months later in humans (Becker et al., 2011). The definition of Th1 responses in this clinical study was a higher ratio of IFN-γ to TGF-β secretion by T-cells when stimulated with a range of self-antigens including myelin basic protein (MBP); however, the magnitude of each of these responses was not reported. Modulation of immunity towards a Th1 phenotype is favoured during the inflammatory response to bacteria; Th1 responses to MBP, in particular, were more prevalent in stroke patients with pneumonia (Becker et al., 2011). It is unclear if these autoreactive cells are involved in short- or long-term pathogenesis or, instead, act as a severity marker or are associated effects of the stroke. Some studies suggest a role of autoreactive Th1 in poor outcome (Zierath et al., 2010), whereas other studies demonstrate no impact (Römer et al., 2015). However, the self-antigen specificity of the response is clear as memory immunity to foreign antigens such as tetanus toxoid did not associate with outcome (Becker et al., 2011). It is possible that a Th1 response could indeed be driving T-cell cytotoxicity in the brain, similar to other autoimmune pathologies, such as type 1 diabetes. Immune-based therapies that modulate the T-cell phenotype away from a cytotoxic response towards a more tolerized response, possibly mediated by Treg, might have application in stroke.

Previous therapies attempted to induce antigen-specific tolerance to E-selectin or to MBP *via* repeated mucosal administration. Induction of a Treg response to MBP in Lewis rats before stroke resulted in an improved outcome at early, but not late (3 months) time points after stroke (Gee et al., 2009). This could be due to the inherent plasticity of T-cell phenotypes, particularly between Treg and Th17, as the latter type is known to be pathogenic in autoimmune CNS diseases [such as the MS mouse model and experimental autoimmune encephalomyelitis (EAE)] (Jadidi-Niaragh and Mirshafiey, 2011). Increased IL-6 expression during infection could promote Treg cells to switch to a more Th17 function (Kimura and Kishimoto 2010). E-selectin is only expressed in blood vessels upon activation. It has therefore been hypothesized that induction of a regulatory T-cell response to E-selectin would be specifically directed to blood vessels undergoing activation in the brain and thereby reduce the risk of stroke (Hallenbeck, 2010). However, induction of mucosal tolerance requires repeated low-dose administration and takes time to develop. Although pre-clinical results provided some proof-of-principle and clinical studies were initiated in 2003 and terminated in 2010 (NCT00069069), no clinical data on safety or potency have yet been published. Overall, induction of antigen-specific Treg using mucosal tolerance has suffered from logistical (repeated doses required) as well as clinical efficacy issues.

Non-antigen-specific approaches are also being evaluated. These cell therapies could act in a more systemic, regenerative manner by targeting reparative, anti-inflammatory processes, which contribute to recovery from disease and co-morbidities and thereby may have a multi-dimensional effect on disease. Phase II/III clinical trials are ongoing in ischaemic stroke patients to assess MultiStem, *in vitro* expanded multipotent adult progenitor bone marrow cells that do not require human leukocyte antigen (HLA) matching (Hess et al., 2014; Osanai et al., 2018). Favourable safety and tolerability have been observed (Hess et al., 2014), with a time window (24–36 h) beyond that of recombinant tissue plasminogen activator (rt-PA) and endovascular thrombectomy. MultiStem treatment did not demonstrate a significant difference to placebo treatment for the primary endpoint of Global Stroke Recovery Assessment or secondary endpoints relating to disability, neurologic deficit, and activities of daily living. However, some (15.4%) patients achieved an improved outcome, and life-threatening adverse events and mortality were lower in the treated group. MultiStem-treated patients showed a significant decrease in the number of circulating CD3+ T-cells, possibly suggesting a decrease in inflammation. Earlier treatment (24–36 h post-stroke) exhibited more favourable outcome than did delayed treatment. Therefore, although the trial failed to achieve the primary or secondary outcomes, it provides positive evidence of the potential of cell-therapy-based approaches, including multipotent adult progenitor cells (MAPCs), while also suggesting that timing is important to success (Mays and Deans, 2016). Elsewhere, various cell immunotherapy strategies are being assessed to treat other autoimmune diseases. Adoptive transfer of *ex vivo* expanded polyclonal Treg for type 1 diabetes, for example, has been demonstrated to be safe, underlying future clinical testing (Bluestone et al., 2015).

Alternatives to adoptive cell transfers are also being developed. Modulating the IL-2/CD25 axis in favour of Treg growth and away from activated and/or effector T-cells has been shown to be safe and potent in clinical trials across 11 autoimmune diseases (Rosenzwajg et al., 2018). It is now being clinically assessed in patients with stable ischaemic heart disease and acute coronary syndromes (NCT03113773) (Zhao et al., 2018). Repeated systemic administration of tolerizing-inducing formulations, such as nanoparticle-based delivery of aryl hydrocarbon receptor ligands and β-cell antigens, has demonstrated pre-clinical efficacy in a mouse model of type 1 diabetes (Yeste et al., 2016). Given that the pathology of ischaemic stroke has clear differences with these more chronic autoimmune diseases, with respect to the involvement of rapid immune depression and infection, successful immunotherapies for other autoimmune disease may not directly translate to AIS. However, lessons learned from all of these cell and immune therapies should be beneficial in developing efficacious immunotherapies that re-establish tolerance for long-term protection against stroke and potentially prevent decreased cognition in the stroke patient.

REGULATORY IMMUNE CELL STRATEGIES

Peripheral immune cells, which may contribute to the repair of the injured brain, include cells of both the innate and adaptive immune systems. M2- but not M1-type macrophages have been considered as promising target to enhance angiogenesis and neurovascular unit remodelling after stroke by producing factors such as vascular endothelial growth factor (VEGF), IL-8, Insulin-like growth factor 1 (IGF-1), and TGF-β (Willenborg et al., 2012; Nakamura et al., 2016). Neutrophils, although typically considered cells that induce damage in the acute phase of stroke (Amulic and Hayes, 2011; Herz et al., 2015), can also be involved in neural network remodelling in the latter stages. Through degradation of extracellular matrix, neutrophils release VEGF and TGF-β. In addition, neutrophils possess the ability to clear dead cells, debris, and bacteria, creating a better microenvironment for repair (Zlokovic, 2006; McDonald et al., 2010; Corps et al., 2015). With the use of genetically modified animals or lymphocyte depletion in animal stroke models ($Rag^{-/-}$ and SCID mice), the important role that lymphocytes play has been shown. Animals lacking lymphocytes had significantly smaller infarcts than had wild-type (WT) mice (Yilmaz et al., 2006; Hurn et al., 2007). Depletion of T-cells (both CD4+ and CD8+ subtypes) significantly reduced infarct volumes. Depletion of B-cells, on the other hand, had no effect on the infarct volumes 24 h after stroke induction (Yilmaz et al., 2006). This could indicate that T-cells but not B-cells play a role in post-stroke neural damage. Interestingly, in a separate study, B-cell knockout mice ($\mu MT^{-/-}$ mice) showed larger infarcts than did WT mice, suggesting that B-cells may have a protective function (Ren et al., 2011). Specifically, one subset of B-cells, IL-10-producing regulatory B-cells, may play an important role in neuroprotection.

Regulatory B-cells were shown to play a protective role in autoimmune animal models such as MS (EAE), rheumatoid arthritis [collagen-induced arthritis (CIA)], type 1 diabetes, and systemic lupus erythematous by dampening pro-inflammatory T-cells and enhancing the expansion of regulatory T-cells (Yang et al., 2013; Tedder, 2015). The main protective effect of regulatory B-cells is mediated through IL-10 production. The role of regulatory B-cells in stroke is still under investigation; however, a study where transfer of WT B-cells into B-cell knockout mice, when compared with mice receiving $IL\text{-}10^{-/-}$ B-cells, 24 h before the induction of stroke showing reduced infarct volume suggests a strong role of IL-10-producing B-cells (Ren et al., 2011). Chen et al. have shown that CD5+CD1dhi B10 cells are enriched in the ipsilateral versus contralateral hemisphere of mice at 48 h post-stroke, as well as circulating regulatory B-cells (Chen et al., 2012). Adoptive transfer of *in vitro*-induced regulatory B-cells to mice 24 h before the induction of stroke resulted in increased regulatory T-cell subsets (CD4+Foxp3+ and CD8+CD122+). Compared with that of animals without stimulated B-cells, infarct volume decreased (Bodhankar et al., 2015). If regulatory B-cells were to be considered for adoptive transfer in stroke, however, the purity of the population would need to be very high. Otherwise, non-regulatory B-cells could exacerbate post-stroke damage through antibody-mediated neurotoxicity (Doyle et al., 2015).

Regulatory T-cells are an important cell subset playing an active regulatory role in the brain after stroke. These cells (CD25+Foxp3+), which constitute approximately 10% of peripheral CD4+ T-cells, are essential for the promotion of immunosuppression through production of cytokines such as IL-10, TGF-β, and IL-35 (Zouggari et al., 2009; Wan, 2010). The protective role of Tregs after cerebral ischaemic injury has been shown in multiple studies (Liesz et al., 2009; Li et al., 2013; Liesz and Kleinschnitz, 2016). Regulatory T-cells function through dampening excessive immune responses and also through promoting the generation of new neuroblasts (Wan, 2010). Induction of immunosuppressive environments by recruitment of suppressive immune cells after ischaemia can reduce inflammation and decrease neural injury. The challenge of the low frequency of regulatory cells, however, has thus far restricted their clinical utility. In addition, questions remain as to how and when Tregs move from the periphery to the brain, a factor that may determine the therapeutic window. Although *in vivo* studies in mice have shown that it is possible to increase the frequency of regulatory cells [e.g., treatment with IL-2/IL-2 antibody complex increased Treg and protected against transient ischaemic attack (TIA)], the safety of this therapy in patients has yet to be established (Zhang et al., 2018). Further studies are needed to fully understand both the timing and frequency of suppressive cell infiltration into the infarcted brain. The methods of regulatory cell induction will also be crucial to evaluate in a clinical setting. Overall, a more comprehensive understanding of regulatory immune responses at different stages of stroke pathology will aid the design of safer and more effective immunomodulatory strategies.

THE ROLE OF THE GUT IN STROKE: TARGETING PERIPHERAL IMMUNE SYSTEMS

The bidirectional brain–gut interaction has received increased attention with respect to several neurologic and psychiatric diseases. Gut microbiota signal to the CNS *via* neural, immunologic, hormonal, and metabolic pathways, whereas the CNS alters the intestine by regulating gut motility and secretion as well as *via* the enteric nervous system. Maintenance of this symbiosis is critical to health; for example, unwanted gut permeability and influx of bacterial components and other danger-signalling molecules (DAMPs) can activate the immune system. At worst, such infiltration can cause bacteraemia, sepsis, and death.

An association between brain autoimmunity and intestinal microbiota was first discussed with respect to EAE (Wekerle, 2017). Pre-clinical studies that assess the impact of the gut microbiota on CNS damage generally involve the use of germ-free (GF) mice or treatment with antibiotic cocktails to deplete drug-sensitive bacterial strains. With respect to stroke, it is proposed that infarcted brain tissue can affect intestinal function and immunity *via* the adrenergic system and/or HPA axis. It has been reported that both T- and B-cell numbers are significantly reduced in Peyer's patches in mice post-stroke, suggesting a link between the CNS and the gut-associated lymphoid tissue (GALT) (Schulte-Herbrüggen et al., 2009). Increased intestinal permeability may promote bacterial invasion to non-gut organs. Increased bacterial load in mesenteric lymph nodes has been reported after MCAO (Caso et al., 2009). In a mouse model of ischaemic stroke, post-stroke infection was not seen in mice born and raised in GF facilities but was observed in those housed from birth in specific-pathogen-free (SPF) facilities. It was demonstrated in the same study that the source of disseminated bacteria in the infected cases was indeed the host small intestine (Stanley et al., 2016). Such bacterial translocation also induces inflammation and promotes Th1 and Th17 responses, all of which are normally required to clear a systemic bacterial infection. As discussed previously, however, these Th1 responses are associated with poorer stroke outcome. An elegant paper by Singh *et al.* showed how large stroke lesions lead to gut microbiota dysbiosis, which in turn worsens stroke outcome *via* immune-mediated mechanisms including intestinal lymphocyte migration to the ischaemic brain (Singh et al., 2016). Faecal microbial transplantation, however, normalizes this stroke-induced dysbiosis and improves stroke outcome. In the same study, it was highlighted that stroke specifically reduces microbiota species diversity and causes overgrowth of Bacteroidetes, a phenomenon associated with intestinal barrier dysfunction and reduced intestinal motility. Effectively, the microbiota composition may impact stroke severity. For example, altering the ratio of Firmicutes to *Bacteroides* in young mice to resemble the ratio observed in old mice before MCAO increased mortality and decreased behavioural performance (Spychala et al., 2018). An "aged" microbiota composition enhanced systemic inflammation when transplanted into young mice. Transplanted mice also had lower levels of short-chain fatty acids (SCFAs). These bacterially produced small molecules are important modulators that stabilize the gut epithelial barrier and modulate immune responses (Spychala et al., 2018). This study again suggests that the gut microbiota can affect stroke outcome in a mouse model. Aberrations to gut microbiota may not only significantly decrease survival, however, but also lead to acute colitis and other post-stroke sequelae (Winek et al., 2016a). However, translational caveats inherent to microbiota research in general are also true for stroke research. The differences in the anatomy, physiology, genetic heterogeneity, diet, and housing of mice compared with humans must be appreciated to prevent incorrect translation of findings in rodent gut microbiota models to human disease (Winek et al., 2016b). Instances where antibiotic-induced alterations to the gut microbiota reduced ischaemic injury should also be further explored (Benakis et al., 2016). Overall, more clinical studies are required to truly evaluate the role of the microbiota in post-stroke responses and to define strategies of how this response can be modified for improved patient outcomes.

ISCHAEMIC PRECONDITIONING

Significant interactions between the stroke and the periphery are also at play in remote ischaemic preconditioning (RIPC). Originally discovered by Murray and colleagues, preconditioning is a procedure by which a noxious stimulus is applied to a tissue or organ below the threshold of damage (Murry et al., 1986). After a recovery period, organs such as the brain develop a tolerance to the same or even different noxious stimuli given above the threshold of damage. Various types of preconditioning stimuli have been used experimentally to protect the brain, heart, liver, kidney, and other organs. Chief among these are ischaemic preconditioning (in which the blood supply to a target organ is temporarily interrupted before introducing a longer infarct) and hypoxic preconditioning (in which animals are exposed to oxygen levels around 8% to 9% for a few hours). However, achieving ischaemic or hypoxic preconditioning in the brain itself would be more challenging and less practical than in other organs. Therefore, experimental and clinical evidence that shows robust tolerance can be achieved in the brain by inducing ischaemia–reperfusion in a distant (remote) non-vital organ has attracted a great deal of attention (Hess et al., 2013; Chen et al., 2018c). Both local preconditioning and RIPC protect the brain either rapidly after stimulation (known as early, first-window, or classical preconditioning) or after a 24-h delay to induce protection lasting at least 48 h (known as delayed or second-window preconditioning). The complex mechanisms underlying early and delayed protection differ, with evidence for both humoral and neurogenic mechanisms (many of which are shared between local preconditioning and RIPC). Most mechanisms (i.e., intracellular signalling cascades, role of mitochondria, and activation of neural pathways) are beyond the scope of this review, and the next section will focus instead on the evidence that inflammation and immunomodulation also play a role.

RIPC prevents BBB breakdown following stroke (Wei et al., 2012) and regulates inflammatory gene expression in the blood

(Konstantinov et al., 2004), whereas blocking pro-inflammatory signalling pathways abolishes ischaemic tolerance to focal stroke in response to hypoxic preconditioning (Stowe et al., 2012; Selvaraj et al., 2017). Molecular inflammatory mechanisms underlying different brain preconditioning modalities were recently reviewed (Garcia-Bonilla et al., 2014), and there is a large body of evidence implicating the innate immune system in preconditioning (Amantea et al., 2015). The adaptive immune response may also play a role, as RIPC results in dramatic changes in T- and B-lymphocyte subsets in the spleen, while splenectomy attenuates the protective effect of RIPC on ischaemic brain injury (Chen et al., 2018b). Because similar neuroinflammatory pathways and lymphocytes underlie the pathophysiology of both MS, a progressive condition, and ischaemic stroke, which occurs more acutely (Paterno and Chillon, 2018), it is interesting to note that local preconditioning and RIPC also seem to be effective in the context of EAE (Camara-Lemarroy et al., 2018). Mice that underwent hypoxic preconditioning show fewer CD4+ T-cells and a delayed Th17-specific cytokine response, as well as increased numbers of Tregs and IL-10 following EAE induction (Esen et al., 2016). This effect on Tregs is reminiscent of observations in the kidney, where local ischaemic preconditioning leads to an increase in CD4+CD25+FoxP3+ and CD4+CD25+IL-10+ Tregs (Cho et al., 2010; Kinsey et al., 2010). These Treg cells seem to be able to suppress conventional T-cells with diverse antigen specificities (Corthay, 2009), suggesting that an increase in Treg number due to preconditioning in one organ might be protective in another and might therefore also play a role in RIPC. Alternatively, preconditioning might affect neutrophils (Shimizu et al., 2010), monocytes/macrophages (McDonough and Weinstein, 2016), or lymphocytes other than Tregs, in particular immunosuppressive B-cells (Monson et al., 2014). RIPC has been shown to alter the CD8+ T-cell, B-cell, NKT-cell, and monocyte response after stroke (Liu et al., 2016). Exercise-induced neuroprotection is another form of preconditioning that also seems to involve immunomodulation (Ding et al., 2005), and multiple reports point to a role of B-cells (reviewed in Selvaraj et al., 2016).

Because of the unpredictable nature of stroke, the clinical relevance of preconditioning is unclear, and RIPC is most likely to be performed under specific circumstances, such as during coronary bypass surgery or in patients undergoing carotid endarterectomy (Walsh et al., 2010). However, the potential clinical effectiveness of hypoxia- and ischaemia-induced tolerance to stroke is supported by the protective effect of living at higher altitude on stroke mortality (Faeh et al., 2009), and by observations that transient ischaemic attacks (TIAs) are associated with reduced severity of subsequent stroke (Weih et al., 1999). Furthermore, remote ischaemic conditioning performed during ("perconditioning") (Schmidt et al., 2007) or after ("postconditioning") (Kerendi et al., 2005) the ischaemic episode in the target organ also seems to be effective in animal models of myocardial infarction, suggesting that mechanisms underlying preconditioning might also be utilized after a stroke has occurred. Indeed, a recent study showing that remote ischaemic postconditioning administered 5 days after stroke reverses peripheral post-stroke immunosuppression and leads to a gradual functional improvement over an observation period of 3 months suggests that this approach not only may be protective but also may in fact promote recovery, lessening the importance of identifying the critical therapeutic time window (Doeppner et al., 2018).

CONCLUSION

Despite the benefits that thrombolysis and mechanical thrombectomy offer in AIS care, new agents are now required both as adjuncts and as separate therapies. **Table 1** highlights various immunomodulatory therapeutic strategies considered in the treatment of AIS to date. In an era of increasingly complex biomedical research, such strategies feature not only small molecule drugs but also monoclonal antibodies and, more recently, cell-based therapies. Although advanced biological therapies offer several advantages over their chemical counterparts (e.g., increased target specificity and reduced toxicity), the issues of cost, patient access, formulation, and unexpected immune reactions still need to be reconciled in the setting of stroke.

A separate dichotomy identifiable in the list of immunomodulatory therapeutic strategies available is whether the mechanism underlying each treatment reduces neurotoxicity or instead promotes neurorestoration and tissue repair. Many of the drugs trialled to date (anakinra and etanercept) target innate immunity, a portion of the immune response responsible for widespread neurotoxicity in the acute phase of the disease. Arguably, however, even if such therapies eventually proved effective, their widespread clinical use could be limited to tPA adjuncts by time alone. Conversely, therapies affecting the adaptive immune response (Tregs and Bregs), involved predominantly in repair processes, could be administered over a longer therapeutic window. In this regard, therapeutic strategies not bound by time constraints (e.g., postconditioning) could offer the most flexibility of all.

One aspect of ischaemic preconditioning, which resonates strongly in current stroke research, is the effect that changes to the periphery could have on both the CNS and the post-stroke organism at large. In this regard, the development of drugs that could abrogate SIID or bolster the host defence against post-stroke infection has received intense focus, especially in the era of antibiotic resistance. Separately, the role of the gut microbiota and the brain–gut axis plays in stroke recovery has been elucidated. Here, novel therapies that could either control post-stroke dysbiosis or modify gut-induced neuroinflammation could improve stroke outcome. The skewing of the peripheral immune response with a view to reduced brain injury could also be exploited through the phenomenon of brain antigen tolerization.

As part of the last several decades of pre-clinical and clinical stroke research, a wealth of information on the immune involvement in AIS has been discovered. As a result, the field has progressed from the initial belief that some innate or adaptive immune components exacerbate ischaemic insult to the current understanding that many immune elements play multi-faceted roles in both stroke-induced damage and post-stroke repair. A greater appreciation of the intimate, bi-directional communication between the CNS and the immune system post-stroke has helped clarify how such functional polarization occurs. Meanwhile, the concept of SIID, potentially responsible for a significant portion of stroke patient mortality, has attracted attention to immunomodulatory therapeutic strategies in AIS. Given the shortcomings of neuroprotection trials, such strategies will no doubt continue to receive increased interest in the future.

AUTHOR CONTRIBUTIONS

KM, SA, AM, and CW wrote the original manuscript. All authors subsequently reviewed, edited, and agreed upon the final draft.

FUNDING

This work was generously supported by a Government of Ireland Postgraduate Scholarship from the Irish Research Council (grant number GOIPG/2017/431), an HRB Health Research Award (HRA-POR-2015-1236), and a Marie Curie Career Integration Grant (631246).

REFERENCES

Abdelnaseer, M. M., Elfauomy, N. M., Esmail, E. H., Kamal, M. M., and Elsawy, E. H. (2017). Matrix metalloproteinase-9 and recovery of acute ischemic stroke. *J. Stroke. Cerebrovasc. Dis.* 26 (4), 733–740. doi: 10.1016/j.jstrokecerebrovasdis.2016.09.043

Alawieh, A., Elvington, A., and Tomlinson, S. (2015a). Complement in the homeostatic and ischemic brain. *Front. Immunol.* 6, 417. doi: 10.3389/fimmu.2015.00417

Alawieh, A., Elvington, A., Zhu, H., Yu, J., Kindy, M. S., Atkinson, C., et al. (2015b). Modulation of post-stroke degenerative and regenerative processes and subacute protection by site-targeted inhibition of the alternative pathway of complement. *J. Neuroinflammation* 12, 247. doi: 10.1186/s12974-015-0464-8

Alawieh, A., Langley, E. F., and Tomlinson, S. (2018). Targeted complement inhibition salvages stressed neurons and inhibits neuroinflammation after stroke in mice. *Sci. Transl. Med.* 10 (441), 1–13. doi: 10.1126/scitranslmed.aao6459

Alawieh, A., and Tomlinson, S. (2016). Injury site-specific targeting of complement inhibitors for treating stroke. *Immunol. Rev.* 274 (1), 270–280. doi: 10.1111/imr.12470

Amantea, D., Bagetta, G., Tassorelli, C., Mercuri, N. B., and Corasaniti, M. T. (2010). Identification of distinct cellular pools of interleukin-1beta during the evolution of the neuroinflammatory response induced by transient middle cerebral artery occlusion in the brain of rat. *Brain Res.* 1313, 259–269. doi: 10.1016/j.brainres.2009.12.017

Amantea, D., Micieli, G., Tassorelli, C., Cuartero, M. I., Ballesteros, I., Certo, M., et al. (2015). Rational modulation of the innate immune system for neuroprotection in ischemic stroke. *Front. Neurosci.* 9, 147. doi: 10.3389/fnins.2015.00147

Amantea, D., Nappi, G., Bernardi, G., Bagetta, G., and Corasaniti, M. T. (2009). Post-ischemic brain damage: pathophysiology and role of inflammatory mediators. *FEBS J.* 276 (1), 13–26. doi: 10.1111/j.1742-4658.2008.06766.x

Amulic, B., and Hayes, G. (2011). Neutrophil extracellular traps. *Curr. Biol.* 21 (9), R297–298. doi: 10.1016/j.cub.2011.03.021

Arumugam, T. V., Salter, J. W., Chidlow, J. H., Ballantyne, C. M., Kevil, C. G., and Granger, D. N. (2004). Contributions of LFA-1 and Mac-1 to brain injury and microvascular dysfunction induced by transient middle cerebral artery occlusion. *Am. J. Physiol. Heart Circ. Physiol.* 287 (6), H2555–2560. doi: 10.1152/ajpheart.00588.2004

Asahi, M., Wang, X., Mori, T., Sumii, T., Jung, J. C., Moskowitz, M. A., et al. (2001). Effects of matrix metalloproteinase-9 gene knock-out on the proteolysis of blood–brain barrier and white matter components after cerebral ischemia. *J. Neurosci.* 21 (19), 7724–7732. doi: 10.1523/JNEUROSCI.21-19-07724.2001

Barreto, G., White, R. E., Ouyang, Y., Xu, L., and Giffard, R. G. (2011). Astrocytes: targets for neuroprotection in stroke. *Cent. Nerv. Syst. Agents Med. Chem.* 11 (2), 164–173. doi: 10.2174/187152411796011303

Baskaya, M. K., Hu, Y., Donaldson, D., Maley, M., Rao, A. M., Prasad, M. R., et al. (1996). Protective effect of the 5-lipoxygenase inhibitor AA-861 on cerebral edema after transient ischemia. *J. Neurosurg.* 85 (1), 112–116. doi: 10.3171/jns.1996.85.1.0112

Basu, A., Lazovic, J., Krady, J. K., Mauger, D. T., Rothstein, R. P., Smith, M. B., et al. (2005). Interleukin-1 and the interleukin-1 type 1 receptor are essential for the progressive neurodegeneration that ensues subsequent to a mild hypoxic/ischemic injury. *J. Cereb. Blood Flow Metab.* 25 (1), 17–29. doi: 10.1038/sj.jcbfm.9600002

Bath, P. M., Krishnan, K., and Appleton, J. P. (2017). Nitric oxide donors (nitrates), l-arginine, or nitric oxide synthase inhibitors for acute stroke. *Cochrane Database Syst. Rev.* 4, CD000398. doi: 10.1002/14651858.CD000398.pub2

Becerra-Calixto, A., and Cardona-Gómez, G. P. (2017). The role of astrocytes in neuroprotection after brain stroke: potential in cell therapy. *Front. Mol. Neurosci.* 10, 88. doi: 10.3389/fnmol.2017.00088

Becker, K. J. (2002). Anti-leukocyte antibodies: LeukArrest (Hu23F2G) and Enlimomab (R6.5) in acute stroke. *Curr. Med. Res. Opin.* 18 Suppl 2, s18–22. doi: 10.1185/030079902125000688

Becker, K. J., Kalil, A. J., Tanzi, P., Zierath, D. K., Savos, A. V., Gee, J. M., et al. (2011). Autoimmune responses to the brain after stroke are associated with worse outcome. *Stroke* 42 (10), 2763–2769. doi: 10.1161/STROKEAHA.111.619593

Benakis, C., Brea, D., Caballero, S., Faraco, G., Moore, J., Murphy, M., et al. (2016). Commensal microbiota affects ischemic stroke outcome by regulating intestinal γδ T cells. *Nat. Med.* 22 (5), 516–523. doi: 10.1038/nm.4068

Bitsch, A., Klene, W., Murtada, L., Prange, H., and Rieckmann, P. (1998). A longitudinal prospective study of soluble adhesion molecules in acute stroke. *Stroke* 29 (10), 2129–2135. doi: 10.1161/01.STR.29.10.2129

Bluestone, J. A., Buckner, J. H., Fitch, M., Gitelman, S. E., Gupta, S., Hellerstein, M. K., et al. (2015). Type 1 diabetes immunotherapy using polyclonal regulatory T cells. *Sci. Transl. Med.* 7 (315), 315ra189. doi: 10.1126/scitranslmed.aad4134

Bodhankar, S., Chen, Y., Lapato, A., Vandenbark, A. A., Murphy, S. J., Saugstad, J. A., et al. (2015). Regulatory CD8(+)CD122 (+) T-cells predominate in CNS after treatment of experimental stroke in male mice with IL-10-secreting B-cells. *Metab. Brain Dis.* 30 (4), 911–924. doi: 10.1007/s11011-014-9639-8

Bodhankar, S., Chen, Y., Vandenbark, A. A., Murphy, S. J., and Offner, H. (2013). IL-10-producing B-cells limit CNS inflammation and infarct volume in experimental stroke. *Metab. Brain Dis.* 28 (3), 375–386. doi: 10.1007/s11011-013-9413-3

Bonventre, J. V., Huang, Z., Taheri, M. R., O'Leary, E., Li, E., Moskowitz, M. A., et al. (1997). Reduced fertility and postischaemic brain injury in mice deficient in cytosolic phospholipase A2. *Nature* 390 (6660), 622–625. doi: 10.1038/37635

Boutin, H., LeFeuvre, R. A., Horai, R., Asano, M., Iwakura, Y., and Rothwell, N. J. (2001). Role of IL-1alpha and IL-1beta in ischemic brain damage. *J. Neurosci.* 21 (15), 5528–5534. doi: 10.1523/JNEUROSCI.21-15-05528.2001

Brait, V. H., Jackman, K. A., Walduck, A. K., Selemidis, S., Diep, H., Mast, A. E., et al. (2010). Mechanisms contributing to cerebral infarct size after stroke: gender, reperfusion, T lymphocytes, and Nox2-derived superoxide. *J. Cereb. Blood Flow Metab.* 30 (7), 1306–1317. doi: 10.1038/jcbfm.2010.14

Brambilla, R., Couch, Y., and Lambertsen, K. L. (2013). The effect of stroke on immune function. *Mol. Cell Neurosci.* 53, 26–33. doi: 10.1016/j.mcn.2012.08.011

Bruce, A. J., Boling, W., Kindy, M. S., Peschon, J., Kraemer, P. J., Carpenter, M. K., et al. (1996). Altered neuronal and microglial responses to excitotoxic and ischemic brain injury in mice lacking TNF receptors. *Nat. Med.* 2 (7), 788–794. doi: 10.1038/nm0796-788

Camara-Lemarroy, C. R., Metz, L., Smith, E. E., Dunn, J. F., and Yong, V. W. (2018). Expanding the potential therapeutic options for remote ischemic preconditioning: use in multiple sclerosis. *Front. Neurol.* 9, 475. doi: 10.3389/fneur.2018.00475

Campos, F., Qin, T., Castillo, J., Seo, J. H., Arai, K., Lo, E. H., et al. (2013). Fingolimod reduces hemorrhagic transformation associated with delayed tissue plasminogen activator treatment in a mouse thromboembolic model. *Stroke* 44 (2), 505–511. doi: 10.1161/STROKEAHA.112.679043

Candelario-Jalil, E., González-Falcón, A., García-Cabrera, M., Alvarez, D., Al-Dalain, S., Martínez, G., et al. (2003). Assessment of the relative contribution of COX-1 and COX-2 isoforms to ischemia-induced oxidative damage and neurodegeneration following transient global cerebral ischemia. *J. Neurochem.* 86 (3), 545–555. doi: 10.1046/j.1471-4159.2003.01812.x

Caso, J. R., Hurtado, O., Pereira, M. P., García-Bueno, B., Menchén, L., Alou, L., et al. (2009). Colonic bacterial translocation as a possible factor in stress-worsening experimental stroke outcome. *Am. J. Physiol. Regul. Integr. Comp. Physiol.* 296 (4), R979–985. doi: 10.1152/ajpregu.90825.2008

Cervera, A., Justicia, C., Reverter, J. C., Planas, A. M., and Chamorro, A. (2004). Steady plasma concentration of unfractionated heparin reduces infarct volume and prevents inflammatory damage after transient focal cerebral ischemia in the rat. *J. Neurosci. Res.* 77 (4), 565–572. doi: 10.1002/jnr.20186

Chamorro, Á., Meisel, A., Planas, A. M., Urra, X., van de Beek, D., and Veltkamp, R. (2012). The immunology of acute stroke. *Nat. Rev. Neurol.* 8 (7), 401–410. doi: 10.1038/nrneurol.2012.98

Che, X., Ye, W., Panga, L., Wu, D. C., and Yang, G. Y. (2001). Monocyte chemoattractant protein-1 expressed in neurons and astrocytes during focal ischemia in mice. *Brain Res.* 902 (2), 171–177. doi: 10.1016/S0006-8993(01)02328-9

Chen, C., Chu, S. F., Liu, D. D., Zhang, Z., Kong, L. L., Zhou, X., et al. (2018a). Chemokines play complex roles in cerebral ischemia. *Neurochem. Int.* 112, 146–158. doi: 10.1016/j.neuint.2017.06.008

Chen, C., Jiang, W., Liu, Z., Li, F., Yang, J., Zhao, Y., et al. (2018b). Splenic responses play an important role in remote ischemic preconditioning-mediated neuroprotection against stroke. *J. Neuroinflammation* 15 (1), 167. doi: 10.1186/s12974-018-1190-9

Chen, G., Thakkar, M., Robinson, C., and Dore, S. (2018c). Limb remote ischemic conditioning: mechanisms, anesthetics, and the potential for expanding therapeutic options. *Front. Neurol.* 9, 40. doi: 10.3389/fneur.2018.00040

Chen, H., Chopp, M., Zhang, R. L., Bodzin, G., Chen, Q., Rusche, J. R., et al. (1994). Anti-CD11b monoclonal antibody reduces ischemic cell damage after transient focal cerebral ischemia in rat. *Ann. Neurol.* 35 (4), 458–463. doi: 10.1002/ana.410350414

Chen, Y., Bodhankar, S., Murphy, S. J., Vandenbark, A. A., Alkayed, N. J., and Offner, H. (2012). Intrastriatal B-cell administration limits infarct size after stroke in B-cell deficient mice. *Metab. Brain Dis.* 27 (4), 487–493. doi: 10.1007/s11011-012-9317-7

Chen, Y., Won, S. J., Xu, Y., and Swanson, R. A. (2014). Targeting microglial activation in stroke therapy: pharmacological tools and gender effects. *Curr. Med. Chem.* 21 (19), 2146–2155. doi: 10.2174/0929867321666131228203906

Chen, Z. Q., Mou, R. T., Feng, D. X., Wang, Z., and Chen, G. (2017). The role of nitric oxide in stroke. *Med. Gas. Res.* 7 (3), 194–203. doi: 10.4103/2045-9912.215750

Chiba, T., and Umegaki, K. (2013). Pivotal roles of monocytes/macrophages in stroke. *Mediators Inflamm.* 2013, 759103. doi: 10.1155/2013/759103

Cho, W. Y., Choi, H. M., Lee, S. Y., Kim, M. G., Kim, H. K., and Jo, S. K. (2010). The role of Tregs and CD11c(+) macrophages/dendritic cells in ischemic preconditioning of the kidney. *Kidney Int.* 78 (10), 981–992. doi: 10.1038/ki.2010.266

Chu, H. X., Kim, H. A. H., Lee, S., Moore, J. P., Chan, C. T., Vinh, A., et al. (2014). Immune cell infiltration in malignant middle cerebral artery infarction: comparison with transient cerebral ischemia. *J. Cereb. Blood Flow Metab.* 34 (3), 450–459. doi: 10.1038/jcbfm.2013.217

Cisbani, G., Le Behot, A., Plante, M. M., Préfontaine, P., Lecordier, M., and Rivest, S. (2018). Role of the chemokine receptors CCR2 and CX3CR1 in an experimental model of thrombotic stroke. *Brain Behav. Immun.* 70, 280–292. doi: 10.1016/j.bbi.2018.03.008

Clausen, B. H., Lambertsen, K. L., Meldgaard, M., and Finsen, B. (2005). A quantitative *in situ* hybridization and polymerase chain reaction study of microglial-macrophage expression of interleukin-1beta mRNA following permanent middle cerebral artery occlusion in mice. *Neuroscience* 132 (4), 879–892. doi: 10.1016/j.neuroscience.2005.01.031

Cojocaru, I. M., Cojocaru, M., Tănăsescu, R., Burcin, C., Atanasiu, A. N., Petrescu, A. M., et al. (2008). Changes in plasma levels of complement in patients with acute ischemic stroke. *Rom. J. Intern. Med.* 46 (1), 77–80.

Connolly, E. S., Winfree, C. J., Springer, T. A., Naka, Y., Liao, H., Yan, S. D., et al. (1996). Cerebral protection in homozygous null ICAM-1 mice after middle cerebral artery occlusion. Role of neutrophil adhesion in the pathogenesis of stroke. *J. Clin. Invest.* 97 (1), 209–216. doi: 10.1172/JCI118392

Corps, K. N., Roth, T. L., and McGavern, D. B. (2015). Inflammation and neuroprotection in traumatic brain injury. *JAMA Neurol.* 72 (3), 355–362. doi: 10.1001/jamaneurol.2014.3558

Corthay, A. (2009). How do regulatory T cells work? *Scand. J. Immunol.* 70 (4), 326–336. doi: 10.1111/j.1365-3083.2009.02308.x

Coughlan, T., Gibson, C., and Murphy, S. (2005). Modulatory effects of progesterone on inducible nitric oxide synthase expression *in vivo* and *in vitro*. *J. Neurochem.* 93 (4), 932–942. doi: 10.1111/j.1471-4159.2005.03068.x

Cui, G., Wang, H., Li, R., Zhang, L., Li, Z., Wang, Y., et al. (2012). Polymorphism of tumor necrosis factor alpha (TNF-alpha) gene promoter, circulating TNF-alpha level, and cardiovascular risk factor for ischemic stroke. *J. Neuroinflammation* 9, 235. doi: 10.1186/1742-2094-9-235

del Zoppo, G. J., Schmid-Schönbein, G. W., Mori, E., Copeland, B. R., and Chang, C. M. (1991). Polymorphonuclear leukocytes occlude capillaries following middle cerebral artery occlusion and reperfusion in baboons. *Stroke* 22 (10), 1276–1283. doi: 10.1161/01.STR.22.10.1276

Ding, Y. H., Young, C. N., Luan, X., Li, J., Rafols, J. A., Clark, J. C., et al. (2005). Exercise preconditioning ameliorates inflammatory injury in ischemic rats during reperfusion. *Acta Neuropathol.* 109 (3), 237–246. doi: 10.1007/s00401-004-0943-y

Doeppner, T. R., Zechmeister, B., Kaltwasser, B., Jin, F., Zheng, X., Majid, A., et al. (2018). Very delayed remote ischemic post-conditioning induces sustained neurological recovery by mechanisms involving enhanced angioneurogenesis and peripheral immunosuppression reversal. *Front. Cell Neurosci.* 12, 383. doi: 10.3389/fncel.2018.00383

Dong, Y., and Benveniste, E. N. (2001). Immune function of astrocytes. *Glia* 36 (2), 180–190. doi: 10.1002/glia.1107

Doré, S., Otsuka, T., Mito, T., Sugo, N., Hand, T., Wu, L., et al. (2003). Neuronal overexpression of cyclooxygenase-2 increases cerebral infarction. *Ann. Neurol.* 54 (2), 155–162. doi: 10.1002/ana.10612

Doyle, K. P., Quach, L. N., Solé, M., Axtell, R. C., Nguyen, T. V., Soler-Llavina, G. J., et al. (2015). B-lymphocyte-mediated delayed cognitive impairment following stroke. *J. Neurosci.* 35 (5), 2133–2145. doi: 10.1523/JNEUROSCI.4098-14.2015

Drieu, A., Levard, D., Vivien, D., and Rubio, M. (2018). Anti-inflammatory treatments for stroke: from bench to bedside. *Ther. Adv. Neurol. Disord.* 11, 1–15. 1756286418789854. doi: 10.1177/1756286418789854

Ducruet, A. F., Mocco, J., Mack, W. J., Coon, A. L., Marsh, H. C., Pinsky, D. J., et al. (2007). Pre-clinical evaluation of an sLe x-glycosylated complement inhibitory protein in a non-human primate model of reperfused stroke. *J. Med. Primatol.* 36 (6), 375–380. doi: 10.1111/j.1600-0684.2007.00213.x

Ducruet, A. F., Zacharia, B. E., Sosunov, S. A., Gigante, P. R., Yeh, M. L., Gorski, J. W., et al. (2012). Complement inhibition promotes endogenous neurogenesis and sustained anti-inflammatory neuroprotection following reperfused stroke. *PLoS One* 7 (6), e38664. doi: 10.1371/journal.pone.0038664

Dziedzic, T., Slowik, A., Pera, J., and Szczudlik, A. (2007). Beta-blockers reduce the risk of early death in ischemic stroke. *J. Neurol. Sci.* 252 (1), 53–56. doi: 10.1016/j.jns.2006.10.007

Elkins, J., Veltkamp, R., Montaner, J., Johnston, S. C., Singhal, A. B., Becker, K., et al. (2017). Safety and efficacy of natalizumab in patients with acute ischaemic stroke (ACTION): a randomised, placebo-controlled, double-blind phase 2 trial. *Lancet Neurol.* 16 (3), 217–226. doi: 10.1016/S1474-4422(16)30357-X

Emsley, H. C., Smith, C. J., Georgiou, R. F., Vail, A., Hopkins, S. J., Rothwell, N. J., et al. (2005). A randomised phase II study of interleukin-1 receptor antagonist in acute stroke patients. *J. Neurol. Neurosurg. Psychiatry.* 76 (10), 1366–1372. doi: 10.1136/jnnp.2004.054882

Engblom, D., Ek, M., Saha, S., Ericsson-Dahlstrand, A., Jakobsson, P. J., and Blomqvist, A. (2002). Prostaglandins as inflammatory messengers across the blood-brain barrier. *J. Mol. Med. (Berl)* 80 (1), 5–15. doi: 10.1007/s00109-001-0289-z

Engelhardt, B., and Sorokin, L. (2009). The blood-brain and the blood-cerebrospinal fluid barriers: function and dysfunction. *Semin. Immunopathol.* 31 (4), 497–511. doi: 10.1007/s00281-009-0177-0

Esen, N., Katyshev, V., Serkin, Z., Katysheva, S., and Dore-Duffy, P. (2016). Endogenous adaptation to low oxygen modulates T-cell regulatory pathways in EAE. *J. Neuroinflammation* 13, 13. doi: 10.1186/s12974-015-0407-4

Faeh, D., Gutzwiller, F., Bopp, M., and Swiss National Cohort Study, G. (2009). Lower mortality from coronary heart disease and stroke at higher altitudes in Switzerland. *Circulation* 120 (6), 495–501. doi: 10.1161/CIRCULATIONAHA.108.819250

Fann, D. Y., Lee, S. Y., Manzanero, S., Chunduri, P., Sobey, C. G., and Arumugam, T. V. (2013). Pathogenesis of acute stroke and the role of inflammasomes. *Ageing Res. Rev.* 12 (4), 941–966. doi: 10.1016/j.arr.2013.09.004

Fu, Y., Hao, J., Zhang, N., Ren, L., Sun, N., Li, Y. J., et al. (2014a). Fingolimod for the treatment of intracerebral hemorrhage: a 2-arm proof-of-concept study. *JAMA Neurol.* 71 (9), 1092–1101. doi: 10.1001/jamaneurol.2014.1065

Fu, Y., Zhang, N., Ren, L., Yan, Y., Sun, N., Li, Y. J., et al. (2014b). Impact of an immune modulator fingolimod on acute ischemic stroke. *Proc. Natl. Acad. Sci. U. S. A.* 111 (51), 18315–18320. doi: 10.1073/pnas.1416166111

Garau, A., Bertini, R., Colotta, F., Casilli, F., Bigini, P., Cagnotto, A., et al. (2005). Neuroprotection with the CXCL8 inhibitor repertaxin in transient brain ischemia. *Cytokine* 30 (3), 125–131. doi: 10.1016/j.cyto.2004.12.014

Garcia-Bonilla, L., Benakis, C., Moore, J., Iadecola, C., and Anrather, J. (2014). Immune mechanisms in cerebral ischemic tolerance. *Front. Neurosci.* 8, 44. doi: 10.3389/fnins.2014.00044

Gasche, Y., Copin, J. C., Sugawara, T., Fujimura, M., and Chan, P. H. (2001). Matrix metalloproteinase inhibition prevents oxidative stress-associated blood–brain barrier disruption after transient focal cerebral ischemia. *J. Cereb. Blood Flow Metab.* 21 (12), 1393–1400. doi: 10.1097/00004647-200112000-00003

Gee, J. M., Zierath, D., Hadwin, J., Savos, A., Kalil, A., Thullbery, M., et al. (2009). Long term immunologic consequences of experimental stroke and mucosal tolerance. *Exp. Transl. Stroke Med.* 1, 3. doi: 10.1186/2040-7378-1-3

Ginis, I., Jaiswal, R., Klimanis, D., Liu, J., Greenspon, J., and Hallenbeck, J. M. (2002). TNF-alpha-induced tolerance to ischemic injury involves differential control of NF-kappaB transactivation: the role of NF-kappaB association with p300 adaptor. *J. Cereb. Blood Flow Metab.* 22 (2), 142–152. doi: 10.1097/00004647-200202000-00002

Gu, Z., Cui, J., Brown, S., Fridman, R., Mobashery, S., Strongin, A. Y., et al. (2005). A highly specific inhibitor of matrix metalloproteinase-9 rescues laminin from proteolysis and neurons from apoptosis in transient focal cerebral ischemia. *J. Neurosci.* 25 (27), 6401–6408. doi: 10.1523/JNEUROSCI.1563-05.2005

Hallenbeck, J. (2010). How inflammation modulates central nervous system vessel activation and provides targets for intervention—a personal perspective. *Ann. N. Y. Acad. Sci.* 1207, 1–7. doi: 10.1111/j.1749-6632.2010.05785.x

Han, H. S., Qiao, Y., Karabiyikoglu, M., Giffard, R. G., and Yenari, M. A. (2002). Influence of mild hypothermia on inducible nitric oxide synthase expression and reactive nitrogen production in experimental stroke and inflammation. *J. Neurosci.* 22 (10), 3921–3928. doi: 10.1523/JNEUROSCI.22-10-03921.2002

Hayakawa, K., Arai, K., and Lo, E. H. (2010). Role of ERK map kinase and CRM1 in IL-1beta-stimulated release of HMGB1 from cortical astrocytes. *Glia* 58 (8), 1007–1015. doi: 10.1002/glia.20982

Herz, J., Sabellek, P., Lane, T. E., Gunzer, M., Hermann, D. M., and Doeppner, T. R. (2015). Role of neutrophils in exacerbation of brain injury after focal cerebral ischemia in hyperlipidemic mice. *Stroke* 46 (10), 2916–2925. doi: 10.1161/STROKEAHA.115.010620

Hess, D. C., Hoda, M. N., and Bhatia, K. (2013). Remote limb perconditioning [corrected] and postconditioning: will it translate into a promising treatment for acute stroke? *Stroke* 44 (4), 1191–1197. doi: 10.1161/STROKEAHA.112.678482

Hess, D. C., Sila, C. A., Furlan, A. J., Wechsler, L. R., Switzer, J. A., and Mays, R. W. (2014). A double-blind placebo-controlled clinical evaluation of MultiStem for the treatment of ischemic stroke. *Int. J. Stroke* 9 (3), 381–386. doi: 10.1111/ijs.12065

Hess, D. C., Zhao, W., Carroll, J., McEachin, M., and Buchanan, K. (1994). Increased expression of ICAM-1 during reoxygenation in brain endothelial cells. *Stroke* 25 (7), 1463–1467. discussion 1468. doi: 10.1161/01.STR.25.7.1463

Hewett, S. J., Jackman, N. A., and Claycomb, R. J. (2012). Interleukin-1β in central nervous system injury and repair. *Eur. J. Neurodegener. Dis.* 1 (2), 195–211.

Huang, H., Al-Shabrawey, M., and Wang, M. H. (2016). Cyclooxygenase- and cytochrome P450-derived eicosanoids in stroke. *Prostaglandins Other Lipid Mediat.* 122, 45–53. doi: 10.1016/j.prostaglandins.2015.12.007

Huang, J., Choudhri, T. F., Winfree, C. J., McTaggart, R. A., Kiss, S., Mocco, J., et al. (2000). Postischemic cerebrovascular E-selectin expression mediates tissue injury in murine stroke. *Stroke* 31 (12), 3047–3053. doi: 10.1161/01.STR.31.12.3047

Huang, J., Kim, L. J., Mealey, R., Marsh, H. C., Zhang, Y., Tenner, A. J., et al. (1999). Neuronal protection in stroke by an sLex-glycosylated complement inhibitory protein. *Science* 285 (5427), 595–599. doi: 10.1126/science.285.5427.595

Huang, J., Upadhyay, U. M., and Tamargo, R. J. (2006). Inflammation in stroke and focal cerebral ischemia. *Surg. Neurol.* 66 (3), 232–245. doi: 10.1016/j.surneu.2005.12.028

Hurn, P. D., Subramanian, S., Parker, S. M., Afentoulis, M. E., Kaler, L. J., Vandenbark, A. A., et al. (2007). T- and B-cell-deficient mice with experimental stroke have reduced lesion size and inflammation. *J. Cereb. Blood Flow Metab.* 27 (11), 1798–1805. doi: 10.1038/sj.jcbfm.9600482

Iadecola, C., and Anrather, J. (2011). The immunology of stroke: from mechanisms to translation. *Nat. Med.* 17 (7), 796–808. doi: 10.1038/nm.2399

Iadecola, C., and Gorelick, P. B. (2005). The Janus face of cyclooxygenase-2 in ischemic stroke: shifting toward downstream targets. *Stroke* 36 (2), 182–185. doi: 10.1161/01.STR.0000153797.33611.d8

Iadecola, C., Sugimoto, K., Niwa, K., Kazama, K., and Ross, M. E. (2001). Increased susceptibility to ischemic brain injury in cyclooxygenase-1-deficient mice. *J. Cereb. Blood Flow Metab.* 21 (12), 1436–1441. doi: 10.1097/00004647-200112000-00008

Iadecola, C., Zhang, F., Xu, S., Casey, R., and Ross, M. E. (1995). Inducible nitric oxide synthase gene expression in brain following cerebral ischemia. *J. Cereb. Blood Flow Metab.* 15 (3), 378–384. doi: 10.1038/jcbfm.1995.47

Investigators, E. A. S. T. (2001). Use of anti-ICAM-1 therapy in ischemic stroke: results of the Enlimomab Acute Stroke Trial. *Neurology* 57 (8), 1428–1434. doi: 10.1212/WNL.57.8.1428

Jadidi-Niaragh, F., and Mirshafiey, A. (2011). Th17 cell, the new player of neuroinflammatory process in multiple sclerosis. *Scand. J. Immunol.* 74 (1), 1–13. doi: 10.1111/j.1365-3083.2011.02536.x

Jauch, E. C., Lindsell, C., Broderick, J., Fagan, S. C., Tilley, B. C., and Levine, S. R. (2006). Association of serial biochemical markers with acute ischemic stroke—The National Institute of Neurological Disorders and Stroke recombinant tissue plasminogen activator Stroke Study. *Stroke* 37 (10), 2508–2513. doi: 10.1161/01.STR.0000242290.01174.9e

Jiang, N., Moyle, M., Soule, H. R., Rote, W. E., and Chopp, M. (1995). Neutrophil inhibitory factor is neuroprotective after focal ischemia in rats. *Ann. Neurol.* 38 (6), 935–942. doi: 10.1002/ana.410380615

Jiang, X., Andjelkovic, A. V., Zhu, L., Yang, T., Bennett, M. V. L., Chen, J., et al. (2018). Blood–brain barrier dysfunction and recovery after ischemic stroke. *Prog. Neurobiol.* 163–164, 144–171. doi: 10.1016/j.pneurobio.2017.10.001

Jickling, G. C., Liu, D., Ander, B. P., Stamova, B., Zhan, X., and Sharp, F. R. (2015). Targeting neutrophils in ischemic stroke: translational insights from experimental studies. *J. Cereb. Blood Flow Metab.* 35 (6), 888–901. doi: 10.1038/jcbfm.2015.45

Jin, A. Y., Tuor, U. I., Rushforth, D., Kaur, J., Muller, R. N., Petterson, J. L., et al. (2010). Reduced blood brain barrier breakdown in P-selectin deficient mice following transient ischemic stroke: a future therapeutic target for treatment of stroke. *BMC Neurosci.* 11, 12. doi: 10.1186/1471-2202-11-12

Justicia, C., Martín, A., Rojas, S., Gironella, M., Cervera, A., Panés, J., et al. (2006). Anti-VCAM-1 antibodies did not protect against ischemic damage either in rats or in mice. *J. Cereb. Blood Flow Metab.* 26 (3), 421–432. doi: 10.1038/sj.jcbfm.9600198

Kamel, H., and Iadecola, C. (2012). Brain-immune interactions and ischemic stroke: clinical implications. *Arch. Neurol.* 69 (5), 576–581. doi: 10.1001/archneurol.2011.3590

Kanazawa, M., Ninomiya, I., Hatakeyama, M., Takahashi, T., and Shimohata, T. (2017). Microglia and monocytes/macrophages polarization reveal novel therapeutic mechanism against stroke. *Int. J. Mol. Sci.* 18 (10), 1–18. doi: 10.3390/ijms18102135

Kanemoto, Y., Nakase, H., Akita, N., and Sakaki, T. (2002). Effects of anti-intercellular adhesion molecule-1 antibody on reperfusion injury induced by late reperfusion in the rat middle cerebral artery occlusion model. *Neurosurgery* 51 (4), 1034–41. discussion 1041-1032. doi: 10.1227/00006123-200210000-00033

Kawabori, M., Kacimi, R., Kauppinen, T., Calosing, C., Kim, J. Y., Hsieh, C. L., et al. (2015). Triggering receptor expressed on myeloid cells 2 (TREM2) deficiency attenuates phagocytic activities of microglia and exacerbates ischemic damage in experimental stroke. *J. Neurosci.* 35 (8), 3384–3396. doi: 10.1523/JNEUROSCI.2620-14.2015

Kawabori, M., and Yenari, M. A. (2015). Inflammatory responses in brain ischemia. *Curr. Med. Chem.* 22 (10), 1258–1277. doi: 10.2174/0929867322666150209154036

Kerendi, F., Kin, H., Halkos, M. E., Jiang, R., Zatta, A. J., Zhao, Z. Q., et al. (2005). Remote postconditioning. Brief renal ischemia and reperfusion applied before coronary artery reperfusion reduces myocardial infarct size *via* endogenous activation of adenosine receptors. *Basic Res. Cardiol.* 100 (5), 404–412. doi: 10.1007/s00395-005-0539-2

Kim, G. H., Mocco, J., Hahn, D. K., Kellner, C. P., Komotar, R. J., Ducruet, A. F., et al. (2008). Protective effect of C5a receptor inhibition after murine reperfused stroke. *Neurosurgery* 63 (1), 122–5. discussion 125–126. doi: 10.1227/01.NEU.0000335079.70222.8D

Kim, J. S., Chopp, M., Chen, H., Levine, S. R., Carey, J. L., and Welch, K. M. (1995a). Adhesive glycoproteins CD11a and CD18 are upregulated in the leukocytes from patients with ischemic stroke and transient ischemic attacks. *J. Neurol. Sci.* 128 (1), 45–50. doi: 10.1016/0022-510X(94)00203-Z

Kim, J. S., Gautam, S. C., Chopp, M., Zaloga, C., Jones, M. L., Ward, P. A., et al. (1995b). Expression of monocyte chemoattractant protein-1 and macrophage inflammatory protein-1 after focal cerebral ischemia in the rat. *J. Neuroimmunol.* 56 (2), 127–134. doi: 10.1016/0165-5728(94)00138-E

Kim, J. Y., Kawabori, M., and Yenari, M. A. (2014). Innate inflammatory responses in stroke: mechanisms and potential therapeutic targets. *Curr. Med. Chem.* 21 (18), 2076–2097. doi: 10.2174/0929867321666131228205146

Kim, J. Y., Park, J., Chang, J. Y., Kim, S. H., and Lee, J. E. (2016). Inflammation after ischemic stroke: the role of leukocytes and glial cells. *Exp. Neurobiol.* 25 (5), 241–251. doi: 10.5607/en.2016.25.5.241

Kimura, A., and Kishimoto, T. (2010). IL-6: regulator of Treg/Th17 balance. *Eur. J. Immunol.* 40 (7), 1830–1835. doi: 10.1002/eji.201040391

Kinsey, G. R., Huang, L., Vergis, A. L., Li, L., and Okusa, M. D. (2010). Regulatory T cells contribute to the protective effect of ischemic preconditioning in the kidney. *Kidney Int.* 77 (9), 771–780. doi: 10.1038/ki.2010.12

Kitagawa, K., Matsumoto, M., and Hori, M. (2004). Cerebral ischemia in 5-lipoxygenase knockout mice. *Brain Res.* 1004 (1–2), 198–202. doi: 10.1016/j.brainres.2004.01.018

Kitagawa, K., Matsumoto, M., Mabuchi, T., Yagita, Y., Ohtsuki, T., Hori, M., et al. (1998). Deficiency of intercellular adhesion molecule 1 attenuates microcirculatory disturbance and infarction size in focal cerebral ischemia. *J. Cereb. Blood Flow Metab.* 18 (12), 1336–1345. doi: 10.1097/00004647-199812000-00008

Kohler, E., Prentice, D. A., Bates, T. R., Hankey, G. J., Claxton, A., van Heerden, J., et al. (2013). Intravenous minocycline in acute stroke: a randomized, controlled pilot study and meta-analysis. *Stroke* 44 (9), 2493–2499. doi: 10.1161/STROKEAHA.113.000780

Konstantinov, I. E., Arab, S., Kharbanda, R. K., Li, J., Cheung, M. M., Cherepanov, V., et al. (2004). The remote ischemic preconditioning stimulus modifies inflammatory gene expression in humans. *Physiol. Genomics* 19 (1), 143–150. doi: 10.1152/physiolgenomics.00046.2004

Kox, M., and Pickkers, P. (2015). Modulation of the innate immune response through the vagus nerve. *Nephron* 131 (2), 79–84. doi: 10.1159/000435843

Kraft, P., Göb, E., Schuhmann, M. K., Göbel, K., Deppermann, C., Thielmann, I., et al. (2013). FTY720 ameliorates acute ischemic stroke in mice by reducing thrombo-inflammation but not by direct neuroprotection. *Stroke* 44 (11), 3202–3210. doi: 10.1161/STROKEAHA.113.002880

Krams, M., Lees, K. R., Hacke, W., Grieve, A. P., Orgogozo, J. M., Ford, G. A., et al. (2003). Acute stroke therapy by inhibition of neutrophils (ASTIN): an adaptive dose-response study of UK-279,276 in acute ischemic stroke. *Stroke* 34 (11), 2543–2548. doi: 10.1161/01.STR.0000092527.33910.89

Krishnamurthi, R. V., Feigin, V. L., Forouzanfar, M. H., Mensah, G. A., Connor, M., Bennett, D. A., et al. (2013). Global and regional burden of first-ever ischaemic and haemorrhagic stroke during 1990–2010: findings from the Global Burden of Disease Study 2010. *Lancet Glob. Health* 1 (5), e259–281. doi: 10.1016/S2214-109X(13)70089-5

Lalancette-Hébert, M., Gowing, G., Simard, A., Weng, Y. C., and Kriz, J. (2007). Selective ablation of proliferating microglial cells exacerbates ischemic injury in the brain. *J. Neurosci.* 27 (10), 2596–2605. doi: 10.1523/JNEUROSCI.5360-06.2007

Lambertsen, K. L., Biber, K., and Finsen, B. (2012). Inflammatory cytokines in experimental and human stroke. *J. Cereb. Blood Flow Metab.* 32 (9), 1677–1698. doi: 10.1038/jcbfm.2012.88

Lampl, Y., Boaz, M., Gilad, R., Lorberboym, M., Dabby, R., Rapoport, A., et al. (2007). Minocycline treatment in acute stroke: an open-label, evaluator-blinded study. *Neurology* 69 (14), 1404–1410. doi: 10.1212/01.wnl.0000277487.04281.db

Lee, S., Chu, H. X., Kim, H. A., Real, N. C., Sharif, S., Fleming, S. B., et al. (2015). Effect of a broad-specificity chemokine-binding protein on brain leukocyte infiltration and infarct development. *Stroke* 46 (2), 537–544. doi: 10.1161/STROKEAHA.114.007298

Lee, S. R., Kim, H. Y., Rogowska, J., Zhao, B. Q., Bhide, P., Parent, J. M., et al. (2006). Involvement of matrix metalloproteinase in neuroblast cell migration from the subventricular zone after stroke. *J. Neurosci.* 26 (13), 3491–3495. doi: 10.1523/JNEUROSCI.4085-05.2006

Lees, K. R., Bluhmki, E., von Kummer, R., Brott, T. G., Toni, D., Grotta, J. C., et al. (2010). Time to treatment with intravenous alteplase and outcome in stroke: an updated pooled analysis of ECASS, ATLANTIS, NINDS, and EPITHET trials. *Lancet* 375 (9727), 1695–1703. doi: 10.1016/S0140-6736(10)60491-6

Li, P., Gan, Y., Sun, B. L., Zhang, F., Lu, B., Gao, Y., et al. (2013). Adoptive regulatory T-cell therapy protects against cerebral ischemia. *Ann. Neurol.* 74 (3), 458–471. doi: 10.1002/ana.23815

Li, W., Xu, H., and Testai, F. D. (2016). Mechanism of action and clinical potential of fingolimod for the treatment of stroke. *Front. Neurol.* 7, 139. doi: 10.3389/fneur.2016.00139

Liesz, A., and Kleinschnitz, C. (2016). Regulatory T cells in post-stroke immune homeostasis. *Transl. Stroke Res.* 7 (4), 313–321. doi: 10.1007/s12975-016-0465-7

Liesz, A., Suri-Payer, E., Veltkamp, C., Doerr, H., Sommer, C., Rivest, S., et al. (2009). Regulatory T cells are key cerebroprotective immunomodulators in acute experimental stroke. *Nat. Med.* 15 (2), 192–199. doi: 10.1038/nm.1927

Liesz, A., Zhou, W., Mracskó, É., Karcher, S., Bauer, H., Schwarting, S., et al. (2011). Inhibition of lymphocyte trafficking shields the brain against deleterious neuroinflammation after stroke. *Brain* 134 (Pt 3), 704–720. doi: 10.1093/brain/awr008

Ling, L., Zhang, S., Ji, Z., Huang, H., Yao, G., Wang, M., et al. (2016). Therapeutic effects of lipo-prostaglandin E1 on angiogenesis and neurogenesis after ischemic stroke in rats. *Int. J. Neurosci.* 126 (5), 469–477. doi: 10.3109/00207454.2015.1031226

Liu, J., Zhang, C., Tao, W., and Liu, M. (2013). Systematic review and meta-analysis of the efficacy of sphingosine-1-phosphate (S1P) receptor agonist FTY720 (fingolimod) in animal models of stroke. *Int. J. Neurosci.* 123 (3), 163–169. doi: 10.3109/00207454.2012.749255

Liu, Z., and Chopp, M. (2016). Astrocytes, therapeutic targets for neuroprotection and neurorestoration in ischemic stroke. *Prog. Neurobiol.* 144, 103–120. doi: 10.1016/j.pneurobio.2015.09.008

Liu, Z. J., Chen, C., Li, X. R., Ran, Y. Y., Xu, T., Zhang, Y., et al. (2016). Remote ischemic preconditioning-mediated neuroprotection against stroke is associated with significant alterations in peripheral immune responses. *CNS Neurosci. Ther.* 22 (1), 43–52. doi: 10.1111/cns.12448

Louveau, A., Harris, T. H., and Kipnis, J. (2015). Revisiting the mechanisms of CNS immune privilege. *Trends Immunol.* 36 (10), 569–577. doi: 10.1016/j.it.2015.08.006

Lucivero, V., Prontera, M., Mezzapesa, D. M., Petruzzellis, M., Sancilio, M., Tinelli, A., et al. (2007). Different roles of matrix metalloproteinases-2 and -9 after human ischaemic stroke. *Neurol. Sci.* 28 (4), 165–170. doi: 10.1007/s10072-007-0814-0

Malone, K., Amu, S., Moore, A. C., and Waeber, C. (2018). The immune system and stroke: from current targets to future therapy. *Immunol. Cell Biol.* 97, 5–16. doi: 10.1111/imcb.12191

Marsh, B. J., Williams-Karnesky, R. L., and Stenzel-Poore, M. P. (2009). Toll-like receptor signaling in endogenous neuroprotection and stroke. *Neuroscience* 158 (3), 1007–1020. doi: 10.1016/j.neuroscience.2008.07.067

Mays, R., and Deans, R. (2016). Adult adherent cell therapy for ischemic stroke: clinical results and development experience using MultiStem. *Transfusion* 56 (4), 6S–8S. doi: 10.1111/trf.13562

McCann, S. K., Cramond, F., Macleod, M. R., and Sena, E. S. (2016). Systematic review and meta-analysis of the efficacy of interleukin-1 receptor antagonist in animal models of stroke: an update. *Transl. Stroke Res.* 7 (5), 395–406. doi: 10.1007/s12975-016-0489-z

McDonald, B., Pittman, K., Menezes, G. B., Hirota, S. A., Slaba, I., Waterhouse, C. C., et al. (2010). Intravascular danger signals guide neutrophils to sites of sterile inflammation. *Science* 330 (6002), 362–366. doi: 10.1126/science.1195491

McDonough, A., and Weinstein, J. R. (2016). Neuroimmune response in ischemic preconditioning. *Neurotherapeutics* 13 (4), 748–761. doi: 10.1007/s13311-016-0465-z

Merali, Z., Huang, K., Mikulis, D., Silver, F., and Kassner, A. (2017). Evolution of blood–brain-barrier permeability after acute ischemic stroke. *PLoS One* 12 (2), 1–11. doi: 10.1371/journal.pone.0171558

Minnerup, J., Wersching, H., Brokinkel, B., Dziewas, R., Heuschmann, P. U., Nabavi, D. G., et al. (2010). The impact of lesion location and lesion size on poststroke infection frequency. *J. Neurol. Neurosurg. Psychiatry* 81 (2), 198–202. doi: 10.1136/jnnp.2009.182394

Mirabelli-Badenier, M., Braunersreuther, V., Viviani, G. L., Dallegri, F., Quercioli, A., Veneselli, E., et al. (2011). CC and CXC chemokines are pivotal mediators of cerebral injury in ischaemic stroke. *Thromb. Haemost.* 105 (3), 409–420. doi: 10.1160/TH10-10-0662

Mocco, J., Choudhri, T., Huang, J., Harfeldt, E., Efros, L., Klingbeil, C., et al. (2002). HuEP5C7 as a humanized monoclonal anti-E/P-selectin neurovascular protective strategy in a blinded placebo-controlled trial of nonhuman primate stroke. *Circ. Res.* 91 (10), 907–914. doi: 10.1161/01.RES.0000042063.15901.20

Mocco, J., Mack, W. J., Ducruet, A. F., King, R. G., Sughrue, M. E., Coon, A. L., et al. (2006a). Preclinical evaluation of the neuroprotective effect of soluble complement receptor type 1 in a nonhuman primate model of reperfused stroke. *J. Neurosurg.* 105 (4), 595–601. doi: 10.3171/jns.2006.105.4.595

Mocco, J., Mack, W. J., Ducruet, A. F., Sosunov, S. A., Sughrue, M. E., Hassid, B. G., et al. (2006b). Complement component C3 mediates inflammatory injury following focal cerebral ischemia. *Circ. Res.* 99 (2), 209–217. doi: 10.1161/01.RES.0000232544.90675.42

Monson, N. L., Ortega, S. B., Ireland, S. J., Meeuwissen, A. J., Chen, D., Plautz, E. J., et al. (2014). Repetitive hypoxic preconditioning induces an immunosuppressed B cell phenotype during endogenous protection from stroke. *J. Neuroinflammation* 11, 22. doi: 10.1186/1742-2094-11-22

Montaner, J., Alvarez-Sabín, J., Molina, C. A., Anglés, A., Abilleira, S., Arenillas, J., et al. (2001). Matrix metalloproteinase expression is related to hemorrhagic transformation after cardioembolic stroke. *Stroke* 32 (12), 2762–2767. doi: 10.1161/hs1201.99512

Mracsko, E., Liesz, A., Karcher, S., Zorn, M., Bari, F., and Veltkamp, R. (2014). Differential effects of sympathetic nervous system and hypothalamic–pituitary–adrenal axis on systemic immune cells after severe experimental stroke. *Brain Behav. Immun.* 41, 200–209. doi: 10.1016/j.bbi.2014.05.015

Mulcahy, N. J., Ross, J., Rothwell, N. J., and Loddick, S. A. (2003). Delayed administration of interleukin-1 receptor antagonist protects against transient cerebral ischaemia in the rat. *Br. J. Pharmacol.* 140 (3), 471–476. doi: 10.1038/sj.bjp.0705462

Muralikrishna Adibhatla, R., and Hatcher, J. F. (2006). Phospholipase A2, reactive oxygen species, and lipid peroxidation in cerebral ischemia. *Free Radic. Biol. Med.* 40 (3), 376–387. doi: 10.1016/j.freeradbiomed.2005.08.044

Murata, Y., Rosell, A., Scannevin, R. H., Rhodes, K. J., Wang, X., and Lo, E. H. (2008). Extension of the thrombolytic time window with minocycline in experimental stroke. *Stroke* 39 (12), 3372–3377. doi: 10.1161/STROKEAHA.108.514026

Murry, C. E., Jennings, R. B., and Reimer, K. A. (1986). Preconditioning with ischemia—a delay of lethal cell injury in ischemic myocardium. *Circulation* 74 (5), 1124–1136. doi: 10.1161/01.CIR.74.5.1124

Nakamura, Y., Sugita, Y., Nakashima, S., Okada, Y., Yoshitomi, M., Kimura, Y., et al. (2016). Alternatively activated macrophages play an important role in vascular remodeling and hemorrhaging in patients with brain arteriovenous malformation. *J. Stroke Cerebrovasc. Dis.* 25 (3), 600–609. doi: 10.1016/j.jstrokecerebrovasdis.2015.11.034

Neuhaus, A. A., Couch, Y., Hadley, G., and Buchan, A. M. (2017). Neuroprotection in stroke: the importance of collaboration and reproducibility. *Brain* 140 (8), 2079–2092. doi: 10.1093/brain/awx126

Ning, M., Furie, K. L., Koroshetz, W. J., Lee, H., Barron, M., Lederer, M., et al. (2006). Association between tPA therapy and raised early matrix metalloproteinase-9 in acute stroke. *Neurology* 66 (10), 1550–1555. doi: 10.1212/01.wnl.0000216133.98416.b4

O'Collins, V. E., Macleod, M. R., Donnan, G. A., Horky, L. L., van der Worp, B. H., and Howells, D. W. (2006). 1,026 experimental treatments in acute stroke. *Ann. Neurol.* 59 (3), 467–477. doi: 10.1002/ana.20741

Osanai, T., Houkin, K., Uchiyama, S., Minematsu, K., Taguchi, A., and Terasaka, S. (2018). Treatment evaluation of acute stroke for using in regenerative cell elements (TREASURE) trial: rationale and design. *Int. J. Stroke* 13 (4), 444–448. doi: 10.1177/1747493017743057

Osthoff, M., Katan, M., Fluri, F., Schuetz, P., Bingisser, R., Kappos, L., et al. (2011). Mannose-binding lectin deficiency is associated with smaller infarction size and favorable outcome in ischemic stroke patients. *PLoS One* 6 (6), e21338. doi: 10.1371/journal.pone.0021338

Padma Srivastava, M. V., Bhasin, A., Bhatia, R., Garg, A., Gaikwad, S., Prasad, K., et al. (2012). Efficacy of minocycline in acute ischemic stroke: a single-blinded, placebo-controlled trial. *Neurol. India* 60 (1), 23–28. doi: 10.4103/0028-3886.93584

Park, E. M., Cho, S., Frys, K. A., Glickstein, S. B., Zhou, P., Anrather, J., et al. (2006). Inducible nitric oxide synthase contributes to gender differences in ischemic brain injury. *J. Cereb. Blood Flow Metab.* 26 (3), 392–401. doi: 10.1038/sj.jcbfm.9600194

Paterno, R., and Chillon, J. M. (2018). Potentially common therapeutic targets for multiple sclerosis and ischemic stroke. *Front. Physiol.* 9, 855. doi: 10.3389/fphys.2018.00855

Perez-de-Puig, I., Miro-Mur, F., Ferrer-Ferrer, M., Gelpi, E., Pedragosa, J., Justicia, C., et al. (2015). Neutrophil recruitment to the brain in mouse and human ischemic stroke. *Acta Neuropathol.* 129 (2), 239–257. doi: 10.1007/s00401-014-1381-0

Petrovic-Djergovic, D., Goonewardena, S. N., and Pinsky, D. J. (2016). Inflammatory disequilibrium in stroke. *Circ. Res.* 119 (1), 142–158. doi: 10.1161/CIRCRESAHA.116.308022

Planas, A. M., Gomez-Choco, M., Urra, X., Gorina, R., Caballero, M., and Chamorro, A. (2012). Brain-derived antigens in lymphoid tissue of patients with acute stroke. *J. Immunol.* 188 (5), 2156–2163. doi: 10.4049/jimmunol.1102289

Pradillo, J. M., Romera, C., Hurtado, O., Cárdenas, A., Moro, M. A., Leza, J. C., et al. (2005). TNFR1 upregulation mediates tolerance after brain ischemic preconditioning. *J. Cereb. Blood Flow Metab.* 25 (2), 193–203. doi: 10.1038/sj.jcbfm.9600019

Prass, K., Meisel, C., Höflich, C., Braun, J., Halle, E., Wolf, T., et al. (2003). Stroke-induced immunodeficiency promotes spontaneous bacterial infections and is mediated by sympathetic activation reversal by poststroke T helper cell type 1-like immunostimulation. *J. Exp. Med.* 198 (5), 725–736. doi: 10.1084/jem.20021098

Prestigiacomo, C. J., Kim, S. C., Connolly, E. S., Liao, H., Yan, S. F., andPinsky, D. J. (1999). CD18-mediated neutrophil recruitment contributes to the pathogenesis of reperfused but not nonreperfused stroke. *Stroke* 30 (5), 1110–1117. doi: 10.1161/01.STR.30.5.1110

Rao, A. M., Hatcher, J. F., Kindy, M. S., and Dempsey, R. J. (1999). Arachidonic acid and leukotriene C4: role in transient cerebral ischemia of gerbils. *Neurochem. Res.* 24 (10), 1225–1232. doi: 10.1023/A:1020916905312

Ren, X., Akiyoshi, K., Dziennis, S., Vandenbark, A. A., Herson, P. S., Hurn, P. D., et al. (2011). Regulatory B cells limit CNS inflammation and neurologic deficits in murine experimental stroke. *J. Neurosci.* 31 (23), 8556–8563. doi: 10.1523/JNEUROSCI.1623-11.2011

Robinson, T. (2018). Reperfusion in the brain: is time important? The DAWN and DEFUSE-3 trials. *Cardiovasc. Res.* 114 (5), e28–e29. doi: 10.1093/cvr/cvy053

Rosas-Ballina, M., Olofsson, P. S., Ochani, M., Valdés-Ferrer, S. I., Levine, Y. A., Reardon, C., et al. (2011). Acetylcholine-synthesizing T cells relay neural signals in a vagus nerve circuit. *Science* 334 (6052), 98–101. doi: 10.1126/science.1209985

Rosell, A., and Lo, E. H. (2008). Multiphasic roles for matrix metalloproteinases after stroke. *Curr. Opin. Pharmacol.* 8 (1), 82–89. doi: 10.1016/j.coph.2007.12.001

Rosenberg, G. A. (2012). Neurological diseases in relation to the blood–brain barrier. *J. Cereb. Blood Flow Metab.* 32 (7), 1139–1151. doi: 10.1038/jcbfm.2011.197

Rosenzwajg, M., Lorenzon, R., Cacoub, P., Pham, H. P., Pitoiset, F., El Soufi, K., et al. (2018). Immunological and clinical effects of low-dose interleukin-2 across 11 autoimmune diseases in a single, open clinical trial. *Ann. Rheum. Dis.* 0, 1–9. doi: 10.1136/annrheumdis-2018-214229

Roy-O'Reilly, M., and McCullough, L. D. (2017). Astrocytes fuel the fire of lymphocyte toxicity after stroke. *Proc. Natl. Acad. Sci. U. S. A.* 114 (3), 425–427. doi: 10.1073/pnas.1619813114

Römer, C., Engel, O., Winek, K., Hochmeister, S., Zhang, T., Royl, G., et al. (2015). Blocking stroke-induced immunodeficiency increases CNS antigen-specific autoreactivity but does not worsen functional outcome after experimental stroke. *J. Neurosci.* 35 (20), 7777–7794. doi: 10.1523/JNEUROSCI.1532-14.2015

Saad, M. A., Abdelsalam, R. M., Kenawy, S. A., and Attia, A. S. (2015). Montelukast, a cysteinyl leukotriene receptor-1 antagonist protects against hippocampal injury induced by transient global cerebral ischemia and reperfusion in rats. *Neurochem. Res.* 40 (1), 139–150. doi: 10.1007/s11064-014-1478-9

Schmidt, M. R., Smerup, M., Konstantinov, I. E., Shimizu, M., Li, J., Cheung, M., et al. (2007). Intermittent peripheral tissue ischemia during coronary ischemia reduces myocardial infarction through a KATP-dependent mechanism: first demonstration of remote ischemic perconditioning. *Am. J. Physiol. Heart Circ. Physiol.* 292 (4), H1883–1890. doi: 10.1152/ajpheart.00617.2006

Schroeter, M., Jander, S., Witte, O. W., and Stoll, G. (1994). Local immune-responses in the rat cerebral-cortex after middle cerebral-artery occlusion. *J. Neuroimmunol.* 55 (2), 195–203. doi: 10.1016/0165-5728(94)90010-8

Schulte-Herbrüggen, O., Quarcoo, D., Meisel, A., and Meisel, C. (2009). Differential affection of intestinal immune cell populations after cerebral ischemia in mice. *Neuroimmunomodulation* 16 (3), 213–218. doi: 10.1159/000205514

Selvaraj, U. M., Ortega, S. B., Hu, R., Gilchrist, R., Kong, X., Plautz, E. J., et al. (2017). Preconditioning-induced CXCL12 upregulation minimizes leukocyte infiltration after stroke in ischemia-tolerant mice. *J. Cereb. Blood Flow Metab.* 37 (3), 801–813. doi: 10.1177/0271678X16639327

Selvaraj, U. M., Poinsatte, K., Torres, V., Ortega, S. B., and Stowe, A. M. (2016). Heterogeneity of B cell functions in stroke-related risk, prevention, injury, and repair. *Neurotherapeutics* 13 (4), 729–747. doi: 10.1007/s13311-016-0460-4

Serlin, Y., Shelef, I., Knyazer, B., and Friedman, A. (2015). Anatomy and physiology of the blood–brain barrier. *Semin. Cell Dev. Biol.* 38, 2–6. doi: 10.1016/j.semcdb.2015.01.002

Shi, K., Wood, K., Shi, F. D., Wang, X., and Liu, Q. (2018). Stroke-induced immunosuppression and poststroke infection. *Stroke Vasc. Neurol.* 3 (1), 34–41. doi: 10.1136/svn-2017-000123

Shimizu, M., Saxena, P., Konstantinov, I. E., Cherepanov, V., Cheung, M. M., Wearden, P., et al. (2010). Remote ischemic preconditioning decreases adhesion and selectively modifies functional responses of human neutrophils. *J. Surg. Res.* 158 (1), 155–161. doi: 10.1016/j.jss.2008.08.010

Singh, V., Roth, S., Llovera, G., Sadler, R., Garzetti, D., Stecher, B., et al. (2016). Microbiota dysbiosis controls the neuroinflammatory response after stroke. *J. Neurosci.* 36 (28), 7428–7440. doi: 10.1523/JNEUROSCI.1114-16.2016

Smith, C. J., Denes, A., Tyrrell, P. J., and Di Napoli, M. (2015). Phase II anti-inflammatory and immune-modulating drugs for acute ischaemic stroke. *Expert Opin. Investig. Drugs* 24 (5), 623–643. doi: 10.1517/13543784.2015.1020110

Smith, C. J., Hulme, S., Vail, A., Heal, C., Parry-Jones, A. R., Scarth, S., et al. (2018). SCIL-STROKE (Subcutaneous Interleukin-1 Receptor Antagonist in Ischemic Stroke): a randomized controlled phase 2 trial. *Stroke* 49 (5), 1210–1216. doi: 10.1161/STROKEAHA.118.020750

Sobowale, O. A., Parry-Jones, A. R., Smith, C. J., Tyrrell, P. J., Rothwell, N. J., and Allan, S. M. (2016). Interleukin-1 in stroke: from bench to bedside. *Stroke* 47 (8), 2160–2167. doi: 10.1161/STROKEAHA.115.010001

Soriano, S. G., Amaravadi, L. S., Wang, Y. F., Zhou, H., Yu, G. X., Tonra, J. R., et al. (2002). Mice deficient in fractalkine are less susceptible to cerebral ischemia-reperfusion injury. *J. Neuroimmunol.* 125 (1–2), 59–65. doi: 10.1016/S0165-5728(02)00033-4

Soriano, S. G., Coxon, A., Wang, Y. F., Frosch, M. P., Lipton, S. A., Hickey, P. R., et al. (1999). Mice deficient in Mac-1 (CD11b/CD18) are less susceptible to cerebral ischemia/reperfusion injury. *Stroke* 30 (1), 134–139. doi: 10.1161/01.STR.30.1.134

Spychala, M. S., Venna, V. R., Jandzinski, M., Doran, S. J., Durgan, D. J., Ganesh, B. P., et al. (2018). Age-related changes in the gut microbiota influence systemic inflammation and stroke outcome. *Ann. Neurol.* 84 (1), 23–36. doi: 10.1002/ana.25250

Sriram, K., and O'Callaghan, J. P. (2007). Divergent roles for tumor necrosis factor-alpha in the brain. *J. Neuroimmune Pharmacol.* 2 (2), 140–153. doi: 10.1007/s11481-007-9070-6

Stanimirovic, D. B., Wong, J., Shapiro, A., and Durkin, J. P. (1997). Increase in surface expression of ICAM-1, VCAM-1 and E-selectin in human cerebromicrovascular endothelial cells subjected to ischemia-like insults. *Acta Neurochir. Suppl.* 70, 12–16. doi: 10.1007/978-3-7091-6837-0_4

Stanley, D., Mason, L. J., Mackin, K. E., Srikhanta, Y. N., Lyras, D., Prakash, M. D., et al. (2016). Translocation and dissemination of commensal bacteria in post-stroke infection. *Nat. Med.* 22 (11), 1277–1284. doi: 10.1038/nm.4194

Stowe, A. M., Wacker, B. K., Cravens, P. D., Perfater, J. L., Li, M. K., Hu, R., et al. (2012). CCL2 upregulation triggers hypoxic preconditioning-induced protection from stroke. *J. Neuroinflammation* 9, 33. doi: 10.1186/1742-2094-9-33

Sugimoto, K., and Iadecola, C. (2003). Delayed effect of administration of COX-2 inhibitor in mice with acute cerebral ischemia. *Brain Res.* 960 (1–2), 273–276. doi: 10.1016/S0006-8993(02)03805-2

Supanc, V., Biloglav, Z., Kes, V. B., and Demarin, V. (2011). Role of cell adhesion molecules in acute ischemic stroke. *Ann. Saudi Med.* 31 (4), 365–370. doi: 10.4103/0256-4947.83217

Sykora, M., Siarnik, P., Diedler, J., and Collaborators, V. A. (2015). β-Blockers, pneumonia, and outcome after ischemic stroke: evidence from Virtual International Stroke Trials Archive. *Stroke* 46 (5), 1269–1274. doi: 10.1161/STROKEAHA.114.008260

Takami, S., Minami, M., Katayama, T., Nagata, I., Namura, S., and Satoh, M. (2002). TAK-779, a nonpeptide CC chemokine receptor antagonist, protects the brain against focal cerebral ischemia in mice. *J. Cereb. Blood Flow Metab.* 22 (7), 780–784. doi: 10.1097/00004647-200207000-00003

Takami, S., Minami, M., Nagata, I., Namura, S., and Satoh, M. (2001). Chemokine receptor antagonist peptide, viral MIP-II, protects the brain against focal cerebral ischemia in mice. *J. Cereb. Blood Flow Metab.* 21 (12), 1430–1435. doi: 10.1097/00004647-200112000-00007

Tedder, T. F. (2015). Introduction: regulatory B cell special issue—making all the pieces fit. *Int. Immunol.* 27 (10), 467–470. doi: 10.1093/intimm/dxv047

Terao, S., Yilmaz, G., Stokes, K. Y., Russell, J., Ishikawa, M., Kawase, T., et al. (2008). Blood cell-derived RANTES mediates cerebral microvascular dysfunction, inflammation, and tissue injury after focal ischemia-reperfusion. *Stroke* 39 (9), 2560–2570. doi: 10.1161/STROKEAHA.107.513150

Terao, Y., Ohta, H., Oda, A., Nakagaito, Y., Kiyota, Y., and Shintani, Y. (2009). Macrophage inflammatory protein-3alpha plays a key role in the inflammatory cascade in rat focal cerebral ischemia. *Neurosci. Res.* 64 (1), 75–82. doi: 10.1016/j.neures.2009.01.017

Tobinick, E., Rodriguez-Romanacce, H., Levine, A., Ignatowski, T. A., and Spengler, R. N. (2014). Immediate neurological recovery following perispinal etanercept years after brain injury. *Clin. Drug Investig.* 34 (5), 361–366. doi: 10.1007/s40261-014-0186-1

Trakhtenberg, E. F., and Goldberg, J. L. (2011). Immunology. Neuroimmune communication. *Science* 334 (6052), 47–48. doi: 10.1126/science.1213099

van Zwam, M., Huizinga, R., Melief, M. J., Wierenga-Wolf, A., van Meurs, M., Voerman, J. S., et al. (2009). Brain antigens in functionally distinct antigen-presenting cell populations in cervical lymph nodes in MS and EAE. *J. Mol. Med.* 87 (3), 273–286. doi: 10.1007/s00109-008-0421-4

Vemuganti, R., Dempsey, R. J., and Bowen, K. K. (2004). Inhibition of intercellular adhesion molecule-1 protein expression by antisense oligonucleotides is neuroprotective after transient middle cerebral artery occlusion in rat. *Stroke* 35 (1), 179–184. doi: 10.1161/01.STR.0000106479.53235.3E

Venkataramana, S., Lourenssen, S., Miller, K. G., and Blennerhassett, M. G. (2015). Early inflammatory damage to intestinal neurons occurs *via* inducible nitric oxide synthase. *Neurobiol. Dis.* 75, 40–52. doi: 10.1016/j.nbd.2014.12.014

Vermeij, J. D., Westendorp, W. F., Dippel, D. W., van de Beek, D., and Nederkoorn, P. J. (2018). Antibiotic therapy for preventing infections in people with acute stroke. *Cochrane Database Syst. Rev.* 1, CD008530. doi: 10.1002/14651858.CD008530.pub3

Walsh, S. R., Nouraei, S. A., Tang, T. Y., Sadat, U., Carpenter, R. H., and Gaunt, M. E. (2010). Remote ischemic preconditioning for cerebral and cardiac protection during carotid endarterectomy: results from a pilot randomized clinical trial. *Vasc. Endovascular Surg.* 44 (6), 434–439. doi: 10.1177/1538574410369709

Wan, Y. Y. (2010). Multi-tasking of helper T cells. *Immunology* 130 (2), 166–171. doi: 10.1111/j.1365-2567.2010.03289.x

Wang, L., Li, Y., Chen, J., Gautam, S. C., Zhang, Z., Lu, M., et al. (2002). Ischemic cerebral tissue and MCP-1 enhance rat bone marrow stromal cell migration in interface culture. *Exp. Hematol.* 30 (7), 831–836. doi: 10.1016/S0301-472X(02)00829-9

Wang, X., Xuan, W., Zhu, Z. Y., Li, Y., Zhu, H., Zhu, L., et al. (2018). The evolving role of neuro-immune interaction in brain repair after cerebral ischemic stroke. *CNS Neurosci. Ther.* 24 (12), 1100–1114. doi: 10.1111/cns.13077

Wang, Y. X., You, Q., Su, W. L., Li, Q., Hu, Z. Q., Wang, Z. G., et al. (2013). A study on inhibition of inflammation *via* p75TNFR signaling pathway activation in mice with traumatic brain injury. *J. Surg. Res.* 182 (1), 127–133. doi: 10.1016/j.jss.2012.07.071

Wattananit, S., Tornero, D., Graubardt, N., Memanishvili, T., Monni, E., Tatarishvili, J., et al. (2016). Monocyte-derived macrophages contribute to spontaneous long-term functional recovery after stroke in mice. *J. Neurosci.* 36 (15), 4182–4195. doi: 10.1523/JNEUROSCI.4317-15.2016

Wei, D., Ren, C., Chen, X., and Zhao, H. (2012). The chronic protective effects of limb remote preconditioning and the underlying mechanisms involved in inflammatory factors in rat stroke. *PLoS One* 7 (2), e30892. doi: 10.1371/journal.pone.0030892

Wei, Y., Yemisci, M., Kim, H. H., Yung, L. M., Shin, H. K., Hwang, S. K., et al. (2011). Fingolimod provides long-term protection in rodent models of cerebral ischemia. *Ann. Neurol.* 69 (1), 119–129. doi: 10.1002/ana.22186

Weih, M., Kallenberg, K., Bergk, A., Dirnagl, U., Harms, L., Wernecke, K. D., et al. (1999). Attenuated stroke severity after prodromal TIA: a role for ischemic tolerance in the brain? *Stroke* 30 (9), 1851–1854. doi: 10.1161/01.STR.30.9.1851

Wekerle, H. (2017). Brain autoimmunity and intestinal microbiota: 100 trillion game changers. *Trends Immunol.* 38 (7), 483–497. doi: 10.1016/j.it.2017.03.008

Westendorp, W. F., Nederkoorn, P. J., Vermeij, J. D., Dijkgraaf, M. G., and van de Beek, D. (2011). Post-stroke infection: a systematic review and meta-analysis. *BMC Neurol.* 11, 110. doi: 10.1186/1471-2377-11-110

Westendorp, W. F., Vermeij, J. D., Brouwer, M. C., Roos, Y. B., Nederkoorn, P. J., van de Beek, D., et al. (2016). Pre-stroke use of beta-blockers does not lower post-stroke infection rate: an exploratory analysis of the preventive antibiotics in stroke study. *Cerebrovasc. Dis.* 42 (5–6), 506–511. doi: 10.1159/000450926

Willenborg, S., Lucas, T., van Loo, G., Knipper, J. A., Krieg, T., Haase, I., et al. (2012). CCR2 recruits an inflammatory macrophage subpopulation critical for angiogenesis in tissue repair. *Blood* 120 (3), 613–625. doi: 10.1182/blood-2012-01-403386

Wilson, E. H., Weninger, W., and Hunter, C. A. (2010). Trafficking of immune cells in the central nervous system. *J. Clin. Invest.* 120 (5), 1368–1379. doi: 10.1172/JCI41911

Winek, K., Engel, O., Koduah, P., Heimesaat, M. M., Fischer, A., Bereswill, S., et al. (2016a). Depletion of cultivatable gut microbiota by broad-spectrum antibiotic pretreatment worsens outcome after murine stroke. *Stroke* 47 (5), 1354–1363. doi: 10.1161/STROKEAHA.115.011800

Winek, K., Meisel, A., and Dirnagl, U. (2016b). Gut microbiota impact on stroke outcome: fad or fact? *J. Cereb. Blood Flow Metab.* 36 (5), 891–898. doi: 10.1177/0271678X16636890

Wong, C. H., Jenne, C. N., Lee, W. Y., Léger, C., and Kubes, P. (2011). Functional innervation of hepatic iNKT cells is immunosuppressive following stroke. *Science* 334 (6052), 101–105. doi: 10.1126/science.1210301

Xu, X., and Jiang, Y. (2014). The yin and yang of innate immunity in stroke. *Biomed. Res. Int.* 2014, 807978. doi: 10.1155/2014/807978

Yagami, T., Koma, H., and Yamamoto, Y. (2016). Pathophysiological roles of cyclooxygenases and prostaglandins in the central nervous system. *Mol. Neurobiol.* 53 (7), 4754–4771. doi: 10.1007/s12035-015-9355-3

Yang, G. Y., Zhao, Y. J., Davidson, B. L., and Betz, A. L. (1997). Overexpression of interleukin-1 receptor antagonist in the mouse brain reduces ischemic brain injury. *Brain Res.* 751 (2), 181–188. doi: 10.1016/S0006-8993(96)01277-2

Yang, M., Rui, K., Wang, S., and Lu, L. (2013). Regulatory B cells in autoimmune diseases. *Cell Mol. Immunol.* 10 (2), 122–132. doi: 10.1038/cmi.2012.60

Yang, Y., Estrada, E. Y., Thompson, J. F., Liu, W., and Rosenberg, G. A. (2007). Matrix metalloproteinase-mediated disruption of tight junction proteins in cerebral vessels is reversed by synthetic matrix metalloproteinase inhibitor in focal ischemia in rat. *J. Cereb. Blood Flow Metab.* 27 (4), 697–709. doi: 10.1038/sj.jcbfm.9600375

Yenari, M. A., Kunis, D., Sun, G. H., Onley, D., Watson, L., Turner, S., et al. (1998). Hu23F2G, an antibody recognizing the leukocyte CD11/CD18 integrin, reduces injury in a rabbit model of transient focal cerebral ischemia. *Exp. Neurol.* 153 (2), 223–233. doi: 10.1006/exnr.1998.6876

Yenari, M. A., Sun, G. H., Kunis, D. M., Onley, D., and Vexler, V. (2001). L-selectin inhibition does not reduce injury in a rabbit model of transient focal cerebral ischemia. *Neurol. Res.* 23 (1), 72–78. doi: 10.1179/016164101101198154

Yeste, A., Takenaka, M. C., Mascanfroni, I. D., Nadeau, M., Kenison, J. E., Patel, B., et al. (2016). Tolerogenic nanoparticles inhibit T cell-mediated autoimmunity through SOCS2. *Sci. Signal* 9 (433), ra61. doi: 10.1126/scisignal.aad0612

Yilmaz, G., Arumugam, T. V., Stokes, K. Y., and Granger, D. N. (2006). Role of T lymphocytes and interferon-gamma in ischemic stroke. *Circulation* 113 (17), 2105–2112. doi: 10.1161/CIRCULATIONAHA.105.593046

Yilmaz, G., and Granger, D. N. (2008). Cell adhesion molecules and ischemic stroke. *Neurol. Res.* 30 (8), 783–793. doi: 10.1179/174313208X341085

Zaremba, J., and Losy, J. (2001). Early TNF-alpha levels correlate with ischaemic stroke severity. *Acta Neurol. Scand.* 104 (5), 288–295. doi: 10.1034/j.1600-0404.2001.00053.x

Zeng, L., Wang, Y., Liu, J., Wang, L., Weng, S., Chen, K., et al. (2013). Pro-inflammatory cytokine network in peripheral inflammation response to cerebral ischemia. *Neurosci. Lett.* 548, 4–9. doi: 10.1016/j.neulet.2013.04.037

Zhang, H., Xia, Y., Ye, Q., Yu, F., Zhu, W., Li, P., et al. (2018). Expansion of regulatory T cells with IL-2/IL-2 antibody complex protects against transient ischemic stroke. *J. Neurosci.* 38 (47), 10168–10179. doi: 10.1523/JNEUROSCI.3411-17.2018

Zhang, L., Zhang, Z. G., Zhang, R. L., Lu, M., Krams, M., and Chopp, M. (2003). Effects of a selective CD11b/CD18 antagonist and recombinant human tissue plasminogen activator treatment alone and in combination in a rat embolic model of stroke. *Stroke* 34 (7), 1790–1795. doi: 10.1161/01.STR.0000077016.55891.2E

Zhang, L. H., and Wei, E. Q. (2003). Neuroprotective effect of ONO-1078, a leukotriene receptor antagonist, on transient global cerebral ischemia in rats. *Acta Pharmacol. Sin.* 24 (12), 1241–1247.

Zhang, R. L., Chopp, M., Jiang, N., Tang, W. X., Prostak, J., Manning, A. M., et al. (1995). Anti-intercellular adhesion molecule-1 antibody reduces ischemic cell damage after transient but not permanent middle cerebral artery occlusion in the Wistar rat. *Stroke* 26 (8), 1438–1442. discussion 1443. doi: 10.1161/01.STR.26.8.1438

Zhao, B. Q., Wang, S., Kim, H. Y., Storrie, H., Rosen, B. R., Mooney, D. J., et al. (2006). Role of matrix metalloproteinases in delayed cortical responses after stroke. *Nat. Med.* 12 (4), 441–445. doi: 10.1038/nm1387

Zhao, T. X., Kostapanos, M., Griffiths, C., Arbon, E. L., Hubsch, A., Kaloyirou, F., et al. (2018). Low-dose interleukin-2 in patients with stable ischaemic heart disease and acute coronary syndromes (LILACS): protocol and study rationale for a randomised, double-blind, placebo-controlled, phase I/II clinical trial. *BMJ Open* 8 (9), e022452. doi: 10.1136/bmjopen-2018-022452

Zhao, X., Haensel, C., Araki, E., Ross, M. E., and Iadecola, C. (2000). Gene-dosing effect and persistence of reduction in ischemic brain injury in mice lacking inducible nitric oxide synthase. *Brain Res.* 872 (1–2), 215–218. doi: 10.1016/S0006-8993(00)02459-8

Zhao, X. J., Larkin, T. M., Lauver, M. A., Ahmad, S., and Ducruet, A. F. (2017). Tissue plasminogen activator mediates deleterious complement cascade activation in stroke. *PLoS One* 12 (7), e0180822. doi: 10.1371/journal.pone.0180822

Zheng, F., Spreckelsen, N. V., Zhang, X., Stavrinou, P., Timmer, M., Dohmen, C., et al. (2017). Should preventive antibiotics be used in patients with acute stroke? A systematic review and meta-analysis of randomized controlled trials. *PLoS One* 12 (10), e0186607. doi: 10.1371/journal.pone.0186607

Zhu, Z., Fu, Y., Tian, D., Sun, N., Han, W., Chang, G., et al. (2015). Combination of the immune modulator fingolimod with alteplase in acute ischemic stroke: a pilot trial. *Circulation* 132 (12), 1104–1112. doi: 10.1161/CIRCULATIONAHA.115.016371

Zierath, D., Thullbery, M., Hadwin, J., Gee, J. M., Savos, A., Kalil, A., et al. (2010). CNS immune responses following experimental stroke. *Neurocrit. Care* 12 (2), 274–284. doi: 10.1007/s12028-009-9270-4

Zlokovic, B. V. (2006). Remodeling after stroke. *Nat. Med.* 12 (4), 390–391. doi: 10.1038/nm0406-390

Zouggari, Y., Ait-Oufella, H., Waeckel, L., Vilar, J., Loinard, C., Cochain, C., et al. (2009). Regulatory T cells modulate postischemic neovascularization. *Circulation* 120 (14), 1415–1425. doi: 10.1161/CIRCULATIONAHA.109.875583

9

Acid-Sensing Ion Channel 1a is Involved in N-Methyl D-Aspartate Receptor-Dependent Long-Term Depression in the Hippocampus

D. Mango[1] and R. Nisticò[1,2*]*

[1] *Laboratory of Neuropharmacology, European Brain Research Institute, Rita Levi-Montalcini Foundation, Rome, Italy,*
[2] *Department of Biology, School of Pharmacy, University of Rome Tor Vergata, Rome, Italy*

Correspondence:
D. Mango
d.mango@ebri.it;
dalilamango@gmail.com
R. Nisticò
r.nistico@ebri.it;
robert.nistico@gmail.com

Acid-sensing ion channels (ASICs), members of the degenerin/epithelial Na^+ channel superfamily, are largely expressed in the mammalian nervous system. ASIC1a is highly permeable to Ca^{2+} and are involved in many physiological processes, including synaptic plasticity, learning, and memory. To clarify the role of ASIC1a in synaptic transmission and plasticity, we investigated N-methyl D-aspartate (NMDA) receptor dependent long-term depression (LTD) in the CA1 region of the hippocampus. We found that: (1) ASIC1a mediates a component of ASIC1a excitatory postsynaptic currents (EPSCs); (2) ASIC1a plays a role in electrical LTD induced by LFS protocol both in P13-18 and P30-40 animals; (3) ASIC1a is involved in chemical LTD induced by brief bath application of NMDA both in P13-18 and P30-40 animals; and finally (4) a functional interaction between ASIC1a and NMDA receptors occurs during LTD. These findings suggest a new role for ASIC1a in specific forms of synaptic plasticity in the mouse hippocampus.

Keywords: ASIC, hippocampus, electrophysiology, LTD, NMDA receptors

INTRODUCTION

Acid-sensing ion channels (ASICs), members of the degenerin/epithelial Na^+ channel superfamily, are largely expressed in the mammalian nervous system (Waldmann et al., 1997a). ASIC1a is highly permeable to Ca^{2+} and localized in different brain regions with high synaptic density, including the hippocampus (Baron et al., 2002; Askwith et al., 2004; Weng et al., 2010; Sherwood et al., 2011). ASIC1a is present at excitatory postsynaptic sites, being activated under normal and pathological conditions (Wemmie et al., 2003, 2006; Zha et al., 2006). In the last years, a growing body of evidence has shown that acidosis, through the activation of ASICs, contributes to synaptic plasticity, i.e., long-term potentiation and dendritic structural plasticity in hippocampal neurons, as well as learning and memory (Wemmie et al., 2002; Xiong et al., 2004; Zha et al., 2006; Arias et al., 2008; Vergo et al., 2011; Du et al., 2014; Kreple et al., 2014; Buta et al., 2015; Mango et al., 2017).

Extracellular acidification occurs in the brain during many different physiological and pathological situations as elevated neural activity, increased metabolism, and neuronal injury. Several works suggested that the acidic pH of synaptic vesicles transiently influences local extracellular pH during neurotrasmitters release (Krishtal et al., 1987; Waldmann et al., 1997b). According with this idea, it has been demonstrated that transient acidification of extracellular pH occurs in synaptic transmission in cultured hippocampal neurons (Miesenböck et al., 1998) and also in hippocampal slices (Krishtal et al., 1987; Wemmie et al., 2003, 2006). In light of these evidences, it has been proposed that ASICs provide a target for protons released in neurotransmission and thus play a role in the physiology of synaptic function (Krishtal et al., 1987; Waldmann et al., 1997b; Du et al., 2014).

Several observations suggest that ASICs contribute to synaptic plasticity in different brain areas. Specifically ASICs facilitate activation of the N-methyl D-aspartate (NMDA) receptor during LTP induction, suggesting a functional interaction between these receptors in the regulation of hippocampal synaptic plasticity (Wemmie et al., 2002; Du et al., 2014; Buta et al., 2015; Liu et al., 2016). Also, the coupling between NMDA receptor and ASIC has been shown to exacerbate acidity-mediated neuronal death occurring during ischemia (Gao et al., 2005, 2015). More recently, our group has suggested a novel function of ASIC1a in the modulation of group I mGlu receptor-dependent synaptic plasticity and intrinsic excitability in the hippocampus (Mango et al., 2017). To shed some light on the role of ASIC1a in another form of synaptic plasticity, here we performed an electrophysiological analysis to explore ASIC1a involvement in excitatory synaptic transmission and in NMDA receptor-dependent LTD in young and adult mice.

MATERIALS AND METHODS

This study was carried out in accordance with the recommendations of international guidelines on the ethical use of animals from the European Communities Council Directive (2010/64/EU). The protocol was approved by the Ministero della Salute.

Slice Preparation

C57BL6/J mice (13–40 days old) were deeply anesthetized with isoflurane and killed by decapitation.

The brain was rapidly removed from the skull and parasagittal hippocampal slices (250 μm) containing the dorsal hippocampus were cut with a vibratome (VT 1200S, Leica) in cold (0°C) artificial cerebrospinal fluid (aCSF) containing (in mM): NaCl (124); KCl (3); $MgSO_4$ (1); $CaCl_2$ (2); NaH_2PO_4 (1.25); $NaHCO_3$ (26); glucose (10); saturated with 95% O_2, 5% CO_2 (pH 7.4), and left to recover for 1 h in ACSF at 33.5°C.

Electrophysiology

Individual slices were placed in a recording chamber, on the stage of an upright microscope (Nikon, Japan) and submerged in a continuously flowing (3 ml/min) solution at 28°C (±0.2°C). Individual neurons were visualized through a 40× water-immersion objective (Nikon, Japan) connected to infrared video microscopy (Hamamatsu, Japan). Borosilicate glass electrodes (3–7 MΩ), pulled with a PP 83 Narishige puller, were filled with a solution containing the following (in mM): CsCl (135), KCl (10), $CaCl_2$ (0.05), EGTA (0.1), Hepes (10), Na3-GTP (0.3), Mg-GTP (4.0), pH adjusted to 7.3 with CsOH or K-Gluconate (135); KCl (10); $MgCl_2$ (2); $CaCl_2$ (0.05); EGTA (0.1); HEPES (10); ATP (4); GTP (0.3), pH 7.3 with KOH as previously published (Mango et al., 2017).

Whole-cell voltage clamp (at −70 mV holding potential) recordings were carried out with a MultiClamp 700B amplifier (Axon Instruments, Foster City, CA), filtered at 1 kHz and digitized (10 kHz).

The excitatory postsynaptic currents (EPSCs) were elicited at 0.033 Hz (EPSCs were elicited by stimulation every 30 s and each plot represents the mean of two consecutive EPSCs) with a glass pipette filled with ACSF, placed in CA1 *stratum radiatum* to stimulate Shaffer collateral fibers and in continuous presence of picrotoxin in bath solution as previously published (Mango et al., 2016). For paired-pulse (PP) experiments, paired-pulse stimuli (50 ms inter-pulse interval) were elicited with stimulating electrode placed close to the recording neuron in the continuous presence of picrotoxin. Paired pulse ratio (PPR) was evaluated as ratio of second EPSC amplitude on first EPSC amplitude.

Low-frequency stimulation (LFS) was obtained by delivering 300 pulses (at 0.75 Hz) at −40 mV.

The ASIC1a inward current was elicited by a CSF buffered to pH 5.5 and pressure-applied (10 psi, 1 s) through a patch electrode connected to Pneumatic Pico-Injector. The puff electrode was positioned above the slice in close proximity to the recorded neuron, and the inward currents were elicited every 3 min.

Electrophysiological data are represented as mean values ± SEM. Statistical significance was evaluated by two-tailed Student's t-test on averaged mean values taken from the last 5 min of each experiment. Statistical significance was set at $p < 0.05$ (indicated in the figures by *).

Drugs

Amiloride; 6-cyano-7-nitroquinoxaline-2,3-dione (CNQX); D-2-amino-5-phosphonovaleric acid (D-AP5); isoflurane; picrotoxin; and N-methyl-d-aspartic acid (NMDA) were purchased from Sigma-Aldrich (Italy); and psalmotoxin-1 was purchased from Alomone Labs. All drugs were dissolved in water.

RESULTS

Acid-Sensing Ion Channel 1a-Mediated Currents in CA1 Pyramidal Neurons

In order to assess whether ASIC1 contributes to basal excitatory transmission, we recorded excitatory postsynaptic currents (EPSCs) elicited by stimulation of the Schaffer collaterals fibers in the presence of PcTx-1, a polypeptide from the venom of spider toxin, that specifically inhibits homomeric ASIC1a currents (Escoubas et al., 2000). Bath application of PcTx-1 (100 ng/ml) did not induce any significant change in EPSC amplitude ($p > 0.05$, $n = 12$; **Figure 1A**). Also PPR, which is used to investigate the probability of neurotransmitter release, was unaffected following bath application of PcTx-1 ($p > 0.05$, $n = 8$; **Figure 1B**), according to a postsynaptic localization of ASIC1a (Fioravante and Regehr, 2011). While protons activate an inward current in different brain areas (Du et al., 2014; Highstein et al., 2014; Kreple et al., 2014), we then investigated the impact of proton-activated current on

Abbreviations: aCSF, artificial cerebrospinal fluid; ASIC, acid sensing ion channel; EPSC, excitatory postsynaptic current; LFS, low-frequency stimulation; LTD, long-term depression; PcTx1, psalmotoxin-1.

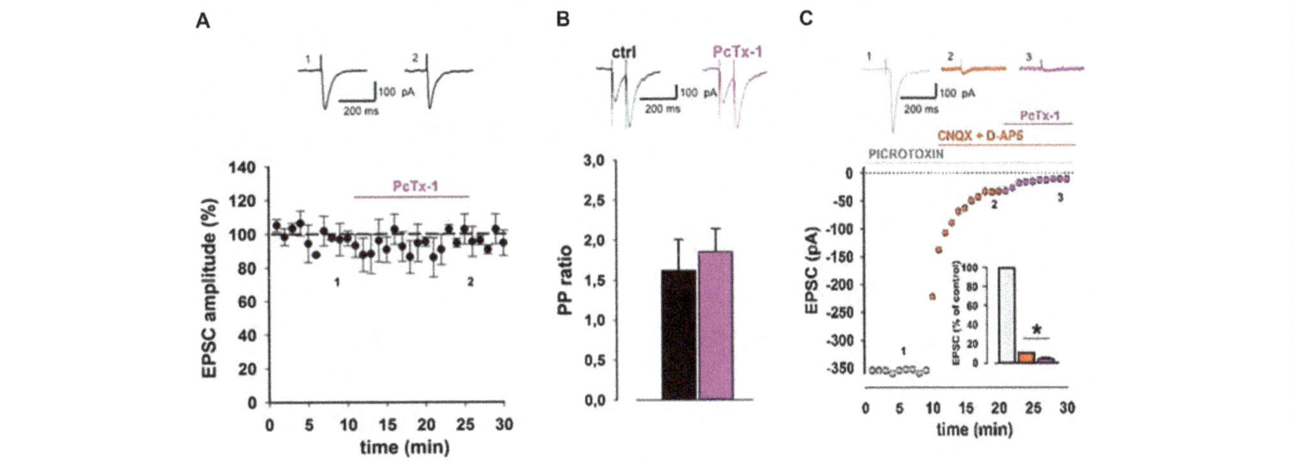

FIGURE 1 | ASIC1a contributes to excitatory synaptic transmission in hippocampal slices. **(A)** Normalized pooled data showing EPSCs in control condition and during PcTx-1 (100 ng/ml) bath application (mean ± SEM, $n = 12$, $p > 0.05$). EPSC was elicited by monopolar electrode placed on Schaffer collateral fibers. On top, representative EPSC traces were taken at the time indicated by number. **(B)** Bar chart illustrates normalized PPR (50 ms inter-pulse interval) in control condition and during PcTx-1 (100 ng/ml) bath application (mean ± SEM, $n = 8$, $p > 0.05$). On top, representative EPSC traces are shown. **(C)** Slices were perfused with picrotoxin ($GABA_A$ receptor antagonist, grey), plus CNQX (30 μM; AMPA receptor antagonist) and D-AP5 (50 μM; NMDA receptors antagonist, red), and subsequently with 100 ng/ml PcTx-1 (pink). Panel shows one representative experiment, bar chart in the inset illustrates the amplitude of EPSC (% of control) in the different conditions (mean ± SEM, $n = 6$, $^*p < 0.05$).

the EPSC in CA1 pyramidal neurons. Application of the ionotropic glutamate receptor antagonists CNQX and D-AP5 strongly reduced EPSC amplitude to 10.6 ± 3% of control ($p < 0.05$, $n = 6$; **Figure 1C**). In this condition, application of PcTx-1 (100 ng/ml) further reduced the current to 4 ± 2% of control ($p < 0.05$, $n = 6$; **Figure 1C**). The amplitude of the ASIC1a-mediated current is very small and this explains why the effect of PcTx-1 is masked in baseline excitatory neurotransmission.

Acid-Sensing Ion Channel 1a Contributes to Hippocampal N-Methyl D-Aspartate Receptor-Dependent Long-Term Depression in Young Mice

We next investigated the involvement of ASIC1a in a specific form of NMDA receptor-dependent synaptic plasticity. It is known that low-frequency stimulation protocol induces a stable long-term depression of synaptic transmission (Dudek and Bear, 1993; Nicolas et al., 2012). The induction of this form of LTD was completely inhibited by the NMDA receptor antagonist D-AP5 (50 μM) (data not shown).

We performed LTD experiments in young mice (P13-18) in the presence of PcTx-1 at different concentrations, applied 10 min before and during LFS protocol. PcTx-1 was able to reduce, in a dose-dependent manner, the magnitude of EPSC-LTD compared to control conditions (control: 32.2 ± 0.9% of baseline, $n = 12$; PcTx-1 30 ng/ml: 44.5 ± 0.9% of baseline, $n = 10$, $p < 0.001$; PcTx-1,100 ng/ml: 59.1 ± 1.3% of baseline, $n = 10$, $p < 0.001$, **Figure 2A**).

To further confirm that ASIC1a is involved in this form of synaptic plasticity, we also performed experiments using the nonselective ASIC blocker amiloride (100 μM). Even under this condition, LTD magnitude was significantly reduced compared to control condition (62.3 ± 1.8% of baseline, $n = 8$, $p < 0.001$, **Figure 2B**).

To distinguish whether ASIC1a plays a role in the induction or rather in the maintenance phase of LTD, we bath applied PcTx-1 10 min after the induction of LTD. Notably, in this condition PcTx-1 did not affect LTD magnitude (44.2 ± 0.8% of baseline, $n = 6$, $p > 0.05$, **Figure 2C**).

Acid-Sensing Ion Channel 1a Contributes to Hippocampal N-Methyl D-Aspartate Receptor-Dependent Long-Term Depression in Adult Mice

Long-term depression is strongly affected by the developmental stages of the brain (Kemp and Bashir, 1997; Kemp et al., 2000). Thus, we extended our electrophysiological analysis also in slices obtained from adult mice (P30-40). Similar to young mice, in adult mice also, LTD magnitude was reduced when PcTx-1 (100 ng/ml) was applied (control: 55.1 ± 1.2% of baseline, $n = 11$, $p < 0.001$, PcTx-1: 79.1 ± 1.5% of baseline, $n = 9$, $p < 0.001$, **Figure 3A**). A comparable effect was also obtained in the presence of amiloride (100 μM) (81 ± 1% of baseline, $n = 7$, $p < 0.001$ **Figure 3B**). Furthermore, we applied PcTx-1 after LTD induction and, as it occurred in young mice, no change was observed in LTD magnitude compared to control (49.7 ± 1.4% of baseline, $n = 8$, $p > 0.05$, **Figure 3C**).

PcTx-1 Inhibits Chemical N-Methyl D-Aspartate Receptor-Dependent Long-Term Depression

To further confirm the role of ASIC1a in NMDA receptor-dependent LTD, we performed experiments using a chemical

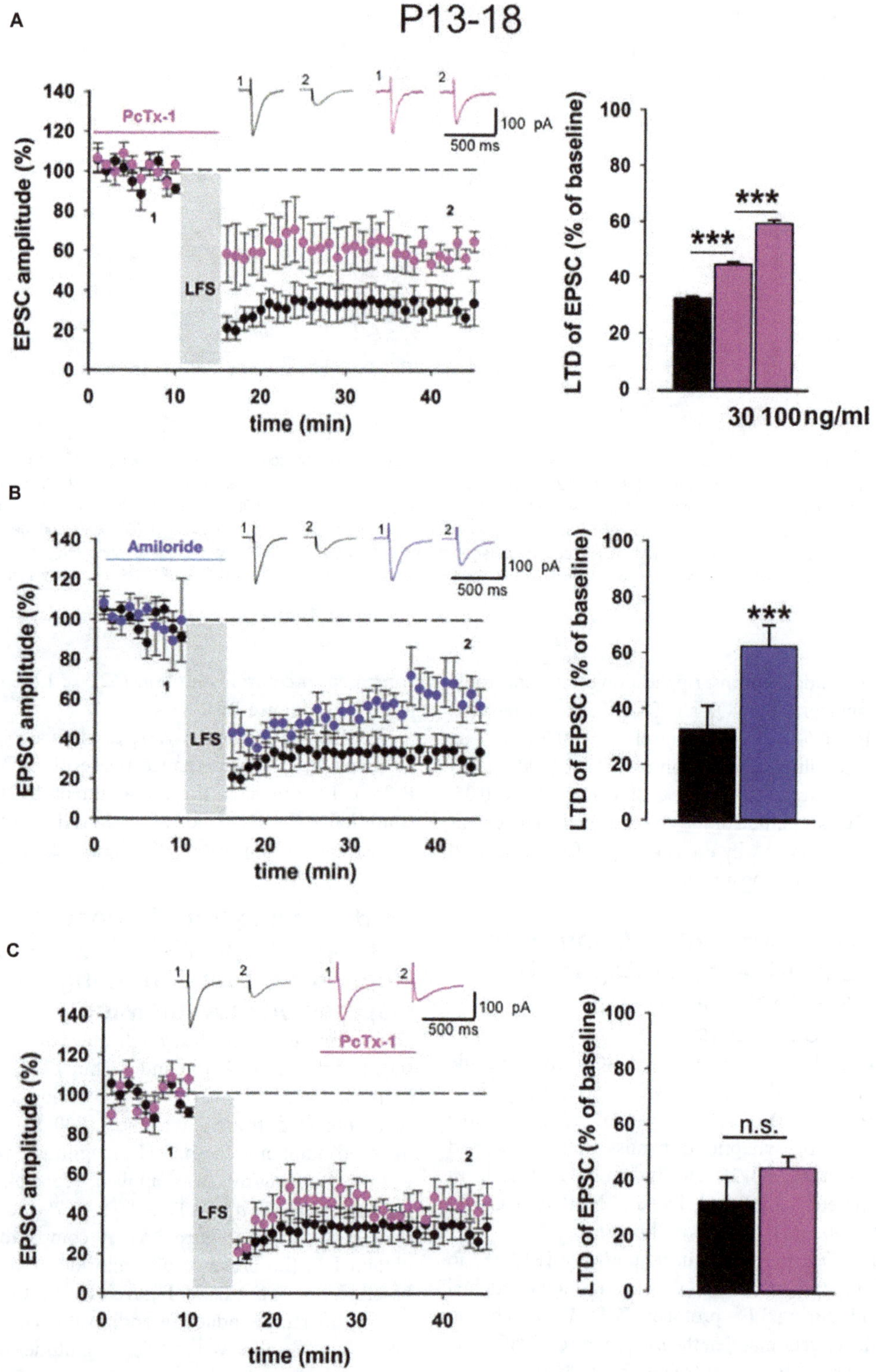

FIGURE 2 | ASIC1a modulates NMDA receptor-dependent LTD in young mice. **(A)** Normalized pooled data showing LTD in control condition (black) and in the presence of Pctx-1 applied before and during LFS (100 ng/ml, pink). Histogram represents the last 5 min of experiment in control ($n = 12$) condition or in the presence of PcTx-1 (30 ng/ml, mean ± SEM, $n = 10$, $^{***}p < 0.001$), (100 ng/ml, mean ± SEM, $n = 10$, $^{***}p < 0.001$). On top, representative traces are shown for each condition. **(B)** Normalized pooled data showing LTD in control condition (black) and in the presence of amiloride (100 μM, blue). Histogram represents the last 5 min of experiment in control condition ($n = 12$) or in presence of amiloride ($n = 8$) (mean ± SEM, $^{***}p < 0.001$). **(C)** Normalized pooled data showing LTD in control condition (black) and in the presence of PcTx-1 (100 ng/ml, pink) applied after LFS protocol. Histogram represents the last 5 min of experiment in control condition ($n = 12$) or in the presence of PcTx-1 ($n = 6$) (mean ± SEM, $p > 0.05$).

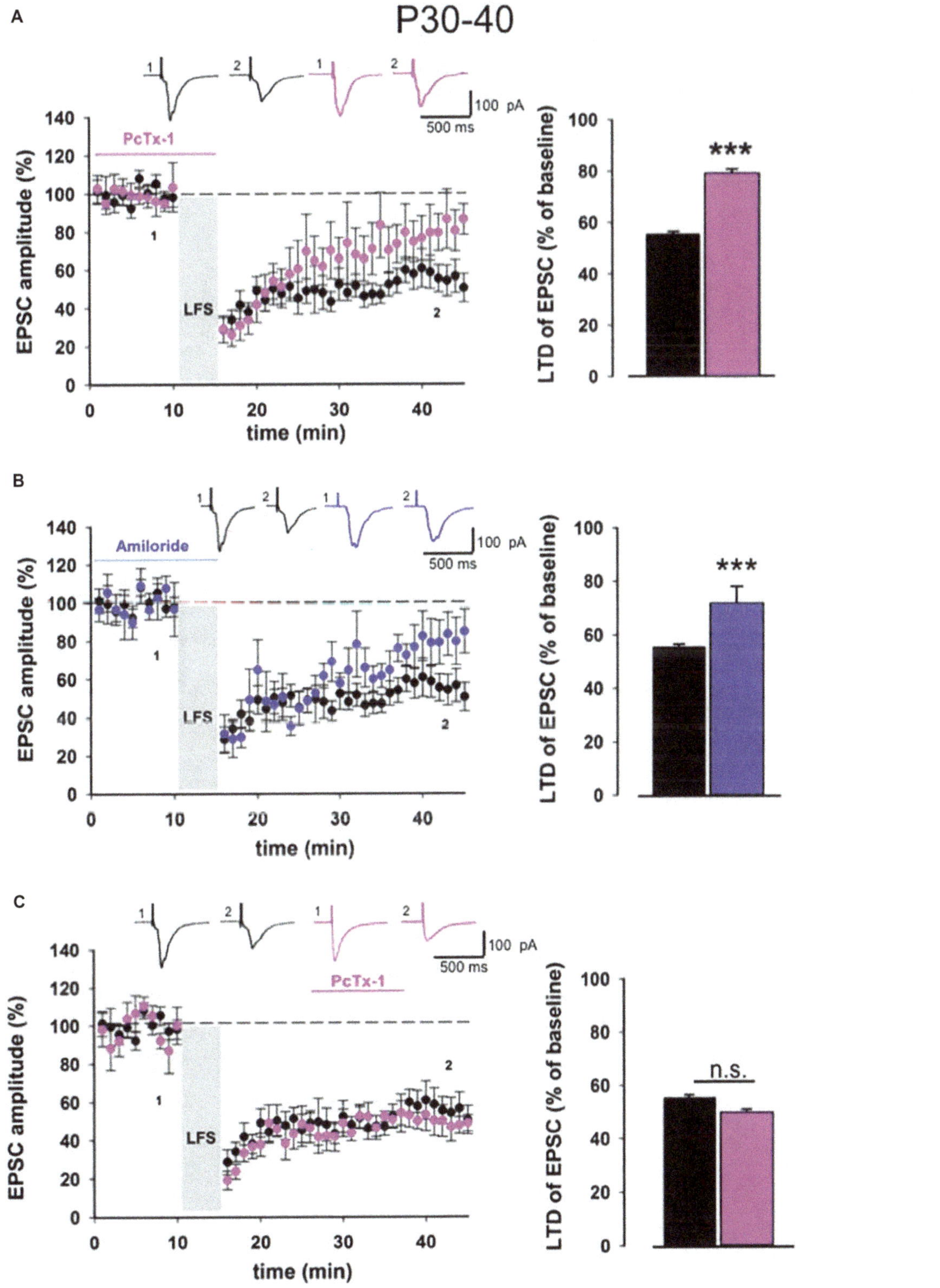

FIGURE 3 | ASIC1a modulates NMDA receptor-dependent LTD in adult mice. **(A)** Normalized pooled data showing LTD in control condition (black) and in the presence of Pctx-1 before and during LFS (100 ng/ml, pink). Histogram represents the last 5 min of experiment in control condition ($n = 11$) or in the presence of PcTx-1 ($n = 9$) (mean ± SEM, $^{***}p < 0.001$). On top, representative traces are shown for each condition. **(B)** Normalized pooled data showing LTD in control condition (black) and in the presence of amiloride (100 μM, blue). Histogram represents the last 5 min of experiment in control condition ($n = 11$) or in the presence of amiloride ($n = 7$) (mean ± SEM, $^{***}p < 0.001$). **(C)** Normalized pooled data showing LTD in control condition (black) and in the presence of PcTx-1 (100 ng/ml, pink) after LFS. Histogram represents the last 5 min of experiment in control condition ($n = 11$) or in the presence of PcTx-1 ($n = 8$) (mean ± SEM, $p > 0.05$).

protocol based on the perfusion of NMDA on hippocampal slices obtained from young and adult mice (Kamal et al., 1999). Bath application of NMDA (20 μM, 3 min) on hippocampal slices from young animals induced a strong EPSC depression that was detectable 30 min after NMDA application (34.1 ± 5.1% of baseline, $n = 9$, **Figure 4A**). Application of PcTx-1 (100 ng/ml) 10 min before and during the perfusion of NMDA partially rescued LTD (72.9 ± 9% of baseline, $n = 7$, $p < 0.001$, **Figure 4A**), suggesting that ASIC1a plays a modulatory role also in this form of LTD. Notably, bath application of PcTx-1 after NMDA-LTD induction did not restore the established depression of EPSC (39.4 ± 5% of baseline, $n = 6$, $p > 0.05$, **Figure 4A**).

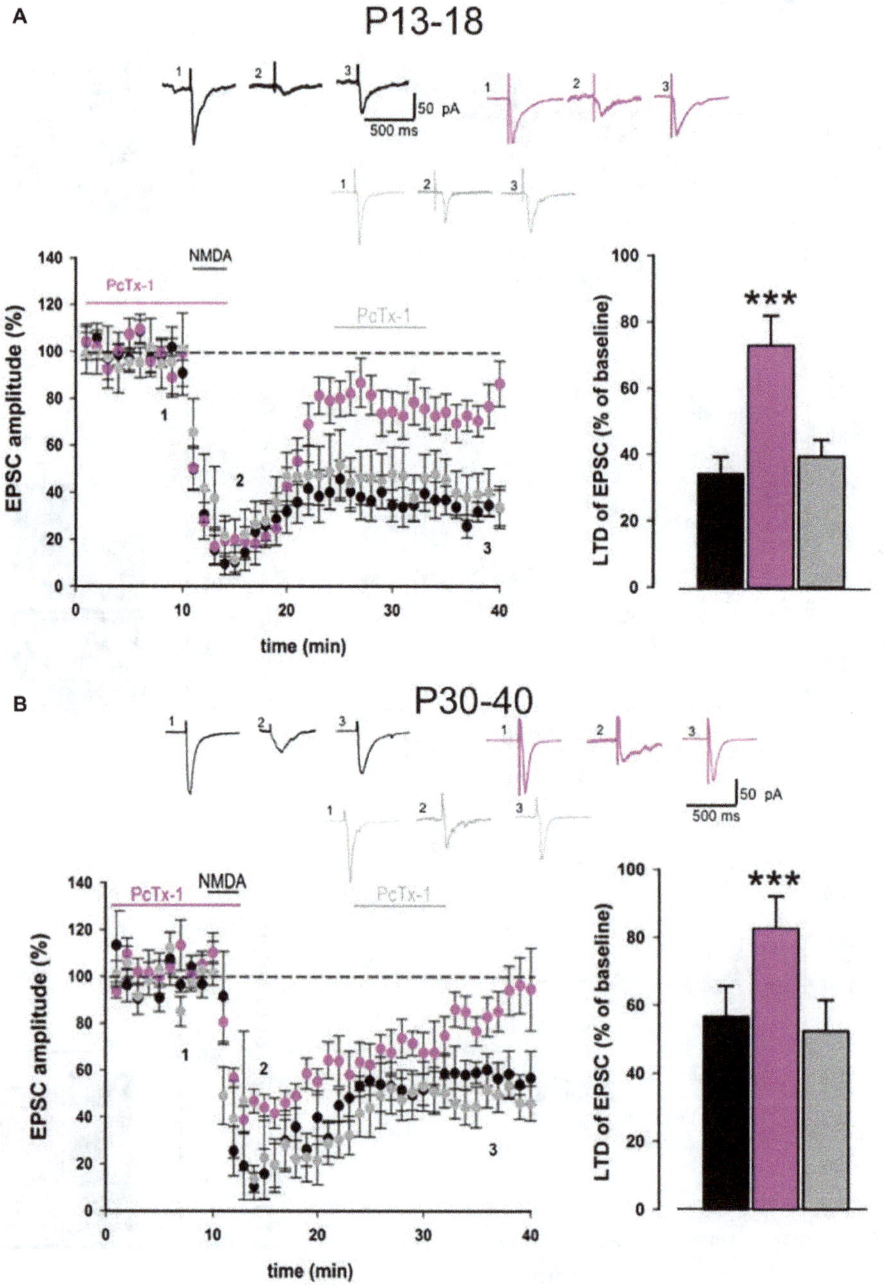

FIGURE 4 | PcTx-1 inhibits chemical NMDA-LTD. **(A)** Pooled data showing LTD induced by NMDA (20 μM) bath applied in slices obtained from young mice in control condition ($n = 9$) (black), in the presence of PcTx-1 ($n = 7$) (100 ng/ml, pink) applied before and during NMDA application, or applied after LTD induction ($n = 6$) (grey). Histogram represents the last 5 min of experiment in each condition (mean ± SEM, ***$p < 0.001$). On the top, representative traces are shown for each condition. **(B)** Pooled data showing LTD induced by NMDA (20 μM) bath applied in slices obtained from adult mice in control condition ($n = 8$) (black), in the presence of PcTx-1 ($n = 7$) (100 ng/ml, pink) applied before and during NMDA application, or applied after LTD induction ($n = 5$) (grey). Histogram represents the last 5 min of experiment in each condition (mean ± SEM, ***$p < 0.001$). On the top, representative traces are shown for each condition.

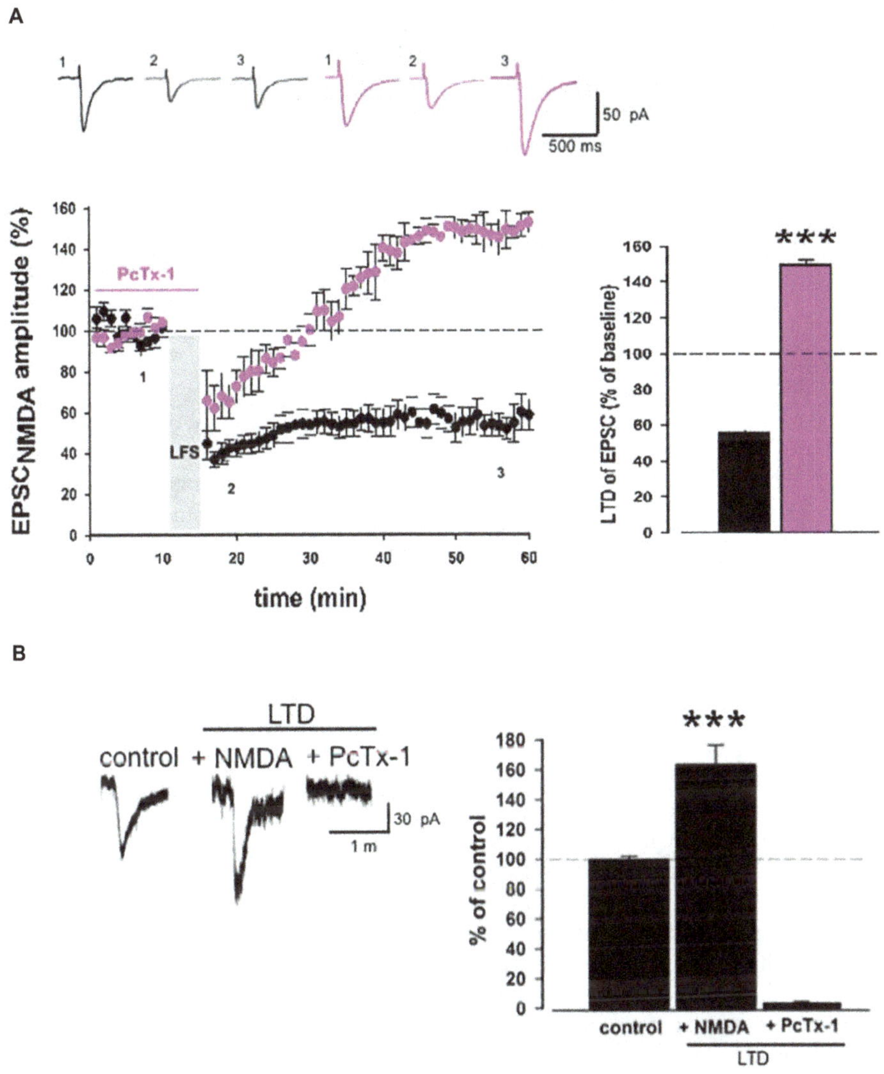

FIGURE 5 | PcTx-1 converts LTD of $EPSC_{NMDA}$ to LTP. **(A)** Normalized pooled data showing LTD of $EPSC_{NMDA}$ in control condition (black) and in the presence of PcTx-1 before and during LFS (100 ng/ml, pink). Histogram represents the last 5 min of experiment in control condition ($n = 9$) or in the presence of PcTx-1 ($n = 7$) (mean ± SEM, $^{***}p < 0.001$). On top, representative traces are shown for each condition. **(B)** Histogram represents the amplitude of ASIC1a-mediated inward current (control condition), in the presence of NMDA up to 10 min later, and in the presence of PcTx-1 ($n = 6$, mean ± SEM, $^{***}p < 0.001$). On the left, representative traces are shown for each condition.

Similar results were obtained also in slices from adult mice. Indeed, NMDA perfusion induced a strong EPSC depression (56.6 ± 9% of baseline, $n = 8$, **Figure 4B**). Pharmacological blockade of ASIC1a before and during NMDA application rescued LTD (82.7 ± 9.5% of baseline, $n = 7$, **Figure 4B**). On the contrary, when PcTx-1 was applied after NMDA-LTD induction, LTD still persisted (52.4 ± 9.2% of baseline, $n = 5$, **Figure 4B**), suggesting that ASIC1a modulates NMDA receptor function *per se*, thereby affecting NMDA receptor-mediated LTD maintenance signaling.

PcTx-1 Converts Long-Term Depression of $EPSC_{NMDA}$ to Potentiation

To explore the functional interplay between ASIC1a and NMDA receptors, we performed LTD experiments on the $EPSC_{NMDA}$, pharmacologically isolated through bath application of picrotoxin and CNQX. Although here we refer to an $EPSC_{NMDA}$ component, we cannot exclude, based on our previous results, that also ASIC1a may be contributing to this current.

Low-frequency stimulation produces a stable long-term depression of $EPSC_{NMDA}$. Surprisingly, PcTx-1 applied before and during LFS was able to convert LTD to LTP (control: 55.4 ± 2.5% of baseline, $n = 9$; PcTx-1,100 ng/ml: 149.3 ± 3.2% of baseline, $n = 7$, $p < 0.001$, **Figure 5A**), even though the mechanisms underlying this effect need to be explored.

To investigate possible changes of ASIC-mediated currents following LTD induction, we performed experiments by delivering puff applications of ACSF at pH 5.5 which elicit inward currents mediated by ASIC1a. Puff applications were applied at a 3-min interval for 10 min before and 10 min after NMDA-LTD induction (NMDA 20 μM, 3 min). Interestingly, we observed an increase in the amplitude of ASIC inward current following NMDA-LTD induction (163 ± 13.2%, $n = 6$, $p < 0.001$, **Figure 5B**), which was then completely abolished by PcTx-1 applied (control: 99.4 ± 2.5% vs. PcTx-1 2.8 ± 1.8%, $n = 6$ $p < 0.001$; **Figure 5B**). Overall, these data confirm that a functional interplay between ASIC1a and NMDA receptors underlies specific forms of synaptic plasticity.

DISCUSSION

In the present study, we have demonstrated that ASIC1a contributes, although to a small extent, to basal excitatory postsynaptic currents in CA1 pyramidal neurons. Indeed in hippocampal slices, the proton-mediated current had a little effect on neurotransmission under basal condition comparable to what was already shown in the amygdala (Du et al., 2014). As previously demonstrated, neurotransmitters glutamate and H^+ are released together during excitatory synaptic transmission bringing a rapid pH drop at synaptic cleft which activates ASICs (Waldmann et al., 1997a,b; DeVries, 2001; Traynelis and Chesler, 2001; Xiong et al., 2004).

Some studies have investigated the involvement of ASIC1a in synaptic plasticity and have shown that this channel was involved in the induction of LTP in different brain areas, such as the hippocampus and amygdala (Wemmie et al., 2002; Du et al., 2014; Buta et al., 2015). In addition, behavioral studies have shown that disrupting or over-expressing ASIC1a in mice might cause alteration in learning and conditioning (Wemmie et al., 2002, 2003, 2004). Recently, we published the researches that demonstrated a role of ASIC1a in metabotropic glutamate (mGlu) receptor-dependent long-term depression (LTD) in the hippocampus (Mango et al., 2017; Mango and Nisticò, 2018). Our results suggest that ASIC1a plays a critical role in intrinsic excitability and mGlu receptor-dependent LTD in CA1 pyramidal neurons of early adult mice. Notably, ASIC1a controls AMPA-GluA1 subunit phosphorylation succeeding mGlu-LTD, suggesting that a functional crosstalk among ASIC1a and AMPA receptors underlies specific forms of synaptic plasticity (Mango et al., 2017).

Here we extend these results by investigating the involvement of ASIC1a in a distinct form of synaptic plasticity. In particular, we studied the NMDA receptor-dependent form of LTD by the use of selective and nonselective ASIC1a blockers, psalmotoxin-1 and amiloride. We have shown that ASIC1a plays a role in NMDA-dependent long-term depression in young and adult hippocampus. Moreover, experiments performed on isolated $EPSC_{NMDA}$ highlight that a functional crosstalk between the two receptors occurs and underlies specific forms of LTD. This interaction was also confirmed by monitoring, during NMDA-LTD experiments, the ASIC1a-mediated currents elicited by puff a pplications o f acidic pH solution. Indeed, ASIC1a currents were increased following chemical LTD induction and were completely abated by PcTx-1 application. It is possible to hypothesize that in the absence of PcTx-1, LFS induces LTD of AMPA-mediated currents; whereas, in the presence of PcTx-1, LFS induces LTP of NMDA- or ASIC1a-mediated currents. Thus, w hen combining the LTD of AMPA-mediated currents and the potentiation of either NMDA-mediated or ASIC1a-mediated currents that occurs following LFS or NMDA application in the presence of PcTx-1, the end result is attenuation of LTD or unmasking of potentiation.

In any case, here we demonstrate that an interplay between ASICs and glutamate receptors (see also Mango et al., 2017) underlies various forms of synaptic plasticity, even though the precise mechanisms mediating these interactions still remain unclear. Gao et al. (2015) have previously demonstrated interplay between ASIC1a and NMDA receptor function. In particular, they show that ASIC1a activity plays a key role in facilitating the opening of NMDA receptor channel, whereas inhibition of ASIC1a impaired NMDA receptor function at physiological pH (Gao et al., 2015). Importantly, a recent paper has shown an increase of the NMDA receptor current following ASIC1a activation, which is mediated by the NR2 subunit (Ma et al., 2019). Based on these results, here we suggest that ASICs' activation is involved in NMDA receptor-dependent LTD. It can be hypothesized that under synaptic activity, the opening of ASIC1a might contribute to depolarize the postsynaptic cell thus allowing Ca^{2+} to flow into the NMDA receptor within the dendritic spine and trigger LTD.

Overall, this work further supports a role for ASICs in regulating synaptic function and potentially cognitive processes. Future studies are required to elucidate how the interplay among ASICs and NMDA receptors might contribute to normal and pathological conditions. Interestingly, it is known that drugs that increase synaptic activity, such as NMDA receptor agonists or modulators, have been extensively explored as treatments to ameliorate memory function (for review see Müller et al., 1994; Chazot, 2004). In this context, also ASICs might be considered as potential therapeutic targets in neurodegenerative disorders (Xiong et al., 2008; Radu et al., 2016).

AUTHOR CONTRIBUTIONS

DM designed the research, performed experiments and wrote the paper. RN designed the research and wrote the paper.

REFERENCES

Arias, R. L., Sung, M. L., Vasylyev, D., Zhang, M. Y., Albinson, K., Kubek, K., et al. (2008). Amiloride is neuroprotective in an MPTP model of Parkinson's disease. *Neurobiol. Dis.* 31, 334–341. doi: 10.1016/j.nbd.2008.05.008

Askwith, C. C., Wemmie, J. A., Price, M. P., Rokhlina, T., and Welsh, M. J. (2004). Acid-sensing ion channel 2 (ASIC2) modulates ASIC1 H+-activated currents in hippocampal neurons. *J. Biol. Chem.* 27, 18296–18305. doi: 10.1074/jbc.M312145200

Baron, A., Waldmann, R., and Lazdunski, M. (2002). ASIC-like, proton-activated currents in rat hippocampal neurons. *J. Physiol.* 539, 485–494. doi: 10.1113/jphysiol.2001.014837

Buta, A., Maximyuk, O., Kovalskyy, D., Sukach, V., Vovk, M., Ievglevskyi, O., et al. (2015). Novel orthosteric antagonist of ASIC1a prevents NMDAR-dependent LTP induction. *J. Med. Chem.* 58, 4449–4461. doi: 10.1021/jm5017329

Chazot, P. L. (2004). The NMDA receptor NR2B subunit: a valid therapeutic target for multiple CNS pathologies. *Curr. Med. Chem.* 11, 389–396. doi: 10.2174/0929867043456061

DeVries, S. H. (2001). Exocytosen protons feedback to suppress the Ca^{2+} current in mammalian cone photoreceptors. *Neuron* 32, 1107–1117. doi: 10.1016/S0896-6273(01)00535-9

Du, J., Reznikov, L. R., Price, M. P., Zha, X. M., Lu, Y., Moninger, T. O., et al. (2014). Protons are a neurotransmitter that regulates synaptic plasticity in the lateral amygdala. *Proc. Natl. Acad. Sci. USA* 111, 8961–8966. doi: 10.1073/pnas1407018111

Dudek, S. M., and Bear, M. F. (1993). Bidirectional long-term modification of synaptic effectiveness in the adult and immature hippocampus. *J. Neurosci.* 13, 2910–2918. doi: 10.1523/JNEUROSCI.13-07-02910.1993

Escoubas, P., De Weille, J. R., Lecoq, A., Diochot, S., Waldmann, R., Champigny, G., et al. (2000). Isolation of a tarantula toxin specific for a class of proton-gated Na+ channels. *J. Biol. Chem.* 275, 25116–25121. doi: 10.1074/jbc.M003643200

Fioravante, D., and Regehr, W. G. (2011). Short-term forms of presynaptic plasticity. *Curr. Opin. Neurobiol.* 21, 269–274. doi: 10.1016/j.conb.2011.02.003

Gao, J., Duan, B., Wang, D. G., Deng, X. H., Zhang, G. Y., Xu, L., et al. (2005). Coupling between NMDA receptor and acid-sensing ion channel contributes to ischemic neuronal death. *Neuron* 48, 635–646. doi: 10.1016/j.neuron.2005.10.011

Gao, S., Yu, Y., Ma, Z. Y., Sun, H., Zhang, Y. L., Wang, X. T., et al. (2015). NMDA-mediated hippocampal neuronal death is exacerbated by activities of ASIC1a. *Neurotox. Res.* 28, 122–137. doi: 10.1007/s12640-015-9530-3

Highstein, S. M., Holstein, G. R., Mann, M. A., and Rabbitt, R. D. (2014). Evidence that protons act as neurotransmitters at vestibular hair cell-calyx afferent synapses. *Proc. Natl. Acad. Sci. USA* 111, 5421–5426. doi: 10.1073/pnas.1319561111

Kamal, A., Ramakers, G. M., Urban, I. J., De Graan, P. N., and Gispen, W. H. (1999). Chemical LTD in the CA1 field of the hippocampus from young and mature rats. *Eur. J. Neurosci.* 11, 3512–3516. doi: 10.1046/j.1460-9568.1999.00769.x

Kemp, N., and Bashir, Z. I. (1997). NMDA receptor-dependent and -independent long-term depression in the CA1 region of the adult rat hippocampus in vitro. *Neuropharmacology* 36, 397–399. doi: 10.1016/S0028-3908(96)90015-5

Kemp, N., McQueen, J., Faulkes, S., and Bashir, Z. I. (2000). Different forms of LTD in the CA1 region of the hippocampus: role of age and stimulus protocol. *Eur. J. Neurosci.* 12, 360–366. doi: 10.1046/j.1460-9568.2000.00903.x

Kreple, C. J., Lu, Y., Taugher, R. J., Schwager-Gutman, A. L., Du, J., Stump, M., et al. (2014). Acid-sensing ion channels contribute to synaptic transmission and inhibit cocaine-evoked plasticity. *Nat. Neurosci.* 17, 1083–1091. doi: 10.1038/nn.3750

Krishtal, O. A., Osipchuk, Y. V., Shelest, T. N., and Smirnoff, S. V. (1987). Rapid extracellular pH transients related to synaptic transmission in rat hippocampal slices. *Brain Res.* 436, 352–356. doi: 10.1016/0006-8993(87)91678-7

Liu, M. G., Li, H. S., Li, W. G., Wu, Y. J., Deng, S. N., Huang, C., et al. (2016). Acid-sensing ion channel 1a contributes to hippocampal LTP inducibility through multiple mechanisms. *Sci. Rep.* 6, 23350–23364. doi: 10.1038/srep39808

Ma, C. L., Sun, H., Yang, L., Wang, X. T., Gao, S., Chen, X. W., et al. (2019). Acid-sensing ion channel 1a modulates NMDA receptor function through targeting NR1/NR2A/NR2B triheteromeric receptors. *Neuroscience* 406, 389–404. doi: 10.1016/j.neuroscience.2019.03.044

Mango, D., Braksator, E., Battaglia, G., Marcelli, S., Mercuri, N. B., Feligioni, M., et al. (2017). Acid-sensing ion channel 1a is required for mGlu receptor dependent long-term depression in the hippocampus. *Pharmacol. Res.* 119, 12–19. doi: 10.1016/j.phrs.2017.01.028

Mango, D., and Nisticò, R. (2018). Role of ASIC1a in Aβ-induced synaptic alterations in the hippocampus. *Pharmacol. Res.* 131, 61–65. doi: 10.1016/j.phrs.2018.03.016

Mango, D., Weisz, F., and Nisticò, R. (2016). Ginkgolic acid protects against Aβ-induced synaptic dysfunction in the hippocampus. *Front. Pharmacol.* 26, 7–401. doi: 10.3389/fphar.2016.00401

Miesenböck, G., De Angelis, D. A., and Rothman, J. E. (1998). Visualizing secretion and synaptic transmission with pH-sensitive green fluorescent proteins. *Nature* 394, 192–195. doi: 10.1038/28190

Müller, W. E., Scheuer, K., and Stoll, S. (1994). Glutamatergic treatment strategies for age-related memory disorders. *Life Sci.* 55, 2147–2153. doi: 10.1016/0024-3205(94)00395-5

Nicolas, C. S., Peineau, S., Amici, M., Csaba, Z., Fafouri, A., Javalet, C., et al. (2012). The Jak/STAT pathway is involved in synaptic plasticity. *Neuron* 73, 374–390. doi: 10.1016/j.neuron.2011.11.024

Radu, B. M., Banciu, A., Banciu, D. D., and Radu, M. (2016). Acid-sensing ion channels as potential pharmacological targets in peripheral and central nervous system diseases. *Adv. Protein Chem. Struct. Biol.* 103, 137–167. doi: 10.1016/bs.apcsb.2015.10.022

Sherwood, T. W., Lee, K. G., Gormley, M. G., and Askwith, C. C. (2011). Heteromeric acid-sensing ion channels (ASICs) composed of ASIC2b and ASIC1a display novel channel properties and contribute to acidosis-induced neuronal death. *J. Neurosci.* 31, 9723–9734. doi: 10.1523/JNEUROSCI.1665-11.2011

Traynelis, S. F., and Chesler, M. (2001). Proton release as a modulator of presynaptic function. *Neuron* 32, 960–962. doi: 10.1016/S0896-6273(01)00549-9

Vergo, S., Craner, M. J., Etzensperger, R., Attfield, K., Friese, M. A., Newcombe, J., et al. (2011). Acid-sensing ion channel 1 is involved in both axonal injury and demyelination in multiple sclerosis and its animal model. *Brain* 134, 571–584. doi: 10.1093/brain/awq337

Waldmann, R., Bassilana, F., de Weille, J., Champigny, G., Heurteaux, C., and Lazdunski, M. (1997b). Molecular cloning of a non-inactivating proton-gated Na+ channel specific for sensory neurons. *J. Biol. Chem.* 272, 20975–20978.

Waldmann, R., Champigny, G., Bassilana, F., Heurteaux, C., and Lazdunski, M. (1997a). A proton-gated cation channel involved in acid-sensing. *Nature* 386, 173–177.

Wemmie, J. A., Askwith, C. C., Lamani, E., Cassell, M. D., Freeman, J. H. Jr., and Welsh, M. J. (2003). Acid-sensing ion channel 1 is localized in brain regions with high synaptic density and contributes to fear conditioning. *J. Neurosci.* 23, 5496–5502. doi: 10.1523/JNEUROSCI.23-13-05496.2003

Wemmie, J. A., Chen, J., Askwith, C. C., Hruska-Hageman, A. M., Price, M. P., Nolan, B. C., et al. (2002). The acid-activated ion channel ASIC contributes to synaptic plasticity, learning, and memory. *Neuron* 34, 463–477. doi: 10.1016/S0896-6273(02)00661-X

Wemmie, J. A., Coryell, M. W., Askwith, C. C., Lamani, E., Leonard, A. S., Sigmund, C. D., et al. (2004). Overexpression of acid-sensing ion channel1a in transgenic mice increases acquired fear-related behavior. *Proc. Natl. Acad. Sci. USA* 101, 3621–3626. doi: 10.1073/pnas.0308753101

Wemmie, J. A., Price, M. P., and Welsh, M. J. (2006). Acid sensing ion channels: advances, questions and therapeutic opportunities. *Trends Neurosci.* 29, 578–586. doi: 10.1016/j.tins.2006.06.014

Weng, J. Y., Lin, Y. C., and Lien, C. C. (2010). Cell type-specific expression of acid-sensing ion channels in hippocampal interneurons. *J. Neurosci.* 30, 6548–6558. doi: 10.1523/JNEUROSCI.0582-10.2010

Xiong, Z. G., Pignataro, G., Li, M., Chang, S. Y., and Simon, R. P. (2008).

10

Repeated Administration of Norbinaltorphimine Produces Cumulative Kappa Opioid Receptor Inactivation

Charles Chavkin, Joshua H. Cohen and Benjamin B. Land*

Department of Pharmacology, University of Washington, Seattle, WA, United States

***Correspondence:**
Charles Chavkin
cchavkin@uw.edu

Kappa receptor activation by dynorphins contributes to the anxiogenic, dysphoric, and cognitive disrupting effects of repeated stress, suggesting that kappa receptor antagonists might have therapeutic utility in the treatment of stress disorders. Three classes of kappa antagonists have been distinguished: non-selective, selective-competitive (readily reversible), and non-competitive (receptor-inactivating); however, which would be the most effective medication has not been established. To assess the utility of receptor inactivating antagonists, we tested the effects of a range of doses in both male and female mice. As previously established, the antinociceptive effects of the kappa agonist U50,488 were blocked by a single injection of the long-acting antagonist norbinatorphimine (norBNI) (10 mg/kg i.p.) in male mice. Ten to 20-fold lower doses of norBNI were ineffective after a single administration, but daily administration of 1.0 or 0.5 mg/kg for 5 days completely blocked U50,488 antinociceptive effects. Daily administration of 0.1 mg/kg norBNI produced slowly accumulating inhibition and completely blocked the antinociceptive effect of U50,488 after 20–30 days. Estrogen reduces female sensitivity to kappa opioid effects, but 30 days of 0.1 mg/kg norBNI completely blocked U50,488 analgesia in ovariectomized mice. Receptor inactivation in both male and female mice treated for 30 days with 0.1 mg/kg norBNI persisted for at least 1-week. These results suggest that receptor-inactivating kappa antagonists are effective in both males and females when given at 100-fold lower doses than typically administered in preclinical studies. The enhanced safety of this low-dosing protocol has important clinical implications if receptor inactivating kappa antagonists advance in medication development.

Keywords: kappa opioid receptor, depression, addiction, receptor inactivation, drug development, sex differences

INTRODUCTION

The physiological stress response provides important metabolic and cardiovascular adaptations that protect the organism and enhance survival; however, sustained stress exposure can produce pathophysiological effects that are ultimately deleterious (Bale and Vale, 2004). For vulnerable individuals, chronic stress can produce mood disorders and increase the risk of substance use disorder (Sinha et al., 2011), and medications able to promote stress-resilience might have important therapeutic utility in the treatment of depression, anxiety, and drug addiction. One type of stress-resilience medication that is currently under clinical development are the kappa opioid receptor antagonists, which block the effects of the endogenous dynorphin opioid peptides (Carroll and Carlezon, 2013). Dynorphins are released by corticotropin releasing factor (CRF) in brain during stress exposure and encode the aversive, anxiogenic, and dysphoric responses to stress (Bruchas et al., 2010). Clinical trials with kappa antagonists show promise (Chavkin and Koob, 2016), but important questions are necessary to resolve at the preclinical level to guide medication development. Specifically, it is not clear which type of kappa antagonist would be most effective. Three classes have been distinguished: (1) ***non-selective antagonists*** that bind to other receptors besides kappa (e.g., buprenorphine, naltrexone, naloxone, and nalmefene), (2) short-acting ***selective competitive antagonists*** that specifically inhibit kappa receptor activation [e.g., PF-04455242, LY2456302 (also called CERC-501, JNJ-67953964), and BTRX-335140], or (3) kappa selective ***receptor-inactivating*** antagonists that produce a long-lasting structural change in the kappa receptor signaling complex by a recently defined c-Jun Kinase mechanism (e.g., norBNI, JDTic, and GNTI) (Schattauer et al., 2017). The latter can be considered as non-competitive antagonists or as a novel class of functionally selective agonists.

There are theoretical advantages and disadvantages of each class of kappa antagonists as potential therapeutics. Receptor-inactivating kappa antagonists may produce more stable stress-resilience, but JNK activation may also produce adverse effects and long-duration of effect would make dose titration problematic. In the present study, we asked if the receptor-inactivating class of kappa antagonist can produce long-acting receptor inactivation in a dose-dependent manner for both male and female mice. Our conjecture is that receptor inactivating kappa antagonists might be safer and more effective than non-selective or competitive kappa antagonists if they can be administered at very low doses that produce accumulating receptor inactivation with minimal off-target effects. In this proof-of-principle study, we found that daily norbinaltorphimine (norBNI) administration at 100-fold lower doses than required for acute receptor antagonism completely blocked kappa receptors in both male and female mice.

METHODS

Drugs

Norbinaltorphimine (norBNI) and U50,488 (NIDA Drug Supply program) were dissolved in sterile saline (0.9%) at injected at 10 mL/kg (i.p.). The GRK2/3 inhibitor CMPD101 (Tocris Bioscience) was used as described (Abraham et al., 2018).

Subjects

Male and female C57BL/6N mice (n = 66) ranging from 8 to 16 weeks of age were used. All experimental procedures were approved by the University of Washington Institutional Animal Use and Care Committee. All testing was during the light phase of the 14-h light/dark cycle. Ovaries were removed from female mice under isoflurane anesthesia as previously described (Smith et al., 2005). Mice were allowed 2 weeks recovery prior to behavioral experiments.

Tail-Flick Analgesia

Mice were administered norBNI or an equivalent volume of saline daily at the specified dose (0.1–10 mg/kg, i.p.) and for the specified duration (1–30 days). 24 h after the norBNI injection on day 2, 6, 11, 21, and 31, the response latency for the mouse to withdraw its tail following immersion into 52.5 +/− 0.2°C water was measured before and 30 min after U50,488 administration (10 mg/kg, i.p.). One additional U50,488 test was performed on day 37, 1 week after the last norBNI injection. Data are expressed as maximum possible effect, normalized to time matched saline/U50,488 controls.

Statistics

Group differences were determined using one-way ANOVA and *post hoc* comparisons analyzed with Dunnett's multiple comparison test (comparison group = saline), or linear trend with α set to 0.05. Data were analyzed with GraphPad Prism 7.

RESULTS

In a typical preclinical study using norBNI, a single injection of 10 mg/kg (i.p.) is administered to the experimental animal to completely inhibit kappa opioid responses. We confirm that when male C57BL/6 mice were given this dose and challenged 24 h later with 10 mg/kg U50,488 (a selective KOR agonist), the analgesic response to U50,488 was fully blocked (**Figure 1A**). For mice given a 10- or 20-fold lower dose of norBNI (1 or 0.5 mg/kg), the response 24 h later to U50,488 was only partially blocked in a dose-dependent manner. However, if male mice are given 1 or 0.5 mg/kg norBNI daily for 5 days, the U50,488 response was fully blocked. When the dose of norBNI was lowered still further and the mice were injected daily with 0.1 mg/kg norBNI, the analgesic response to U50,488 challenge was slowly reduced and was fully blocked only after 20–30 days of dosing.

Female mice and rats have been reported to be less sensitive than males in their responses to kappa opioid agonists and antagonists (Russell et al., 2014; Abraham et al., 2018; Laman-Maharg et al., 2018; Williams and Trainor, 2018). These sex differences raise important questions about the utility of kappa antagonists in the treatment of stress-disorders in women. Additionally, U50,488 treatment does not produce analgesia in female mice when their estrogen levels are high. Estrogen was found to activate G protein Receptor Kinase 2 (GRK2), which blocked $G\beta\gamma$ mediated analgesia (Abraham et al., 2018). Similar to results using kappa agonists, female mice respond to receptor inactivating KOR antagonists in an estrogen-sensitive manner; norBNI is not long lasting in females when administered during high estrogen phases of their estrus cycle, and inhibition of GRK2 by CMPD101 (15 mg/kg, 30 min prior) made 10 mg/kg norBNI long-lasting (data not shown). After ovariectomy, female mice respond to the analgesic effects of U50,488 similarly to

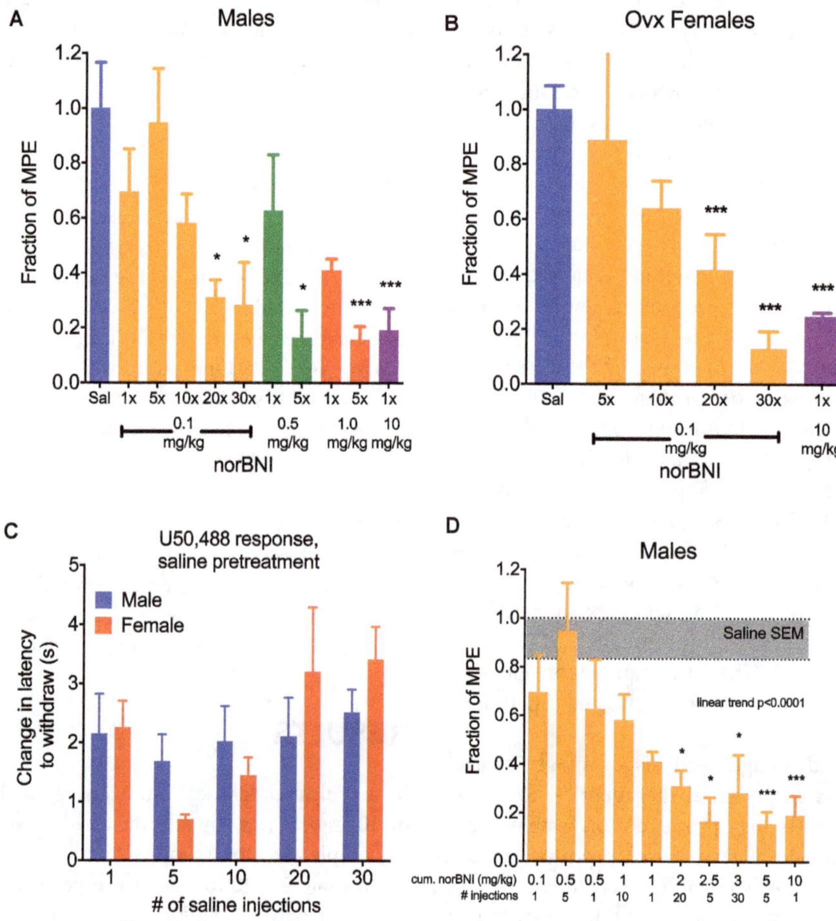

FIGURE 1 | Daily administration of low doses of norBNI produced accumulating receptor inactivation. **(A)** Male C57BL/6 mice were injected with norBNI at the doses and number of daily administrations listed on the *x*-axis and the fraction of the maximal possible analgesic effect in the tail flick latency assay (MPE, determined from saline-pretreated animals) after U50,488 (10 mg/kg) is shown on the *y*-axis; (n = 4–18, ANOVA F = 4.377, $^*p < 0.05$, $^{***}p < 0.001$) **(B)** Ovariectomized female C57BL/6 mice were injected with norBNI at the doses and number of daily administrations listed on the *x*-axis and the fraction of the MPE of tail flick latency was determined after U50,488 (n = 4–5, ANOVA F = 17.16, $^{***}p < 0.001$) **(C)**. The analgesic effect of U50,488 does not significantly change over the course of the experiment in either males or females. *Y*-axis represents the change in latency to remove tail post-U50,488 (10 mg/kg) subtracted from the latency pre-U50,488; (n = 3–8, 2-way ANOVA $F_{\text{interaction}} = 0.9131$, $p = 0.47$; $F_{\text{day}} = 2.21$, $p = 0.09$; $F_{,\text{sex}} = 0.06$, $p = 0.80$) **(D)**. Cumulative dosing of norBNI in males shows that significant effects are apparent at 2 mg/kg equivalence. Bars are reorganized from panel A in increasing cumulative dosing of norBNI; (n = 4–18, ANOVA F = 4.377, *post hoc* for linear trend).

males. In this study, U50,488 (10 mg/kg) produced significant antinociceptive effects in female mice that were blocked by a single injection of 10 mg/kg norBNI (**Figure 1B**). Consistent with the effects observed with males, daily administration of 0.1 mg/kg norBNI also significantly blocked U50,488 effects after 20–30 days. In this protocol, mice were each injected with U50,488 five times: first 24 h after the single norBNI injection (1×), then after 5, 10, 20, and 30 days. Daily treatment of ovariectomized females with 0.1 mg/kg norBNI fully blocked U50,488-induced analgesia along the same time course as males. There was no evidence of analgesic tolerance to U50,488 caused by this injection protocol; the response to U50,488 did not significantly change during the course of the injection series for either male or female mice (**Figure 1C**).

As expected in this dosing protocol, the effects of norBNI accumulated with each injection. This result is predicted by the long effective duration of norBNI effects, which have been shown to reverse with a half-life of approximately 14 days in male mice (Bruchas et al., 2007). To visualize this cumulative effect, we replotted the blockade of analgesia as the total amount of norBNI injected at the time of U50,488 administration (**Figure 1D**). The degree of kappa receptor inhibition clearly depended on the history of norBNI administration, following a linear trend, with a cumulative dose of about 2 mg/kg as the point where significant block of analgesia is produced.

To further characterize the effects of this dosing scheme, we challenged mice with U50,488 1 week after receiving daily low doses of norBNI (0.1 mg/kg) for 30 days and found that in both male and female mice the kappa receptors remained inactivated (**Figure 2**). Thus, clinical efficacy may be achieved at doses 100-fold lower than

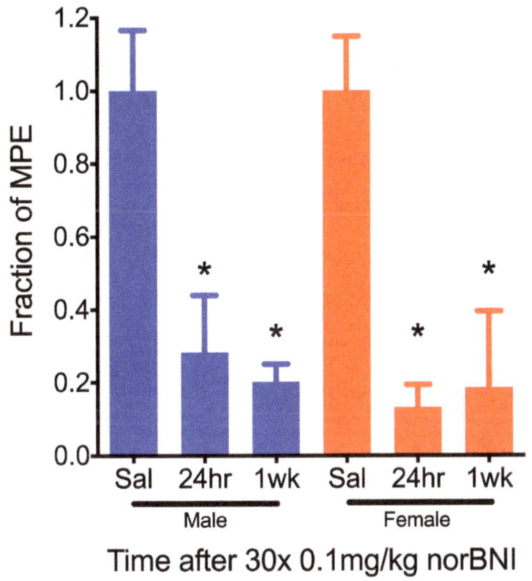

FIGURE 2 | The effects of repeated, low-dose norBNI are long-lasting. Male and female mice were tested 24 h and 1 week after the last of 30 daily injections of 0.01 mg/kg norBNI or saline. *Y*-axis represents the fraction of the MPE in the tail flick latency assay after U50,488 (10 mg/kg) [$n = 4–9$, ANOVA $F = 5.234$ (male), $F = 5.407$ (female), $^*p < 0.05$].

required for acute receptor saturation, and both males and ovariectomized female mice exhibited long-duration of kappa receptor inactivation after administration of low doses of norBNI.

DISCUSSION

The principal findings of the study are that receptor-inactivating kappa antagonists may be effective at 100-fold lower doses than required for acute antagonism. While sex differences are important to consider in kappa receptor directed medications, receptor inactivation by norBNI was evident in both male and female mice. The key implication of this study is that receptor inactivating antagonists may be more selective and safer medications when used at these low doses. The 3–4 weeks required for optimization of effect would not be expected to be a significant limitation for clinical treatment since antidepressants and other mood stabilizing medications often require slow titration and months of treatment before clinical efficacy is established. Whether c-Jun Kinase activation by receptor-inactivating antagonists is a safety concern is not yet clear, but it should be noted that kappa opioid receptor activation by dynorphin and mu opioid receptor activation by morphine also activate c-Jun Kinase (Schattauer et al., 2017) without documented adverse effects. Thus, physiological levels of c-Jun Kinase activation at the low pharmacological doses necessary may not have the toxic effects noted with intense activation (Bubici and Papa, 2014).

There are theoretical advantages and disadvantages of each class of kappa antagonists as potential therapeutics: non-selective antagonists have the advantage that their safety has been established by a long clinical history, and they are already FDA approved for human use. Non-selective medications can be more effective in treatment of psychiatric disorders (e.g., clinically effective antipsychotic medications lack receptor selectivity), and this may also be true in stress-disorders if resilience requires the block of multiple stress systems. However, the off-target effects of non-selective antagonists might be problematic or unnecessary. Kappa selective, competitive antagonists are conventional medications whose selectivity would theoretically reduce their off-target effects. The short acting effects could be readily titrated by dose adjustment. However, a significant concern with competitive antagonists is that they may lack clinical efficacy if they are not given at doses that adequately block the kappa receptors during an unanticipated stress event. High antagonist doses (resulting in off-target effects) and frequent dosing (resulting in challenging medications compliance issues) may be required to block stress-induced dynorphin effects. In contrast, receptor-inactivating kappa antagonists may produce more stable stress-resilience with off-target effects minimized by the low doses required. While the utility of receptor inactivating kappa antagonists in women remains to be established, we predict that these drugs would be effective during the normal menstrual cycle while estrogen levels are low and that kappa receptor inactivation will accumulate with daily administration of low doses of antagonist. In support of this conjecture, the recovery rate of kappa receptors in rhesus monkeys treated with norBNI required more than 20 weeks (Ko et al., 2003), suggesting that receptor half-life in primates is even longer than rodents.

Therapeutic efficacy of antagonists requires adequate receptor blockade to prevent the endogenous agonist effects. While the degree of receptor block required for kappa system is not yet known, clinical trials of conventional competitive CRF R1 receptor antagonists failed to demonstrate efficacy (Spierling and Zorrilla, 2017), and we suggest that this may have been a consequence of R1 receptor occupancy by the antagonist doses used that was insufficient to block endogenous CRF effects. Because dynorphin is a highly efficacious agonist and spare kappa receptors are evident (Chavkin and Goldstein, 1981), dynorphin may be able to produce robust dysphoric effects at very low receptor occupancy. If true, complete kappa receptor inactivation may be necessary for clinical efficacy. This remains to be established in human stress disorders, but is an important aspect to consider in medication development. Unlike the CRF – CRF R1 receptor system where complete inactivation would produce Addison's Disease-like symptoms, complete kappa-receptor inactivation does not affect viability (as demonstrated by the viability of prodynorphin or kappa receptor gene deletion).

The present study was done in mice and using tail flick antinociception assay as a readout. This is useful in a proof of principle study; however, receptor-inactivating antagonists are also known to have long durations of effect in the preclinical models for anxiety, depression, and addiction (Carroll and Carlezon, 2013). Thus, the results of this study support the conjecture that low doses of kappa-receptor inactivating antagonists may show greater safety, selectivity, and clinical efficacy than the alternatives.

AUTHOR CONTRIBUTIONS

CC designed the experiment and wrote the paper. JC performed the experiment. BL analyzed the data and generated the figures.

FUNDING

This research was supported by a USPHS grant P50 MH106428 from the National Institute on Mental Health.

REFERENCES

Abraham, A. D., Schattauer, S. S., Reichard, K. L., Cohen, J. H., Fontaine, H. M., Song, A. J., et al. (2018). Estrogen regulation of GRK2 inactivates kappa opioid receptor signaling mediating analgesia. but not aversion. *J. Neurosci.* 38, 8031–8043. doi: 10.1523/JNEUROSCI.0653-18.2018

Bale, T. L., and Vale, W. W. (2004). CRF and CRF receptors: role in stress responsivity and other behaviors. *Annu. Rev. Pharmacol. Toxicol.* 44, 525–557. doi: 10.1146/annurev.pharmtox.44.101802.121410

Bruchas, M. R., Land, B. B., and Chavkin, C. (2010). The dynorphin/kappa opioid system as a modulator of stress-induced and pro-addictive behaviors. *Brain Res.* 1314, 44–55. doi: 10.1016/j.brainres.2009.08.062

Bruchas, M. R., Yang, T., Schreiber, S., Defino, M., Kwan, S. C., Li, S., et al. (2007). Long-acting kappa opioid antagonists disrupt receptor signaling and produce noncompetitive effects by activating c-Jun N-terminal kinase. *J. Biol. Chem.* 282, 29803–29811. doi: 10.1074/jbc.M705540200

Bubici, C., and Papa, S. (2014). JNK signalling in cancer: in need of new, smarter therapeutic targets. *Br. J. Pharmacol.* 171, 24–37. doi: 10.1111/bph.12432

Carroll, F. I., and Carlezon, W. A. Jr. (2013). Development of κ opioid receptor antagonists. *J. Med. Chem.* 56, 2178–2195. doi: 10.1021/jm301783x

Chavkin, C., and Goldstein, A. (1981). Demonstration of a specific dynorphin receptor in guinea pig ileum myenteric plexus. *Nature* 291, 591–593. doi: 10.1038/291591a0

Chavkin, C., and Koob, G. F. (2016). Dynorphin, dysphoria, and dependence: the stress of addiction. *Neuropsychopharmacology* 41, 373–374. doi: 10.1038/npp.2015.258

Ko, M. C., Willmont, K. J., Lee, H., Flory, G. S., and Woods, J. H. (2003). Ultra-long antagonism of kappa opioid agonist-induced diuresis by intracisternal nor-binaltorphimine in monkeys. *Brain Res.* 982, 38–44. doi: 10.1016/S0006-8993(03)02938-X

Laman-Maharg, A., Williams, A. V., Zufelt, M. D., Minie, V. A., Ramos-Maciel, S., Hao, R., et al. (2018). Sex differences in the effects of a kappa opioid receptor antagonist in the forced swim test. *Front. Pharmacol.* 9:93. doi: 10.3389/fphar.2018.00093

Russell, S. E., Rachlin, A. B., Smith, K. L., Muschamp, J., Berry, L., Zhao, Z., et al. (2014). Sex differences in sensitivity to the depressive-like effects of the kappa opioid receptor agonist U-50488 in rats. *Biol. Psychiatry* 76, 213–222. doi: 10.1016/j.biopsych.2013.07.042

Schattauer, S. S., Land, B. B., Reichard, K. L., Abraham, A. D., Burgeno, L. M., Kuhar, J. R., et al. (2017). Peroxiredoxin 6 mediates Gαi protein-coupled receptor inactivation by cJun kinase. *Nat. Commun.* 8:743. doi: 10.1038/s41467-017-00791-2

Sinha, R., Shaham, Y., and Heilig, M. (2011). Translational and reverse translational research on the role of stress in drug craving and relapse. *Psychopharmacology* 218, 69–82. doi: 10.1007/s00213-011-2263-y

Smith, J. T., Cunningham, M. J., Rissman, E. F., Clifton, D. K., and Steiner, R. A. (2005). Regulation of Kiss1 gene expression in the brain of the female mouse. *Endocrinology* 146, 3686–3692. doi: 10.1210/en.2005-0488

Spierling, S. R., and Zorrilla, E. P. (2017). Don't stress about CRF: assessing the translational failures of CRF1antagonists. *Psychopharmacology* 234, 1467–1481. doi: 10.1007/s00213-017-4556-2

Williams, A. V., and Trainor, B. C. (2018). The impact of sex as a biological variable in the search for novel antidepressants. *Front. Neuroendocrinol.* 50:107–117. doi: 10.1016/j.yfrne.2018.05.003

11

Bone Mesenchymal Stem Cell-Derived Extracellular Vesicles Promote Recovery Following Spinal Cord Injury via Improvement of the Integrity of the Blood-Spinal Cord Barrier

Yanhui Lu[1,2†], Yan Zhou[3†‡], Ruiyi Zhang[1,2], Lulu Wen[1], Kaimin Wu[1], Yanfei Li[1], Yaobing Yao[1], Ranran Duan[1] and Yanjie Jia[1]*

[1] Department of Neurology, The First Affiliated Hospital of Zhengzhou University, Zhengzhou, China, [2] Academy of Medical Sciences, Zhengzhou University, Zhengzhou, China, [3] Department of Radiology, The First Affiliated Hospital of Zhengzhou University, Zhengzhou, China

***Correspondence:**
Yanjie Jia
jiayanjie1971@zzu.edu.cn

† These two authors contributed equally to the work

‡ Co-first author

Mesenchymal stem cell (MSC) transplantation has been shown to represent a potential treatment for traumatic spinal cord injury (SCI). However, there are several obstacles that need to be overcome before MSCs can be considered for clinical application, such as failure of MSCs to reach the spinal cord lesion core and possible tumor formation. Recent studies have suggested that MSC treatment is beneficial owing to paracrine-secreted factors. Extracellular vesicles are considered to be some of the most valuable paracrine molecules. However, the therapeutic mechanism of extracellular vesicles on spinal cord injury has not been studied clearly. Therefore, our study investigated the effect of systemic administration of extracellular vesicles on the loss of motor function after SCI and examined the potential mechanisms underlying their effects. Disruption of the blood-spinal cord barrier (BSCB) is a crucial factor that can be detrimental to motor function recovery. Pericytes are an important component of the neurovascular unit, and play a pivotal role in maintaining the structural integrity of the BSCB. Our study demonstrated that administration of bone mesenchymal stem cell-derived extracellular vesicles (BMSC-EV) reduced brain cell death, enhanced neuronal survival and regeneration, and improved motor function compared with the administration of BMSC-EV free culture media (EV-free CM). Besides, the BSCB was attenuated and pericyte coverage was significantly decreased *in vivo*. Furthermore, we found that exosomes reduced pericyte migration via downregulation of NF-κB p65 signaling, with a consequent decrease in the permeability of the BSCB. In summary, we identified that extracellular vesicles treatment suppressed the migration of pericytes and further improved the integrity of the BSCB via NF-κB p65 signaling in pericytes. Our data suggest that extracellular vesicles may serve as a promising treatment strategy for SCI.

Keywords: extracellular vesicles, bone mesenchymal stromal cells, spinal cord injury, blood spinal cord barrier, pericytes, migration, NF-κB

INTRODUCTION

Traumatic spinal cord injury (SCI) causes permanent motor/sensory dysfunction, and even paralysis and death, resulting in a considerable reduction in the quality of life of the patient (Eckert and Martin, 2017). Many studies have shown that the failure of regeneration following SCI relates to molecular and cellular factors, such as the absence of phosphatase and tensin homolog (PTEN) and mammalian target of rapamycin (mTOR), and the presence of Nogo associated with myelin debris, debris-clearing inflammatory cells, and scar-forming cells (Schwab, 2004; Sun et al., 2011). Although considerable research has been carried out on the mechanisms involved, there are still no effective treatments for SCI.

For many years, MSCs have been exploited as an experimental therapy for SCI because of their multidirectional differentiation and potential neuroprotective properties (Xu and Yang, 2018). Although research has shown that MSCs extenuate lesions and improve axon regeneration, several obstacles need to be overcome. For example, it is reported that the majority of MSCs fail to reach the lesion and survive, but accumulate in lung tissue. Thus, the effectiveness of this treatment strategy is limited unless MSCs are directly transplanted into the spinal cord lesion. Fortunately, recent research has suggested that MSCs may play a therapeutic role via the release of paracrine factors and stimulation of host cells, instead of through their differentiation (Caplan and Dennis, 2006; Caplan and Correa, 2011). EV, which are composed of lipid bilayer, are regarded as an important component of MSC-induced paracrine factor secretion. Depending on the size of diameter, EV was divided into exosomes, microvesicles and apoptotic bodies, of which the diameter of exosomes is the smallest, 30–150 nm (Tkach and Thery, 2016; Juan and Furthauer, 2018). EV have the capacity to carry intracellular sorted cargoes, including various proteins, lipids, mRNA, and microRNA, and further target select cells in various ways including delivering functional substances and so on (Camussi et al., 2010; Phinney and Pittenger, 2017).

Several studies have demonstrated that EV participate in therapeutic effects, such as wound regeneration and reduction of neuronal cell death following cerebral ischemia (Goodarzi et al., 2018; Zagrean et al., 2018). However, it is unclear how EV promote motor recovery post-SCI. Therefore, to get a better understanding of the potential mechanisms involved in EV therapy, we further studied how EV protect the BSCB following SCI.

MATERIALS AND METHODS

Isolation and Identification of Extracellular Vesicles

Total bone marrow cells were flushed from the tibias of rats (3-months-old) with Dulbecco's modified Eagle medium (DMEM; GIBCO). Complete DMEM containing 15% fetal bovine serum (FBS), 100 U/ml penicillin, and 100 U/ml streptomycin was used to culture the bone mesenchymal stem cells (BMSCs). Extracellular vesicles were harvested from passage (P) 3 to P5 of the BMSCs as previously described (Wang et al., 2018). Briefly, exosome-depleted FBS was made by ultra-centrifuging FBS at 120,000 × *g* for 18 h. The culture medium was replaced with an exosome-depleted medium 48 h prior to the isolation of exosomes. The culture supernatants were collected and differently centrifuged at 300 × *g* for 10 min, 2000 × *g* for 10 min, and then 10,000 × *g* for 70 min to remove cells and debris. This was followed by ultracentrifugation at 100,000 × *g* for 70 min to obtain exosomes as pellets. The collected exosomes were resuspended with phosphate buffered saline (PBS) and then ultracentrifuged (110,000 × *g* for 70 min) again to refine the purity of the extracellular vesicles (BMSC-derived extracellular vesicles; BMSC-EV). The remaining medium was extracellular vesicles-free culture medium (EV-free CM). The morphology of the acquired EV was observed by transmission electron microscopy (TEM; Tecnai 12, Philips, Netherlands). Western blot was performed to verify the specific exosome surface markers, including CD9, CD63, and CD81.

BMSC-EV Labeling

PKH26 dye (Sigma-Aldrich, St. Louis, MO, United States) with a final concentration of 2×10^6 M was incubated with BMSC-EV at 25°C for 20 min followed by an equal amount of 5% bovine serum albumin (BSA; Sigma-Aldrich) to stop the staining reaction. Then, the mixture was resuspended in PBS and the EV were extracted again by ultracentrifugation as described above.

Animals

All procedures and operations complied with the National Guidelines for the Care and Use of Laboratory Animals and were authorized by the Ethics Committee of the First Affiliated Hospital of Zhengzhou University and the Ethics Committee of Zhengzhou University. Adult male Sprague–Dawley (SD) rats (200–250 g) were raised in separated cages and provided with water and food. One hundred SD rats were randomly assigned to four groups: Sham, SCI rats treated with PBS (SCI+PBS), SCI rats treated with EV-free CM (SCI+ EV-free CM), and SCI rats treated with BMSC- EV (SCI+BMSC-EV). SCI SD rats were anesthetized with 4% isoflurane and anesthesia was maintained with 2% isoflurane for 2 min (1 L/min). When the rats were unconscious, the skin, fascia, and muscle were bluntly separated to allow a laminectomy to be performed at the level of T10. The exposed spinal cord underwent a contusive injury (200 kilodyne) with a spinal cord impactor (IH Impactor; Precision Systems and Instrumentation, Lexington, KY, United States). After surgery, rats were given bladder care until they could urinate spontaneously. The sham group was subjected to laminectomy without contusive injury.

BMSC-EV and EV-Free CM Injection

In the SCI+ EV-free CM group, 200 μL EV-free CM derived from 1×10^6 MSCs were injected via the tail vein (200 μL/min) 30 min after SCI. At 1-day post-injury (dpi), 200 μL of EV-free CM was injected in the same manner. In the SCI+BMSC-EV group, 200 μL of EV derived from 1×10^6 BMSCs was injected into the tail vein (200 μL/min) at 30 min post-SCI. Subsequently, 200 μL of EV (200 μg/mL) were injected in the same manner at 1 dpi. In the SCI group, 200 μL PBS was injected at the same timepoints mentioned above.

TUNEL Assay

At 1 dpi, spinal cord cell apoptosis within the lesion was identified and quantified with an *in situ* cell death detection kit (Roche, Mannheim, Germany) according to the manufacturer's protocol. First, tissue slides were dewaxed and rehydrated, and this was followed by pre-treatment of the tissue slides with proteinase-K for 30 min. Then, tissue slides were equilibrated with the kit's equilibration buffer for 1 h at 37°C. After incubation with converter POD, tissue slides were incubated with diaminobenzidine and imaged using a microscope at 200× magnification (Olympus, Tokyo, Japan).

Nissl Staining

Nissl staining was used to assess neuronal survival. Briefly, the tissue slides were incubated with 1% thionine solution at 50°C for 40 min, and subsequently differentiated with 70% alcohol for 3 min.

Immunofluorescence

First passage pericytes were grown in culture dishes with a cell creep plate. At 28 dpi the rats were sacrificed and perfused with warm PBS and subsequently with 4% paraformaldehyde in PBS solution. 5% BSA was applied for 1 h to block non-specific antibody binding, followed by 0.3% Triton X-100 in PBS for 30 min. All paraffin sections of tissues and cell creep plates were incubated with primary antibodies at 4°C overnight. These included: rabbit anti-platelet-derived growth factor receptor beta (PDGFR-β; 1:200; Abcam), mouse p65 (1:200; Cell Signaling Technology, Danvers, MA, United States), rabbit anti-Type I collagen (Col-I; 1:200; Abcam), and mouse anti-NF200 (1:100; Abcam). All paraffin sections of tissues and cell creep plates were rewashed with PBS three times and subsequently incubated with their corresponding secondary antibodies, including red cyanine-3-conjugated goat anti-rabbit IgG (1:500; Beyotime Biotechnology, Shanghai, China) and green 488-conjugated goat anti-mouse IgG (1:500; Beyotime Biotechnology) for 2 h at 37°C. The cell nuclei were stained with diamidino-2-phenylindole (DAPI) and imaged using microscopy (Olympus, Tokyo, Japan).

Basso, Beattie, and Bresnahan (BBB) Locomotor Rating Scale

Basso, Beattie, and Bresnahan scores were detected to assess the locomotor function of the hindlimbs after SCI. According to the BBB open-field 21-point locomotor rating scale (Basso et al., 1995), the assessment was conducted weekly and scores were recorded by two independent observers blinded to the treatment groups.

Assessment of BSCB Permeability With Evans Blue (EB)

According to a well-established protocol adapted from He et al., EB extravasation leakage was performed to evaluate BSCB integrity (He et al., 2017). Briefly, EB (2% in normal saline, 4 mL/kg; Sigma-Aldrich) was injected into uninjured control animals or SCI rats through the tail vein 1 day post-SCI. Rats were anesthetized 2 h later and extensively perfused with saline until the EB dye no longer flowed out of the right atrium to remove the intravascular EB. After isolation of the spinal cord, the meninges were stripped off and the dye distribution was evaluated via photographs taken using a digital camera. The injured spinal cord tissues were weighed and then homogenized in 50% trichloroacetic solution and centrifuged for 20 min at 20,000 × *g*. The supernatant was collected and mixed with absolute ethanol (1:3). EB extravasation was quantified by measuring fluorescence from the supernatant (620 excitation, 680 emission). Ipsilateral/contralateral ratios were calculated and analyzed.

Cell Isolation and Culture

According to an established protocol (He et al., 2013; Wan et al., 2018), rat spinal cord microvascular pericytes were isolated from SD rats (3–5 weeks old) with some modifications. In brief, the rat spinal cord was separated and minced in ice-cold PBS, followed by digestion in 10 mL Dulbecco's Modified Eagle's Medium (DMEM) containing collagenase type 2 (1 mg/mL; Worthington, Lakewood, NJ, United States) and DNase I (15 g/mL; Sigma) for 1.5 h at 37°C. After adding 10 mL DMEM to the cell suspension and centrifuging it at 500 × *g* for 5 min at 4°C, the sediment was suspended with 20% BSA-DMEM and centrifuged (1000 × *g*, 20 min) to adsorb the neurons and myelin. The sediment containing microvessels were digested with collagenase/dispase (1 mg/mL; Roche, Basel, Switzerland) and DNase I (6.7 mg/mL) in DMEM for 1 h at 37°C. A 33% continuous Percoll (GE Healthcare, Buckinghamshire, United Kingdom) gradient was used to discard endothelial cells and purify pericytes. After centrifugation at 1000 × *g* for 10 min, the pellet was collected for plating in culture dishes coated with collagen type IV (both 0.1 mg/mL; Sigma-Aldrich). Pure rat spinal cord pericytes were obtained by a prolonged 2-week culture protocol, during which endothelial cells disappeared. Cells were incubated in suitable conditions (5% CO_2, 95% O_2) at 37°C and the culture medium was changed every 3 days. The fourth to sixth passages of purity exceeding 95% were used.

Oxygen-Glucose-Deprivation/Reperfusion (OGD/R)

Cells were exposed to oxygen-glucose-deprivation/reperfusion (OGD) conditions as per a previously reported protocol with modifications. Briefly, the glucose-free medium was placed in a hypoxia chamber (37°C, 1% O_2, 5% CO_2, and 94% N_2) for 30 min to remove oxygen from the medium. Cells were washed with glucose-free medium twice and then incubated in the prepared hypoxia medium for 2 h in the hypoxia chamber. After 2 h of OGD exposure, cells were reperfused with oxygen and the corresponding medium according to a previous protocol (Wan et al., 2018).

Migration Assay

A *trans*-well assay was used to assess the migration capacity of pericytes. Briefly, a volume of 200 μL (1×10^5 cells/cm^2) of pericytes were seeded into the upper chamber with 600 μL/well of 0 or 100 μg/mL of BMSC-EV added to the lower chamber. After OGD/R exposure, cells on the upper surface of the filter membranes were removed gently by a cotton swab, while cells migrating to the lower surface of the filter membrane were fixed with 4% paraformaldehyde for 15 min before staining with 0.1% crystal violet for 30 min. The number of stained cells was counted under an optical microscope (Olympus, Tokyo, Japan).

Pericytes (2×10^5 cells/well) were seeded into 6-well plates for 48 h until the cells had grown to 100% confluence. A uniform scratch was made by sterile 200 ml pipette tip in the well. The eliminated cells were washed away with PBS three times and then BMSC-EV was added. Initial images were acquired microscopically. Images were taken at 0 and 6h after OGD/R exposure. The migration was determined using Image Pro Plus 6.0 (IPP, Media Cybernetics, Carlsbad, CA, United States) as an average closed width of the wound relative to the initial wound width.

Drug Treatment

Pyrrolidine dithiocarbamate (PDTC; Sigma-Aldrich) was dissolved to 10 μM with dimethyl sulfoxide (DMSO) and added to pericytes 3 h before OGD exposure to inhibit the nuclear factor kappa-light-chain-enhancer of activated B cells (NF-kB) signaling pathway.

Western Blot Analysis

Total protein was extracted with the RIPA lysis buffer (Beyotime Biotechnology) containing 1% phenylmethane sulfonyl fluoride (PMSF). Proteins from the cytoplasm and nuclear fraction were separately extracted using a nuclear protein extraction kit (R0050; Solarbio). A BCA Protein Assay Kit (23227; Solarbio) was used to quantify protein concentrations. Subsequently, proteins were denatured by boiling, separated with 10% sodium dodecyl sulfate polyacrylamide gel electrophoresis (SDS-PAGE), and transferred onto a polyvinylidene fluoride (PVDF) membrane. This was immersed in non-fat milk powder (5%) for 2 h at room temperature to block non-specific binding sites on the membrane. Next, the PVDF membrane was incubated with primary antibodies against p65 (1:1000; #8242; Cell Signaling Technology), phosphorylated-p65 (1:1000; #3033; Cell Signaling Technology), IKBα (1:1000; #4812; Cell Signaling Technology), p-NF-KB inhibitor alpha (p-IKBα; 1:1000; #2859; Cell Signaling Technology), β-actin (1:1000; 20536-1-AP; Proteintech), and Histone H3 (1:1000; #9715; Cell Signaling Technology) at 4°C overnight, followed by the secondary goat anti-mouse or rabbit HRP–linked antibodies. Target bands were visualized by enhanced chemiluminescence reagent (Thermo Fisher Scientific, United States) and analyzed using Image J.

Statistical Analysis

Statistical analyses were performed using Graph Pad Prism 5.0 (San Diego, CA, United States) in triplicate. Differences with $P < 0.05$ were considered statistically significant. All data are presented as mean ± standard error of the mean (SEM). BBB scores were analyzed using a two-way analysis of variance with repeated measures. Statistical analysis between two groups was conducted using Student's *t*-tests and Bonferroni *post hoc* tests.

RESULTS

Extracellular Vesicles Attenuated Neuronal Cell Death and Improved Motor Recovery After SCI *in vivo*

BMSC-EV were isolated in BMSC-culture supernatant as previously described and further identified by TEM and western blot analysis (**Figures 1A,B**). Under the TEM, BMSC-EV had a round-shaped morphology. Unique exosome markers, including CD63, CD9, and CD81 were also confirmed by western blot analysis, while exosome-specific proteins were not detected in EV-free CM. To trace BMSC-EV to their target tissue, BMSC-EV were labeled in red with PKH-26 before injection (**Figure 1C**). As shown in **Figures 1D,E**, numerous BMSC-EV were taken up by pericytes and reached the spinal cord lesion.

To explore the role of BMSC-EV, we performed a series of histology analyses. First, TUNEL assays were used to assess neuronal cell death in the traumatic area of the spinal cord *in vivo*. At 1 dpi, a dramatic reduction in the number of TUNEL-positive cells was found in the BMSC-EV group compared with the SCI+PBS group and EV-free CM treated group (**Figures 2A,D**). Next, we assessed the survival of motor neurons in the lesion core using Nissl staining. After BMSC-EV treatment, the number of Nissl-positive neurons significantly increased. This is suggestive of functional recovery (**Figure 2B**). In summary, these data indicated that BMSC-EV exert an anti-cell death effect.

In addition to glial scars around the lesion, stromal scars at the core of the lesion can also obstruct axon regeneration. Therefore, we further explored the density of neurons and axons in the injured lesion core. Neurofilaments are proteins that specifically exist in neuronal cell bodies and axons and play an important role in maintaining neuronal function and axoplasmic transport. Col-I is produced by pericytes in the core of the lesion, hindering neuronal regeneration. Immunostaining analysis of the 200 kDa subunit of a neurofilament (NF200) and Col-I was performed to assess the density of neurons and axons. At 28 dpi, the staining intensity of NF200 was dramatically reduced while that of Col-I was increased. Interestingly, BMSC-EV administration increased the immunostaining for NF200 but decreased that for Col-I. However, EV-free CM treatment did not alter this effect, indicating that BMSC-EV improved axonal regeneration (**Figures 2C,E,F**).

To further investigate the effect of BMSC-EV on motor function, hindlimb locomotor behavior was assessed using the 21-point BBB locomotor rating scale in an open-field arena. Both hindlimbs were totally paralyzed (BBB score = 0) at 3 dpi. However, rats in the BMSC-EV group exhibited significant improvements in locomotor function compared with rats in

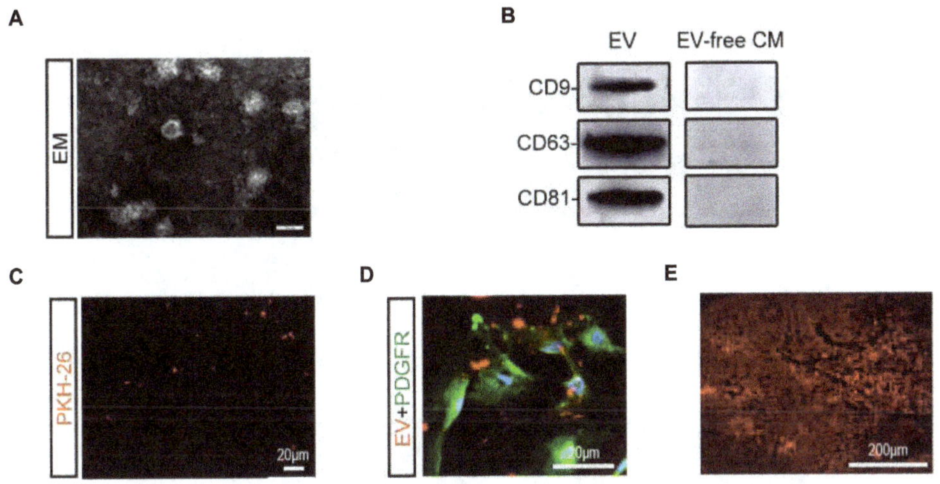

FIGURE 1 | Characterization and labeling of BMSC-EV. **(A)** Morphological observation of BMSC-derived extracellular vesicles (BMSC-EV) by TEM. Scale bar = 100 nm. **(B)** Expression of BMSC-EV markers (CD9, CD63, CD81) was detected using western blot analysis. **(C)** Immunofluorescence image showing the PKH26-stained BMSC-EV (red). Scale bar = 20 μm. **(D)** Immunofluorescence image showing the PKH26-stained BMSC-EV (red) were taken up by pericytes (green). Scale bar = 20 μm. **(E)** Immunofluorescence image showing PKH26-labeled BMSC-EV (red) reaching the SCI lesion. Scale bar = 200 μm.

the SCI+PBS and EV-free CM groups from the second week post-SCI (**Figure 2G**).

BMSC-EV Administration Increases BSCB Pericyte Coverage and Decreases BSCB Permeability

Extracellular vesicles promoted functional recovery by directly acting on neurons, in addition to other effects. The microvasculature and the BSCB were damaged immediately after SCI, peaking in the first week and persisting for up to 6 weeks. Therefore, we measured EB infiltration to determine BSCB permeability. The results proved that the amount of EB in the surrounding tissue was significantly increased after SCI compared to the sham group, and that BMSC-EV reduced the EB extravasation, indicating preservation of BSCB integrity (**Figures 3A,C**).

To further investigate the mechanisms underlying the protection of BSCB integrity by BMSC-EV, we examined pericytes. Pericytes occupy a strategic position in the neurovascular unit, crucially contributing to the structure and function of the vascular bed. Previous studies showed that 5 days after SCI, some pericytes had detached from the vascular wall. Thus, we quantified the percentage of vessels with PDGFRβ-positive pericyte coverage to assess pericyte/vessel contact 5 days after SCI. First, the morphology of PDGFRβ-positive cells after SCI differed from pericytes in the uninjured sham control group. Consistent with previous studies, the vascular wall showed a loss of pericyte coverage, and the morphology of the pericytes differed from those in the uninjured sham controls. Interestingly, our findings demonstrated greater preservation of vascular pericyte coverage after BMSC-exo administration. In contrast, there was no significant effect of exo-free CM treatment (**Figures 3B,D**).

BMSC-EV Inhibit Pericyte Migration via the NF-κB p65 Pathway

Based on the *in vivo* results, we further explored the effect of BMSC-EV on pericytes *in vitro*. Many studies have shown that abnormal migration of pericytes results in an increase in BBB permeability (Pfister et al., 2008; Wan et al., 2018). Thus, we used OGD/R to simulate the pathological environment of SCI *in vitro*. Our data revealed that pericyte migration was enhanced after OGD/R exposure. This migration could be partly attenuated by BMSC-EV administration, as assessed by a wound healing assay and transwell migration assay (**Figure 4**).

We further explored the molecular mechanisms underlying BMSC-EV-mediated migration of pericytes. Numerous studies have confirmed that the NF-kB signaling pathway regulates the migration of various cancer cells (Shostak and Chariot, 2015). Thus, we hypothesized that BMSC-EV regulate pericytes migration through NF-kB signaling. To confirm that the NF-kB signaling pathway participates in the migration of pericytes, we pre-treated pericytes with PDTC, an NF-kB inhibitor before subjecting them to OGD/R. PDTC dramatically decreased the activation of the NF-kB signaling pathway in pericytes as well as the migration of pericytes after OGD/R exposure, as assessed by the Transwell migration and wound healing assay (**Figures 5A–D**). Our results demonstrated that the total protein expression of p-p65 and p65 were enhanced after OGD/R. At the same time, the expression of the nuclear protein NF-kB p65 was increased in pericytes. Compared with EV-free CM treatment, BMSC-EV caused greater inhibition of this increase in pericytes (**Figures 5F–H**). Similarly, immunofluorescence staining revealed the rate at which p65 entered the nucleus was decreased via BMSC-EV treatment (**Figure 5E**). This indicated that pericyte migration was enhanced through activation of the NF-kB signaling pathway and that BMSC-EV inhibited pericytes migration

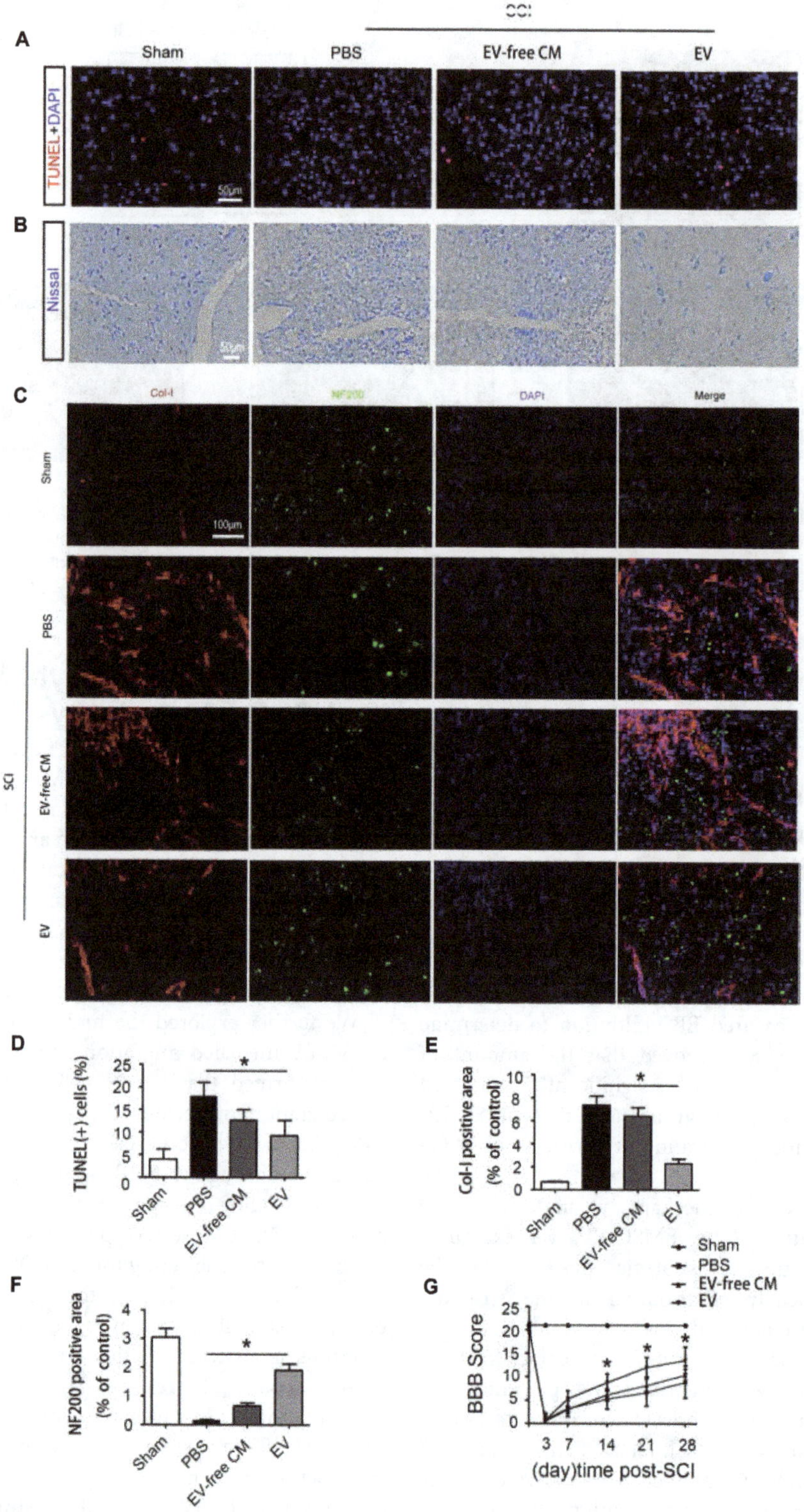

FIGURE 2 | Exosomes improve cell morphology and motor function recovery after SCI *in vivo*. **(A)** TUNEL assay showing fluorescence images of TUNEL-positive apoptotic cells (red) after SCI treated with EV-free CM or BMSC-EV. Cell nuclei were stained with DAPI. Scale bar = 50 μm. **(B)** Nissl staining showing the transverse sections of the spinal cord at 28 dpi ($n = 6$). Scale bar = 50 μm. **(C)** Immunofluorescence staining for Col-I (red) and NF200 (green) in the transverse sections at 28 dpi from different groups. Scale bar = 100 μm. **(D)** Comparison of the number of TUNEL-positive cells with EV-free CM or BMSC-EV treatment ($n = 6$). $^*P < 0.05$. **(E,F)** Semi-quantitative analysis of the percentage of Col-I (red) and NF200 (green) positive areas in each group ($n = 6$). $^*P < 0.05$. **(G)** Representative Basso, Beattie, and Bresnahan (BBB) scores of rats from different groups at different timepoints ($n = 10$). $^*P < 0.05$.

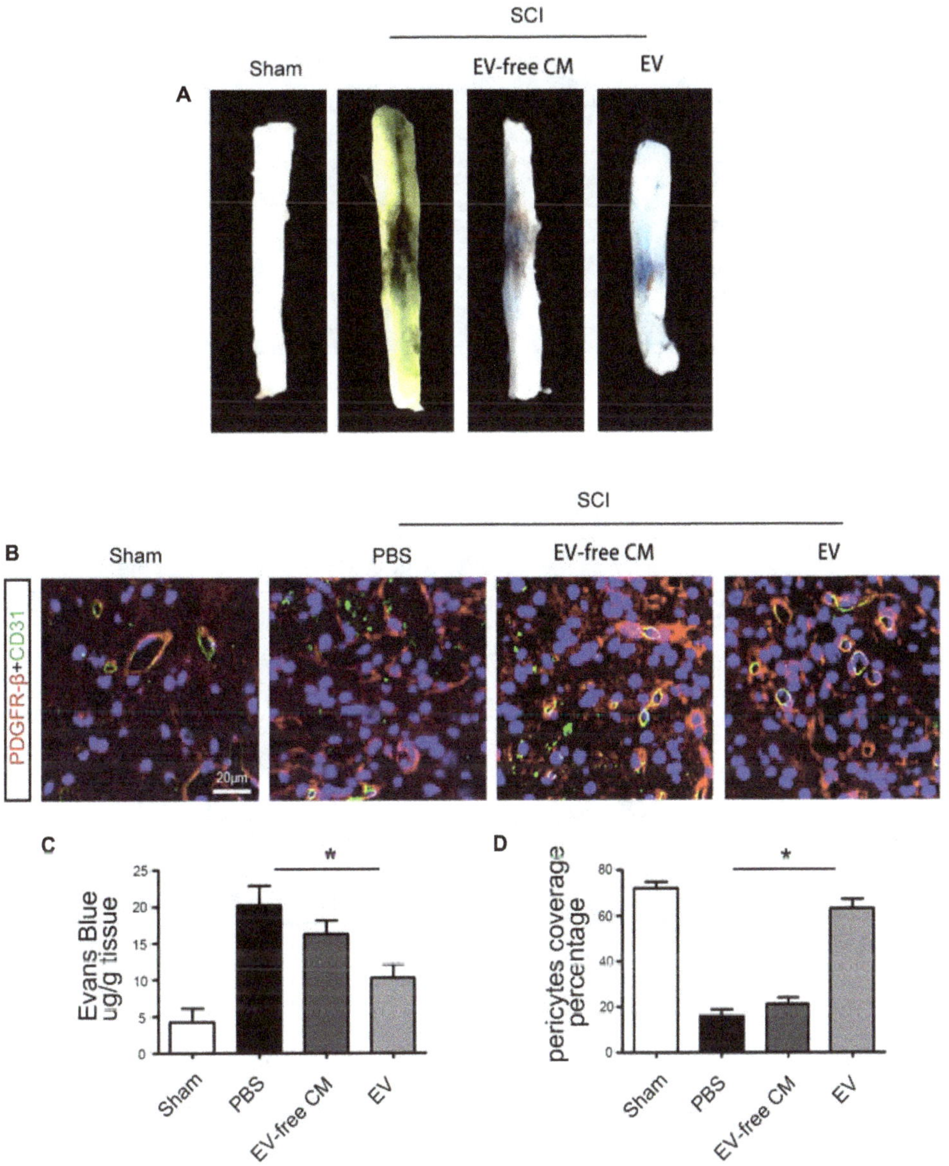

FIGURE 3 | BMSC-EV administration protects the Blood-Spinal Cord Barrier (BSCB). **(A)** Representative gross morphology of Evans Blue (EB) extravasation from different groups. **(B)** Immunolocalization microscopy analysis of CD31+ endothelial cells and PBGFRβ+ pericytes after SCI and treatment with BMSC-EV. Scale bar = 20 μm. **(C)** The effects of BMSC-EV on BSCB permeability represented by quantification of extravascular EB after SCI ($n = 6$). $^{*}P < 0.05$. **(D)** Quantification of regional PDGFRβ-positive pericytes coverage of endothelial cells in spinal cord capillaries ($n = 6$). $^{*}P < 0.05$.

after OGD/R treatment, while EV-free CM did not have this beneficial effect. Collectively, our data suggest that BMSC-EV improve the integrity of BSCB and protect neuronal cells (**Figure 6**).

DISCUSSION

Spinal cord injury can result in paralysis, bladder dysfunction, and even death. However, functional recovery is impeded by neuronal necrosis, ongoing neuroinflammation, the altered microenvironment, and a dysfunctional BSCB (Kjell and Olson, 2016). This highlights the need for effective treatments. Exosomes are essential components of the paracrine factors released by MSCs (Ren, 2018). Our findings demonstrate that BMSC-EV administration critically improves neuronal regeneration and attenuates nerve cell death, which is beneficial for motor function recovery after SCI. Furthermore, pericyte migration could be prohibited by BMSC-EV administration via suppression of the activation of the NF-kB signaling pathway. This led to an improvement in the integrity of the BSCB.

Due to their potential capacity to self-reproduce and undergo multidirectional differentiation, alongside their low immunogenicity and regenerative secretion profile, MSCs have attracted a great deal of attention. Furthermore, cell transplantation treatments have been applied in clinical trials

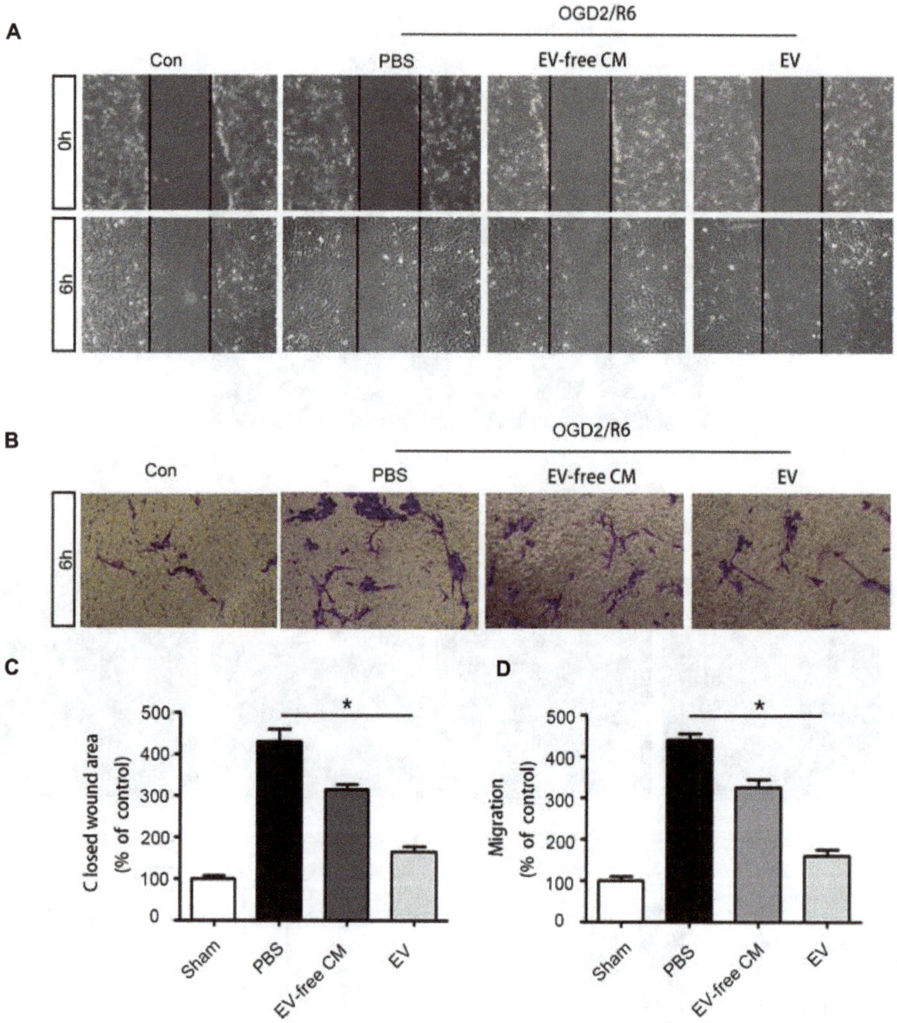

FIGURE 4 | BMSC-EV regulate pericyte migration. **(A,C)** Pericyte migration was detected by healing assay initial images (0 h) and after OGD/R treatment (original magnification 200×) (n = 6). $^*P < 0.05$. **(B,D)** Pericyte migration was detected by a Transwell migration assay after (Oxygen-glucose-deprivation/reperfusion) OGD/R treatment (original magnification 100×) (n = 6). $^*P < 0.05$.

of Parkinson's disease (Cizkova et al., 2011; Venkatesh and Sen, 2017). In addition, MSC therapy in animal models of SCI promoted recovery of motor function (Shende and Subedi, 2017). However, in this study a large number of transplanted BMSCs got trapped in the lung or liver, meaning that few of the MSCs were transferred to the target lesion (Phinney and Prockop, 2007). Thus, there are several limitations and difficulties that need to be addressed before wide clinical application of MSCs. However, recent studies have shown that one potential mechanism driving the beneficial effects of MSCs administration may be the secretion of a large spectrum of molecules rather than the transplanted-MSCs directly differentiating into desired cells (Ratajczak et al., 2014).

EV are one of the most important components of this paracrine secretion. MSC-derived EV contain several important active components, and their double lipid membrane also protects the inner contents from degradation and digestion (Marote et al., 2016; Yang et al., 2017). Furthermore, EV can freely pass through the BSCB, which facilitates their ability to reach the lesion. All of these are beneficial for functional recovery after SCI (Liu et al., 2018). Therefore, we chose BMSC-EV for SCI in this study. We successfully isolated EV from BMSCs, which was confirmed by TEM and labeling with specific exosome surface markers, including CD9, CD63, and CD81. Furthermore, our results demonstrate that BMSC-EV administration contributed to neuronal survival, with less apoptosis and promotion of functional recovery observed.

The BSCB plays an essential role in supporting proper nervous system function and is modulated by neurovascular unit cells to maintain its unique properties and function (Bartanusz et al., 2011). Pericytes, part of the neurovascular unit, play a vital role in vascular integrity and barrier properties during development

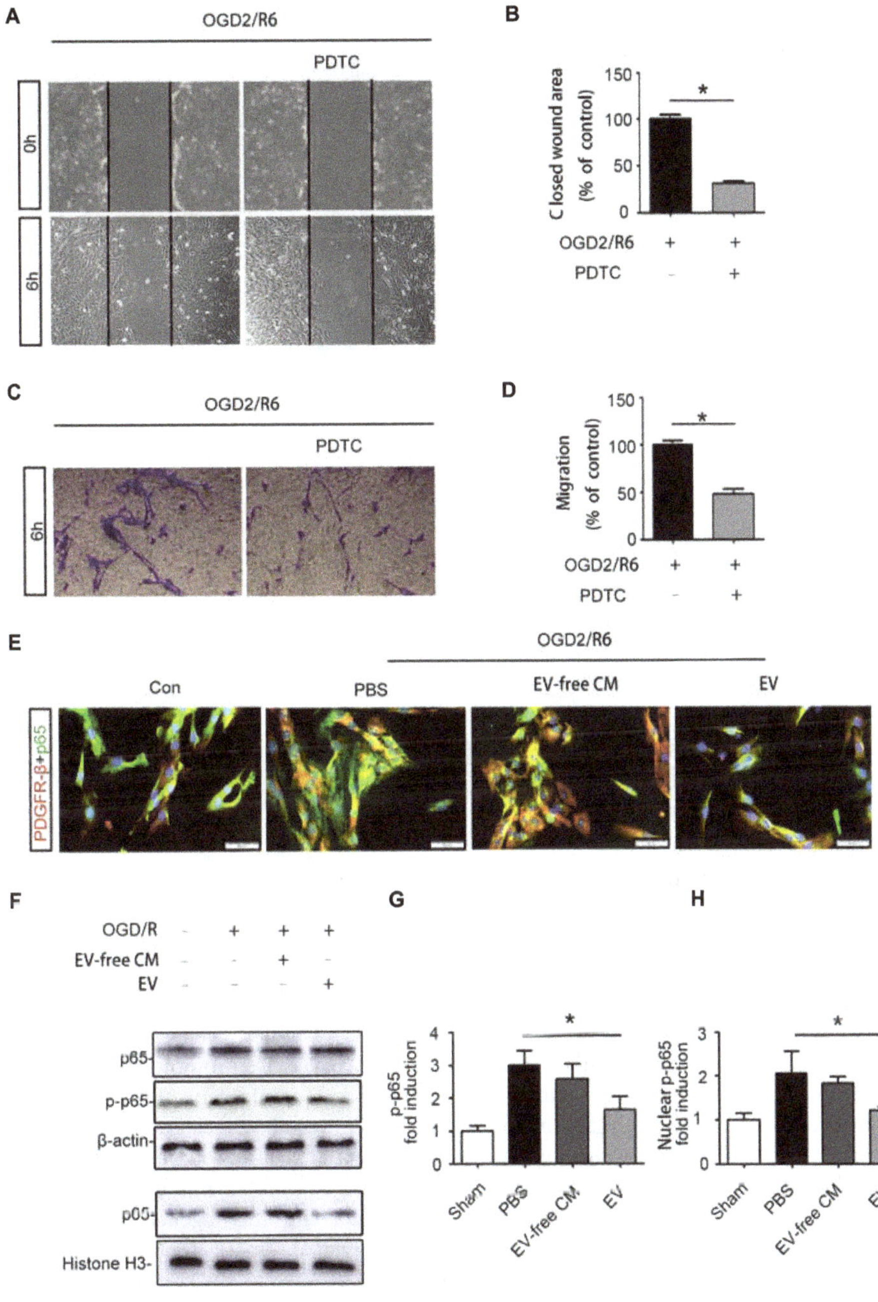

FIGURE 5 | BMSC-EV regulate pericyte migration via NF-kB p65 signaling. **(A,B)** Pericyte migration was prohibited by PDTC under the OGD/R condition, as determined by the wound healing assay (original magnification 200×) (n = 6). $^*P < 0.05$. **(C,D)** Pericyte migration was prohibited by PDTC under the OGD/R condition, as detected by a Transwell migration assay (original magnification 100×) (n = 6). $^*P < 0.05$. **(E)** Immunofluorescence images showing the proportion of p65 entering the nuclei of pericytes in different groups (original magnification 400×). $^*P < 0.05$. **(F,G,H)** Western blot analysis of the total protein expression of p-NF-kB p65 and NF-kB p65 in pericytes from different groups (n = 6). $^*P < 0.05$.

and physiological conditions (Sweeney et al., 2016). Previous studies demonstrated that pericytes participate in maintaining microvascular stability mainly via three potential mechanisms: regulation of vesicular transport and bulk flow transcytosis, promotion of endothelial tight junction protein expression (i.e., ZO-1 and occludin), and moderate tight junctional alignment (Jo et al., 2013). In neurological conditions, such as stroke and amyotrophic lateral sclerosis (ALS), mounting evidence has demonstrated that abnormal migration of pericytes contributes to further enlargement of the lesion (Winkler et al., 2013; Cheng et al., 2018). Blood vessels at the injury site are immediately destroyed after SCI and even the BSCB distant from the injury core was permanently disrupted (Figley et al., 2014). SCI causes pericytes to detach from the vascular wall, leading

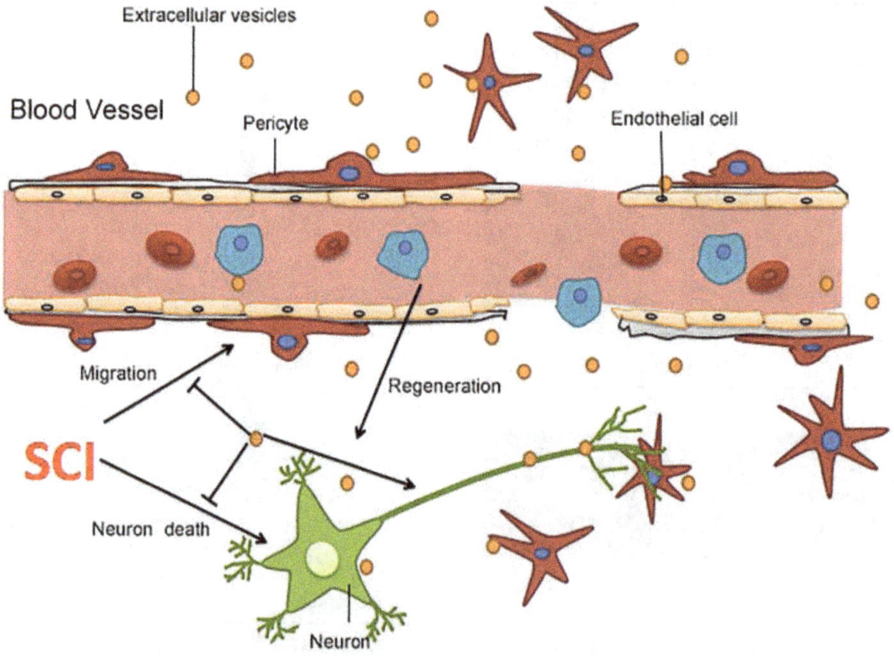

FIGURE 6 | Summary of the proposed mechanism of BMSC-EV-induced protection after SCI. BMSC-EV have the capacity to repress neuronal cell death, promote neuronal survival, improve axonal regeneration, and therefore boost locomotor recovery after SCI. Moreover, BMSC-EV protected the BSCB through suppression of pericytes detaching from the microvascular wall.

to microvascular stability disruption and an increase in BSCB permeability. Here, our findings demonstrate that extracellular vesicles from BMSCs improve the structural integrity of the BSCB by inhibiting the migration of pericytes and improving the rate of pericyte coverage. As a result, better functional recovery after SCI was obtained by BMSC-EV treatment.

In the resting state, NF-κB signaling participates in the regulation of proliferation, differentiation, migration, survival, and other key cellular activities. Multitudinous pro-inflammatory agents induced by SCI, such as cytokines, free radicals, and reactive oxygen species, can activate NF-κB, which leads to an inflammatory response and neurotoxic effects by glial cells (Rahimifard et al., 2017). Neuroinflammation and ischemia induce two different types of reactive astrocytes, namely "A1" and "A2" (analogy to the "M1"/"M2" macrophage nomenclature), and A1 astrocytes might be harmful to synapses (Liddelow et al., 2017). Previous studies demonstrated that A1 astrocytes that are activated via NF-κB signaling impede functional recovery after SCI (Wang et al., 2018). Furthermore, activation of NF-κB in BV2 microglia leads to the production of multiple pro-inflammatory cytokines (Blasi et al., 1990; Zhou et al., 2016). In our study, NF-kB p65 in pericytes was increasingly phosphorylated and the amount of NF-kB p65 within the nucleus was elevated after exposure to OGD/R. At the same time, OGD/R promoted pericyte migration, while PDTC inhibited it. Thus, all of this demonstrates that the pericytes migrate away from the vascular wall via activation of NF-κB signaling. In addition, we have shown for the first time that exosome administration could significantly suppress abnormal migration of pericytes via inhibition of the NF-kB signaling pathway. This suggests a potential mechanism whereby pericyte coverage is enhanced at an early stage of SCI, as assessed via the number of pericytes adhering to endothelial cells.

Overall, our findings are in accordance with results reported by previous studies, which have revealed that MSC-derived extracellular vesicles promote neurovascular remodeling as well as reducing neuroinflammation after SCI or traumatic brain injury (Kim et al., 2016; Zhang et al., 2017; Liu et al., 2018). Furthermore, Li and colleagues found that exosomes derived from microRNA-133b-modified MSCs improved the survival of neurons and the regeneration of axons via extracellular signal-regulated kinase 1/2 (ERK1/2), signal transducer and activator of transcription 3 (STAT3), and cAMP response element binding protein (CREB) signaling pathways (Li et al., 2018). The extracellular vesicles components involved in the regulation of pericyte migration remain to be elucidated. Moreover, we only detected the migration of pericytes 6 h after OGD exposure. Such a time period makes it impossible to identify the exact effect of BMSC-EV. Thus, observations at longer timepoints should be performed in future experiments.

In summary, our study provides the first evidence that BMSC-EV can effectively inhibit the migration of pericytes, thereby maintaining the integrity of the BSCB after SCI. This was accompanied by a reduction in neuronal cell apoptosis, axonal regeneration, and locomotor recovery. Therefore, our results suggest that extracellular vesicles may serve as a promising treatment strategy for SCI.

AUTHOR CONTRIBUTIONS

YJ conceived and supervised the research. YLu and YZ designed and planned the experiments. YLu, YZ, LW, and KW performed the experiments. YLi, RD, and YY were involved in collecting the data and statistical analyses. YLu drafted the manuscript and figures. YZ, RZ, and KW reviewed the manuscript.

FUNDING

This study was supported by National Natural Science Foundation of China (U1604170).

REFERENCES

Bartanusz, V., Jezova, D., Alajajian, B., and Digicaylioglu, M. (2011). The blood-spinal cord barrier: morphology and clinical implications. *Ann. Neurol.* 70, 194–206. doi: 10.1002/ana.22421

Basso, D. M., Beattie, M. S., and Bresnahan, J. C. (1995). A sensitive and reliable locomotor rating scale for open field testing in rats. *J. Neurotrauma* 12, 1–21. doi: 10.1089/neu.1995.12.1

Blasi, E., Barluzzi, R., Bocchini, V., Mazzolla, R., and Bistoni, F. (1990). Immortalization of murine microglial cells by a v-raf/v-myc carrying retrovirus. *J. Neuroimmunol.* 27, 229–237. doi: 10.1016/0165-5728(90)90073-V

Camussi, G., Deregibus, M. C., Bruno, S., Cantaluppi, V., and Biancone, L. (2010). Exosomes/microvesicles as a mechanism of cell-to-cell communication. *Kidney Int.* 78, 838–848. doi: 10.1038/ki.2010.278

Caplan, A. I., and Correa, D. (2011). The MSC: an injury drugstore. *Cell Stem Cell* 9, 11–15. doi: 10.1016/j.stem.2011.06.008

Caplan, A. I., and Dennis, J. E. (2006). Mesenchymal stem cells as trophic mediators. *J. Cell. Biochem.* 98, 1076–1084. doi: 10.1002/jcb.20886

Cheng, J., Korte, N., Nortley, R., Sethi, H., Tang, Y., and Attwell, D. (2018). Targeting pericytes for therapeutic approaches to neurological disorders. *Acta Neuropathol.* 136, 507–523. doi: 10.1007/s00401-018-1893-0

Cizkova, D., Novotna, I., Slovinska, L., Vanicky, I., Jergova, S., Rosocha, J., et al. (2011). Repetitive intrathecal catheter delivery of bone marrow mesenchymal stromal cells improves functional recovery in a rat model of contusive spinal cord injury. *J. Neurotrauma* 28, 1951–1961. doi: 10.1089/neu.2010.1413

Eckert, M. J., and Martin, M. J. (2017). Trauma: spinal cord injury. *Surg. Clin. North Am.* 97, 1031–1045. doi: 10.1016/j.suc.2017.06.008

Figley, S. A., Khosravi, R., Legasto, J. M., Tseng, Y. F., and Fehlings, M. G. (2014). Characterization of vascular disruption and blood-spinal cord barrier permeability following traumatic spinal cord injury. *J. Neurotrauma* 31, 541–552. doi: 10.1089/neu.2013.3034

Goodarzi, P., Larijani, B., Alavi-Moghadam, S., Tayanloo-Beik, A., Mohamadi-Jahani, F., Ranjbaran, N., et al. (2018). Mesenchymal stem cells-derived exosomes for wound regeneration. *Adv. Exp. Med. Biol.* 1119, 119–131. doi: 10.1007/5584_2018_251

He, Q. W., Xia, Y. P., Chen, S. C., Wang, Y., Huang, M., Huang, Y., et al. (2013). Astrocyte-derived sonic hedgehog contributes to angiogenesis in brain microvascular endothelial cells via RhoA/ROCK pathway after oxygen-glucose deprivation. *Mol. Neurobiol.* 47, 976–987. doi: 10.1007/s12035-013-8396-8

He, Z., Zhou, Y., Wang, Q., Li, J., Zheng, Z., Chen, J., et al. (2017). Inhibiting endoplasmic reticulum stress by lithium chloride contributes to the integrity of blood-spinal cord barrier and functional recovery after spinal cord injury. *Am. J. Transl. Res.* 9, 1012–1024.

Jo, D. H., Kim, J. H., Heo, J. I., Kim, J. H., and Cho, C. H. (2013). Interaction between pericytes and endothelial cells leads to formation of tight junction in hyaloid vessels. *Mol. Cells* 36, 465–471. doi: 10.1007/s10059-013-0228-1

Juan, T., and Furthauer, M. (2018). Biogenesis and function of ESCRT-dependent extracellular vesicles. *Semin. Cell Dev. Biol.* 74, 66–77. doi: 10.1016/j.semcdb.2017.08.022

Kim, D. K., Nishida, H., An, S. Y., Shetty, A. K., Bartosh, T. J., and Prockop, D. J. (2016). Chromatographically isolated CD63+CD81+ extracellular vesicles from mesenchymal stromal cells rescue cognitive impairments after TBI. *Proc. Natl. Acad. Sci. U.S.A.* 113, 170–175. doi: 10.1073/pnas.1522297113

Kjell, J., and Olson, L. (2016). Rat models of spinal cord injury: from pathology to potential therapies. *Dis. Model. Mech.* 9, 1125–1137. doi: 10.1242/dmm.025833

Li, D., Zhang, P., Yao, X., Li, H., Shen, H., Li, X., et al. (2018). Exosomes derived from MIR-133b-modified mesenchymal stem cells promote recovery after spinal cord injury. *Front. Neurosci.* 12:845. doi: 10.3389/fnins.2018.00845

Liddelow, S. A., Guttenplan, K. A., Clarke, L. E., Bennett, F. C., Bohlen, C. J., Schirmer, L., et al. (2017). Neurotoxic reactive astrocytes are induced by activated microglia. *Nature* 541, 481–487. doi: 10.1038/nature21029

Liu, W., Wang, Y., Gong, F., Rong, Y., Luo, Y., Tang, P., et al. (2018). Exosomes derived from bone mesenchymal stem cells repair traumatic spinal cord injury by suppressing the activation of A1 neurotoxic reactive astrocytes. *J. Neurotrauma* 36, 469–484. doi: 10.1089/neu.2018.5835

Marote, A., Teixeira, F. G., Mendes-Pinheiro, B., and Salgado, A. J. (2016). MSCs-derived exosomes: cell-secreted nanovesicles with regenerative potential. *Front. Pharmacol.* 7:231. doi: 10.3389/fphar.2016.00231

Pfister, F., Feng, Y., vom Hagen, F., Hoffmann, S., Molema, G., Hillebrands, J. L., et al. (2008). Pericyte migration: a novel mechanism of pericyte loss in experimental diabetic retinopathy. *Diabetes* 57, 2495–2502. doi: 10.2337/db08-0325

Phinney, D. G., and Pittenger, M. F. (2017). Concise review: MSC-derived exosomes for cell-free therapy. *Stem Cells* 35, 851–858. doi: 10.1002/stem.2575

Phinney, D. G., and Prockop, D. J. (2007). Concise review: mesenchymal stem/multipotent stromal cells: the state of transdifferentiation and modes of tissue repair–current views. *Stem Cells* 25, 2896–2902. doi: 10.1634/stemcells.2007-0637

Rahimifard, M., Maqbool, F., Moeini-Nodeh, S., Niaz, K., Abdollahi, M., Braidy, N., et al. (2017). Targeting the TLR4 signaling pathway by polyphenols: a novel therapeutic strategy for neuroinflammation. *Ageing Res. Rev.* 36, 11–19. doi: 10.1016/j.arr.2017.02.004

Ratajczak, M. Z., Jadczyk, T., Pedziwiatr, D., and Wojakowski, W. (2014). New advances in stem cell research: practical implications for regenerative medicine. *Pol. Arch. Med. Wewn.* 124, 417–426. doi: 10.20452/pamw.2355

Ren, K. (2018). Exosomes in perspective: a potential surrogate for stem cell therapy. *Odontology* doi: 10.1007/s10266-018-0395-9 [Epub ahead of print].

Schwab, M. E. (2004). Nogo and axon regeneration. *Curr. Opin. Neurobiol.* 14, 118–124. doi: 10.1016/j.conb.2004.01.004

Shende, P., and Subedi, M. (2017). Pathophysiology, mechanisms and applications of mesenchymal stem cells for the treatment of spinal cord injury. *Biomed. Pharmacother.* 91, 693–706. doi: 10.1016/j.biopha.2017.04.126

Shostak, K., and Chariot, A. (2015). EGFR and NF-kappaB: partners in cancer. *Trends Mol. Med.* 21, 385–393. doi: 10.1016/j.molmed.2015.04.001

Sun, F., Park, K. K., Belin, S., Wang, D., Lu, T., Chen, G., et al. (2011). Sustained axon regeneration induced by co-deletion of PTEN and SOCS3. *Nature* 480, 372–375. doi: 10.1038/nature10594

Sweeney, M. D., Ayyadurai, S., and Zlokovic, B. V. (2016). Pericytes of the neurovascular unit: key functions and signaling pathways. *Nat. Neurosci.* 19, 771–783. doi: 10.1038/nn.4288

Tkach, M., and Thery, C. (2016). Communication by extracellular vesicles: where we are and where we need to go. *Cell* 164, 1226–1232. doi: 10.1016/j.cell.2016.01.043

Venkatesh, K., and Sen, D. (2017). Mesenchymal stem cells as a source of dopaminergic neurons: a potential cell based therapy for Parkinson's disease. *Curr. Stem Cell Res. Ther.* 12, 326–347. doi: 10.2174/1574888X12666161114122059

Wan, Y., Jin, H. J., Zhu, Y. Y., Fang, Z., Mao, L., He, Q., et al. (2018). MicroRNA-149-5p regulates blood-brain barrier permeability after transient middle cerebral artery occlusion in rats by targeting S1PR2 of pericytes. *FASEB J.* 32, 3133–3148. doi: 10.1096/fj.201701121R

Wang, Y., Zhao, R., Liu, D., Deng, W., Xu, G., Liu, W., et al. (2018). Exosomes Derived from miR-214-enriched bone marrow-derived mesenchymal stem cells regulate oxidative damage in cardiac stem cells by targeting CaMKII. *Oxid. Med. Cell. Longev.* 2018:4971261. doi: 10.1155/2018/4971261

Winkler, E. A., Sengillo, J. D., Sullivan, J. S., Henkel, J. S., Appel, S. H., and Zlokovic, B. V. (2013). Blood-spinal cord barrier breakdown and pericyte reductions in amyotrophic lateral sclerosis. *Acta Neuropathol.* 125, 111–120. doi: 10.1007/s00401-012-1039-8

Xu, P., and Yang, X. (2018). The efficacy and safety of mesenchymal stem cell transplantation for spinal cord injury patients: a meta-analysis and systematic review. *Cell Transplant.* 28, 36–46. doi: 10.1177/0963689718808471

Yang, Y., Ye, Y., Su, X., He, J., Bai, W., and He, X. (2017). MSCs-derived exosomes and neuroinflammation, neurogenesis and therapy of traumatic brain injury. *Front. Cell Neurosci.* 11:55. doi: 10.3389/fncel.2017.00055

Zagrean, A. M., Hermann, D. M., Opris, I., Zagrean, L., and Popa-Wagner, A. (2018). Multicellular crosstalk between exosomes and the neurovascular unit after cerebral ischemia. Therapeutic Implications. *Front. Neurosci.* 12:811. doi: 10.3389/fnins.2018.00811

Zhang, Y., Chopp, M., Zhang, Z. G., Katakowski, M., Xin, H., Qu, C., et al. (2017). Systemic administration of cell-free exosomes generated by human bone marrow derived mesenchymal stem cells cultured under 2D and 3D conditions improves functional recovery in rats after traumatic brain injury. *Neurochem. Int.* 111, 69–81. doi: 10.1016/j.neuint.2016.08.003

Zhou, H. J., Wang, L. Q., Xu, Q. S., Fan, Z. X., Zhu, Y., Jiang, H., et al. (2016). Downregulation of miR-199b promotes the acute spinal cord injury through IKKbeta-NF-kappaB signaling pathway activating microglial cells. *Exp. Cell Res.* 349, 60–67. doi: 10.1016/j.yexcr.2016.09.020

12

Fluoxetine and Vortioxetine Reverse Depressive-Like Phenotype and Memory Deficits Induced by $A\beta_{1-42}$ Oligomers in Mice: A Key Role of Transforming Growth Factor-β1

Sebastiano Alfio Torrisi[1†], Federica Geraci[1†], Maria Rosaria Tropea[1†], Margherita Grasso[2,3], Giuseppe Caruso[3], Annamaria Fidilio[2], Nicolò Musso[4], Giulia Sanfilippo[1], Fabio Tascedda[5], Agostino Palmeri[1], Salvatore Salomone[1], Filippo Drago[1], Daniela Puzzo[1,3], Gian Marco Leggio[1‡] and Filippo Caraci[2,3‡]*

[1] Department of Biomedical and Biotechnological Sciences, University of Catania, Catania, Italy, [2] Department of Drug Sciences, University of Catania, Catania, Italy, [3] Oasi Research Institute—IRCCS, Troina, Italy, [4] Bio-nanotech Research and Innovation Tower (BRIT), University of Catania, Catania, Italy, [5] Department of Life Sciences and Center for Neuroscience and Neurotechnology, University of Modena and Reggio Emilia, Modena, Italy

***Correspondence**
Filippo Caraci
carafil@hotmail.com

†These authors have contributed equally to this work.

‡These authors share last co-authorship.

Depression is a risk factor for the development of Alzheimer's disease (AD), and the presence of depressive symptoms significantly increases the conversion of mild cognitive impairment (MCI) into AD. A long-term treatment with antidepressants reduces the risk to develop AD, and different second-generation antidepressants such as selective serotonin reuptake inhibitors (SSRIs) are currently being studied for their neuroprotective properties in AD. In the present work, the SSRI fluoxetine and the new multimodal antidepressant vortioxetine were tested for their ability to prevent memory deficits and depressive-like phenotype induced by intracerebroventricular injection of amyloid-β (1-42) ($A\beta_{1-42}$) oligomers in 2-month-old C57BL/6 mice. Starting from 7 days before Aβ injection, fluoxetine (10 mg/kg) and vortioxetine (5 and 10 mg/kg) were intraperitoneally injected daily for 24 days. Chronic treatment with fluoxetine and vortioxetine (both at the dose of 10 mg/kg) was able to rescue the loss of memory assessed 14 days after Aβ injection by the passive avoidance task and the object recognition test. Both antidepressants reversed the increase in immobility time detected 19 days after Aβ injection by forced swim test. Vortioxetine exerted significant antidepressant effects also at the dose of 5 mg/kg. A significant deficit of transforming growth factor-β1 (TGF-β1), paralleling memory deficits and depressive-like phenotype, was found in the hippocampus of Aβ-injected mice in combination with a significant reduction of the synaptic proteins synaptophysin and PSD-95. Fluoxetine and vortioxetine completely rescued hippocampal TGF-β1 levels in Aβ-injected mice as well as synaptophysin and PSD-95 levels. This is the first evidence that a chronic treatment with fluoxetine or vortioxetine can prevent both cognitive deficits and depressive-like phenotype in a non-transgenic animal model of AD with a key contribution of TGF-β1.

Keywords: Alzheimer's disease, amyloid-β, vortioxetine, antidepressants, fluoxetine, memory, TGF-β1, depression

INTRODUCTION

Alzheimer's disease (AD) is a neurodegenerative disorder characterized by memory loss, cognitive decline, and neuropsychiatric symptoms, such as depression and psychotic signs, which strongly interfere with normal daily activities (Lanctôt et al., 2017). Different neurobiological and clinical links have been found between depression and AD (Caraci et al., 2018). Depression is a risk factor for the development of AD, and the presence of depressive symptoms significantly increases the conversion of mild cognitive impairment (MCI) into AD (Modrego and Ferrández, 2004). Common pathophysiological events have been identified in depression and AD, including activation of the hypothalamic–pituitary–adrenal (HPA) axis with increased glucocorticoid levels, neuroinflammation with an aberrant tumor necrosis factor-α (TNF-α) signaling, and an impairment of transforming growth factor-β1 (TGF-β1) signaling (Caraci et al., 2018).

Intracerebroventricular (i.c.v.) injection of oligomers of amyloid-β (1-42) ($A\beta_{1\text{-}42}$), the most toxic form of amyloid aggregates in AD brain, can induce both memory deficits and depressive-like phenotype in rats (Colaianna et al., 2010; Schiavone et al., 2017) and mice (Ledo et al., 2013; Ledo et al., 2016), while an acute treatment with the selective reuptake inhibitor (SSRI) fluoxetine can revert this phenotype (Ledo et al., 2013; Ledo et al., 2016; Schiavone et al., 2017). Evidence also exists that fluoxetine prevents amyloid pathology and reverses memory impairment in different AD animal models (Wang et al., 2014; Jin et al., 2016). Interestingly, a continued long-term treatment with antidepressants is known to reduce the risk to develop AD (Kessing et al., 2009; Kessing, 2012). It has been hypothesized that a chronic treatment with second-generation antidepressants can exert relevant neuroprotective effects in depressed MCI patients with a high risk to develop AD, but the molecular mechanisms underlying the neuroprotective effects of antidepressants are not yet completely understood (Caraci et al., 2018).

Deficit of TGF-β1 signaling is a common pathophysiological event in both depression and AD (Caraci et al., 2018). Among SSRIs, fluoxetine increases circulating TGF-β1 levels in depressed patients (Lee and Kim, 2006; Sutcigil et al., 2007) and prevents Aβ-induced toxicity in neuronal cultures by increasing the release of TGF-β1 (Caraci et al., 2016). However, it is presently unknown whether a chronic treatment with fluoxetine or other second-generation antidepressant drugs can prevent memory deficits and depressive-like phenotype in animal models of AD.

Vortioxetine is a third-generation antidepressant with a novel, multimodal, mechanism of action, directly acting on several serotonin (5-hydroxytryptamine, 5-HT) receptors (as an agonist on 5-HT_{1A} receptor, a partial agonist on 5-HT_{1B}, and an antagonist on 5-HT_{1D}, 5-HT_3, and 5-HT_7) besides inhibiting the serotonin transporter (SERT; Mørk et al., 2012). Several preclinical studies have clearly demonstrated robust pro-cognitive effects of vortioxetine in different animal models of depression (Pehrson et al., 2015). In particular, vortioxetine displays a superior efficacy on visuospatial memory and depressive-like behavior, than does fluoxetine, in aged mice (Li et al., 2015; Li et al., 2017). Recent clinical studies also suggest an improved efficacy of vortioxetine on specific clinical domains, where SSRIs are less effective, such as cognitive deficits associated with major depressive disorder (MDD; Thase et al., 2016), in particular in elderly patients (McIntyre et al., 2016).

No studies have been conducted so far to examine the preclinical efficacy of vortioxetine compared with fluoxetine in treating depressive-like behavior and memory impairment induced by the i.c.v. injection of $A\beta_{1\text{-}42}$ oligomers.

The aim of the present study is to assess whether a chronic treatment with fluoxetine or vortioxetine can prevent memory deficits and depressive-like phenotype in a non-Tg model of AD obtained by i.c.v. injection of $A\beta_{1\text{-}42}$ oligomers.

We show that a chronic (24 days) treatment with fluoxetine or vortioxetine in young (2-month-old) C57BL/6 mice can revert both Aβ-induced depressive-like behavior and memory impairment with a key contribute played by TGF-β1.

MATERIALS AND METHODS

Animals

Eight-week-old male C57BL/6 mice, from Envigo RMS s.r.l. laboratories (San Pietro al Natisone, Italy), were individually housed, with free access to chow and water, in an air-conditioned room, with a 12-h light–dark cycle and with constant temperature (23 ± 1°C) and humidity (57 ± 3%) conditions. Animals were left undisturbed for 1 week before beginning any behavioral procedure. All animal experiments were carried out in accordance with Italian (D.M. 116192) and EEC (O.J. of E.C.L 358/1 12/18/1986) regulations on protection of animals. Every effort has been made to minimize animal suffering and to reduce the number of animals used.

Preparation of Human $A\beta_{1\text{-}42}$ Oligomers and i.c.v. Injection in Mice

Synthetic human $A\beta_{1\text{-}42}$ oligomers were prepared according to the original protocol of Klein's group (Gong et al., 2003). Briefly, the $A\beta_{1\text{-}42}$ lyophilized peptide, purchased from Bachem Distribution Services GmbH (Weil am Rhein, Germany), was dissolved in trifluoroacetic acid (TFA) (1 mg/ml) and sonicated in a water bath sonicator for 10 min. Then, TFA was evaporated under a gentle stream of argon, and 1 ml of 1,1,1,3,3,3-hexafluoro-2-propanol (HFIP) was added to the peptide. After 1-h incubation at 37°C, the peptide solution was dried under a stream of argon and then solubilized again by adding 2 ml of HFIP. Finally, HFIP was removed by argon streaming followed by further drying in a lyophilizer for 1 h, and then $A\beta_{1\text{-}42}$ was suspended in 5 mM of anhydrous dimethyl sulfoxide (DMSO), before dilution to 100 μM in ice-cold cell culture medium Dulbecco's Modified Eagle Medium/Nutrient Mixture F-12 (DMEM/F12). Samples of $A\beta_{1\text{-}42}$ at the concentration of 100 μM were incubated for 72 h at 4°C and then stored at −20°C until use.

To obtain a non-transgenic (non-Tg) AD model, animals were anesthetized for 7 min with 2.5% isoflurane using a vaporizer system and gently restrained only during the injection procedure. $A\beta_{1\text{-}42}$ oligomers were administered i.c.v. into the brain. Synthetic human $A\beta_{1\text{-}42}$ oligomers were diluted from the stock in DMEM solution (100 μM) in sterile 0.1 M phosphate buffered saline (PBS) (pH 7.4) at a final concentration of 10 μM and then injected i.c.v. Sterile 0.1 M PBS was injected i.c.v. into control animals (vehicle). Intracerebroventricular injection was used because of its simplicity with respect to stereotaxis in mice and to ensure diffusion of $A\beta_{1-42}$ in the whole brain (Maurice et al., 1996; Leggio et al., 2016). Two microliters was injected using a microsyringe with a 28-gauge 3.0-mm-long stainless steel needle (Hamilton); 2 μL of the 10 μM Aβ solution corresponds to 20 pmol of Aβ monomer equivalent, e.g., 0.09 μg Aβ per mouse brain (weighing around 500 mg). Assuming that soluble Aβ oligomers are freely diffusing in cerebrospinal fluid and then in the brain, their final concentration would be approximately 0.18 μg/g of tissue.

Drugs and Treatment

Vortioxetine hydrobromide [purity > 98.0% (HPLC)] was provided by H. Lundbeck A/S (Denmark) according to the MTA N.417394 signed by University of Catania (Department of Drug Sciences) and H. Lundbeck A/S and Lundbeck Italia S.p.A. Fluoxetine hydrochloride [product number: F132; purity > 98.0% (TLC)] was purchased from Sigma-Aldrich (St Louis, MO). Both compounds were dissolved in DMSO and further diluted with a final concentration of 1% of DMSO. Fluoxetine was administered intraperitoneally (i.p.) at the dose of 10 mg/kg (100 μL/10 g body weight), while vortioxetine was administered i.p. at two different doses (5 and 10 mg/kg; 100 μL/10 g body weight). Control animals received the vehicle i.p. (100 μL/10 g, DMSO 1%). The fluoxetine dose and the two vortioxetine doses were selected on the basis of previous studies where these antidepressant drugs were administered in animal models of depression (Pehrson et al., 2015).

Experimental Design

In order to assess the effects of fluoxetine and vortioxetine on depressive-like behavior and memory impairment induced by Aβ oligomers, three different cohorts of animals were used, according to the following experimental design.

Experiment 1 (first cohort): No i.c.v. injection of $A\beta_{1-42}$ oligomers was performed in this cohort. Mice were randomly divided into four experimental groups (n = 7–10 mice per treatment group): vehicle, fluoxetine (FLX) 10 mg/kg, vortioxetine (VTX) 5 mg/kg, and VTX 10 mg/kg. All drugs were administered i.p. for 21 days. To assess the antidepressant activity of fluoxetine and vortioxetine, mice were tested in the forced swim test (FST) on day 22.

Experiment 2 (second cohort): $A\beta_{1-42}$ oligomers or PBS i.c.v. injection was performed in this cohort of mice 7 days after the beginning of antidepressant treatment (day 7). The treatment with antidepressants lasted until day 26, when all behavioral tests were completed. Mice were randomly allocated to five experimental groups (n = 7–8 animals/group): PBS i.c.v. + vehicle i.p., Aβ i.c.v. + vehicle i.p., Aβ i.c.v. + FLX 10 mg/kg i.p., Aβ i.c.v. + VTX 5 mg/kg i.p., and Aβ i.c.v. + VTX 10 mg/kg i.p. Memory deficits were evaluated after 24 days of chronic treatment with FLX or VTX in the passive avoidance test (PAT), 15–17 days after Aβ injection, whereas depressive-like behavior was evaluated with FST after 26 days of treatment with antidepressant drugs.

Experiment 3 (third cohort): Animals received 3 weeks of treatment with antidepressants and $A\beta_{1-42}$ oligomers or PBS. Intracerebroventricular injection was performed 7 days after the beginning of antidepressant treatment (day 7). Experimental groups were not only those described in Experiment 2 but also those included the following four experimental groups: vehicle, FLX 10 mg/kg, VTX 5 mg/kg, and VTX 10 mg/kg. This third cohort of animals was tested in the object recognition test (ORT), after 21 days of chronic treatment with FLX or VTX.

Forced Swim Test

The FST protocol employed here was adapted from Porsolt et al., (1978). Mice were placed for 6 min in a 4-L Pyrex glass beaker containing 3 L of water at 24 ± 1°C. Water was changed between animals. After a habituation period of 2 min, mobility and immobility were recorded during the last 4 min of the 6-min testing period. A trained researcher blinded to group assignment recorded immobility time using a stopwatch. An increase in immobility time indicates depressive-like behavior. A mouse was judged immobile when it floated in an upright position and displayed only small movements to keep its head above water.

Passive Avoidance Test

PAT was performed as previously described (Leggio et al., 2016). The apparatus for the step-through PAT was an automated shuttle box divided into an illuminated compartment and a dark compartment of the same size by a wall with a guillotine door. In the experimental session, each mouse was trained to adapt to the step-through passive avoidance apparatus. In the adaptation trial, the animal was placed into the illuminated compartment. After 10 s, the door between these two boxes was opened, and the mouse was allowed to freely move into the dark compartment. The learning trial was similar to the adaptation trial except that the door was closed automatically as soon as the mouse stepped into the dark compartment and an inescapable foot shock (0.2 mA, 2 s) was delivered through the grid floor. Following the shock, the mouse was removed and returned to its home cage. The retention of the step-through passive avoidance response was measured the day after the learning trial, and the latency to re-enter into the dark compartment was recorded. In the retention test, no foot shock was delivered. Adaptation trial, learning trial, and retention test were performed 15, 16, and 17 days, respectively, after PBS or Aβ i.c.v. injections (see above for details regarding the experimental design).

Object Recognition Test

ORT was performed as previously described (Gulisano et al., 2018). The apparatus consisted in the arena (a plastic white box 50 × 35 × 45 cm) being placed on a lab bench with a webcam connected to the computer and was fixed on the wall, with objects of different colors and shapes (e.g., pyramid, cube, truncated sphere, cylinder, prism, and star) designed by SolidWorks software and 3D printed in polylactic acid by a Prusa-inspired 3D printer of our design. Three days before training (from day 21 to day 23), mice were habituated to the new context (empty arena and arena containing one or two objects) and allowed to freely explore it for 10 min. On day 24, mice, previously treated for 24 days with i.p. injections of antidepressants or vehicle, 45 min after the last injection of FLX or VTX, underwent the first trial (T1) of ORT consisting in exploring two identical objects (randomly chosen among our collection) placed in the central part of the box, equally distant from the perimeter. T1 lasted 10 min, a time sufficient to learn the task. The second trial (T2) was performed 24 h after T1 (day 25) to test memory retention for 10 min. Mice were presented with two objects, a "familiar" (i.e., the one used for T1) and a "novel" object. The latter was placed on the left or the right side of the box in a randomly but balanced manner, to minimize potential biases due to a preference for particular locations. To avoid olfactory cues, the objects and the apparatus were cleaned with 70% ethanol after each trial. Exploration, defined as the mouse pointing its nose toward the object from a distance not >2 cm (as marked by a reference circle), was manually evaluated by an investigator blind with respect to treatment. In particular, the following parameters were studied: i) discrimination index (D), calculated as "exploration of novel object minus exploration of familiar object/total exploration time," and ii) total exploration time. We excluded from the analyses mice with a total exploration time < 5 s.

Western Blot

Western blot analysis was performed as previously described (Caraci et al., 2015) on hippocampi of mice from the different experimental groups (n = 4 per group). Tissues were harvested at 4°C in radioimmunoprecipitation assay (RIPA) buffer, in the presence of a cocktail of protease inhibitors (Sigma-Aldrich, P2714), serine/threonine phosphatase inhibitors (Sigma-Aldrich, P0044), and tyrosine protein phosphatase inhibitors (Sigma-Aldrich, P5726), followed by sonication. Protein concentrations were determined by Bradford's method using bovine serum albumin as a standard. After being blocked, membranes were incubated with the following primary antibodies, overnight at 4°C: rabbit anti-TGF-β1 (Abcam 92486, Cambridge, UK; 1:1,000), mouse anti-GAPDH (Millipore MAB374, Burlington, MA, USA; 1:1,000), rabbit anti-PSD-95 (3450S Cell Signaling Technology Inc., Danvers, MA, USA; 1:1,000), mouse anti-synaptophysin (SC-17750 Sunta Cruz Biotechnology Inc., CA, USA; 1:40.000), and rabbit anti-actin (A2066, Sigma-Aldrich, St Louis, MO; 1:5.000). Secondary goat anti-rabbit labeled with IRDye 680 (Li-COR Biosciences; 1:20.000) and goat anti-mouse labeled with IRDye 800 (Li-COR Biosciences; 1:20.000) were used at room temperature for 45 min. Hybridization signals were detected with the Odyssey Infrared Imaging System (LI-COR Biosciences). Western blot data were quantified by densitometry analysis of the hybridization signals in four different blots per experiment.

Gene Expression Analysis by Real-Time RT-PCR

Gene expression analysis by quantitative qRT-PCR was performed as previously described (Caruso et al., 2019b) with slight modifications. In brief, the concentration of total RNA recovered by using RNeasy Mini Kit from 10 mg of hippocampus tissue was determined by measuring the absorbance at 260 nm with a Nano Drop® ND-1000 (Thermo Fisher Scientific, Waltham, MA, USA). SuperScript III First-Strand Synthesis SuperMix (Thermo Fisher Scientific) was used to carry out the reverse transcription (100 ng of total RNA for each sample), by random priming. All samples were then quantified with a NanoDrop® ND-1000, diluted to a final concentration of 25 ng/μL, and the gene expression was simultaneously measured for all the samples by using a 384-well plates and a LightCycler® 480 System (Roche Molecular Systems, Inc., Pleasanton, CA, USA). The QuantiTect Primer Assays (Qiagen, Hilden, Germany) employed for gene expression analysis along with official name, official symbol, alternative titles/symbols, detected transcript, amplicon length, and primers catalogue number are shown in **Table 1**.

For each sample amplification, performed in quadruplicate, a total reaction volume of 10 μL, consisting of 6 μL of amplification mixture (5 μL PCR Master Mix + 1 μL specific primers) plus 4 μL of cDNA (100 ng), was used. Amplification conditions and fluorescence data collection included a first cycle at 95°C (15 min) followed by 50 cycles at 94°C (15 s), an annealing step at

TABLE 1 | List of primers used for quantitative real-time PCR (qRT-PCR).

Official name[#]	Official symbol	Alternative titles/symbols	Detected transcript	Amplicon length	Cat. no.[§]
Interleukin 1 beta	Il1b	Il-1b; IL-1beta; IL-1β	NM_008361 XM_006498795	150 682	QT01048355
Tumor necrosis factor	Tnf	DIF; Tnfa; TNF-a; TNFSF2; Tnlg1f; Tnfsf1a; TNFalpha; TNF-alpha; TNF-α	NM_013693 NM_001278601	112 bp 112 bp	QT00104006
Interleukin 4	IL4	Il-4; BSF-1	NM_021283	132 bp	QT02418311
Transforming growth factor, beta 1	Tgfb1	Tgfb; Tgfb-1; TGFbeta1; TGF-beta1	NM_011577	145 bp	QT00145250
Glyceraldehyde-3-phosphate dehydrogenase	Gapdh	Gapd	NM_008084 XM_001003314 XM_990238 NM_001289726	144 bp	QT01658692

[#]*https://www.ncbi.nlm.nih.gov/gene/*
[§]*https://www.qiagen.com/it/shop/pcr/real-time-pcr-enzymes-and-kits/two-step-qrt-pcr/quantitect-primer-assays/*

56°C (30 s), and a final cycle at 72°C (30 s). As a negative control, a reaction in absence of cDNA (no template control, NTC) was performed. The relative RNA expression level for each sample was calculated using the $2^{-\Delta\Delta CT}$ method by comparing the threshold cycle (CT) value of the gene of interest with the CT value of our selected internal control (GAPDH gene).

Statistics

All experiments were blind with respect to treatment. Data were expressed as mean ± standard error mean (SEM). Statistical analysis was performed using dedicated software (GraphPad Prism, La Jolla, CA; Systat 9 Software, Chicago, IL). The within-group comparison was performed by a one-way analysis of variance (ANOVA). The *post hoc* Bonferroni test was used for multiple comparisons. One-sample *t*-test was used to compare D index with zero in ORT.

Study Approval

The study was authorized by the Institutional Animal Care and Use Committee (IACUC) of the University of Catania and by the Italian Ministry of Health (DDL 26/2014 and previous legislation; OPBA Project #266/2016). Animal care followed Italian (D.M. 116192) and EEC (O.J. of E.C.L 358/1 12/18/1986) regulations on protection of animals used for experimental and scientific purposes.

RESULTS

Fluoxetine and Vortioxetine Showed Similar Antidepressant Efficacy in Young Mice

We first examined the effects of FLX and VTX on depressive-like behavior in the first cohort of mice (Experiment 1) in the FST, a well-established behavioral test used to evaluate the preclinical efficacy of antidepressant drugs (Castagné et al., 2011; Li et al., 2017). Depressive-like behavior was assessed at day 22 by scoring immobility time (expressed in seconds) for each animal (**Figure 1A**). As depicted in **Figure 1B**, both FLX and VTX, at the dose of 10 mg/kg, gave comparable results, reducing the immobility time [$p < 0.001$ and $p < 0.01$ for FLX and VTX vs. vehicle (VEH), respectively]. VTX was able to significantly reduce the immobility time also at the dose of 5 mg/kg ($p < 0.01$ vs. VEH).

Fluoxetine and Vortioxetine Prevented Memory Retention Loss and Depressive-Like Behavior Induced by Aβ Oligomers

We then investigated the effects of FLX and VTX on the memory retention loss in mice treated with Aβ oligomers (second cohort of mice, Experiment 2). The treatment with antidepressants started 7 days before $A\beta_{1-42}$ oligomers or PBS i.c.v. injection, and memory deficits were evaluated in the PAT with memory retention test after 24 days of chronic treatment with FLX or VTX (i.e., 17 days after Aβ injection, **Figure 2A**). As observed in our previous studies (Leggio et al., 2016), mice treated with $A\beta_{1-42}$ showed a lower latency time in PAT than did vehicle-treated controls ($p < 0.01$ vs. VEH; **Figure 2B**). Interestingly, a chronic treatment with FLX (10 mg/kg) and VTX (10 mg/kg) was able to rescue Aβ-induced memory loss ($p < 0.01$ vs. Aβ + VEH and $p < 0.05$ vs. Aβ + VEH, respectively) (**Figure 2B**).

Depressive-like behavior was then evaluated in FST, in the same cohort of mice, 26 days after treatment with antidepressant drugs (19 days after Aβ injection; **Figure 2C**). We show, for the first time, that Aβ injection was able to induce a long-lasting significant increase in immobility time 19 days after i.c.v. Aβ injection ($p < 0.05$ vs. VEH). Chronic i.p. treatment with VTX or FLX, administered at the same dose of 10 mg/kg for 26 days, was able to revert $A\beta_{1-42}$-induced depressive-like behavior ($p < 0.001$ and $p < 0.01$ for FLX and VTX vs. Aβ + VEH, respectively). Interestingly, VTX at the low dose of 5 mg/kg was also effective in preventing depressive-like behavior in Aβ-injected mice ($p < 0.01$ vs. Aβ + VEH).

Fluoxetine and Vortioxetine Improved Object Recognition Memory in Aβ-Treated Mice

We then evaluated recognition memory by ORT, a task based on the natural tendency of rodents to explore unfamiliar objects, which depends upon integrity of the perirhinal cortex, the hippocampus, and the medial temporal lobe (Barker et al., 2007; Broadbent et al., 2009). We measured the exploration time of both the familiar and novel objects at T2, i.e., 24 h after training, in Aβ-injected mice; and we calculated the discrimination index (D = exploration of novel object minus exploration of familiar object/total exploration time) (**Figure 3A**). Aβ-injected mice, compared with vehicle-injected mice, showed an impairment of recognition memory, as they did not discriminate between the familiar and novel objects ($p < 0.05$; **Figure 3B**). Comparison of D with zero confirmed that Aβ-injected mice were not able to learn ($p > 0.05$). The chronic treatment with FLX (10 mg/kg) or VTX (10 mg/kg) was effective in rescuing Aβ-induced memory impairment ($p < 0.01$ vs. Aβ + VEH for both treatments). Results were not affected by differences in total exploration time between the animal groups (**Figure 3C**). Treatment with FLX or VTX *per se* did not modify discrimination index (**Figure 3D**) nor (**Figure 3E**) total exploration index.

Molecular Mechanisms Underlying the Antidepressant and Procognitive Effects of Fluoxetine and Vortioxetine: A Key Role of TGF-β1

Neuroinflammation plays a central role in the pathogenesis of depression (Bhattacharya et al., 2016) and AD (Businaro et al., 2018; Knezevic and Mizrahi, 2018). Previous studies have demonstrated that Aβ oligomers promote neuroinflammation and neurodegeneration in AD brain and in animal models of AD by eliciting the release of pro-inflammatory cytokines from microglia (Ledo et al., 2016; Businaro et al., 2018) and also by interfering with the synthesis of TGF-β1 (Diniz et al., 2017). We therefore examined the effects of $A\beta_{1-42}$ oligomers

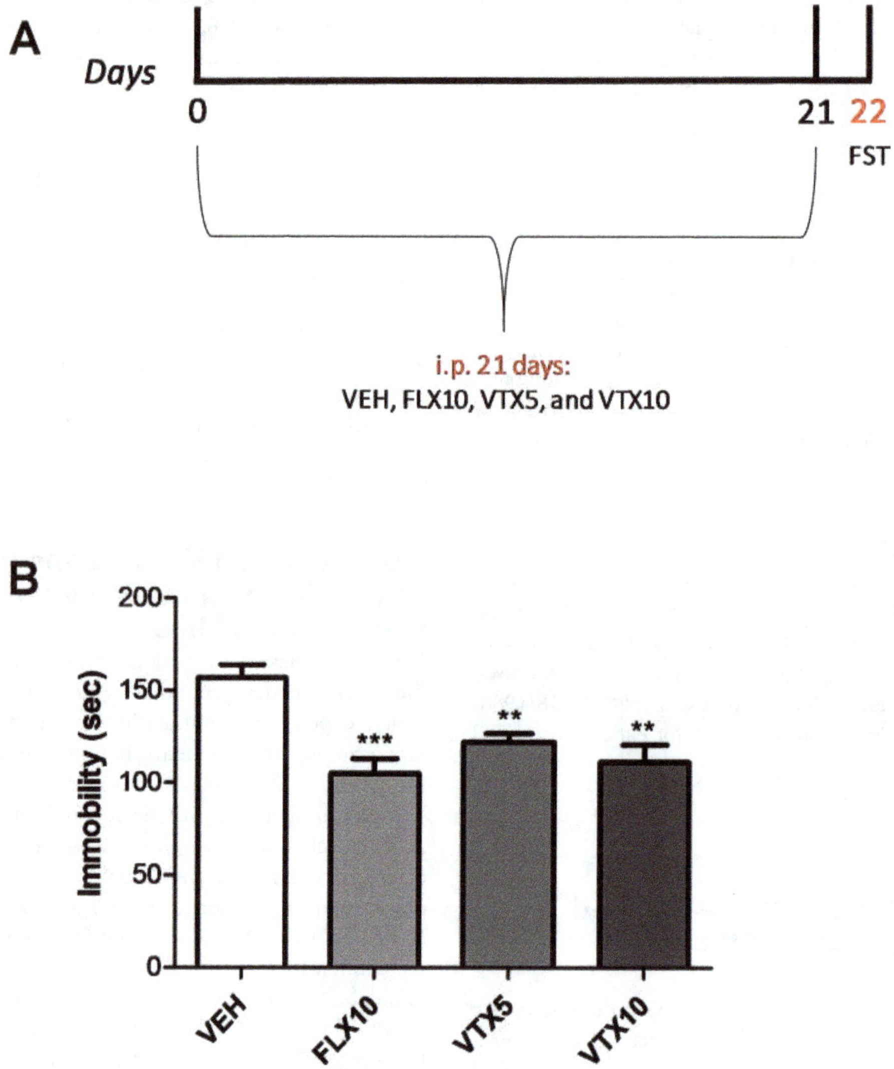

FIGURE 1 | Vortioxetine decreases depressive-like behavior in a concentration-dependent manner. Forced swim test (FST), carried out to evaluate the depressive-like behavior, was performed the day after the last injection. VEH = vehicle (i.p.), FLX10 = fluoxetine 10 mg/kg, (i.p.), VTX5 = vortioxetine 5 mg/kg (i.p.), and VTX10 = vortioxetine 10 mg/kg (i.p.) were administered chronically for 21 days. i.p. = intraperitoneal injection. **(A)** Schematic representation of the experimental design. **(B)** Immobility time displayed by groups treated with FLX10 (n = 9), VTX5 (n = 10), and VTX10 (n = 7) was significantly reduced if compared with that of vehicle-treated group (n = 9) over a 4-min test period. Immobility time measures are expressed in seconds. Data are shown as mean ± SEM. $^{**}p < 0.01$, $^{***}p < 0.001$ vs. VEH; ANOVA among all: $F_{(3,31)} = 10.04$.

i.c.v. injection on the mRNA levels of pro-inflammatory cytokines (IL-1β and TNF-α) and anti-inflammatory cytokines (IL-4 and TGF-β1) in the hippocampus (**Figure 4**), a brain area of primary relevance in the pathogenesis of depression (Villa et al., 2016). Aβ injection did not affect the expression level of IL-1β and TNF-α mRNA (**Figure 4A** and **B**), and the expression level of IL-4 (**Figure 4C**), whereas it induced a statistically significant decrease in the expression level of TGF-β1 mRNA in the hippocampus of Aβ-injected mice compared with vehicle-treated controls ($p < 0.05$ vs. VEH; **Figure 4D**). Interestingly, VTX at the low dose (5 mg/kg) was able to completely rescue hippocampal TGF-β1 mRNA levels compared with those in Aβ-injected mice ($p < 0.01$ vs. Aβ + VEH), and it further increased TGF-β1 mRNA levels at the dose of 10 mg/kg ($p < 0.001$ vs. Aβ + VEH). FLX at the dose of 10 mg/kg rescued hippocampal TGF-β1 mRNA levels with an efficacy comparable with that of VTX 5 mg/kg ($p < 0.05$ vs. Aβ + VEH). These antidepressant drugs *per se* did not increase hippocampal TGF-β1 mRNA (**Figure 4E**).

TGF-β1 is an anti-inflammatory cytokine whose final activity is regulated not only at a transcriptional level but also at a post-transcriptional level and primarily regulated through the conversion of latent TGF-β1 to active TGF-β1 by a variety of proteases (Annes et al., 2003). Interestingly, western blot analysis

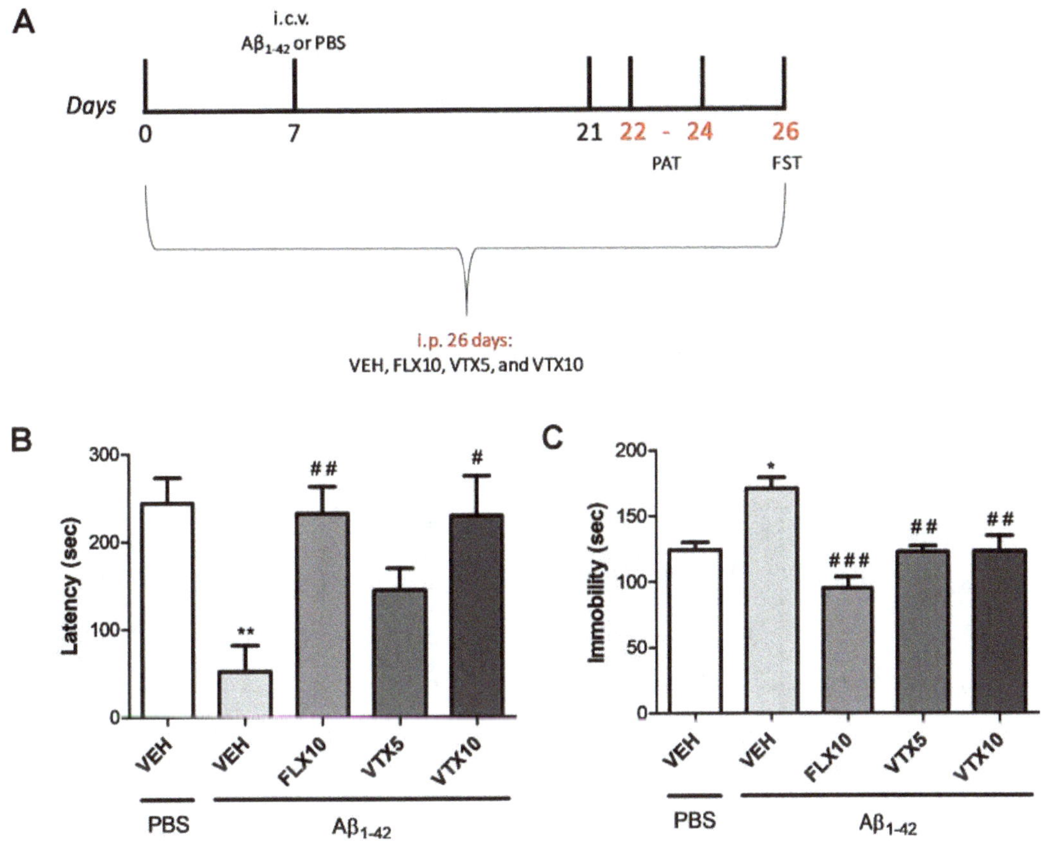

FIGURE 2 | Vortioxetine decreases depressive-like behavior and memory impairment $A\beta_{1-42}$-induced. Forced swim test (FST) and passive avoidance test (PAT) were used to evaluate depressive-like behavior and memory impairment, respectively. VEH, FLX10, VTX5, and VTX10 were administered chronically for 26 days. Sterile PBS or $A\beta_{1-42}$ was administered i.c.v. 7 days after the first i.p. injection. i.c.v. = intracerebroventricular injection. **(A)** Schematic representation of the experimental design. **(B)** Latency time to re-enter the dark box during the retention test is expressed in seconds. **(C)** Immobility time measures are expressed in seconds. PBS + VEH ($n = 8$), $A\beta_{1-42}$ + VEH ($n = 5$), $A\beta_{1-42}$ + FLX10 ($n = 7$), $A\beta_{1-42}$ + VTX5 ($n = 7$), and $A\beta_{1-42}$ + VTX10 ($n = 6$). FST and PAT were performed on the same experimental animal groups. Data are shown as mean ± SEM. $^{*}p < 0.05$, $^{**}p < 0.01$ vs. PBS + VEH; $^{\#}p < 0.05$, $^{\#\#}p < 0.01$, $^{\#\#\#}p < 0.001$ vs. $A\beta_{1-42}$ + VEH; $F_{(4,28)} = 10.44$ for **(B)** and $F_{(4,28)} = 5.59$ for **(C)**.

carried out in the hippocampus of these mice confirmed that i.c.v. Aβ injection was able to induce a significant decrease of active TGF-β1 levels ($p < 0.05$ vs. PBS + VEH) and, most importantly, that both FLX and VTX (at both doses) were able to completely rescue hippocampal TGF-β1 levels when compared with those in Aβ-injected mice treated with vehicle ($p < 0.01$ vs. Aβ + VEH for FLX and VTX at 5 mg/kg; $p < 0.001$ vs. Aβ + VEH for VTX at 10 mg/kg; **Figure 5A** and **B**). Since it is known that TGF-β1 protects synapses against Aβ oligomers toxicity (Diniz et al., 2017), we examined the expression levels of two established synaptic protein markers, synaptophysin and PSD-95, in the hippocampus of Aβ-injected mice. Aβ injection significantly decreased both synaptophysin (**Figure 5C** and **D**) and PSD-95 levels (**Figure 5E** and **F**) ($p < 0.05$ vs. PBS + VEH); and, interestingly, both FLX and VTX (at 10 mg/kg) rescued hippocampal synaptophysin ($p < 0.01$ vs. Aβ + VEH for FLX and VTX at 10 mg/kg) and PSD-95 ($p < 0.05$ vs. Aβ + VEH for FLX and $p < 0.01$ vs. Aβ + VEH for VTX at 10 mg/kg) levels when compared with those in Aβ-injected mice treated with vehicle.

DISCUSSION

In this paper, we have demonstrated for the first time that a long-term treatment with fluoxetine (10 mg/kg/day) or with the multimodal antidepressant vortioxetine (5 and 10 mg/kg/day) was able to prevent the loss of memory and the $A\beta_{1-42}$ oligomer-induced depressive-like phenotype with a key contribute played by TGF-β1 in the mouse hippocampus.

We have used a non-Tg model of AD obtained by i.c.v. injection of $A\beta_{1-42}$ oligomers, known to play a primary role in synaptic loss and progressive cognitive decline in AD (Ferretti et al., 2012; Klein, 2013). Synthetic human $A\beta_{1-42}$ oligomers were prepared according to the original protocol of Klein's group as modified and characterized in Giuffrida et al. (2009). An open question in the field remains to establish whether $A\beta_{1-42}$ oligomers can induce transient or long-term memory deficits in mice (Balducci and Forloni, 2014; Epelbaum et al., 2015). Different groups have demonstrated that, in the field of translational neuropharmacology, this model represents

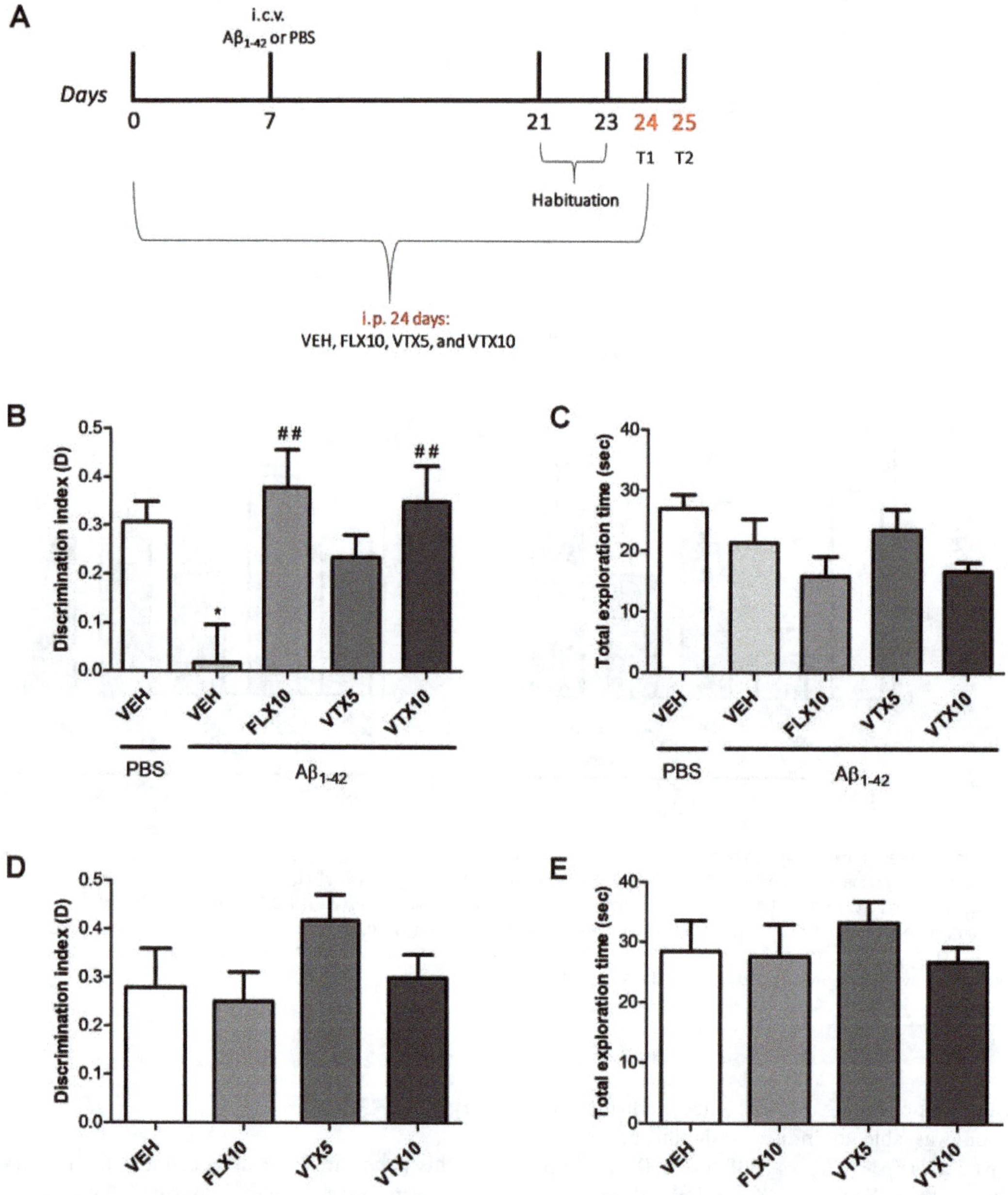

FIGURE 3 | Vortioxetine reduces the $A\beta_{1\text{-}42}$-induced impairment of recognition memory. Object recognition test (ORT) was used to evaluate recognition memory by assessing the discrimination index (D). **(A)** Schematic representation of the experimental design. **(B)** The impairment of recognition memory induced by i.c.v. administration of $A\beta_{1\text{-}42}$ ($t_{(9)} = 0.221$, $p > 0.05$ for $A\beta_{1\text{-}42}$ group vs. zero) is completely rescued by FLX10 and VTX10 treatments (ANOVA among all: $F_{(5,54)} = 4.4$; Bonferroni's $p < 0.05$ between PBS + VEH and $A\beta_{1\text{-}42}$ + VEH; $p < 0.01$ between $A\beta_{1\text{-}42}$ + VEH and VTX10 and FLX10). **(C)** Total exploration time is similar among the different conditions (ANOVA among all: $F_{(5,54)} = 2.274$). PBS + VEH ($n = 14$), $A\beta_{1\text{-}42}$ + VEH ($n = 10$), $A\beta_{1\text{-}42}$ + FLX10 ($n = 7$), $A\beta_{1\text{-}42}$ + VTX5 ($n = 11$), and $A\beta_{1\text{-}42}$ + VTX10 ($n = 11$). **(D)** FLX10, VTX5, or VTX10 treatments *per se* do not modify discrimination index ($F_{(3,28)} = 1.409$) nor **(E)** total exploration time ($F_{(3,28)} = 0.467$). $^{*}p < 0.05$ vs. PBS + VEH, $^{\#\#}p < 0.01$ vs. $A\beta_{1\text{-}42}$ + VEH.

a simple and reliable paradigm, useful to investigate the molecular mechanisms through which Aβ oligomers interfere with cognitive processes and finally to test the efficacy of new therapeutic approaches (Balducci and Forloni, 2014). We have adopted this non-Tg AD model because we know from our previous work that i) the amount of injected oligomers reaches a cerebral concentration comparable with the concentration of soluble Aβ observed in AD brains, e.g., close to 1 μg/g (Leggio et al., 2016); and ii) i.c.v. injection of Aβ induces a memory deficit that persists for 14–21 days, as assessed by using two well-validated tasks in AD field, the passive avoidance task and the object recognition test (Leggio et al., 2016). We used this non-Tg model of AD to study the neurobiological links between depression and AD and the role of Aβ oligomers in

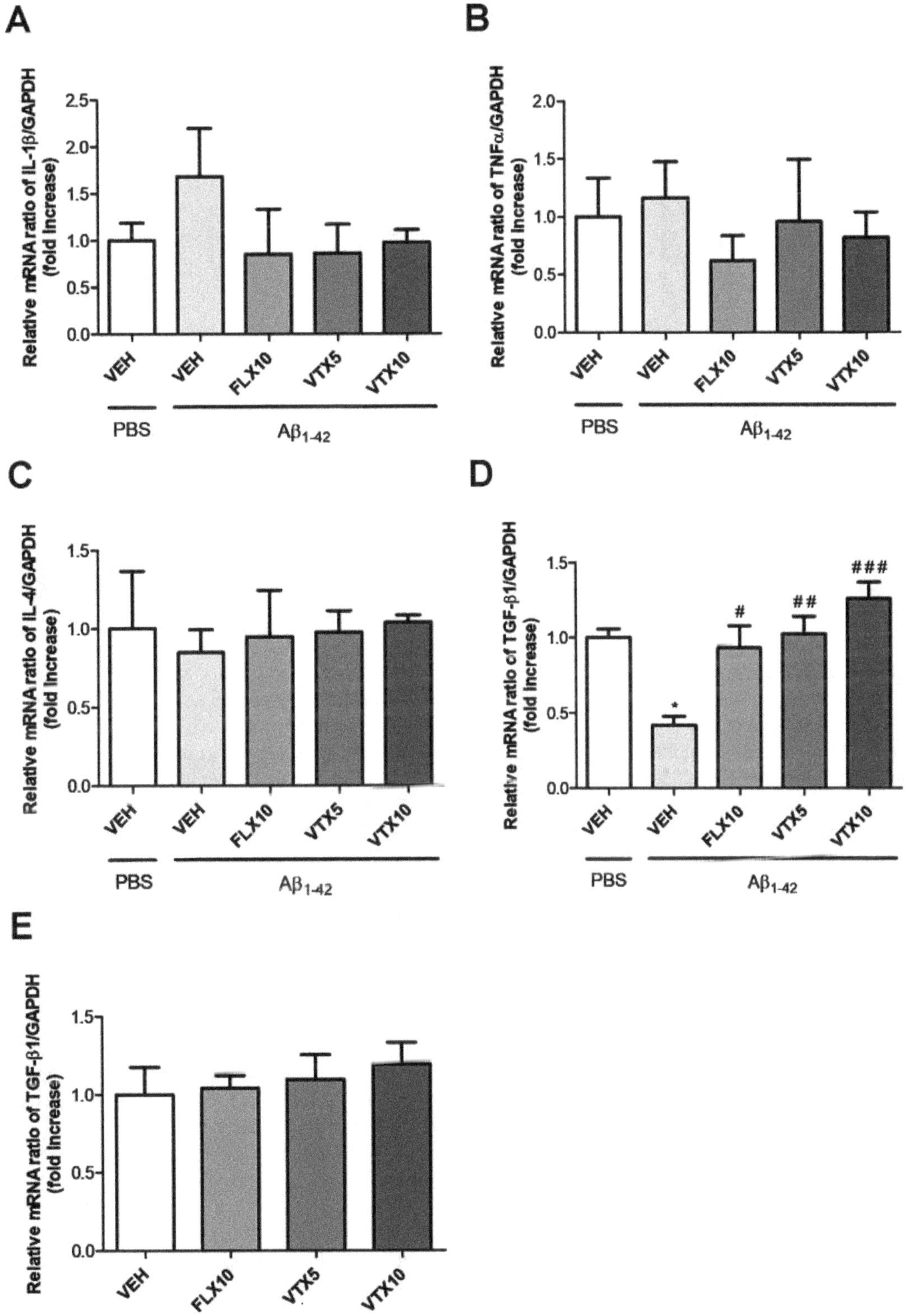

FIGURE 4 | Fluoxetine and vortioxetine increase the expression of TGF-β1 mRNA. Effects induced by i.c.v. administration of $A\beta_{1-42}$ ($A\beta_{1-42}$ + VEH) in absence or presence of FLX10, VTX5, or VTX10 on IL-1β **(A)**, TNF-α **(B)**, IL-4 **(C)**, and **(D)** TGF-β1 mRNAs expression examined by qRT-PCR (Experiment 2). **(E)** Effects of drugs on TGF-β1 mRNA expression in absence of $A\beta_{1-42}$ treatment (Experiment 3). The abundance of each mRNA of interest was expressed relative to the abundance of GAPDH-mRNA, as an internal control. As a negative control, a reaction in absence of cDNA (no template control, NTC) was performed. qRT-PCR amplifications were performed in quadruplicate. Data are shown as mean ± SEM. $^{*}p < 0.05$ vs. PBS + VEH, $^{\#}p < 0.05$ vs. $A\beta_{1-42}$ + VEH, $^{\#\#}p < 0.01$ vs. $A\beta_{1-42}$ + VEH, $^{\#\#\#}p < 0.001$ vs. $A\beta_{1-42}$ + VEH; $F_{(4,14)} = 0.86$ for **(A)**, $F_{(4,10)} = 0.35$ for **(B)**, $F_{(4,10)} = 0.06$ for **(C)**, $F_{(4,15)} = 10.23$ for **(D)**, and $F_{(3,19)} = 0.35$ for **(E)**.

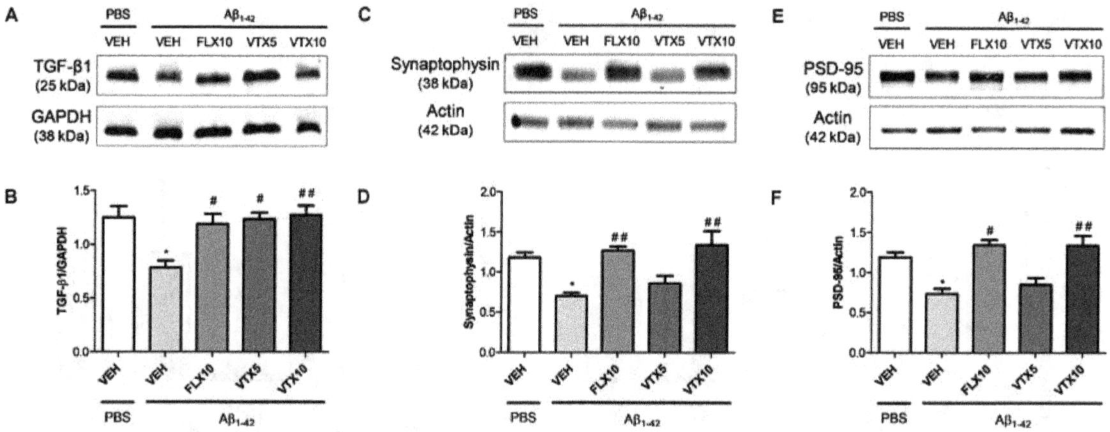

FIGURE 5 | Fluoxetine and vortioxetine rescue TGF-β1, synaptophysin, and PSD-95 levels in $A\beta_{1-42}$-treated mice. Effects induced by i.c.v. administration of $A\beta_{1-42}$ ($A\beta_{1-42}$ + VEH) in absence or presence of FLX10, VTX5, or VTX10 on TGF-β1, synaptophysin and PSD-95 levels examined by western blot. **(A)** Representative immunoblots of active TGF-β1 (about 25 kDa) in total protein extracts from hippocampus tissues. **(B)** Histograms refer to the means ± SEM of the densitometric values of active TGF-β1 bands normalized against GAPDH. Each experiment was repeated four times. $^{*}p < 0.05$ vs. PBS + VEH, $^{\#}p < 0.05$ vs. $A\beta_{1-42}$ + VEH, $^{\#\#}p < 0.01$ vs. $A\beta_{1-42}$ + VEH; $F_{(4,15)} = 5.91$ for **(B)**. **(C)** Representative immunoblots of synaptophysin (about 38 kDa) in total protein extracts from hippocampus tissues. **(D)** Histograms refer to the means ± SEM of the densitometric values of synaptophysin bands normalized against actin. Each experiment was repeated four times. $^{*}p < 0.05$ vs. PBS + VEH, $^{\#\#}p < 0.01$ vs. $A\beta_{1-42}$ + VEH; $F_{(4,17)} = 7.91$ for **(D)**. **(E)** Representative immunoblots of PSD-95 (about 95 kDa) in total protein extracts from hippocampus tissues. **(D)** Histograms refer to the means ± SEM of the densitometric values of PSD-95 bands normalized against actin. Each experiment was repeated four times. $^{*}p < 0.05$ vs. PBS + VEH, $^{\#}p < 0.05$ vs. $A\beta_{1-42}$ + VEH, $^{\#\#}p < 0.01$ vs. $A\beta_{1-42}$ + VEH; $F_{(4,17)} = 8.21$ for **(F)**.

the pathophysiology of amyloid-related depression, a recently identified clinical phenotype characterized by a low response to "monoaminergic antidepressants in depressed patients with an high risk to develop AD" (Li et al., 2017). Mimicking this clinical phenotype in rodents is a difficult challenge (Nyarko et al., 2019) but also an essential step to improve drug discovery processes in AD and explore the disease-modifying potential of antidepressant drugs in AD (Caraci et al., 2018).

Previous studies have been conducted in rodents where a depressive-like phenotype was detected by FST only 7 days after a single Aβ injection in rats (Colaianna et al., 2010; Schiavone et al., 2017) or 24 h after Aβ infusion in mice (Ledo et al., 2016). In the present work, we demonstrate for the first time that Aβ injection can induce a long-lasting depressive-like phenotype, with a significant reduction in immobility time detectable with FST until 19 days after Aβ injection (**Figure 2C**). Interestingly, this depressive-like phenotype co-exists in our Aβ-injected mice with a severe impairment of reference memory (assessed by PAT) (**Figure 2B**) and object recognition memory (assessed by ORT) (**Figure 3A** and **B**). In the present work, only one memory test was conducted in each cohort of mice (second and third) to minimize potential effect of behavioral testing on FST. Future studies should be conducted in the same model to assess whether depressive-like phenotype precedes the onset of cognitive deficits as recently observed in late-life depressed patients with an increased risk to develop AD (Chung et al., 2015; Yasuno et al., 2016).

In the present work, we measured the antidepressant-like efficacy of fluoxetine and vortioxetine in FST, in the second cohort of Aβ-injected mice, after a 26-day treatment. Drug doses for both fluoxetine and vortioxetine were chosen to reach a reliable occupancy of SERT in brain, as reported in previous studies (Pehrson et al., 2015). For the present study, we selected these specific antidepressants because fluoxetine is a SSRI known to revert cognitive deficits in different transgenic animal models of AD (Wang et al., 2014; Jin et al., 2016; Ma et al., 2017; Sun et al., 2017), and it is also able to rescue memory deficits in MCI patients (Mowla et al., 2007), while vortioxetine is a novel multimodal antidepressant endowed with strong pro-cognitive effects in preclinical models of depression (Pehrson et al., 2015) with a high clinical efficacy in the treatment of elderly patients with late-life depression and cognitive symptoms, a clinical subgroup that shows an increased risk to develop AD (Lauriola et al., 2018).

Interestingly, when comparing the effects of a chronic treatment (26 days) of fluoxetine and vortioxetine in our non-Tg AD model, we found for the first time that these two drugs have a similar preclinical efficacy at a dose of 10 mg/kg/day in preventing memory deficits, as assessed by PAT and ORT. Other studies have shown that fluoxetine can impair recognition memory in rats (Valluzzi and Chan, 2007) and in middle-aged mice (Castañé et al., 2015; Li et al., 2017), whereas vortioxetine does not affect object recognition memory in middle-aged mice (Li et al., 2017) but significantly improves the performance in this task in different animal models of cognitive dysfunction (Westrich et al., 2015; Pehrson et al., 2018). Surprisingly, 5 mg/kg vortioxetine exerted a significant antidepressant effect as detected in FST (without a further increase at a dose of 10 mg/kg), which was comparable with that of fluoxetine 10 mg/kg. Considering that vortioxetine at the dose of 5 mg/kg nearly saturates all 5-HT_3 receptors, but only partially occupies the SERT (Sanchez et al., 2015), these data seem to suggest an increased, and probably SERT-independent, antidepressant efficacy of vortioxetine compared with fluoxetine in our model of amyloid-related depression. We cannot exclude that the young age of our cohorts of mice can affect our results in behavioral tests, but we should also consider that in this study we have adopted a secondary prevention strategy to prevent the onset of amyloid-related depression, starting the treatment with antidepressants 7 days before Aβ injection. This approach was also settled moving from the evidence that second-generation antidepressants, such as fluoxetine, exert relevant neuroprotective effects *in vitro* in experimental models of Aβ-induced neurodegeneration (Caraci et al., 2016; Caraci et al., 2018). We also believe that this approach might be helpful in the future to assess the disease-modifying efficacy of antidepressants in animal models of AD, independently from their symptomatic efficacy against the depressive-like phenotype.

To understand the molecular mechanisms underlying the precognitive and antidepressant effects of vortioxetine and fluoxetine, we focused on neuroinflammatory phenomena in the hippocampus of Aβ-injected mice, because previous studies in the same model found aberrant TNF-α signaling with increases in hippocampal levels of TNF-α 24 h after Aβ infusion (Ledo et al., 2016). In order to correlate the preclinical efficacy of antidepressants with the effects on neuroinflammatory phenomena, we examined the mRNA levels of different pro-inflammatory (IL-1β and TNF-α) and anti-inflammatory (IL-4 and TGF-β1) cytokines in the hippocampus of the second cohort mice only after completing behavioral tests (26 days). We did not detect a significant increase in hippocampal levels of TNF-α and IL-1β (**Figure 4A** and **B**), but we found a significant decrease in hippocampal levels of TGF-β1 (**Figure 4D**), further confirmed by western blot analysis (**Figure 5A** and **B**). Our data are in accordance with a previous study conducted in 3-month-old male Swiss mice, where reduced TGF-β1 levels were found in the hippocampus 24 h after Aβ injection (Diniz et al., 2017). Interestingly, we found that the deficit of hippocampal TGF-β1 is a long-lasting molecular marker associated with depressive-like phenotype and memory deficits in our non-Tg model of AD. TGF-β1 is an anti-inflammatory cytokine that exerts neuroprotective effects in different models of amyloid-induced neurodegeneration (Caraci et al., 2008; Caruso et al., 2019a; reviewed by Caraci et al., 2011). We have recently identified a key role for TGF-β1 in recognition memory formation, demonstrating that it is essential for the transition from early to late long-term potentiation (Caraci et al., 2015). Deficit of TGF-β1 signaling is a primary event in AD pathogenesis, and a reduced expression of type 2 TGF-β1 receptor specifically correlates with cognitive decline in early AD patients (Tesseur et al., 2006). TGF-β1 plays a key role in synaptic plasticity (Caraci et al., 2015), and it also protects synapses against Aβ oligomers toxicity (Diniz et al., 2017). Interestingly, we found, in our non-Tg model of AD, a significant reduction of the synaptic proteins synaptophysin and PSD-95 paralleling the deficit of TGF-β1 detected in the hippocampus of Aβ-injected mice. Aβ oligomers are known to exert synaptotoxic effects (Musardo and Marcello, 2017), and our data are in accordance with previous studies where i.c.v. Aβ injection in mice caused both memory deficits and a significant decrease of PSD-95 and synaptophysin levels in the hippocampus (Morroni et al., 2016; Wu et al., 2018). In the present work, for the first time, we found a correlation between the synaptotoxic effects of Aβ oligomers and the deficit of TGF-β1 in the hippocampus of Aβ-injected mice.

The deficit of TGF-β1 signaling has been hypothesized to contribute to inflammaging and cognitive decline in both depression and AD (Caraci et al., 2018). The +10 CC genotype of TGF-β1 gene, which affects the levels of expression of TGF-β1, is associated with depressive symptoms in AD (>5-fold risk) (Caraci et al., 2012), and an impairment of TGF-β1 signaling can promote the onset of a depressive-like phenotype in mice (Depino et al., 2011). TGF-β1 plasma levels are reduced in MDD patients, correlate with depression severity, and significantly contribute to treatment resistance in MDD patients (Musil et al., 2011; Caraci et al., 2018), a clinical subgroup with an increased risk to develop AD (Chung et al., 2015, Li et al., 2017).

Our work identified for the first time a selective deficit of TGF-β1 in a non-Tg model of AD that mimics what was observed in AD brain and, most importantly, showed that vortioxetine (5 mg/kg) and fluoxetine (10 mg/kg) completely rescue hippocampal TGF-β1 levels. Interestingly, fluoxetine and vortioxetine completely rescued hippocampal synaptophysin and PSD-95 levels in Aβ-injected mice only at the dose of 10 mg/kg, suggesting a protective effect of these drugs against the synaptotoxic effects of Aβ oligomers. Fluoxetine was known to induce TGF-β1 release from cortical astrocytes (Caraci et al., 2016), but this is the first demonstration that a chronic treatment with the multimodal antidepressant vortioxetine promotes TGF-β1 synthesis at hippocampal level in an animal model of amyloid-related depression. Future studies should be conducted in transgenic animal models of AD to assess whether fluoxetine or vortioxetine can prevent amyloid-induced depression and cognitive deficits by rescue of TGF-β1 signaling.

Overall, our data, obtained in a non-Tg model of AD, indicate that a deficit in TGF-β1 might represent one of the neurobiological links between depression and AD and also that rescue of TGF-β1 signaling with second-generation antidepressants might represent a new pharmacological strategy to prevent both amyloid-induced depression and cognitive decline in AD.

AUTHOR CONTRIBUTIONS

FC gave substantial contributions to the conception and design of the work. ST, FG, MT, MG, AF, NM, GS, and GC performed the experiments. FC, SS, DP, and GL analyzed the data. GL, FT, AP, SS, DP, and FD participated in the design of the study. FC and GL drafted the work. All authors approved the version to be published.

FUNDING

This research was conducted with the unrestricted support of Lundbeck.

REFERENCES

Annes, J. P., Munger, J. S., and Rifkin, D. B. (2003). Making sense of latent TGFbeta activation. *J. Cell Sci.* 116 (Pt 2), 217–224.

Balducci, C., and Forloni, G. (2014). In vivo application of beta amyloid oligomers: a simple tool to evaluate mechanisms of action and new therapeutic approaches. *Curr. Pharm. Des.* 20, 2491–2505. doi: 10.2174/13816128113199990497

Barker, G. R., Bird, F., Alexander, V., and Warburton, E. C. (2007). Recognition memory for objects, place, and temporal order: a disconnection analysis of the role of the medial prefrontal cortex and perirhinal cortex. *J. Neurosci.* 27, 2948–2957. doi: 10.1523/JNEUROSCI.5289-06.2007

Bhattacharya, A., Derecki, N. C., Lovenberg, T. W., and Drevets, W. C. (2016). Role of neuro-immunological factors in the pathophysiology of mood disorders. *Psychopharmacology (Berl).* 233, 1623–1636. doi: 10.1007/s00213-016-4214-0

Broadbent, N. J., Gaskin, S., Squire, L. R., and Clark, R. E. (2009). Object recognition memory and the rodent hippocampus. *Learn. Mem.* 17, 5–11. doi: 10.1101/lm.1650110

Businaro, R., Corsi, M., Asprino, R., Di Lorenzo, C., Laskin, D., Corbo, R. M., et al. (2018). Modulation of inflammation as a way of delaying Alzheimer's disease progression: the diet's role. *Curr. Alzheimer Res.* 15, 363–380. doi: 10.2174/1567205014666170829100100

Caraci, F., Battaglia, G., Busceti, C., Biagioni, F., Mastroiacovo, F., Bosco, P., et al. (2008). TGF-β1 protects against Aβ-neurotoxicity via the phosphatidylinositol-3-kinase pathway. *Neurobiol. Dis.* 30, 234–242. doi: 10.1016/j.nbd.2008.01.007

Caraci, F., Battaglia, G., Bruno, V., Bosco, P., Carbonaro, V., Giuffrida, M. L., et al. (2011). TGF-β1 pathway as a new target for neuroprotection in Alzheimer's disease. *CNS Neurosci. Ther.* 17, 237–249. doi: 10.1111/j.1755-5949.2009.00115.x

Caraci, F., Bosco, P., Signorelli, M., Spada, R. S., Cosentino, F. I., Toscano, G., et al. (2012). The CC genotype of transforming growth factor-β1 increases the risk of late-onset Alzheimer's disease and is associated with AD-related depression. *Eur. Neuropsychopharmacol.* 22, 281–289. doi: 10.1016/j.euroneuro.2011.08.006

Caraci, F., Gulisano, W., Guida, A. C., Impellizzeri, A. R., Drago, F., Puzzo, D., et al. (2015). A key role for TGF-β1 in hippocampal synaptic plasticity and memory. *Sci. Rep.* 5, 11252. doi: 10.1038/srep11252

Caraci, F., Tascedda, F., Merlo, S., Benatti, C., Spampinato, S. F., Munafò, A., et al. (2016). Fluoxetine prevents Aβ(1-42)-induced toxicity via a paracrine signaling mediated by transforming-growth-factor-β1. *Front. Pharmacol.* 7, 389. doi: 10.3389/fphar.2016.00389

Caraci, F., Spampinato, S. F., Morgese, M. G., Tascedda, F., Salluzzo, M. G., Giambirtone, M. C., et al. (2018). Neurobiological links between depression and AD: the role of TGF-β1 signaling as a new pharmacological target. *Pharmacol. Res.* 130, 374–384. doi: 10.1016/j.phrs.2018.02.007

Caruso, G., Caraci, F., and Jolivet, R.B. (2019a). Pivotal role of carnosine in the modulation of brain cells activity: Multimodal mechanism of action and therapeutic potential in neurodegenerative disorders. *Prog. Neurobiol.* 175, 35–53. doi: 10.1016/j.pneurobio.2018.12.004

Caruso, G., Fresta, C. G., Musso, N., Giambirtone, M., Grasso, M., Spampinato, S. F., et al. (2019b). Carnosine prevents Aβ-induced oxidative stress and inflammation in microglial cells: a key role of TGF-β1. *Cells* 8, E64. doi: 10.3390/cells8010064

Castagné, V., Moser, P., Roux, S., and Porsolt, R. D. (2011). Rodent models of depression: forced swim and tail suspension behavioral despair tests in rats and mice. *Curr. Protoc. Neurosci.* 55 (1), 8.10A.1–8.10A.14. doi: 10.1002/0471142301.ns0810as55

Castañé, A., Kargieman, L., Celada, P., Bortolozzi, A., and Artigas, F. (2015). 5-HT2A receptors are involved in cognitive but not antidepressant effects of fluoxetine. *Eur. Neuropsychopharmacol.* 25, 1353–1361. doi: 10.1016/j.euroneuro.2015.04.006

Chung, J. K., Plitman, E., Nakajima, S., Chow, T., Chakravarty, M. M., Caravaggio, F., et al. (2015). Alzheimer's Disease Neuroimaging Initiative. Lifetime history of depression predicts increased amyloid-β accumulation in patients with mild cognitive impairment. *J. Alzheimers Dis.* 45, 907–919. doi: 10.3233/JAD-142931

Colaianna, M., Tucci, P., Zotti, M., Morgese, M. G., Schiavone, S., Govoni, S., et al. (2010). Soluble beta amyloid(1-42): a critical player in producing behavioural and biochemical changes evoking depressive-related state? *Br. J. Pharmacol.* 159, 1704–1715. doi: 10.1111/j.1476-5381.2010.00669.x

Depino, A. M., Lucchina, L., and Pitossi, F. (2011). Early and adult hippocampal TGF-β1 overexpression have opposite effects on behavior. *Brain Behav. Immun.* 25, 1582–1591. doi: 10.1016/j.bbi.2011.05.007

Diniz, L. P., Tortelli, V., Matias, I., Morgado, J., BérgamoAraujo, A. P., Melo, H. M., et al. (2017). Astrocyte transforming growth factor beta 1 protects synapses against Aβ oligomers in Alzheimer's disease model. *J. Neurosci.* 37, 6797–6809. doi: 10.1523/JNEUROSCI.3351-16.2017

Epelbaum, S., Youssef, I., Lacor, P. N., Chaurand, P., Duplus, E., Brugg, B., et al. (2015). Acute amnestic encephalopathy in amyloid-β oligomer-injected mice is due to their widespread diffusion *in vivo*. *Neurobiol. Aging* 36, 2043–2052. doi: 10.1016/j.neurobiolaging.2015.03.005

Ferretti, M. T., Bruno, M. A., Ducatenzeiler, A., Klein, W. L., and Cuello, A. C. (2012). Intracellular Abeta-oligomers and early inflammation in a model of Alzheimer's disease. *Neurobiol. Aging* 33, 1329–1342. doi: 10.1016/j.neurobiolaging.2011.01.007

Giuffrida, M. L., Caraci, F., Pignataro, B., Cataldo, S., De Bona, P., Bruno, V., et al. (2009). Beta-amyloid monomers are neuroprotective. *J. Neurosci.* 29, 10582–10587. doi: 10.1523/JNEUROSCI.1736-09.2009

Gong, Y., Chang, L., Viola, K. L., Lacor, P. N., Lambert, M. P., Finch, C. E., et al. (2003). Alzheimer's disease-affected brain: presence of oligomeric A beta ligands (ADDLs) suggests a molecular basis for reversible memory loss. *Proc. Natl. Acad. Sci. U.S.A.* 100, 10417–10422. doi: 10.1073/pnas.1834302100

Gulisano, W., Tropea, M. R., Arancio, O., Palmeri, A., and Puzzo, D. (2018). Sub-efficacious doses of phosphodiesterase 4 and 5 inhibitors improve memory in a mouse model of Alzheimer's disease. *Neuropharmacology* 138, 151–159. doi: 10.1016/j.neuropharm.2018.06.002

Jin, L., Gao, L. F., Sun, D. S., Wu, H., Wang, Q., Ke, D., et al. (2016). Long-term ameliorative effects of the antidepressant fluoxetine exposure on cognitive deficits in 3×TgAD mice. *Mol. Neurobiol.* 54 (6), 4160–4171. doi: 10.1007/s12035-016-9952-9

Kessing, L. V. (2012). Depression and the risk for dementia. *Curr. Opin. Psychiatry* 25, 457–461. doi: 10.1097/YCO.0b013e328356c368

Kessing, L. V., Søndergård, L., Forman, J. L., and Andersen, P. K. (2009). Antidepressants and dementia. *J. Affect. Disord.* 117, 24–29. doi: 10.1016/j.jad.2008.11.020

Klein, W. L. (2013). Synaptotoxic amyloid-β oligomers: a molecular basis for the cause, diagnosis, and treatment of Alzheimer's disease? *J. Alzheimers Dis.* 33 Suppl 1, S49–65. doi: 10.3233/JAD-2012-129039

Knezevic, D., and Mizrahi, R. (2018). Molecular imaging of neuroinflammation in Alzheimer's disease and mild cognitive impairment. *Prog. Neuropsychopharmacol. Biol. Psychiatry* 80, 123–131. doi: 10.1016/j.pnpbp.2017.05.007

Lanctôt, K. L., Amatniek, J., Ancoli-Israel, S., Arnold, S. E., Ballard, C., Cohen-Mansfield, J., et al. (2017). Neuropsychiatric signs and symptoms of Alzheimer's disease: new treatment paradigms. *Alzheimers Dement (N Y).* 3, 440–449. doi: 10.1016/j.trci.2017.07.001

Lauriola, M., Mangiacotti, A., D'Onofrio, G., Cascavilla, L., Paris, F., Ciccone, F., et al. (2018). Late-life depression versus amnestic mild cognitive impairment: Alzheimer's disease incidence in 4 years of follow-up. *Dement. Geriatr. Cogn. Disord.* 46, 140–153. doi: 10.1159/000492489

Ledo, J. H., Azevedo, E. P., Clarke, J. R., Ribeiro, F. C., Figueiredo, C. P., Foguel, D., et al. (2013). Amyloid-β oligomers link depressive-like behavior and cognitive deficits in mice. *Mol. Psychiatry* 18, 1053–1054. doi: 10.1038/mp.2012.168

Ledo, J. H., Azevedo, E. P., Beckman, D., Ribeiro, F. C., Santos, L. E., Razolli, D. S., et al. (2016). Cross talk between brain innate immunity and serotonin signaling underlies depressive-like behavior induced by Alzheimer's amyloid-β oligomers in mice. *J. Neurosci.* 36, 12106–12116. doi: 10.1523/JNEUROSCI.1269-16.2016

Lee, K. M., and Kim, Y. K. (2006). The role of IL-12 and TGF-beta1 in the pathophysiology of major depressive disorder. *Int. Immunopharmacol.* 6, 1298–1304. doi: 10.1016/j.intimp.2006.03.015

Leggio, G. M., Catania, M. V., Puzzo, D., Spatuzza, M., Pellitteri, R., Gulisano, W., et al. (2016). The antineoplastic drug flavopiridol reverses memory impairment induced by amyloid-β1-42 oligomers in mice. *Pharmacol. Res.* 106, 10–20. doi: 10.1016/j.phrs.2016.02.007

Li, Y., Sanchez, C., and Gulinello, M. (2017). Distinct antidepressant-like and cognitive effects of antidepressants with different mechanisms of action in middle-aged female mice. *Int. J. Neuropsychopharmacol.* 20, 510–515. doi: 10.1093/ijnp/pyx004

Li, Y., Abdourahman, A., Tamm, J. A., Pehrson, A. L., Sánchez, C., and Gulinello, M. (2015). Reversal of age-associated cognitive deficits is accompanied by increased plasticity-related gene expression after chronic antidepressant administration in middle-aged mice. *Pharmacol. Biochem. Behav.* 135, 70–82. doi: 10.1016/j.pbb.2015.05.013

Li, P., Hsiao, I. T., Liu, C. Y., Chen, C. H., Huang, S. Y., Yen, T. C., et al. (2017). Beta-amyloid deposition in patients with major depressive disorder with differing levels of treatment resistance: a pilot study. *EJNMMI Res.* 7, 24. doi: 10.1186/s13550-017-0273-4

Ma, J., Gao, Y., Jiang, L., Chao, F. L., Huang, W., Zhou, C. N., et al. (2017). Fluoxetine attenuates the impairment of spatial learning ability and prevents neuron loss in middle-aged APPswe/PSEN1dE9 double transgenic Alzheimer's disease mice. *Oncotarget* 8, 27676–27692. doi: 10.18632/oncotarget.15398

Maurice, T., Lockhart, B. P., and Privat, A. (1996). Amnesia induced in mice by centrally administered beta-amyloid peptides involves cholinergic dysfunction. *Brain Res.* 706, 181–193. doi: 10.1016/0006-8993(95)01032-7

McIntyre, R. S., Harrison, J., Loft, H., Jacobson, W., and Olsen, C. K. (2016). The effects of vortioxetine on cognitive function in patients with major depressive disorder: a meta-analysis of three randomized controlled trials. *Int. J. Neuropsychopharmacol.* 19 (10), pyw055. doi: 10.1093/ijnp/pyw055

Modrego, P. J., and Ferrández, J. (2004). Depression in patients with mild cognitive impairment increases the risk of developing dementia of Alzheimer type: a prospective cohort study. *Arch. Neurol.* 61, 1290–1203. doi: 10.1001/archneur.61.8.1290

Morroni, F., Sita, G., Tarozzi, A., Rimondini, R., and Hrelia, P. (2016). Early effects of Abeta1-42 oligomers injection in mice: involvement of PI3K/Akt/GSK3 and MAPK/ERK1/2 pathways. *Behav. Brain. Res.* 314, 106–115. doi: 10.1016/j.bbr.2016.08.002

Mørk, A., Pehrson, A., Brennum, L. T., Nielsen, S. M., Zhong, H., Lassen, A. B., et al. (2012). Pharmacological effects of Lu AA21004: a novel multimodal compound for the treatment of major depressive disorder. *J. Pharmacol. Exp. Ther.* 340, 666–675. doi: 10.1124/jpet.111.189068

Mowla, A., Mosavinasab, M., and Pani, A. (2007). Does fluoxetine have any effect on the cognition of patients with mild cognitive impairment? A double-blind placebo-controlled, clinical trial. *J. Clin. Psychopharmacol.* 27, 67–70. doi: 10.1097/JCP.0b013e31802e0002

Musardo, S., and Marcello, E. (2017). Synaptic dysfunction in Alzheimer's disease: from the role of amyloid β-peptide to the α-secretase ADAM10. *Eur. J. Pharmacol.* 817, 30–37. doi: 10.1016/j.ejphar.2017.06.018

Musil, R., Schwarz, M. J., Riedel, M., Dehning, S., Cerovecki, A., Spellmann, I., et al. (2011). Elevated macrophage migration inhibitory factor and decreased transforming growth factor-beta levels in major depression—no influence of celecoxib treatment. *J. Affect. Disord.* 134, 217–225. doi: 10.1016/j.jad.2011.05.047

Nyarko, J. N. K., Quartey, M. O., Baker, G. B., and Mousseau, D. D. (2019). Can animal models inform on the relationship between depression and Alzheimer disease? *Can. J. Psychiatry* 64, 18–29. doi: 10.1177/0706743718772514

Pehrson, A. L., Pedersen, C. S., Tølbøl, K. S., and Sanchez, C. (2018). Vortioxetine treatment reverses subchronic PCP treatment-induced cognitive impairments: a potential role for serotonin receptor-mediated regulation of GABA neurotransmission. *Front. Pharmacol.* 9, 162. doi: 10.3389/fphar.2018.00162

Pehrson, A. L., Leiser, S. C., Gulinello, M., Dale, E., Li, Y., Waller, J. A., et al. (2015). Treatment of cognitive dysfunction in major depressive disorder—a review of the preclinical evidence for efficacy of selective serotonin reuptake inhibitors, serotonin-norepinephrine reuptake inhibitors and the multimodal-acting antidepressant vortioxetine. *Eur. J. Pharmacol.* 753, 19–31. doi: 10.1016/j.ejphar.2014.07.044

Porsolt, R. D., Bertin, A., and Jalfre, M. (1978). "Behavioural despair" in rats and mice: strain differences and the effects of imipramine. *Eur. J. Pharmacol.* 51 (3), 291–294.

Sanchez, C., Asin, K. E., and Artigas, F. (2015). Vortioxetine, a novel antidepressant with multimodal activity: review of preclinical and clinical data. *Pharmacol. Ther.* 145, 43–57. doi: 10.1016/j.pharmthera.2014.07.001

Schiavone, S., Tucci, P., Mhillaj, E., Bove, M., Trabace, L., and Morgese, M. G. (2017). Antidepressant drugs for beta amyloid-induced depression: a new standpoint? *Prog. Neuropsychopharmacol. Biol. Psychiatry* 78, 114–122. doi: 10.1016/j.pnpbp.2017.05.004

Sun, D. S., Gao, L. F., Jin, L., Wu, H., Wang, Q., Zhou, Y., et al. (2017). Fluoxetine administration during adolescence attenuates cognitive and synaptic deficits in adult 3× TgAD mice. *Neuropharmacology* 126, 200–212. doi: 10.1016/j.neuropharm.2017.08.037

Sutcigil, L., Oktenli, C., Musabak, U., Bozkurt, A., Cansever, A., Uzun, O., et al. (2007). Pro- and anti-inflammatory cytokine balance in major depression: effect of sertraline therapy. *Clin. Dev. Immunol.* 2007, 76396. doi: 10.1155/2007/76396

Tesseur, I., Zou, K., Esposito, L., Bard, F., Berber, E., Can, J. V., et al. (2006). Deficiency in neuronal TGF-beta signaling promotes neurodegeneration and Alzheimer's pathology. *J. Clin. Invest.* 116, 3060–3069. doi: 10.1172/JCI27341

Thase, M. E., Mahableshwarkar, A. R., Dragheim, M., Loft, H., and Vieta, E. (2016). A meta-analysis of randomized, placebo-controlled trials of vortioxetine for the treatment of major depressive disorder in adults. *Eur. Neuropsychopharmacol.* 26, 979–993. doi: 10.1016/j.euroneuro.2016.03.007

Valluzzi, J. A., and Chan, K. (2007). Effects of fluoxetine on hippocampal-dependent and hippocampal-independent learning tasks. *Behav. Pharmacol.* 18, 507–513. doi: 10.1097/FBP.0b013e3282ee2a91

Villa, R. F., Ferrari, F., Gorini, A., Brunello, N., and Tascedda, F. (2016). Effect of desipramine and fluoxetine on energy metabolism of cerebral mitochondria. *Neuroscience* 330, 326–334. doi: 10.1016/j.neuroscience.2016.05.051

Wang, J., Zhang, Y., Xu, H., Zhu, S., Wang, H., He, J., et al. (2014). Fluoxetine improves behavioral performance by suppressing the production of soluble β-amyloid in APP/PS1 mice. *Curr. Alzheimer Res.* 11, 672–680. doi: 10.2174/1567205011666140812114715

Westrich, L., Haddjeri, N., Dkhissi-Benyahya, O., and Sánchez, C. (2015). Involvement of 5-HT7 receptors in vortioxetine's modulation of circadian rhythms and episodic memory in rodents. *Neuropharmacology* 89, 382–390. doi: 10.1016/j.neuropharm.2014.10.015

Wu, X., Lv, Y. G., Du, Y. F., Chen, F., Reed, M. N., Hu, M., et al. (2018). Neuroprotective effects of INT-777 against Abeta1-42-induced cognitive impairment, neuroinflammation, apoptosis, and synaptic dysfunction in mice. *Brain. Behav. Immun.* 73, 533–545. doi: 10.1016/j.bbi.2018.06.018

Yasuno, F., Kazui, H., Morita, N., Kajimoto, K., Ihara, M., Taguchi, A., et al. (2016). High amyloid-β deposition related to depressive symptoms in older individuals with normal cognition: a pilot study. *Int. J. Geriatr. Psychiatry* 31, 920–928. doi: 10.1002/gps.4409

13

Biomarker-Drug and Liquid Biopsy Co-Development for Disease Staging and Targeted Therapy: Cornerstones for Alzheimer's Precision Medicine and Pharmacology

Harald Hampel[1,2,3,4]*, Edward J. Goetzl[5], Dimitrios Kapogiannis[6], Simone Lista[1,2,3,4] and Andrea Vergallo[1,2,3,4]* on behalf of Alzheimer Precision Medicine Initiative (APMI)

[1] AXA Research Fund & Sorbonne University Chair, Paris, France, [2] Sorbonne University, GRC n° 21, Alzheimer Precision Medicine (APM), AP-HP, Pitié-Salpêtrière Hospital, Paris, France, [3] Brain & Spine Institute (ICM), INSERM U 1127, CNRS UMR 7225, Boulevard de l'Hôpital, Paris, France, [4] Department of Neurology, Institute of Memory and Alzheimer's Disease (IM2A), Pitié-Salpêtrière Hospital, AP-HP, Boulevard de l'Hôpital, Paris, France, [5] Department of Medicine, University of California, San Francisco, San Francisco, CA, United States, [6] Laboratory of Neurosciences, Intramural Research Program, National Institute on Aging, Baltimore, MD, United States

****Correspondence:***
Harald Hampel
harald.hampel@med.uni-muenchen.de
Andrea Vergallo
andrea.vergallo@icm-institute.org

Systems biology studies have demonstrated that different (epi)genetic and pathophysiological alterations may be mapped onto a single tumor's clinical phenotype thereby revealing commonalities shared by cancers with divergent phenotypes. The success of this approach in cancer based on analyses of traditional and emerging body fluid-based biomarkers has given rise to the concept of liquid biopsy enabling a non-invasive and widely accessible precision medicine approach and a significant paradigm shift in the management of cancer. Serial liquid biopsies offer clues about the evolution of cancer in individual patients across disease stages enabling the application of individualized genetically and biologically guided therapies. Moreover, liquid biopsy is contributing to the transformation of drug research and development strategies as well as supporting clinical practice allowing identification of subsets of patients who may enter pathway-based targeted therapies not dictated by clinical phenotypes alone. A similar liquid biopsy concept is emerging for Alzheimer's disease, in which blood-based biomarkers adaptable to each patient and stage of disease, may be used for positive and negative patient selection to facilitate establishment of high-value drug targets and counter-measures for drug resistance. Going beyond the "one marker, one drug" model, integrated applications of genomics, transcriptomics, proteomics, receptor expression and receptor cell biology and conformational status assessments during biomarker-drug co-development may lead to a new successful era for Alzheimer's disease therapeutics. We argue that the time is now for implementing a liquid biopsy-guided strategy for the development of drugs that precisely target Alzheimer's disease pathophysiology in individual patients.

Keywords: Alzheimer's disease, liquid biopsy, exosomes, systems pharmacology, precision medicine

CHALLENGES IN BIOMARKER-BASED ALGORITHM FOR DRUG R&D PROGRAMS

The dramatic rate of Alzheimer's disease (AD) clinical trial failures for putative disease-modifying therapies (DmT) calls for a shift in Research and Development (R&D) strategies. The drug development field needs to advance to a more comprehensive scrutinization of AD-related pathophysiology, an earlier detection and definition of appropriate preclinical target subpopulations, taking interindividual biological variability into account (Cummings, 2011; Hampel et al., 2018a).

Particularly during early disease stages, evolving decompensating molecular pathways may be effectively regulated (Hampel et al., 2018a,b). At specific time points during the long preclinical stage, brain network homeostasis as well as adaptive responses and compensatory mechanisms may still be restorable, thus ensuring resilience and ultimately prolonging brain health-span (Hampel et al., 2018a,b).

An agnostic hypothesis-independent biomarker-driven classification system (the A/T/N system) has been proposed to stratify individuals according to core AD-related pathological and pathophysiological hallmarks (brain overaccumulation of both amyloid-β and tau proteins aggregates, and neurodegeneration) (Jack et al., 2016). The A/T/N system is aligned with the established conceptual framework and is based on much-researched and largely-validated CSF and PET biomarkers of AD. The A/T/N system is expected to provide consistent subject enrollment and target engagement among different sites in AD clinical trials.

Although the ATN system provides key pathophysiological insights, it only partially reflects the expanding *spectrum* of pathomechanistic alterations occurring in AD (Hampel et al., 2018c; Molinuevo et al., 2018). Newly identified disease mechanisms may represent relevant therapeutic targets and an increasing number of such innovative compounds are currently investigated by industry-led R&D programs (Hampel et al., 2018a; Molinuevo et al., 2018).

A growing number of candidate biomarkers, capable of charting a wider set of age- and AD-related pathophysiological pathways is currently available, for instance: upstream regulators of amyloidogenic pathways and axonal sprouting such as β-site amyloid precursor protein (APP) cleaving enzyme 1 (BACE1) (Shen et al., 2018), TAR DNA binding protein-43 (TDP-43) (Molinuevo et al., 2018), regulators of astrocyte- and microglia-mediated dysfunction and neuroinflammation (such as the human cartilage glycoprotein-39 and chitinase-like protein 1, [YKL-40] and TREM2) (Hampel et al., 2018c; Molinuevo et al., 2018), damage of large-caliber myelinated axons [reflected by release of neurofilament light chain (NFL)] (Mattsson et al., 2017; Preische et al., 2019), synaptic dysfunction (reflected by release of synaptic proteins, such as neurogranin and alpha-synuclein) (Kvartsberg et al., 2015; Vergallo et al., 2018).

Besides biological and pathophysiological issues, a number of challenges remain to reach the objective of translating these criteria into an operational biomarker-based algorithm for drug R&D programs as well as for broad clinical diagnostic practice.

First, there is a need to better understand the role that established, and newly identified biomarkers may play for distinctive contexts-of-use (COU), such as for clinical diagnosis, preclinical risk assessment and participant selection (O'Bryant et al., 2017).

With the global epidemic rise of AD and with the exponential increase in the number of individuals at risk and or individuals with preclinical disease, it is urgent to step up the development of comprehensive blood-based biomarker panels which are widely accessible, minimally invasive, and less time- and cost-consuming compared with CSF and neuroimaging assessment.

The collection, processing, and storage of blood is globally accessible from biotech and pharmaceutical industry, to academic research, until primary health care facilities. All advantages of blood-based biomarkers compared with CSF or PET biomarkers are essential in clinical research studies investigating large-scale heterogeneous populations of cognitive normal individuals at risk of AD and when time series are part of the study design.

The roadmap to ultimately validating and qualifying blood-based biomarkers for different COU and to set up a liquid biopsy for AD still requires an enormous worldwide-scaled effort for the standardization and harmonization of preanalytical and analytical protocols.

In this regard, a professional interest area focused on Blood Based Biomarkers (BBB-PIA), as a part of the Alzheimer's Association's International Society to Advance Alzheimer's Research and Treatment (ISTAART) as well as the European Union-North American Clinical Trials in Alzheimer's Disease Task Force (EU/US CTAD Task Force) are intensely supporting the achievement of a field-wide consensus on the harmonization of pre-analytic and analytic protocols in order to speed up the analytical and clinical validation of blood-based biomarkers (Snyder et al., 2014).

In the last 5 years, several population-based studies demonstrated correlation between CSF and blood concentrations of different candidate markers. Moreover, several mono- and multi-centric studies have proven a significant predictive power of blood-based biomarkers of brain amyloidosis and tau-related neuronal injury using PET and/or MRI imaging as a standard of truth (Fandos et al., 2017; Mielke et al., 2018; Nakamura et al., 2018; Park et al., 2019).

Therefore, a blood-based matrix would help overcome the invasive and time-consuming profile of lumbar puncture and would display an intrinsic superiority compared with PET-based methods that can capture only a single molecular mechanism at a time.

Such a comprehensive blood-based biomarker matrix has already become reality in more advanced biomedical areas including Oncology and clinical Immunology constituting the liquid biopsy approach (Wan et al., 2017; Heitzer et al., 2019; Pantel and Alix-Panabieres, 2019).

The U.S. National Cancer Institute (NCI) defines liquid biopsy (LB) as "a test done on a sample of blood to look for cancer cells from a tumor that are circulating in the blood or for pieces of DNA from tumor cells that are in the blood".

The progressive field of Oncology is increasingly benefiting from breakthrough high-resolution biomarker technologies generating liquid biopsy-driven patient health care algorithms and successfully implementing anti-cancer drug R&D pipelines.

Anti-cancer clinical trials are increasingly employing the exhaustive biological tumor profiling facilitated by liquid biopsy, which paves the way toward a paradigmatic shift to precision medicine and pathway-based medicine. In 2017 the U.S. Food and Drug Administration (FDA) had accelerated the approval of two tumor type- and site- agnostic therapy approaches, pembrolizumab and nivolumab (Goldberg et al., 2018).

We argue that the right time to develop liquid biopsy-guided strategies for AD drug R&D pipelines is clearly approaching.

In our model we suggest that the term liquid biopsy would equally account for any trackable bioindicators originating in brain tissue inflicted by the pathophysiological processes of AD. Liquid biopsy of AD will enable an early biological stratification of large-scale heterogeneous populations of asymptomatic individuals at risk and patients with preclinical AD. In a future multi-stage risk-population screening strategy, liquid biopsies may identify individuals at higher risk for AD who may be further investigated with more specific, cost-intensive, and invasive methods (such as CSF or PET investigations) (Hampel et al., 2018c; Molinuevo et al., 2018).

Several blood-based candidate biomarkers reflecting distinct pathophysiological mechanisms of AD as well as unbiased exploratory quantitative high-throughput "omics" biomarker platforms are increasingly gaining *momentum*. We hypothesize that Neural-Derived Exosome Protein and MicroRNAs (miRNAs) may constitute the scaffolding of a single standardized workflow to (I) expand the current research criteria of AD with additional molecular biomarkers belonging to the wider spectrum of the pathophysiological landscape of polygenic late-onset AD, (II) expand the unbiased A/T/N biomarker classification system to integrate comprehensive pathophysiological blood-based biomarker information, making real-world application of this application more feasible, cost- and time-effective and globally accessible.

NEURAL-DERIVED EXOSOME PROTEIN ABNORMALITIES REVEAL TARGETS FOR PREVENTION AND THERAPY OF CNS DISEASES IN THE ELDERLY: NEURAL EXOSOME PROTEIN THERAPEUTIC TARGETS

An emerging possibility for prediction of preclinical Alzheimer disease (AD), other neurodegenerative diseases and cerebrovascular disease is quantification of pathogenic proteins in plasma neural cell-derived exosomes (Mustapic et al., 2017). We will review recent progress in neural exosome analysis, advances in clinical applications, and examples of exosome protein biomarker candidates that may become targets for preventative or therapeutic approaches to CNS diseases.

Exosomes derived from any type of CNS cell may be harvested efficiently from human plasma by initial physical precipitation followed by immunoabsorption with antibodies that selectively recognize a surface antigen on that CNS cell-type (Mustapic et al., 2017). This two-step process permits separate enrichment of exosomes secreted by neurons, astrocytes, microglia and chondroitin sulfate proteoglycan type 4 (CSPG4) cells.

The evidence for CNS cell-origin of exosomes recovered through this process continues to accumulate. Briefly, co-authors in this paper and others have demonstrated many-fold higher levels for multiple known neuronal and astrocytic markers using Western Blot and ELISA-type analyses (Goetzl et al., 2016; Mustapic et al., 2017); enrichment for multiple neuronal proteins based on targeted and untargeted proteomics (Pulliam et al., 2019) and demonstration of high-yield immunocapture of known neuronal exosomes from the plasma matrix [see Supplementary Material in Athauda et al. (2019)]. Efforts to directly determine the relationship between brain pathology and circulating exosomes in animal models and humans are currently underway.

In steady-states of chronic CNS degeneration, the plasma concentration of exosomes from each cell-type are unchanged by disease and neuropathological effects are seen predominantly in the concentrations of cargo proteins per exosome (Mustapic et al., 2017). Variations in efficiency of neural exosome isolation from individual plasma are determined using constitutive protein markers present at uniform levels irrespective of disease. Normalization of biomarker levels to the same number of exosomes with constitutive markers [such as CD81 (Fiandaca et al., 2015) or Alix (Pulliam et al., 2019)] delineates effects of CNS diseases. Progress using this approach includes the following findings:

(1) Higher levels of P-T181-tau, P-S396-tau and Aβ42 in neuronally-derived exosomes (NDEs) of patients with AD compared to age-matched controls, that were detected as early as 10 years before overt clinical disease (Fiandaca et al., 2015).
(2) NDE protein abnormalities characteristic of defective autophagy, insulin resistance, synaptic dysfunction, and reduced protection against cellular stress in AD (Goetzl et al., 2018a).
(3) Substantially lower intracellular levels of the Aβ peptide-generating proteins, such as β-secretase cleaving enzyme 1 (BACE-1) γ-secretase and APP in astrocytes compared to neurons, but much higher secreted concentrations of these proteins in astrocyte-derived exosomes (ADEs) compared to NDEs, with ADEs of AD patients having higher levels compared to controls (Goetzl et al., 2016).
(4) Higher concentrations of neurotoxic complement proteins, such as C3b, Bb and C5b-C9, and lower levels of endogenous complement inhibitors, such as CD59, in ADEs of AD patients compared to controls (Goetzl et al., 2018b).
(5) Higher NDE concentrations of P-T181-tau, P-S396-tau and Aβ42, and ADE levels of complement proteins in subjects with mild cognitive impairment (MCI) predictive

of conversion to AD dementia in three years with high sensitivity.

(6) Higher endothelial cell-derived exosome (EDE) concentrations of CNS-specific endothelial proteins in patients with clinical cerebrovascular disease compared to controls (Goetzl et al., 2017).

(7) Higher EDE levels of CNS-specific endothelial proteins and cytotoxic complement proteins in asymptomatic subjects with MRI signs of small vessels cerebrovascular disease compared to age-matched controls having normal MRIs.

Tentative evaluation of our neural-derived exosome biomarker data suggests potential value of some cargo proteins as therapeutic targets (**Table 1**). In AD, the highest value may be assigned to blocking astrocyte complement-mediated neurotoxicity and to restoring growth and regenerative factors of the small, but widespread, set of CSPG4 cells. Altering activities of various kinases and proteases and restoring levels of excitatory synaptic proteins may also be useful efforts, but lack of specificity is a deterrent. In cerebrovascular disease, similar efforts to block complement-mediated endothelial toxicity are promising. Enhancing eNOS activity in endothelial cells by suppressing the level of NOSTRIN and enhancing angiogenesis of collateral vessels by increasing endothelial P-YAP-1 transcriptional activity provide optimism.

MicroRNA–MESSENGER RNA (miRNA–mRNA) SIGNALLING IN ALZHEIMER'S DISEASE

MicroRNAs (miRNAs) constitute a large family of small non-coding RNA, consisting of maximum 24 nucleotides, that exert an inhibitory function of gene expression, by destabilizing messenger RNAs and down-regulating the translation process (Alexandrov et al., 2012; Zhao et al., 2016). Consequently, miRNAs may play a key regulatory role for all intracellular signals.

The deregulation of miRNAs turn-over is associated with the development of a broad *spectrum* of diseases such as cancer, diabetes, and several pathological brain conditions including multiple sclerosis and sporadic AD (Alexandrov et al., 2012; Bergman et al., 2016; Sorensen et al., 2016; Zhao et al., 2016).

Research work to date has defined a small ~5-membered family of NF-kB-inducible miRNAs including miRNA-9, miRNA-34a, miRNA-125b, miRNA-146a and miRNA-155 which have been found to be up-regulated in the extracellular and cerebrospinal fluid contiguous to AD-affected brain regions (Alexandrov et al., 2012; Bergman et al., 2016; Sorensen et al., 2016; Zhao et al., 2016). These results have been found in independent studies conducted on autopsy-confirmed AD patients, transgenic murine models of AD (TgAD), and stressed human brain cells derived from primary cultures. These up-regulated miRNAs appear to slow down their mRNA targets, providing a mechanistic explanation for several interactive AD-related failures involving phagocytosis, synaptogenesis, bioenergetic homeostasis, modulation of inflammatory signaling, and amyloidogenesis (Alexandrov et al., 2012; Bergman et al., 2016; Sorensen et al., 2016; Zhao et al., 2016). For example, the up-regulation of both miRNA-9 and miRNA-146a in AD has been shown to down-regulate the expression of the innate-immune glycoprotein complement factor H (CFH), and this stimulates runaway innate-immune and inflammatory signalling in AD that directly impacts mitochondrial-based energy-generating capacities (Alexandrov et al., 2012; Bergman et al., 2016; Sorensen et al., 2016; Zhao et al., 2016).

Whether these circulating miRNAs predict highly specific genetic-epigenetic signalling pathways involved in the

TABLE 1 | Experimental therapeutic targets suggested by neural exosome protein abnormalities.

Disease	Protein(s)	Neural cell source	Desired effect	Estimated feasibility as an approachable target
AD	P-tau species	Neurons	Suppress kinase(s) (CDK5, GSK3b, ERK2) Enhance phosphatase(s)	1
	P-S-IRS-1	Neurons	Suppress kinase(s)	2
	Excitatory pathway synaptic proteins	Neurons	Restore protein levels	2
	Aβ-generating BACE-1 and γ-secretase	Astrocytes	Selective protease inhibitors	2
	Complement (C) system [C3b, Bb, C5b-C9]	Astrocytes	Suppress complement activation; block C receptors	3
	Growth and regenerative factors (HGF, FGF-13, IGF-1)	CSPG4 cells	Restore CSPG4 proteins	3
CeVD	Regulators of vascular tone and repair/regeneration (NOSTRIN, YAP-1/P-YAP-1)	Endothelial cells	Decrease NOSTRIN, increase active YAP-1	2
	Complement (C) system [C3b, Bb, C5b-C9]	Endothelial cells	Suppress complement activation; block C receptors	3

AD, Alzheimer disease; CeVD, cerebrovascular disease; P-S-IRS-1, serine phosphorylated type 1 insulin receptor substrate; Aβ, amyloid β peptide; BACE-1, type 1 β-secretase or type 1 β site-amyloid precursor protein cleaving enzyme; CSPG4 cell, neural cell type expressing high levels of chondroitin sulfate proteoglycan; HGF, hepatic growth factor; FGF-13, type 13 fibroblast growth factor; IGF-1, type 1 insulin growth factor; NOSTRIN, nitric oxide synthase traffic inducer; YAP-1, type 1 Yes-associated protein; P-YAP, S127-phosphorylated YAP1. The estimated feasibility scale is: 1 = unlikely to succeed, 2 = likely to succeed if technical obstacles are overcome, 3 = likely to be a useful approach.

pathophysiology of sporadic AD as well as already established fluid and neuroimaging biomarkers, will be clarified in the coming years and may open up a therapeutic avenue to molecular miRNA-targeted therapies.

LIQUID BIOPSY-GUIDED DRUG DEVELOPMENT

Systems biology derived exploratory biomarkers are beginning to bridge the historically developed separation between medical specialties and the deconstructed disease concepts as well as traditionally delineated drug development programs (e.g., within and between the different fields) (Hampel et al., 2018a,b). Indeed, biomarker panels are untangling shared pathways (pathophysiological and pathological commonalities) between nosologically diverse diseases which are differently conceptualized across different medical fields, such as Neurology, Oncology, and clinical Immunology.

Liquid biopsies will define stage- and individual-specific thresholds for AD pathophysiological dynamics and will constitute the core of future disease modeling paradigms in which different biological levels can be explored simultaneously (Roukos, 2017; Hampel et al., 2018c). Indeed, we hypothesize that liquid biopsy will enable to untangle the spatial and temporal dynamics between molecular-cellular pathways and brain large-scale brain network functional shifts, from adaptation to resilience until systems failure and cognitive decline. Hypothesis-independent identification and quantification of evolving risk of detrimental mechanisms of AD will be facilitated through a multi-purpose biomarker *armamentarium* (see **Figure 1**).

A liquid biopsy-guided stratification approach based on upcoming clustering and other artificial intelligence methods will create novel patient strata aggregating subjects which have similar biomarker profiles and segregating patients which do not.

To follow, the clinical trajectories of each biological cluster will be mapped out, hence, providing an innovative liquid biopsy-based risk prediction matrix of AD pathophysiology in asymptomatic at-risk individuals. Moreover, liquid biopsies may inform a staging framework from very early pathophysiological alterations to later preclinical and clinical manifestations. To achieve these objectives, it is necessary to trace and model

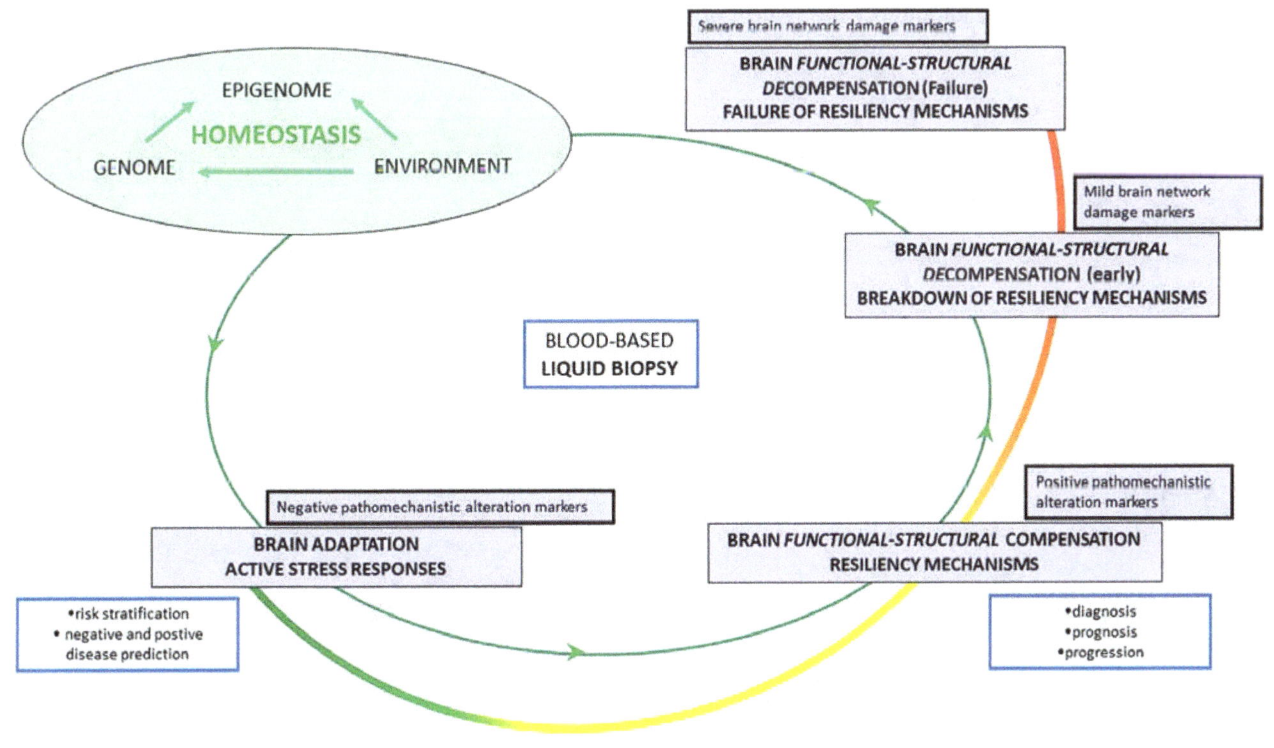

FIGURE 1 | Liquid biopsy-guided management of Alzheimer's disease according to a hypothetical model of spatial-temporal system-wide shifts: from adaptation to irreversible failure. Homeostasis is ensured by adaptive responses and compensatory mechanisms scaled in time and space across multi-level system networks: from molecular pathways, to cellular stress responses, to brain cell-to-cell and synaptic dynamics, to large-scale brain network activity, to brain-periphery cross-talks. If a decompensatory cascade occurs, homeostasis progressively breaks down until final systems failure. *Functional stage – adaptation stage – stress responses*: Metabolic and energetic reconfiguration associated with functional switch in molecular/cellular/tissue/brain systems/body system network activity. *Functional–structural stage – compensation stage – resiliency mechanisms*: Structural and functional counterbalancing of one or more initial pathomechanistic alterations. *Early decompensation stage – breakdown of resiliency mechanisms*: Initial and progressive loss of compensatory effect (resilience) or over sustained compensation which may be neither protective nor homeostatic. *Late decompensation stage (failure stage) – failure of resiliency mechanisms*: Hypothetical point of no-return. The colored curve line from green to red indicates a decreasing magnitude of drugs efficacy. The colored curve from green to red indicates a decreasing magnitude of drugs efficacy. The blue rectangles indicate the different context-of-use of biomarkers according to the pathophysiological evolution.

individual longitudinal trajectories and dynamics for each biomarker taking into account age ranges, sex, and common genetic variants associated with increased risk of developing AD (Nho et al., 2013; Ferretti et al., 2018; Pimenova et al., 2018).

The catalyzing impact of systems theory, systems biology, systems pharmacology, and precision pharmacology-oriented drug R&D programs will ultimately support more precise future medical strategies (Hampel et al., 2018a,b).

Systems pharmacology is a novel conceptual framework that models traditional pharmacological parameters, derived from pharmacodynamics and pharmacokinetics, operating under the theoretical background of systems medicine (Geerts et al., 2015, 2018). Systems pharmacology allows modeling a drug effects through key biological factors such as the genetic background, sexual dimorphism and age-related pathomechanistic alterations (Geerts et al., 2015; Roberts et al., 2016). Precision pharmacology is a biomarker-based approach providing pathway-based therapies through exploratory and predictive outcomes, from initial proof-of-pharmacology to all subsequently relevant decision-making processes (Hampel et al., 2018d).

We argue that liquid biopsy will support the proof of pharmacology for a putative DmT which requires successful demonstration of the capacity of a compound on several critical levels. This means clear indication of engagement of the intended biological target (i.e., druggability: the capacity of a molecular target to be modulated by a small-molecule drug), with predictable downstream alterations in pathophysiological mechanisms, in association with clinically relevant benefits (Geerts et al., 2015; Kozakov et al., 2015; Wu et al., 2016). For instance, recent studies have provided proof of principle for using protein cargo in neural-derived exosomes to demonstrate engagement of a specific target intracellular signaling cascade (e.g., the insulin cascade) by an experimental treatment (Eitan et al., 2017; Athauda et al., 2019). In particular, signaling mediators manifesting different functionality depending on their phosphorylation state may be particularly revealing for the effects of a drug when consistent changes are revealed in neural-derived exosomes after treatment. Such a signal has been likened to a "message in a bottle" (Dubal and Pleasure, 2019).

It is well established that multifactorial polygenic diseases such as several cancers, diabetes and AD, show non-linear pathophysiological dynamics likely due to evolutionary conserved pathways with complex molecular cross-talks and feedback loops and may also manifest individual differences in drug response (Rask-Andersen et al., 2014; Mitsopoulos et al., 2015; Deng and Nakamura, 2017; Roukos, 2017). Thus, in cancer as well diabetes and brain diseases, the magnitude of the improvement in clinical outcomes attained by a given

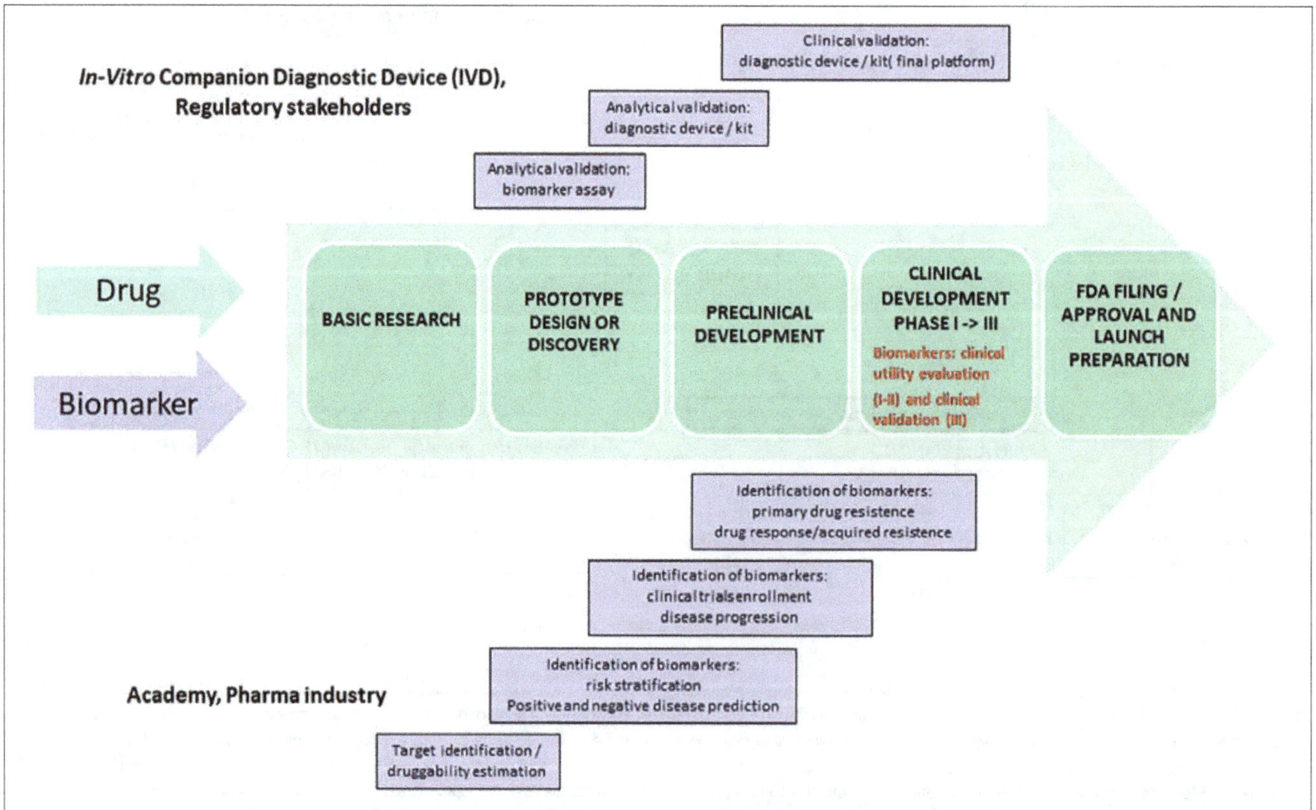

FIGURE 2 | Ideally, biomarkers should be carried through all phases of drug development and validated and qualified in agreement with regulators. The picture shows one possible model for biomarker-drug co-development program: a regulatory scenario for a single test that would be used in conjunction with a single drug in the clinical management of a patient. The figure highlights key events for both the diagnostic test and drug regulation with overall coordination of the regulatory processes governing them so that the products launch together.

small molecule may substantially change over time depending on the stage of the disease and the individual (epi)genetic biological background. Indeed, the likelihood of a positive biological effect induced by specific drug on a specific target may change over time, being related to the spatial-temporal target druggability patterns (dynamic evolution of the ligand binding affinity) as well as to mechanisms of drug resistance (Rask-Andersen et al., 2014; Mitsopoulos et al., 2015; Deng and Nakamura, 2017; Roukos, 2017). Drug-resistance refers to the presence of gene variants that impact drug target pathways through downstream effectors with either gain or loss of function. Within biomarker-positive populations entering a trial of a molecularly targeted treatment identified as druggable, some individuals are expected to display primary or acquired resistance (Schubbert et al., 2007; Deng and Nakamura, 2017; Drilon et al., 2018).

Temporary patterns of target druggability may be tightly linked to some key spatial and temporal pathophysiological coordinates that today can be deciphered through experimental and computational innovation integrated in the systems medicine approach (Roberts et al., 2016; Geerts et al., 2018). Likewise, cancer also in AD, liquid-biopsy will serve to accomplish druggability and drug-resistance profiling, from *in silico* computational prediction to *in vivo* biomarkers-drug co-development programs with the approval of both *in vitro* companion diagnostic device (IVD) and hopefully effective pharmacological compounds (see **Figure 2**) (Jorgensen and Hersom, 2016; Twomey et al., 2017). The feasibility profile of liquid-biopsy (minimally invasive, cost and time effective) seems to perfectly match the requirements of academic researchers, pharma companies, and regulatory stakeholders to successfully inform biomarker-drug co-development programs (Nicolaides et al., 2014; Jorgensen and Hersom, 2016; Twomey et al., 2017; Hampel et al., 2018c). This process will hopefully translate into discovering novel targets, including some currently considered non-druggable due to the lack of adequate surrogate outcomes. Consequently, liquid-biopsy related biomarker-drug co-development will improve the blueprints of clinical trials for AD by facilitating adaptive designs.

We assume that liquid biopsy may represent a key tool of systems pharmacology to dynamically and adaptively prioritize potential drug targets consistent with the pathophysiological evolution of the disease. Such focused breakthrough will support the precise treatment of the right patient, the best druggable target(s) at a defined time point of the disease based on a biologically identified and classified stage.

CONCLUSION

Biomarker panels critically support objective clinical decision-making processes in health facilities, academic research settings, payor organizations, and pharma/biotech development programs (O'Bryant et al., 2017; Hampel et al., 2018a).

Current efforts to re-define diagnostic criteria and bolster programs for biomarker discovery and drug development based on liquid-biopsy-guided disease modelling show promise to lead us to precision medicine for AD (Nicolaides et al., 2014; Jorgensen and Hersom, 2016; Twomey et al., 2017; Hampel et al., 2018c).

Clinical cancer studies investigating pathway-based therapies have shown, however, that not all biomarker-positive patients respond to a given compound (Drilon et al., 2018). Both positive and negative predictive biomarkers are required for detecting and quantifying target druggability and drug resistance, guiding the selection of patient subsets for specific treatments, and for dynamically treating AD as its pathophysiology evolves (Geerts et al., 2018; Gibson, 2019). To validation, qualification, and standardization of a comprehensive liquid biopsy for AD, blood-based biomarker panels should be subjected to rigorous testing using large-scale observational and longitudinal studies of cognitively intact individuals at risk of AD.

Toward this end, consequent academic-industry blood-based biomarker- drug co-development collaboration programs through all development stages and with strong regulatory science consideration are required. The Interest Area focused on Blood Based Biomarkers (BBB-PIA) - integrated in the Alzheimer's Association's ISTAART, in close collaboration with the Alzheimer Precision Medicine Initiative (APMI[1]) – will continue to facilitate the stepwise identification, validation, and standardization process of biomarker candidates (O'Bryant et al., 2017; Hampel et al., 2018c).

These advances are required to facilitate the emerging precision pharmacology and precision medicine paradigms in neuroscience and neurology, as already successfully established in other medical fields.

The emerging liquid biopsy framework is by definition not restricted to any disease field or specialty, it is an approach facilitated by technological and conceptual advances in the discovery and validation of blood-based biomarkers indicative of pathophysiological mechanisms underlying any disease. Therefore, it becomes inherently clear that the current substantial advances in blood-based biomarker development in AD will subsequently lead into practical and useful liquid biopsy solutions as part of early detection and screening as well as drug discovery programs. These solutions are currently on the horizon, based on strong evolving biomarker evidence.

MEMBERS OF THE ALZHEIMER PRECISION MEDICINE INITIATIVE – WORKING GROUP (APMI–WG)

Mohammad Afshar (Paris), Lisi Flores Aguilar (Montréal), Leyla Akman-Anderson (Sacramento), Joaquín Arenas (Madrid), Claudio Babiloni (Rome), Filippo Baldacci (Pisa), Richard Batrla (Rotkreuz), Norbert Benda (Bonn), Keith L. Black (Los Angeles), Arun L. W. Bokde (Dublin), Ubaldo Bonuccelli (Pisa), Karl Broich (Bonn), Francesco Cacciola (Siena), Filippo Caraci (Catania), Juan Castrillo (deceased) (Derio), Enrica Cavedo (Paris), Roberto Ceravolo (Pisa), Patrizia A. Chiesa (Paris),

[1] www.apmiscience.com

Jean-Christophe Corvol (Paris), Augusto Claudio Cuello (Montréal), Jeffrey L. Cummings (Las Vegas), Herman Depypere (Gent), Bruno Dubois (Paris), Andrea Duggento (Rome), Enzo Emanuele (Pavia), Valentina Escott-Price (Cardiff), Howard Federoff (Irvine), Maria Teresa Ferretti (Zurich), Massimo Fiandaca (Irvine), Richard A. Frank (Malvern), Francesco Garaci (Rome), Hugo Geerts (Berwyn), Filippo S. Giorgi (Pisa), Edward J. Goetzl (San Francisco), Manuela Graziani (Roma), Marion Haberkamp (Bonn), Marie-Odile Habert (Paris), Harald Hampel (Paris), Karl Herholz (Manchester), Dimitrios Kapogiannis (Baltimore), Eric Karran (Cambridge), Steven J. Kiddle (Cambridge), Seung H. Kim (Seoul), Yosef Koronyo (Los Angeles), Maya Koronyo-Hamaoui (Los Angeles), Todd Langevin (Minneapolis-Saint Paul), Stéphane Lehéricy (Paris), Alejandro Lucía (Madrid), Simone Lista (Paris), Jean Lorenceau (Paris), Dalila Mango (Rome), Mark Mapstone (Irvine), Christian Neri (Paris), Robert Nisticò (Rome), Sid E. O'Bryant (Fort Worth), Giovanni Palermo (Pisa), George Perry (San Antonio), Craig Ritchie (Edinburgh), Simone Rossi (Siena), Amira Saidi (Rome), Emiliano Santarnecchi (Siena), Lon S. Schneider (Los Angeles), Olaf Sporns (Bloomington), Nicola Toschi (Rome), Steven R. Verdooner (Sacramento), Andrea Vergallo (Paris), Nicolas Villain (Paris), Lindsay A. Welikovitch (Montréal), Janet Woodcock (Silver Spring), Erfan Younesi (Esch-sur-Alzette).

AUTHOR CONTRIBUTIONS

HH conceptualized the study, wrote the article, and provided a critical review of the literature. SL, EG, and DK contributed to the writing of the article and provided a critical review of the literature. AV conceptualized the study, contributed to the writing of the article, and provided a critical review of the literature.

FUNDING

This research benefited from the support of the Program "PHOENIX" led by the Sorbonne University Foundation and sponsored by la *Fondation pour la Recherche sur Alzheimer*. This research was supported in part (DK) by the Intramural Research Program of the National Institute on Aging, NIH. HH was supported by the AXA Research Fund, the "Fondation partenariale Sorbonne Université" and the "Fondation pour la Recherche sur Alzheimer", Paris, France.

REFERENCES

Alexandrov, P. N., Dua, P., Hill, J. M., Bhattacharjee, S., Zhao, Y., and Lukiw, W. J. (2012). MicroRNA (miRNA) speciation in Alzheimer's disease (AD) cerebrospinal fluid (CSF) and extracellular fluid (ECF). *Int. J. Biochem. Mol. Biol.* 3, 365–373.

Athauda, D., Gulyani, S., Karnati, H., Li, Y., Tweedie, D., Mustapic, M., et al. (2019). Utility of neuronal-derived exosomes to examine molecular mechanisms that affect motor function in patients with parkinson disease: a secondary analysis of the exenatide-pd trial. *JAMA Neurol.* doi: 10.1001/jamaneurol.2018.4304 [Epub ahead of print].

Bergman, P., Piket, E., Khademi, M., James, T., Brundin, L., Olsson, T., et al. (2016). Circulating miR-150 in CSF is a novel candidate biomarker for multiple sclerosis. *Neurol. Neuroimmunol. Neuroinflamm.* 3:e219. doi: 10.1212/NXI.0000000000000219

Cummings, J. L. (2011). Biomarkers in Alzheimer's disease drug development. *Alzheimers Dement* 7, e13–e44. doi: 10.1016/j.jalz.2010.06.004

Deng, X., and Nakamura, Y. (2017). Cancer precision medicine: from cancer screening to drug selection and personalized immunotherapy. *Trends Pharmacol. Sci.* 38, 15–24. doi: 10.1016/j.tips.2016.10.013

Drilon, A., Laetsch, T. W., Kummar, S., DuBois, S. G., Lassen, U. N., Demetri, G. D., et al. (2018). Efficacy of larotrectinib in trk fusion-positive cancers in adults and children. *N. Engl. J. Med.* 378, 731–739. doi: 10.1056/NEJMoa1714448

Dubal, D. B., and Pleasure, S. J. (2019). Neural-derived extracellular vesicles in clinical trials: message in a bottle. *JAMA Neurol.* doi: 10.1001/jamaneurol.2018.4325 [Epub ahead of print].

Eitan, E., Tosti, V., Suire, C. N., Cava, E., Berkowitz, S., Bertozzi, B., et al. (2017). In a randomized trial in prostate cancer patients, dietary protein restriction modifies markers of leptin and insulin signaling in plasma extracellular vesicles. *Aging Cell* 16, 1430–1433. doi: 10.1111/acel.12657

Fandos, N., Perez-Grijalba, V., Pesini, P., Olmos, S., Bossa, M., Villemagne, V. L., et al. (2017). Plasma amyloid beta 42/40 ratios as biomarkers for amyloid beta cerebral deposition in cognitively normal individuals. *Alzheimer's Dement* 8, 179–187.

Ferretti, M. T., Iulita, M. F., Cavedo, E., Chiesa, P. A., Schumacher Dimech, A., Santuccione Chadha, A., et al. (2018). Sex differences in Alzheimer disease - the gateway to precision medicine. *Nat. Rev. Neurol.* 14, 457–469. doi: 10.1038/s41582-018-0032-9

Fiandaca, M. S., Kapogiannis, D., Mapstone, M., Boxer, A., Eitan, E., Schwartz, J. B., et al. (2015). Identification of preclinical Alzheimer's disease by a profile of pathogenic proteins in neurally derived blood exosomes: a case-control study. *Alzheimers Dement* 11, 600-607.e1. doi: 10.1016/j.jalz.2014.06.008

Geerts, H., Gieschke, R., and Peck, R. (2018). Use of quantitative clinical pharmacology to improve early clinical development success in neurodegenerative diseases. *Expert Rev. Clin. Pharmacol.* 11, 789–795. doi: 10.1080/17512433.2018.1501555

Geerts, H., Roberts, P., and Spiros, A. (2015). Assessing the synergy between cholinomimetics and memantine as augmentation therapy in cognitive impairment in schizophrenia. A virtual human patient trial using quantitative systems pharmacology. *Front. Pharmacol.* 6:198. doi: 10.3389/fphar.2015.00198

Gibson, G. (2019). Going to the negative: genomics for optimized medical prescription. *Nat. Rev. Genet.* 20, 1–2. doi: 10.1038/s41576-018-0061-7

Goetzl, E. J., Mustapic, M., Kapogiannis, D., Eitan, E., Lobach, I. V., Goetzl, L., et al. (2016). Cargo proteins of plasma astrocyte-derived exosomes in Alzheimer's disease. *FASEB J.* 30, 3853–3859. doi: 10.1096/fj.201600756R

Goetzl, E. J., Schwartz, J. B., Mustapic, M., Lobach, I. V., Daneman, R., Abner, E. L., et al. (2017). Altered cargo proteins of human plasma endothelial cell-derived exosomes in atherosclerotic cerebrovascular disease. *FASEB J.* 31, 3689–3694. doi: 10.1096/fj.201700149

Goetzl, E. J., Abner, E. L., Jicha, G. A., Kapogiannis, D., and Schwartz, J. B. (2018a). Declining levels of functionally specialized synaptic proteins in plasma neuronal exosomes with progression of Alzheimer's disease. *FASEB J.* 32, 888–893. doi: 10.1096/fj.201700731R

Goetzl, E. J., Schwartz, J. B., Abner, E. L., Jicha, G. A., and Kapogiannis, D. (2018b). High complement levels in astrocyte-derived exosomes of Alzheimer disease. *Ann. Neurol.* 83, 544–552. doi: 10.1002/ana.25172

Goldberg, K. B., Blumenthal, G. M., McKee, A. E., and Pazdur, R. (2018). The FDA oncology center of excellence and precision medicine. *Exp. Biol. Med.* 243, 308–312. doi: 10.1177/1535370217740861

Hampel, H., O'Bryant, S. E., Molinuevo, J. L., Zetterberg, H., Masters, C. L., Lista, S., et al. (2018a). Blood-based biomarkers for Alzheimer disease: mapping the road to the clinic. *Nat. Rev. Neurol.* 14, 639–652. doi: 10.1038/s41582-018-0079-7

Hampel, H., Toschi, N., Babiloni, C., Baldacci, F., Black, K. L., Bokde, A. L. W., et al. (2018b). Revolution of alzheimer precision neurology. passageway of systems biology and neurophysiology. *J. Alzheimers. Dis.* 64, S47–S105. doi: 10.3233/JAD-179932

Hampel, H., Toschi, N., Baldacci, F., Zetterberg, H., Blennow, K., Kilimann, I., et al. (2018c). Alzheimer's disease biomarker-guided diagnostic workflow using the added value of six combined cerebrospinal fluid candidates: abeta1-42, total-tau, phosphorylated-tau, NFL, neurogranin, and YKL-40. *Alzheimers Dement* 14, 492–501. doi: 10.1016/j.jalz.2017.11.015

Hampel, H., Vergallo, A., Aguilar, L. F., Benda, N., Broich, K., Cuello, A. C., et al. (2018d). Precision pharmacology for Alzheimer's disease. *Pharmacol. Res.* 130, 331–365. doi: 10.1016/j.phrs.2018.02.014

Heitzer, E., Haque, I. S., Roberts, C. E. S., and Speicher, M. R. (2019). Current and future perspectives of liquid biopsies in genomics-driven oncology. *Nat. Rev. Genet.* 20, 71–88. doi: 10.1038/s41576-018-0071-5

Jack, C. R. J., Bennett, D. A., Blennow, K., Carrillo, M. C., Feldman, H. H., Frisoni, G. B., et al. (2016). A/T/N: an unbiased descriptive classification scheme for Alzheimer disease biomarkers. *Neurology* 87, 539–547. doi: 10.1212/WNL.0000000000002923

Jorgensen, J. T., and Hersom, M. (2016). Companion diagnostics-a tool to improve pharmacotherapy. *Ann. Transl. Med.* 4:482. doi: 10.21037/atm.2016.12.26

Kozakov, D., Hall, D. R., Napoleon, R. L., Yueh, C., Whitty, A., and Vajda, S. (2015). New frontiers in druggability. *J. Med. Chem.* 58, 9063–9088. doi: 10.1021/acs.jmedchem.5b00586

Kvartsberg, H., Duits, F. H., Ingelsson, M., Andreasen, N., Ohrfelt, A., Andersson, K., et al. (2015). Cerebrospinal fluid levels of the synaptic protein neurogranin correlates with cognitive decline in prodromal Alzheimer's disease. *Alzheimers Dement* 11, 1180–1190. doi: 10.1016/j.jalz.2014.10.009

Mattsson, N., Andreasson, U., Zetterberg, H., and Blennow, K. (2017). Association of plasma neurofilament light with neurodegeneration in patients with alzheimer disease. *JAMA Neurol.* 74, 557–566. doi: 10.1001/jamaneurol.2016.6117

Mielke, M. M., Hagen, C. E., Xu, J., Chai, X., Vemuri, P., Lowe, V. J., et al. (2018). Plasma phospho-tau181 increases with Alzheimer's disease clinical severity and is associated with tau- and amyloid-positron emission tomography. *Alzheimers Dement* 14, 989–997. doi: 10.1016/j.jalz.2018.02.013

Mitsopoulos, C., Schierz, A. C., Workman, P., and Al-Lazikani, B. (2015). Distinctive behaviors of druggable proteins in cellular networks. *PLoS Comput. Biol.* 11:e1004597. doi: 10.1371/journal.pcbi.1004597

Molinuevo, J. L., Ayton, S., Batrla, R., Bednar, M. M., Bittner, T., Cummings, J., et al. (2018). Current state of Alzheimer's fluid biomarkers. *Acta Neuropathol.* 136, 821–853. doi: 10.1007/s00401-018-1932-x

Mustapic, M., Eitan, E., Werner, J. K. J., Berkowitz, S. T., Lazaropoulos, M. P., Tran, J., et al. (2017). Plasma extracellular vesicles enriched for neuronal origin: a potential window into brain pathologic processes. *Front. Neurosci.* 11:278. doi: 10.3389/fnins.2017.00278

Nakamura, A., Kaneko, N., Villemagne, V. L., Kato, T., Doecke, J., Dore, V., et al. (2018). High performance plasma amyloid-beta biomarkers for Alzheimer's disease. *Nature* 554, 249–254. doi: 10.1038/nature25456

Nho, K., Corneveaux, J. J., Kim, S., Lin, H., Risacher, S. L., Shen, L., et al. (2013). Whole-exome sequencing and imaging genetics identify functional variants for rate of change in hippocampal volume in mild cognitive impairment. *Mol. Psychiatry* 18, 781–787. doi: 10.1038/mp.2013.24

Nicolaides, N. C., O'Shannessy, D. J., Albone, E., and Grasso, L. (2014). Co-development of diagnostic vectors to support targeted therapies and theranostics: essential tools in personalized cancer therapy. *Front. Oncol.* 4:141. doi: 10.3389/fonc.2014.00141

O'Bryant, S. E., Mielke, M. M., Rissman, R. A., Lista, S., Vanderstichele, H., Zetterberg, H., et al. (2017). Blood-based biomarkers in Alzheimer disease: current state of the science and a novel collaborative paradigm for advancing from discovery to clinic. *Alzheimers Dement* 13, 45–58. doi: 10.1016/j.jalz.2016.09.014

Pantel, K., and Alix-Panabieres, C. (2019). Liquid biopsy and minimal residual disease - latest advances and implications for cure. *Nat. Rev. Clin. Oncol.* doi: 10.1038/s41571-019-0187-3 [Epub ahead of print].

Park, J. C., Han, S. -H., Yi, D., Byun, M. S., Lee, J. H., Jang, S., et al. (2019). Plasma tau/amyloid-beta1-42 ratio predicts brain tau deposition and neurodegeneration in Alzheimer's disease. *Brain* 142, 771–786. doi: 10.1093/brain/awy347

Pimenova, A. A., Raj, T., and Goate, A. M. (2018). Untangling genetic risk for Alzheimer's Disease. *Biol. Psychiatry* 83, 300–310. doi: 10.1016/j.biopsych.2017.05.014

Preische, O., Schultz, S. A., Apel, A., Kuhle, J., Kaeser, S. A., Barro, C., et al. (2019). Serum neurofilament dynamics predicts neurodegeneration and clinical progression in presymptomatic Alzheimer's disease. *Nat. Med.* 25, 277–283. doi: 10.1038/s41591-018-0304-3

Pulliam, L., Sun, B., Mustapic, M., Chawla, S., and Kapogiannis, D. (2019). Plasma neuronal exosomes serve as biomarkers of cognitive impairment in HIV infection and Alzheimer's disease. *J. Neurovirol.* doi: 10.1007/s13365-018-0695-4 [Epub ahead of print].

Rask-Andersen, M., Masuram, S., and Schioth, H. B. (2014). The druggable genome: evaluation of drug targets in clinical trials suggests major shifts in molecular class and indication. *Annu. Rev. Pharmacol. Toxicol.* 54, 9–26. doi: 10.1146/annurev-pharmtox-011613-135943

Roberts, P., Spiros, A., and Geerts, H. (2016). A humanized clinically calibrated quantitative systems pharmacology model for hypokinetic motor symptoms in parkinson's disease. *Front. Pharmacol.* 7:6. doi: 10.3389/fphar.2016.00006

Roukos, D. H. (2017). Spatiotemporal diversification of intrapatient genomic clones and early drug development concepts realize the roadmap of precision cancer medicine. *Drug Discov. Today* 22, 1148–1164. doi: 10.1016/j.drudis.2017.03.014

Schubbert, S., Bollag, G., Lyubynska, N., Nguyen, H., Kratz, C. P., Zenker, M., et al. (2007). Biochemical and functional characterization of germ line KRAS mutations. *Mol. Cell. Biol.* 27, 7765–7770. doi: 10.1128/MCB.00965-07

Shen, Y., Wang, H., Sun, Q., Yao, H., Keegan, A. P., Mullan, M., et al. (2018). increased plasma beta-secretase 1 may predict conversion to Alzheimer's disease dementia in individuals with mild cognitive impairment. *Biol. Psychiatry* 83, 447–455. doi: 10.1016/j.biopsych.2017.02.007

Snyder, H. M., Carrillo, M. C., Grodstein, F., Henriksen, K., Jeromin, A., Lovestone, S., et al. (2014). Developing novel blood-based biomarkers for Alzheimer's disease. *Alzheimers Dement* 10, 109–114. doi: 10.1016/j.jalz.2013.10.007

Sorensen, S. S., Nygaard, A. B., and Christensen, T. (2016). MiRNA expression profiles in cerebrospinal fluid and blood of patients with Alzheimer's disease and other types of dementia - an exploratory study. *Transl. Neurodegener.* 5:6. doi: 10.1186/s40035-016-0053-5

Twomey, J. D., Brahme, N. N., and Zhang, B. (2017). Drug-biomarker co-development in oncology - 20 years and counting. *Drug Resist. Updat.* 30, 48–62. doi: 10.1016/j.drup.2017.02.002

Vergallo, A., Bun, R. -S., Toschi, N., Baldacci, F., Zetterberg, H., Blennow, K., et al. (2018). Association of cerebrospinal fluid alpha-synuclein with total and phospho-tau181 protein concentrations and brain amyloid load in cognitively normal subjective memory complainers stratified by Alzheimer's disease biomarkers. *Alzheimers Dement* 14, 1623–1631. doi: 10.1016/j.jalz.2018.06.3053

Wan, J. C. M., Massie, C., Garcia-Corbacho, J., Mouliere, F., Brenton, J. D., Caldas, C., et al. (2017). Liquid biopsies come of age: towards implementation of circulating tumour DNA. *Nat. Rev. Cancer* 17, 223–238. doi: 10.1038/nrc.2017.7

Wu, F., Ma, C., and Tan, C. (2016). Network motifs modulate druggability of cellular targets. *Sci. Rep.* 6:36626. doi: 10.1038/srep36626

Zhao, Y., Alexandrov, P. N., and Lukiw, W. J. (2016). Anti-microRNAs as novel therapeutic agents in the clinical management of Alzheimer's Disease. *Front. Neurosci.* 10:59. doi: 10.3389/fnins.2016.00059

14

Experimental Pharmacology in Transgenic Rodent Models of Alzheimer's Disease

A. Claudio Cuello[1,2,3†], Hélène Hall[1†] and Sonia Do Carmo[1]*

[1] Department of Pharmacology and Therapeutics, McGill University, Montreal, QC, Canada, [2] Department of Neurology and Neurosurgery, McGill University, Montreal, QC, Canada, [3] Department of Anatomy and Cell Biology, McGill University, Montreal, QC, Canada

***Correspondence:**
A. Claudio Cuello
claudio.cuello@mcgill.ca

† These authors have contributed equally to this work

This Mini Review discusses the merits and shortfalls of transgenic (tg) rodents modeling aspects of the human Alzheimer's disease (AD) pathology and their application to evaluate experimental therapeutics. It addresses some of the differences between mouse and rat tg models for these investigations. It relates, in a condensed fashion, the experience of our research laboratory with the application of anti-inflammatory compounds and S-adenosylmethionine (SAM) at the earliest stages of AD-like amyloid pathology in tg mice. The application of SAM was intended to revert the global brain DNA hypomethylation unleashed by the intraneuronal accumulation of amyloid-β-immunoreactive material, an intervention that restored levels of DNA methylation including of the *bace1* gene. This review also summarizes experimental pharmacology observations made in the McGill tg rat model of AD-like pathology by applying "nano-lithium" or a drug with allosteric M1 muscarinic and sigma 1 receptor agonistic properties (AF710B). Extremely low doses of lithium (up to 400 times lower than used in the clinic) had remarkable beneficial effects on lowering pathology and improving cognitive functions in tg rats. Likewise, AF710B treatment, even at advanced stages of the pathology, displayed remarkable beneficial effects. This drug, in experimental conditions, demonstrated possible "disease-modifying" properties as pathology was frankly diminished and cognition improved after a month of "wash-out" period. The Mini-Review ends with a discussion on the predictive value of similar experimental pharmacological interventions in current rodent tg models. It comments on the validity of some of these approaches for early interventions at preclinical stages of AD, interventions which may be envisioned once definitive diagnosis of AD before clinical presentation is made possible.

Keywords: Alzheimer's disease, cholinergic, DNA hypomethylation, experimental therapy, neuroinflammation, lithium, muscarinic/sigma1 receptors, S-adenosyl methionine

INTRODUCTION

Alzheimer's disease (AD) is a progressive neurodegenerative disease and the leading cause of dementia in the elderly (Hardy et al., 2014; Aisen et al., 2017). Postmortem brains from AD patients display characteristic pathological hallmarks, defined as extracellular amyloid plaques and intracellular neurofibrillary tangles made of hyper-phosphorylated tau protein. In addition, the cholinergic system is severely compromised. The vast majority of AD cases is sporadic, while $<1\%$ of cases corresponds to autosomal dominant forms, or familial AD (FAD), in which specific genetic mutations drive disease onset (Bateman et al., 2011; Ryman et al., 2014).

To date, there is no treatment to cure or prevent the development of the disease. Patients only have access to a few therapeutic options which offer limited symptomatic relief. Three of the four drugs approved by the Food and Drug Administration (FDA) for AD are cholinesterase inhibitors (AChEI). They enhance cholinergic synaptic transmission by preventing the breakdown of acetylcholine, a neurotransmitter essential for learning and memory. The fourth drug is memantine, an NMDA-receptor antagonist, while an additional pharmacological option combines one of the AChEI (donepezil) and memantine (Alzheimer's Association, 2018).

Although studies would indicate a decrease in the incidence of AD in high-income countries over the past 10 years (Langa, 2015; Derby et al., 2017; Seblova et al., 2018), it is unlikely to offset the aging population. In fact, AD prevalence is increasing worldwide and is reaching near-epidemic proportions (Hickman et al., 2016). In that context, it is urgent to develop new drugs that can halt or prevent the progression of the disease. As of January 30, 2018, there were 112 agents in the AD treatment pipeline registered on clinicaltrial.gov, 63% of which are disease-modifying therapies (Cummings et al., 2018), illustrating the current efforts devoted to finding a cure for AD. Preclinical studies constitute an important cornerstone in drug development; validation of drug safety and efficacy in animal models is a necessary step before moving a drug into clinical trials. As such, animal models are a critical component to move the research field forward.

In this review, we will provide a concise overview of transgenic (tg) rodent models mimicking key aspects of the AD pathology and discuss their value in the drug development pipeline, as well as the challenges to predict drug efficacy in AD patients based on animal studies. In particular, we will focus on our experience with our transgenic mouse and rat models and describe experimental pharmacology studies using these models.

OVERVIEW OF TRANSGENIC MODELS OF ALZHEIMER'S DISEASE

A large number of tg mice and rats reproducing key features of the AD pathology have been generated. As of December 2018, the Alzheimer Forum Website lists 160 tg rodent models in its online database[1] (Kinoshita and Clark, 2007), 156 of which are mice and only 4 are rats. The majority of these models express human genes bearing mutations described in FAD cases and human tauopathies, as well as human genes identified by Genome Wide Association Studies as susceptibility genes increasing the risk of developing AD (Tosto and Reitz, 2013). As such, they mostly mimic rare familial forms of AD and may not provide data translatable to sporadic AD. The most popular models are based on overexpression of human amyloid precursor protein (APP), presenilin (PSEN) [part of the γ-secretase complex involved in the cleavage of APP into amyloid-β (Aβ)] and tau, alone or in combination, to trigger accumulation of high levels of Aβ into plaques as well as the development of tauopathy (Spires and Hyman, 2005).

In particular, the most frequently used mouse models have been mice overexpressing human APP with the double Swedish (K670N and M671L) (Mullan et al., 1992) and the Indiana (V717F) (Murrell et al., 1991) mutations, such as the PDAPP (Games et al., 1995), tg2576 (Hsiao et al., 1996) and J20 (Mucke et al., 2000) models, as well as mice overexpressing mutant human APP and PSEN such as the APP/PS1 (Holcomb et al., 1998) and 5xFAD (Oakley et al., 2006) mice. One of the most popular mouse models to date is the 3xTg model harboring mutated APP, PSEN and tau genes (Oddo et al., 2003). In parallel, mouse models of tauopathies, in particular the hTauP301S (Allen et al., 2002) and PS19 mice (Yoshiyama et al., 2007), have become popular to study the tau component of the AD pathology (Gotz et al., 2007), although their main limitation resides in the expression of human tau harboring mutations seen in frontotemporal dementia and parkinsonism linked to chromosome 17 and not in AD. The particular characteristics and merits of tg mice for AD research have been discussed in several reviews (Hsiao, 1998; Bales, 2012; LaFerla and Green, 2012; Puzzo et al., 2015; Ameen-Ali et al., 2017; Jankowsky and Zheng, 2017; Sasaguri et al., 2017).

The most frequently used tg rats modeling the AD-like amyloid pathology are the McGill-R-Thy1-APP (Leon et al., 2010) and TgF344-AD (Cohen et al., 2013) rats. The clear imbalance in the ratio of mouse/rat models of AD reflects the inherent difficulty of producing tg rats in the early years of transgenesis, rather than an advantage of mice over rats. However, advances in transgenesis techniques have had a substantial impact on the development of tg rats (Filipiak and Saunders, 2006). In fact, rats are better suited than mice for biomedical research relevant to human. The increased value of rats over mice to study, in particular, human neurodegenerative conditions has been highlighted in recent reviews, with an emphasis on cognitive outcomes (Do Carmo and Cuello, 2013) and brain imaging (Zimmer et al., 2014). More recently, Drummond and Wisniewski (2017) discussed the relative characteristics of diverse species for a better representation of the human AD pathology and the challenges ahead.

Tg rodent models of AD have undoubtedly provided invaluable insights into the pathological processes of AD. They have also been instrumental in moving experimental therapy into clinical trials, following reports of positive therapeutic outcomes in rodent models. In this context, tg models played a pivotal role in the development of immunotherapy for AD, following the first experimental evidence that immunization of PDAPP mice with fibrillary $A\beta_{42}$ decreased amyloid pathology (Schenk et al., 1999). Subsequent studies demonstrated that vaccination with Aβ also prevented memory loss in tg mouse models of AD (Janus et al., 2000; Morgan et al., 2000), which rapidly led to clinical trials. The first of these trials was unfortunately prematurely halted after a subset of patients developed acute meningoencephalitis (Orgogozo et al., 2003). Since then, more than one thousand publications have emerged illustrating efficacy, in varying degrees, of a large range of

[1] https://www.alzforum.org/research-models/alzheimers-disease

compounds. Some of these experimental attempts have been reviewed in LaFerla and Green (2012) and Sasaguri et al. (2017).

PHARMACOLOGICAL THERAPY IN MOUSE AND RAT MODELS OF THE AD-LIKE AMYLOID PATHOLOGY – INSIGHTS FROM OUR EXPERIENCE

Our laboratory has developed tg lines expressing human APP with the double Swedish and the Indiana mutations under the Thy1 promoter, which recapitulate key features of the AD-like amyloid pathology in mice and rats. The McGill-Thy1-APP mice (Ferretti et al., 2011) and McGill-R-Thy1-APP rats (Leon et al., 2010) have been extensively studied by us (Cuello et al., 2010, 2012; Ferretti et al., 2012a,b; Hanzel et al., 2014; Iulita et al., 2014, 2017; Pimentel et al., 2015; Do Carmo et al., 2016, 2018; Wilson et al., 2017a,b, 2018; Hall et al., 2018) and others (Nilsen et al., 2012, 2014a,b; Galeano et al., 2014, 2018; Qi et al., 2014, 2018; Heggland et al., 2015; Martino Adami et al., 2017a,b; Parent et al., 2017; Zhang et al., 2017; Prestia et al., 2018). In the following section, we will discuss the particular value of these specific models in experimental pharmacology.

McGill-Thy1-APP Mice

In the McGill-Thy1-APP mouse model, overexpression of mutant human APP triggers intraneuronal accumulation of Aβ material, including Aβ oligomers and fibrillary oligomers in cortical and hippocampal pyramidal neurons. Cognitive deficits are present prior to deposition of extracellular amyloid plaques at 4 months of age. At the same time, cholinergic alterations are detected in the cerebral cortex. Levels of insulin degrading enzyme, a well-established Aβ degrading enzyme, are downregulated in the cerebral cortex, suggesting that an impaired clearance of Aβ material likely contributes to the Aβ accumulation (Ferretti et al., 2011). In addition, microglial activation and recruitment toward Aβ-burdened neurons is present before plaque formation, along with an upregulation in major histocompatibility complex II, inducible nitric oxide (i-NOS) and CD40. This pre-plaque proinflammatory process is also accompanied by neuronal cyclooxygenase-2 (COX-2) upregulation (Ferretti et al., 2012b).

Minocycline

At late, clinical stages of AD, there is well-characterized chronic CNS inflammation. This late neuroinflammatory process is characterized by a strong immune response and phagocytic removal of Aβ material (McGeer and Rogers, 1992; McGeer and McGeer, 2013). These findings and the evidence that long term NSAIDs treatment for rheumathoid arthritis diminished AD prevalence (McGeer et al., 1990) sparked the idea that therapeutic agents directed at lowering inflammation could be of benefit for AD patients. However, studies showed that anti-inflammatories administered after AD clinical presentation did not improve cognitive decline (Jaturapatporn et al., 2012). In contrast, a large number of epidemiological studies confirmed that cognitively normal individuals receiving long term anti-inflammatory medication had a reduced risk of developing AD when compared to the general population (Breitner et al., 2011; McGeer and McGeer, 2013; Zhang et al., 2018). Taken together, these apparent contradictory findings support the idea that CNS inflammation at early (preclinical) and late (clinical) stages of AD are fundamentally distinct processes and suggest that blunting the early disease-aggravating inflammatory process may be of benefit for AD patients, concepts that have been further discussed in an opinion paper in TIPS (Cuello, 2017) and in a "white paper" in Alzheimer's and Dementia by Rogers (2018).

As detailed in the previous section, McGill-Thy1-APP mice display an early pre-plaque disease-aggravating neuroinflammatory process (Ferretti et al., 2011) which, according to the above, may constitute an interesting target for therapeutic intervention. To test this hypothesis, and supported by prior observations (Seabrook et al., 2006), tg mice were treated with minocycline, a tetracyclic derivative with anti-inflammatory properties, at a young, pre-plaque stage, for one month. Minocycline treatment corrected the upregulation of i-NOS and COX-2, lowered interleukin-1β levels and decreased microglial activation. The reduction in inflammation was accompanied by changes in the APP processing, namely a decrease in full length APP and Aβ trimer levels, while the activity of the β-site APP cleaving enzyme 1 (BACE1) was normalized (Ferretti et al., 2012a). Overall this study demonstrates that the early, pre-plaque, disease aggravating neuroinflammatory process triggered by the AD-like amyloid pathology can be dampened by the pharmacological application of minocycline.

These findings would support the notion that targeting inflammation early in the disease process should have a beneficial outcome in individuals with preclinical AD pathology. Successful implementation of such a strategy will, however, rely on the unequivocal identification of biomarkers of AD preclinical stages.

S-Adenosylmethionine (SAM)

There is growing evidence revealing that epigenetic deregulations and dysregulated DNA methylation may unleash disease-aggravating mechanisms in several neuropathologies. AD patients and AD animal models display global and gene-specific DNA hypomethylation within the brain (West et al., 1995; Mastroeni et al., 2010; Bakulski et al., 2012; Chouliaras et al., 2013; Cadena-del-Castillo et al., 2014; De Jager et al., 2014; Iwata et al., 2014; Smith et al., 2016; Nicolia et al., 2017; Zhao et al., 2017), likely contributing to the AD pathology and associated memory deficits. We have demonstrated the occurrence of global DNA hypomethylation, which is prominent in neurons, at early pathological stages in McGill-Thy1-APP mice. Importantly, the *bace1* promoter is hypomethylated in our tg mice. This was associated with higher levels of BACE1 protein and BACE1 activity, and in consequence increased Aβ peptides in the CNS (Do Carmo et al., 2016).

The cause of global hypomethylation in AD remains unclear. However, we found that early intraneuronal accumulation of Aβ is sufficient to provoke global DNA hypomethylation (Do Carmo et al., 2016). Importantly, in AD patients the levels of the ubiquitous methyl donor S-adenosylmethionine (SAM) are low in the brain and cerebrospinal fluid (Bottiglieri et al., 1991; Morrison et al., 1996). This prompted us to administer systemically SAM to McGill-Thy1-APP mice, starting at early stages of the pathology. This straightforward therapy was sufficient to abolish the pre-existing global hypomethylation, as well as *bace1* hypomethylation. BACE1 protein levels and activity were restored to control levels and brain amyloid pathology decreased. This strategy was sufficient to fully revert the cognitive impairment consequent to the CNS amyloid pathology, as revealed by the novel object recognition (NOR) and the Morris water maze (MWM) tests (Do Carmo et al., 2016). The findings, in our model, of an early neuronal demethylation and its rescue by SAM treatment reinforce a causal link between Aβ accumulation and impaired DNA methylation, rather than the consequence of stochastic events.

In addition, in human brains from the Religious Orders Study cohorts, we also found correlations between *bace1* methylation levels and amyloid and tangle load as well as measures of cognition (Do Carmo et al., 2016). Overall, our observations in tg mice and AD patients suggest that DNA hypomethylation should be considered as a drugable target for the treatment of AD, and that, in consequence, SAM-based therapy might constitute a promising therapeutic avenue. Of note, the use of SAM in the treatment of multiple neuropsychiatric disorders is currently being explored (Sharma et al., 2017).

McGill-R-Thy1-APP Rats

The McGill-R-Thy1-APP rats display early intraneuronal accumulation of Aβ in the hippocampus and cerebral cortex, evident one week after birth. As the amyloid pathology progresses with age, extracellular plaques start to develop. The first plaques are observed in the subiculum at 6–9 months of age (Leon et al., 2010) and later spread through anatomically connected regions (Heggland et al., 2015). Cognitive deficits are apparent at 3 months of age and worsen as the pathology progresses (Leon et al., 2010). This evolving pathology is accompanied by an early, disease-aggravating, pre-plaque neuroinflammatory process (Hanzel et al., 2014). Deficits in synaptic plasticity are evident at the pre-plaque stage and appear to be inflammasome-dependent (Qi et al., 2014, 2018). Similarly, deficits in synaptosomal bioenergetics are reported before the appearance of plaques (Martino Adami et al., 2017b). At the post-plaque stage, the NGF metabolic pathway is dysregulated and shows impairment in neurotrophin expression (Iulita et al., 2017), as seen during the progression of AD in patients (Iulita and Cuello, 2016). These changes are accompanied by a reduction in cholinergic synaptic boutons (Iulita et al., 2017). Moderate neuronal loss in the subiculum (Heggland et al., 2015), hippocampal shrinkage and glucose hypometabolism further characterize the post-plaque stage (Parent et al., 2017). Overall, in the McGill-R-Thy1-APP rat model, a slowly evolving amyloid pathology triggers a cascade of events reminiscent of what is seen in AD brains, thereby offering an array of targets possibly amenable to therapeutic intervention.

NP03-Lithium

The complex nature of the human AD pathology, which involves multiple processes such as abnormal Aβ and tau processing, CNS inflammation, mitochondrial dysfunction and calcium dyshomeostasis, calls for the use of multi-target drugs rather than a compound targeting a single molecule. In that context, lithium is of interest as it reportedly has the ability to modulate several of these pathways (Malhi and Outhred, 2016).

Lithium salts are widely used in the treatment of psychiatric conditions such as bipolar disorder. A limited number of studies have also examined the potential use of lithium in amnestic mild cognitive impairment and clinical AD populations, and have reported promising but often conflicting results (Havens and Cole, 1982; Terao et al., 2006; Macdonald et al., 2008; Hampel et al., 2009; Leyhe et al., 2009; Forlenza et al., 2011, 2016; Nunes et al., 2013; Mauer et al., 2014; Morris and Berk, 2016; Kessing et al., 2017). Unfortunately, lithium has a narrow therapeutic window and a low brain penetration. It elicits with some frequency severe side effects which limit its long-term use in the elderly population (Gelenberg and Jefferson, 1995; Livingstone and Rampes, 2006; Azab et al., 2015). Coincidently with the finding that trace amounts of lithium in drinking water are associated with a reduced incidence of dementia (Mauer et al., 2014; Kessing et al., 2017; McGrath and Berk, 2017; Fajardo et al., 2018), there has been a growing interest for low-dose lithium in the treatment of AD (Nunes et al., 2013, 2015; Zhao et al., 2014). Treatment with microdose lithium was shown to prevent cognitive decline in AD patients and in AD tg models (Nunes et al., 2013, 2015).

NP03 is a novel formulation of lithium, in which microdose lithium is encapsulated in a water-in-oil microemulsion (Aonys technology developed by Medesis Pharma, Montpellier, France). This formulation can enhance the CNS penetration of significantly lower amounts of lithium, with doses 100 to 400 times lower than what is usually prescribed for bipolar disorder. Such doses can most likely avoid the adverse effects associated with classical, higher dosage, lithium formulations. Treatment of young, pre-plaque McGill-R-Thy1-APP rats with NP03 resulted in cognitive improvements as measured by the NOR, MWM and fear conditioning tests. Unexpectedly, NP03 treatment also reduced BACE1 levels and activity, leading to a decrease in levels of soluble Aβ42. NP03 treatment was also shown to inactivate GSK-3β, rescue impaired CRTC1 promoter binding of synaptic plasticity genes and restore hippocampal neurogenesis in tg rats (Wilson et al., 2017b). In addition, NP03 reduced oxidative stress and inflammation markers in tg rats, as evidenced by decreased levels of protein-bound 4-hydroxynonenal and protein-resident 3-nitrotyrosine, as well as reduced production of cytokines such as TNF-α, IFN-γ, IL-10, and IL-5. Finally, NP03 downregulated transcripts levels of the microglia surface receptor TREM2 concomitantly with a reduced recruitment of microglia toward Aβ-burden neurons in the hippocampus (Wilson et al., 2018). These findings highlight the value of novel formulations of non-toxic microdose lithium NP03 in the treatment of AD at its early, preclinical, stages.

Combined M1 Muscarinic/Sigma 1 Receptor Agonist

In the early 1990s, a pivotal study demonstrated that activation of muscarinic cholinergic receptors could modulate the APP processing toward a non-amyloidogenic pathway (Nitsch et al., 1992), thereby reducing the production of toxic Aβ. It was later shown that the M1 muscarinic receptors in particular played a key role in modulating the AD-like amyloid pathology *in vivo* (Caccamo et al., 2006). Following these seminal discoveries, it was hypothesized that M1 receptor agonists could extend the cholinergic-based therapeutic arsenal for AD: they should, not only enhance the cholinergic tone for the cognitive benefits of AD patients, but also provide disease-modifying properties. Unfortunately, first generation muscarinic agonists lacked specificity for the M1 receptors, and activation of other receptor subtypes led to major side effects (Fisher, 2008). However, the generation of novel subtype specific muscarinic agonists has renewed the interest for this type of compounds (Fisher, 2012).

Given the complexity of AD pathophysiology, drugs that can target multiple receptors or impaired signaling pathways would likely offer a therapeutic advantage over more conventional single-target drug, as illustrated in the previous section. In that regards, the novel compound AF710B (aka ANAVEX 3-71) merits further attention. It is a combined selective allosteric M1 muscarinic and sigma 1 receptor agonist (Fisher et al., 2016). Targeting sigma 1 receptor has been shown to provide neuroprotection and anti-amnestic properties (Marrazzo et al., 2005; Maurice and Su, 2009; Villard et al., 2011). Combined with M1 muscarinic receptor-mediated effects on APP metabolism, it would confer AF710B a pharmacological profile of interest to tackle various pathological aspects of AD.

AF710B can rescue synapse loss *in vitro*, while low doses of the compound can attenuate cognitive deficits and alleviate hallmarks of the established AD-like pathology in 3xTg-AD mice (Fisher et al., 2016). In order to validate the putative disease-modifying effect of the drug, AF710B was administered (in the micromolar range) *per os* daily to post-plaque McGill-R-Thy1-APP rats for 5 months. Completion of the treatment was followed by a wash-out phase of 5 weeks, a unique experimental design key to discriminate true disease-modifying effects from symptomatic effects. The former should disappear after treatment cessation while the latter would be persistent (Ploeger and Holford, 2009). This treatment regimen was sufficient to fully restore cognition in the McGill tg rats. It also led to a substantial decrease in the production of cortical Aβ and in the amount of mature amyloid plaques. Interestingly, the reduction in Aβ load was accompanied by an increase in CSF Aβ42 levels, suggesting that the drug could not only lower Aβ production but also increase its clearance (Hall et al., 2018). Of note, this finding may be of translational value to non-invasively follow treatment response in a human population. Further to it, CNS inflammation was decreased, as mirrored by the abolishment of microglia recruitment toward Aβ-burdened neurons in the hippocampus and the normalization of hippocampal Iba1 protein levels and cortical IL-10 mRNA expression levels. Finally, these changes were accompanied by an increase in synaptophysin levels, suggesting possible synaptogenic activity (Hall et al., 2018).

In summary, with M1/sigma-1 activity as well as putative disease-modifying properties at very low dose, AF710B is well positioned for therapeutic interventions in AD. The case of AF710B as detailed above provides interesting clues pertaining to potentially increasing the predictive value of preclinical studies. In this particular case, results from the study in McGill-R-Thy1-APP tg rats complemented the initial findings of AF710B beneficial effects in trihexyphenidyl rats and tg mice, by offering new insights into the properties of the drug (Fisher et al., 2016; Hall et al., 2018). Such approach, where efficacy of a drug is validated in several models and under different conditions, should be encouraged before translation to human trials. This is particularly important considering that no single model can recapitulate all aspects of the human disease.

GENERAL CONSIDERATIONS: TRANSLATIONAL VALUE OF EXPERIMENTAL PHARMACOLOGY IN RODENT MODELS

Despite the growing list of compounds that have demonstrated positive therapeutic effects in tg rodent models, none of these experimental leads have yet reached FDA-approval for the treatment of AD in humans, highlighting a clear deficit in translational research. In line with these failures, the question that arises is: how can we better predict drug efficacy in humans based on animal studies?

Although tg APP rodent models have been instrumental in increasing our understanding of Aβ-driven pathogenic processes in AD, it is challenging to ascertain whether the phenotypes observed in these tg animals can be solely attributed to elevated Aβ levels or result from overexpression of APP. To address this concern, single humanized APP knock-in (KI) mice have been recently developed (Saito et al., 2014), paving the way toward more physiological models of the disease. Evidently, one of the main shortcomings of the current tg AD models is that they express genes carrying mutations seen in FAD, whereas most AD cases are sporadic. It remains an open question whether the findings obtained from FAD-like models can in fact be translated to heterogeneous sporadic cases, in which a multitude of susceptibility factors likely drive disease onset (genetic, environmental or lifestyle) (Rocchi et al., 2003; Mattson, 2004).

Mouse has been the species of choice since the inception of tg models, mostly for technical and economic reasons. Several characteristics unique to rats would, however, indicate that they may be better suited than mice for research relevant to humans, especially in the neuroscience field [reviewed in Do Carmo and Cuello (2013); Zimmer et al. (2014) and Ellenbroek and Youn (2016)]. Indeed, rats have a more complex CNS than mice and their brain development in postnatal life is more similar to humans than mice (Wood et al., 2003; Pressler and Auvin, 2013). Although the rat and mouse brains are anatomically similar, there are important functional differences between the two, including substantial differences in neuronal plasticity. For example, recent studies indicate that in adult rats, the rate of hippocampal neurogenesis is faster than in mice and new neurons are more likely to be recruited during learning than in mice (Snyder et al., 2009). Rats display a richer behavior including more complex social behavior (such a juvenile play) compared to mice, allowing for a larger range of cognitive analyses (Whishaw et al., 2001; Do Carmo and Cuello, 2013). Genetically, they also resemble humans more than mice do. For example, the rat apolipoprotein E (ApoE) gene bears more homology with human ApoE than mouse ApoE (Rajavashisth et al., 1985; Tran et al., 2013). This is of significance considering that polymorphism in ApoE is a strong genetic risk factor for AD, with ApoE4 showing the strongest association with the disease (Poirier et al., 1993; Strittmatter et al., 1993; Roses et al., 1994). As the genetic toolbox for rats is growing, the number of tg rat models will likely increase in the future. Whether rat-based models will better predict the human condition and the efficacy of experimental therapeutics remains to be established.

One important aspect of current tg models is that they likely mimic early disease stage when the focus of most current clinical trials has been mild-moderate AD. It is therefore highly likely that some of the therapeutic leads emerging from experimentation in tg mice and rats might have an important impact in slowing or diminishing the AD pathology at the preclinical stage. Such opportunity would have a consequential impact on the global AD prevalence since it has been estimated that a 5-year delay in the onset of clinical AD would decrease the total number of affected individuals by 50% at the end of a 25 year period (Alzheimer's Association, 2015). However, adequate identification and selection of human participants for such trials remains challenging and is pending on the discovery of novel biomarkers that can unequivocally identify preclinical AD stage. In the meantime, some clinical trials have been focusing on individuals with a high risk of developing AD dementia due to a family history of AD. These individuals have been recruited and enrolled before they develop any sign of cognitive decline (Cummings et al., 2018). Results from these ongoing prevention trials such as the DIAN-TU, DEPEND or HEART studies (which have enrolled individuals with a family history of autosomal dominant AD, a family history of AD or a parental history of AD, respectively) are highly anticipated and may indicate whether pharmacological interventions at preclinical AD stages could prevent or delay cognitive decline.

CONCLUSION

Over the past decades, our understanding of AD has grown tremendously, owing for a large part to the contribution of tg models mimicking various aspects of the AD pathology. However, despite intensive research, there is still no cure for this devastating disease. As the prevalence of AD increases worldwide, it is crucial to identify bottlenecks in the drug development pipeline, which may slow down progress toward the market approval of promising drug candidates. The shortcomings of current tg models of AD are well-acknowledged by the research community. In response, there is a growing effort to provide better predictive animal models of the disease. Along these lines, current efforts toward the identification of biomarkers that would identify an ongoing AD process before clinical presentation will most likely culminate in refined clinical trial design. These initiatives are much needed to translate positive preclinical studies into efficacy in human clinical trials. An optimist outlook regarding successful preclinical studies is that they might offer novel therapeutic avenues with probable tangible benefits if applied at the earliest, preclinical stages of the disease. A favorable future scenario in which diagnosis of AD pathology is made about 10 years before dementia could help radically change the currently disappointing therapeutic arsenal.

AUTHOR CONTRIBUTIONS

ACC and HH designed the structure and contents of the review. All authors contributed to the writing of the manuscript.

FUNDING

This work was funded by the Canadian Institute of Health and Research Project Grant (201603PJT-364544) and the National Institute of Health and Aging Operating Grant (R01-AG056850) to ACC.

ACKNOWLEDGMENTS

ACC is the holder of the Charles E. Frosst/Merck endowed Chair in Pharmacology and a member of the Canadian Consortium on Neurodegeneration in Aging. The authors are grateful for the unrestricted support provided by Merck Canada.

REFERENCES

Aisen, P. S., Cummings, J., Jack, C. R. Jr., Morris, J. C., Sperling, R., Frölich, L., et al. (2017). On the path to 2025: understanding the Alzheimer's disease continuum. *Alzheimers Res. Ther.* 9:60. doi: 10.1186/s13195-017-0283-5

Allen, B., Ingram, E., Takao, M., Smith, M. J., Jakes, R., Virdee, K., et al. (2002). Abundant tau filaments and nonapoptotic neurodegeneration in transgenic mice expressing human P301S tau protein. *J. Neurosci.* 22, 9340–9351. doi: 10.1523/JNEUROSCI.22-21-09340.2002

Alzheimer's Association (2015). *Changing the Trajectory of Alzheimer's Disease: How Treatment by 2025 Saves Lives and Dollars.* Chicago, IL: Alzheimer's Association, 1–16.

Alzheimer's Association (2018). *Alzheimer's Disease Facts and Figures.* Chicago, IL: Alzheimer's Association.

Ameen-Ali, K. E., Wharton, S. B., Simpson, J. E., Heath, P. R., Sharp, P., and Berwick, J. (2017). Review: neuropathology and behavioural features of transgenic murine models of Alzheimer's disease. *Neuropathol. Appl. Neurobiol.* 43, 553–570. doi: 10.1111/nan.12440

Azab, A. N., Shnaider, A., Osher, Y., Wang, D., Bersudsky, Y., and Belmaker, R. H. (2015). Lithium nephrotoxicity. *Int. J. Bipolar Disord.* 3:28. doi: 10.1186/s40345-015-0028-y

Bakulski, K. M., Dolinoy, D. C., Sartor, M. A., Paulson, H. L., Konen, J. R., Lieberman, A. P., et al. (2012). Genome-wide DNA methylation differences between late-onset Alzheimer's disease and cognitively normal controls in human frontal cortex. *J. Alzheimers Dis.* 29, 571–588. doi: 10.3233/JAD-2012-111223

Bales, K. R. (2012). The value and limitations of transgenic mouse models used in drug discovery for Alzheimer's disease: an update. *Expert Opin. Drug Discov.* 7, 281–297. doi: 10.1517/17460441.2012.666234

Bateman, R. J., Aisen, P. S., De Strooper, B., Fox, N. C., Lemere, C. A., Ringman, J. M., et al. (2011). Autosomal-dominant Alzheimer's disease: a review and proposal for the prevention of Alzheimer's disease. *Alzheimers Res. Ther.* 3:1. doi: 10.1186/alzrt59

Bottiglieri, T., Reynolds, E. H., Toone, B. K., and Carney, M. W. (1991). CSF S-adenosylmethionine in neuropsychiatric disorders. *Lancet* 338:121. doi: 10.1016/0140-6736(91)90114-5

Breitner, J. C., Baker, L. D., Montine, T. J., Meinert, C. L., Lyketsos, C. G., Ashe, K. H., et al. (2011). Extended results of the Alzheimer's disease anti-inflammatory prevention trial. *Alzheimers Dement.* 7, 402–411. doi: 10.1016/j.jalz.2010.12.014

Caccamo, A., Oddo, S., Billings, L. M., Green, K. N., Martinez-Coria, H., Fisher, A., et al. (2006). M1 receptors play a central role in modulating AD-like pathology in transgenic mice. *Neuron* 49, 671–682. doi: 10.1016/j.neuron.2006.01.020

Cadena-del-Castillo, C., Valdes-Quezada, C., Carmona-Aldana, F., Arias, C., Bermudez-Rattoni, F., and Recillas-Targa, F. (2014). Age-dependent increment of hydroxymethylation in the brain cortex in the triple-transgenic mouse model of Alzheimer's disease. *J. Alzheimers Dis.* 41, 845–854. doi: 10.3233/JAD-132285

Chouliaras, L., Mastroeni, D., Delvaux, E., Grover, A., Kenis, G., Hof, P. R., et al. (2013). Consistent decrease in global DNA methylation and hydroxymethylation in the hippocampus of Alzheimer's disease patients. *Neurobiol. Aging* 34, 2091–2099. doi: 10.1016/j.neurobiolaging.2013.02.021

Cohen, R. M., Rezai-Zadeh, K., Weitz, T. M., Rentsendorj, A., Gate, D., Spivak, I., et al. (2013). A transgenic Alzheimer rat with plaques, tau pathology, behavioral impairment, oligomeric abeta, and frank neuronal loss. *J. Neurosci.* 33, 6245–6256. doi: 10.1523/JNEUROSCI.3672-12.2013

Cuello, A. C. (2017). Early and late CNS inflammation in Alzheimer's disease: two extremes of a continuum? *Trends Pharmacol. Sci.* 38, 956–966. doi: 10.1016/j.tips.2017.07.005

Cuello, A. C., Ferretti, M. T., and Iulita, M. F. (2012). Preplaque ('Preclinical') a beta-induced inflammation and nerve growth factor deregulation in transgenic models of Alzheimer's disease-like amyloid pathology. *Neurodegener. Dis.* 10, 104–107. doi: 10.1159/000333339

Cuello, A. C., Ferretti, M. T., Leon, W. C., Iulita, M. F., Melis, T., Ducatenzeiler, A., et al. (2010). Early-stage inflammation and experimental therapy in transgenic models of the Alzheimer-like amyloid pathology. *Neurodegener. Dis.* 7, 96–98. doi: 10.1159/000285514

Cummings, J., Lee, G., Ritter, A., and Zhong, K. (2018). Alzheimer's disease drug development pipeline: 2018. *Alzheimers Dement.* 4, 195–214. doi: 10.1016/j.trci.2018.03.009

De Jager, P. L., Srivastava, G., Lunnon, K., Burgess, J., Schalkwyk, L. C., Yu, L., et al. (2014). Alzheimer's disease: early alterations in brain DNA methylation at ANK1, BIN1, RHBDF2 and other loci. *Nat. Neurosci.* 17, 1156–1163. doi: 10.1038/nn.3786

Derby, C. A., Katz, M. J., Lipton, R. B., and Hall, C. B. (2017). Trends in dementia incidence in a birth cohort analysis of the Einstein aging study. *JAMA Neurol.* 74, 1345–1351. doi: 10.1001/jamaneurol.2017.1964

Do Carmo, S., Crynen, G., Paradis, T., Reed, J., Iulita, M. F., Ducatenzeiler, A., et al. (2018). Hippocampal proteomic analysis reveals distinct pathway deregulation profiles at early and late stages in a rat model of Alzheimer's-like amyloid pathology. *Mol. Neurobiol.* 55, 3451–3476. doi: 10.1007/s12035-017-0580-9

Do Carmo, S., and Cuello, A. C. (2013). Modeling Alzheimer's disease in transgenic rats. *Mol. Neurodegener.* 8:37. doi: 10.1186/1750-1326-8-37

Do Carmo, S., Hanzel, C. E., Jacobs, M. L., Machnes, Z., Iulita, M. F., Yang, J., et al. (2016). Rescue of early bace-1 and global DNA demethylation by S-adenosylmethionine reduces amyloid pathology and improves cognition in an Alzheimer's model. *Sci. Rep.* 6:34051. doi: 10.1038/srep34051

Drummond, E., and Wisniewski, T. (2017). Alzheimer's disease: experimental models and reality. *Acta Neuropathol.* 133, 155–175. doi: 10.1007/s00401-016-1662-x

Ellenbroek, B., and Youn, J. (2016). Rodent models in neuroscience research: is it a rat race? *Dis. Model. Mech.* 9, 1079–1087. doi: 10.1242/dmm.026120

Fajardo, V. A., Fajardo, V. A., LeBlanc, P. J., and MacPherson, R. E. K. (2018). Examining the relationship between trace lithium in drinking water and the rising rates of age-adjusted Alzheimer's disease mortality in Texas. *J. Alzheimers Dis.* 61, 425–434. doi: 10.3233/JAD-170744

Ferretti, M. T., Allard, S., Partridge, V., Ducatenzeiler, A., and Cuello, A. C. (2012a). Minocycline corrects early, pre-plaque neuroinflammation and inhibits BACE-1 in a transgenic model of Alzheimer's disease-like amyloid pathology. *J. Neuroinflammation* 9:62. doi: 10.1186/1742-2094-9-62

Ferretti, M. T., Bruno, M. A., Ducatenzeiler, A., Klein, W. L., and Cuello, A. C. (2012b). Intracellular Abeta-oligomers and early inflammation in a model of Alzheimer's disease. *Neurobiol. Aging* 33, 1329–1342. doi: 10.1016/j.neurobiolaging.2011.01.007

Ferretti, M. T., Partridge, V., Leon, W. C., Canneva, F., Allard, S., Arvanitis, D. N., et al. (2011). Transgenic mice as a model of pre-clinical Alzheimer's disease. *Curr. Alzheimer Res.* 8, 4–23. doi: 10.2174/156720511794604561

Filipiak, W. E., and Saunders, T. L. (2006). Advances in transgenic rat production. *Transgenic Res.* 15, 673–686. doi: 10.1007/s11248-006-9002-x

Fisher, A. (2008). Cholinergic treatments with emphasis on m1 muscarinic agonists as potential disease-modifying agents for Alzheimer's disease. *Neurotherapeutics* 5, 433–442. doi: 10.1016/j.nurt.2008.05.002

Fisher, A. (2012). Cholinergic modulation of amyloid precursor protein processing with emphasis on M1 muscarinic receptor: perspectives and challenges in treatment of Alzheimer's disease. *J. Neurochem.* 120(Suppl. 1), 22–33. doi: 10.1111/j.1471-4159.2011.07507.x

Fisher, A., Bezprozvanny, I., Wu, L., Ryskamp, D. A., Bar-Ner, N., Natan, N., et al. (2016). AF710B, a novel M1/sigma1 agonist with therapeutic efficacy in animal models of Alzheimer's disease. *Neurodegener. Dis.* 16, 95–110. doi: 10.1159/000440864

Forlenza, O. V., Aprahamian, I., de Paula, V. J., and Hajek, T. (2016). Lithium, a therapy for AD: current evidence from clinical trials of neurodegenerative disorders. *Curr. Alzheimer Res.* 13, 879–886. doi: 10.2174/1567205013666160219112854

Forlenza, O. V., Diniz, B. S., Radanovic, M., Santos, F. S., Talib, L. L., and Gattaz, W. F. (2011). Disease-modifying properties of long-term lithium treatment for amnestic mild cognitive impairment: randomised controlled trial. *Br. J. Psychiatry* 198, 351–356. doi: 10.1192/bjp.bp.110.080044

Galeano, P., Leal, M. C., Ferrari, C. C., Dalmasso, M. C., Martino Adami, P. V., Farias, M. I., et al. (2018). Chronic hippocampal expression of notch intracellular domain induces vascular thickening, reduces glucose availability, and exacerbates spatial memory deficits in a rat model of early Alzheimer. *Mol. Neurobiol.* 55, 8637–8650. doi: 10.1007/s12035-018-1002-3

Galeano, P., Martino Adami, P. V., Do Carmo, S., Blanco, E., Rotondaro, C., Capani, F., et al. (2014). Longitudinal analysis of the behavioral phenotype in a novel transgenic rat model of early stages of Alzheimer's disease. *Front. Behav. Neurosci.* 8:321. doi: 10.3389/fnbeh.2014.00321

Games, D., Adams, D., Alessandrini, R., Barbour, R., Berthelette, P., Blackwell, C., et al. (1995). Alzheimer-type neuropathology in transgenic mice overexpressing V717F beta-amyloid precursor protein. *Nature* 373, 523–527. doi: 10.1038/373523a0

Gelenberg, A. J., and Jefferson, J. W. (1995). Lithium tremor. *J. Clin. Psychiatry* 56, 283–287.

Gotz, J., Deters, N., Doldissen, A., Bokhari, L., Ke, Y., Wiesner, A., et al. (2007). A decade of tau transgenic animal models and beyond. *Brain Pathol.* 17, 91–103. doi: 10.1111/j.1750-3639.2007.00051.x

Hall, H., Iulita, M. F., Gubert, P., Flores Aguilar, L., Ducatenzeiler, A., Fisher, A., et al. (2018). AF710B, an M1/sigma-1 receptor agonist with long-lasting disease-modifying properties in a transgenic rat model of Alzheimer's disease. *Alzheimers Dement.* 14, 811–823. doi: 10.1016/j.jalz.2017.11.009

Hampel, H., Ewers, M., Burger, K., Annas, P., Mortberg, A., Bogstedt, A., et al. (2009). Lithium trial in Alzheimer's disease: a randomized, single-blind, placebo-controlled, multicenter 10-week study. *J. Clin. Psychiatry* 70, 922–931. doi: 10.4088/JCP.08m04606

Hanzel, C. E., Pichet-Binette, A., Pimentel, L. S., Iulita, M. F., Allard, S., Ducatenzeiler, A., et al. (2014). Neuronal driven pre-plaque inflammation in a transgenic rat model of Alzheimer's disease. *Neurobiol. Aging* 35, 2249–2262. doi: 10.1016/j.neurobiolaging.2014.03.026

Hardy, J., Bogdanovic, N., Winblad, B., Portelius, E., Andreasen, N., Cedazo-Minguez, A., et al. (2014). Pathways to Alzheimer's disease. *J. Intern. Med.* 275, 296–303. doi: 10.1111/joim.12192

Havens, W. W. II, and Cole, J. (1982). Successful treatment of dementia with lithium. *J. Clin. Psychopharmacol.* 2, 71–72. doi: 10.1097/00004714-198202000-00013

Heggland, I., Storkaas, I. S., Soligard, H. T., Kobro-Flatmoen, A., and Witter, M. P. (2015). Stereological estimation of neuron number and plaque load in the hippocampal region of a transgenic rat model of Alzheimer's disease. *Eur. J. Neurosci.* 41, 1245–1262. doi: 10.1111/ejn.12876

Hickman, R. A., Faustin, A., and Wisniewski, T. (2016). Alzheimer disease and its growing epidemic: risk factors, biomarkers, and the urgent need for therapeutics. *Neurol. Clin.* 34, 941–953. doi: 10.1016/j.ncl.2016.06.009

Holcomb, L., Gordon, M. N., McGowan, E., Yu, X., Benkovic, S., Jantzen, P., et al. (1998). Accelerated Alzheimer-type phenotype in transgenic mice carrying both mutant amyloid precursor protein and presenilin 1 transgenes. *Nat. Med.* 4, 97–100. doi: 10.1038/nm0198-097

Hsiao, K. (1998). Transgenic mice expressing Alzheimer amyloid precursor proteins. *Exp. Gerontol.* 33, 883–889. doi: 10.1016/S0531-5565(98)00045-X

Hsiao, K., Chapman, P., Nilsen, S., Eckman, C., Harigaya, Y., Younkin, S., et al. (1996). Correlative memory deficits, Abeta elevation, and amyloid plaques in transgenic mice. *Science* 274, 99–102. doi: 10.1126/science.274.5284.99

Iulita, M. F., Allard, S., Richter, L., Munter, L.-M., Ducatenzeiler, A., Weise, C., et al. (2014). Intracellular Aβ pathology and early cognitive impairments in a transgenic rat overexpressing human amyloid precursor protein: a multidimensional study. *Acta Neuropathol. Commun.* 2:61. doi: 10.1186/2051-5960-2-61

Iulita, M. F., Bistue Millon, M. B., Pentz, R., Aguilar, L. F., Do Carmo, S., Allard, S., et al. (2017). Differential deregulation of NGF and BDNF neurotrophins in a transgenic rat model of Alzheimer's disease. *Neurobiol. Dis.* 108, 307–323. doi: 10.1016/j.nbd.2017.08.019

Iulita, M. F., and Cuello, A. C. (2016). The NGF metabolic pathway in the CNS and its dysregulation in down syndrome and Alzheimer's disease. *Curr. Alzheimer Res.* 13, 53–67. doi: 10.2174/1567205012666150921100030

Iwata, A., Nagata, K., Hatsuta, H., Takuma, H., Bundo, M., Iwamoto, K., et al. (2014). Altered CpG methylation in sporadic Alzheimer's disease is associated with APP and MAPT dysregulation. *Hum. Mol. Genet.* 23, 648–656. doi: 10.1093/hmg/ddt451

Jankowsky, J. L., and Zheng, H. (2017). Practical considerations for choosing a mouse model of Alzheimer's disease. *Mol. Neurodegener.* 12:89. doi: 10.1186/s13024-017-0231-7

Janus, C., Pearson, J., McLaurin, J., Mathews, P. M., Jiang, Y., Schmidt, S. D., et al. (2000). A beta peptide immunization reduces behavioural impairment and plaques in a model of Alzheimer's disease. *Nature* 408, 979–982. doi: 10.1038/35050110

Jaturapatporn, D., Isaac, M. G., McCleery, J., and Tabet, N. (2012). Aspirin, steroidal and non-steroidal anti-inflammatory drugs for the treatment of Alzheimer's disease. *Cochrane Database Syst. Rev.* 2:CD006378. doi: 10.1002/14651858.CD006378.pub2

Kessing, L. V., Gerds, T. A., Knudsen, N. N., Jorgensen, L. F., Kristiansen, S. M., Voutchkova, D., et al. (2017). Association of lithium in drinking water with the incidence of dementia. *JAMA Psychiatry* 74, 1005–1010. doi: 10.1001/jamapsychiatry.2017.2362

Kinoshita, J., and Clark, T. (2007). Alzforum. *Methods Mol. Biol.* 401, 365–381. doi: 10.1007/978-1-59745-520-6_19

LaFerla, F. M., and Green, K. N. (2012). Animal models of Alzheimer disease. *Cold Spring Harb. Perspect. Med.* 2:a006320. doi: 10.1101/cshperspect.a006320

Langa, K. M. (2015). Is the risk of Alzheimer's disease and dementia declining? *Alzheimers Res. Ther.* 7:34. doi: 10.1186/s13195-015-0118-1

Leon, W. C., Canneva, F., Partridge, V., Allard, S., Ferretti, M. T., DeWilde, A., et al. (2010). A novel transgenic rat model with a full Alzheimer's-like amyloid pathology displays pre-plaque intracellular amyloid-β-associated cognitive impairment. *J. Alzheimers Dis.* 20, 113–126. doi: 10.3233/JAD-2010-1349

Leyhe, T., Eschweiler, G. W., Stransky, E., Gasser, T., Annas, P., Basun, H., et al. (2009). Increase of BDNF serum concentration in lithium treated patients with early Alzheimer's disease. *J. Alzheimers Dis.* 16, 649–656. doi: 10.3233/JAD-2009-1004

Livingstone, C., and Rampes, H. (2006). Lithium: a review of its metabolic adverse effects. *J. Psychopharmacol.* 20, 347–355. doi: 10.1177/0269881105057515

Macdonald, A., Briggs, K., Poppe, M., Higgins, A., Velayudhan, L., and Lovestone, S. (2008). A feasibility and tolerability study of lithium in Alzheimer's disease. *Int. J. Geriatr. Psychiatry* 23, 704–711. doi: 10.1002/gps.1964

Malhi, G. S., and Outhred, T. (2016). Therapeutic mechanisms of lithium in bipolar disorder: recent advances and current understanding. *CNS Drugs* 30, 931–949. doi: 10.1007/s40263-016-0380-1

Marrazzo, A., Caraci, F., Salinaro, E. T., Su, T. P., Copani, A., and Ronsisvalle, G. (2005). Neuroprotective effects of sigma-1 receptor agonists against beta-amyloid-induced toxicity. *Neuroreport* 16, 1223–1226. doi: 10.1097/00001756-200508010-00018

Martino Adami, P. V., Galeano, P., Wallinger, M. L., Quijano, C., Rabossi, A., Pagano, E. S., et al. (2017a). Worsening of memory deficit induced by energy-dense diet in a rat model of early-Alzheimer's disease is associated to neurotoxic Abeta species and independent of neuroinflammation. *Biochim. Biophys. Acta* 1863, 731–743. doi: 10.1016/j.bbadis.2016.12.014

Martino Adami, P. V., Quijano, C., Magnani, N., Galeano, P., Evelson, P., Cassina, A., et al. (2017b). Synaptosomal bioenergetic defects are associated with cognitive impairment in a transgenic rat model of early Alzheimer's disease. *J. Cereb. Blood Flow Metab.* 37, 69–84. doi: 10.1177/0271678X15615132

Mastroeni, D., Grover, A., Delvaux, E., Whiteside, C., Coleman, P. D., and Rogers, J. (2010). Epigenetic changes in Alzheimer's disease: decrements in DNA methylation. *Neurobiol. Aging* 31, 2025–2037. doi: 10.1016/j.neurobiolaging.2008.12.005

Mattson, M. P. (2004). Pathways towards and away from Alzheimer's disease. *Nature* 430, 631–639. doi: 10.1038/nature02621

Mauer, S., Vergne, D., and Ghaemi, S. N. (2014). Standard and trace-dose lithium: a systematic review of dementia prevention and other behavioral benefits. *Aust. N. Z. J. Psychiatry* 48, 809–818. doi: 10.1177/0004867414536932

Maurice, T., and Su, T. P. (2009). The pharmacology of sigma-1 receptors. *Pharmacol. Ther.* 124, 195–206. doi: 10.1016/j.pharmthera.2009.07.001

McGeer, P. L., McGeer, E., Rogers, J., and Sibley, J. (1990). Anti-inflammatory drugs and Alzheimer disease. *Lancet* 335:1037. doi: 10.1016/0140-6736(90)91101-F

McGeer, P. L., and McGeer, E. G. (2013). The amyloid cascade-inflammatory hypothesis of Alzheimer disease: implications for therapy. *Acta Neuropathol.* 126, 479–497. doi: 10.1007/s00401-013-1177-7

McGeer, P. L., and Rogers, J. (1992). Anti-inflammatory agents as a therapeutic approach to Alzheimer's disease. *Neurology* 42, 447–449. doi: 10.1212/WNL.42.2.447

McGrath, J. J., and Berk, M. (2017). Could lithium in drinking water reduce the incidence of dementia? *JAMA Psychiatry* 74, 983–984. doi: 10.1001/jamapsychiatry.2017.2336

Morgan, D., Diamond, D. M., Gottschall, P. E., Ugen, K. E., Dickey, C., Hardy, J., et al. (2000). A beta peptide vaccination prevents memory loss in an animal model of Alzheimer's disease. *Nature* 408, 982–985. doi: 10.1038/35050116

Morris, G., and Berk, M. (2016). The putative use of lithium in Alzheimer's disease. *Curr. Alzheimer Res.* 13, 853–861. doi: 10.2174/1567205013666160219113112

Morrison, L. D., Smith, D. D., and Kish, S. J. (1996). Brain S-adenosylmethionine levels are severely decreased in Alzheimer's disease. *J. Neurochem.* 67, 1328–1331. doi: 10.1046/j.1471-4159.1996.67031328.x

Mucke, L., Masliah, E., Yu, G. Q., Mallory, M., Rockenstein, E. M., Tatsuno, G., et al. (2000). High-level neuronal expression of abeta 1-42 in wild-type human amyloid protein precursor transgenic mice: synaptotoxicity without plaque formation. *J. Neurosci.* 20, 4050–4058. doi: 10.1523/JNEUROSCI.20-11-04050.2000

Mullan, M., Crawford, F., Axelman, K., Houlden, H., Lilius, L., Winblad, B., et al. (1992). A pathogenic mutation for probable Alzheimer's disease in the APP gene at the N-terminus of beta-amyloid. *Nat. Genet.* 1, 345–347. doi: 10.1038/ng0892-345

Murrell, J., Farlow, M., Ghetti, B., and Benson, M. D. (1991). A mutation in the amyloid precursor protein associated with hereditary Alzheimer's disease. *Science* 254, 97–99. doi: 10.1126/science.1925564

Nicolia, V., Cavallaro, R. A., Lopez-Gonzalez, I., Maccarrone, M., Scarpa, S., Ferrer, I., et al. (2017). DNA methylation profiles of selected pro-inflammatory cytokines in Alzheimer disease. *J. Neuropathol. Exp. Neurol.* 76, 27–31. doi: 10.1093/jnen/nlw099

Nilsen, L. H., Melo, T. M., Saether, O., Witter, M. P., and Sonnewald, U. (2012). Altered neurochemical profile in the McGill-R-Thy1-APP rat model of Alzheimer's disease: a longitudinal in vivo 1 H MRS study. *J. Neurochem.* 123, 532–541. doi: 10.1111/jnc.12003

Nilsen, L. H., Melo, T. M., Witter, M. P., and Sonnewald, U. (2014a). Early differences in dorsal hippocampal metabolite levels in males but not females in a transgenic rat model of Alzheimer's disease. *Neurochem. Res.* 39, 305–312. doi: 10.1007/s11064-013-1222-x

Nilsen, L. H., Witter, M. P., and Sonnewald, U. (2014b). Neuronal and astrocytic metabolism in a transgenic rat model of Alzheimer's disease. *J. Cereb. Blood Flow Metab.* 34, 906–914. doi: 10.1038/jcbfm.2014.37

Nitsch, R. M., Slack, B. E., Wurtman, R. J., and Growdon, J. H. (1992). Release of Alzheimer amyloid precursor derivatives stimulated by activation of muscarinic acetylcholine receptors. *Science* 258, 304–307. doi: 10.1126/science.1411529

Nunes, M. A., Schowe, N. M., Monteiro-Silva, K. C., Baraldi-Tornisielo, T., Souza, S. I., Balthazar, J., et al. (2015). Chronic microdose lithium treatment prevented memory loss and neurohistopathological changes in a transgenic mouse model of Alzheimer's disease. *PLoS One* 10:e0142267. doi: 10.1371/journal.pone.0142267

Nunes, M. A., Viel, T. A., and Buck, H. S. (2013). Microdose lithium treatment stabilized cognitive impairment in patients with Alzheimer's disease. *Curr. Alzheimer Res.* 10, 104–107.

Oakley, H., Cole, S. L., Logan, S., Maus, E., Shao, P., Craft, J., et al. (2006). Intraneuronal beta-amyloid aggregates, neurodegeneration, and neuron loss in transgenic mice with five familial Alzheimer's disease mutations: potential factors in amyloid plaque formation. *J. Neurosci.* 26, 10129–10140. doi: 10.1523/JNEUROSCI.1202-06.2006

Oddo, S., Caccamo, A., Shepherd, J. D., Murphy, M. P., Golde, T. E., Kayed, R., et al. (2003). Triple-transgenic model of Alzheimer's disease with plaques and tangles: intracellular Abeta and synaptic dysfunction. *Neuron* 39, 409–421. doi: 10.1016/S0896-6273(03)00434-3

Orgogozo, J. M., Gilman, S., Dartigues, J. F., Laurent, B., Puel, M., Kirby, L. C., et al. (2003). Subacute meningoencephalitis in a subset of patients with AD after Abeta42 immunization. *Neurology* 61, 46–54. doi: 10.1212/01.WNL.0000073623.84147.A8

Parent, M. J., Zimmer, E. R., Shin, M., Kang, M. S., Fonov, V. S., Mathieu, A., et al. (2017). Multimodal imaging in rat model recapitulates Alzheimer's disease biomarkers abnormalities. *J. Neurosci.* 37, 12263–12271. doi: 10.1523/JNEUROSCI.1346-17.2017

Pimentel, L. S., Allard, S., Do Carmo, S., Weinreb, O., Danik, M., Hanzel, C. E., et al. (2015). The multi-target drug M30 shows pro-cognitive and anti-inflammatory effects in a rat model of Alzheimer's disease. *J. Alzheimers Dis.* 47, 373–383. doi: 10.3233/JAD-143126

Ploeger, B. A., and Holford, N. H. (2009). Washout and delayed start designs for identifying disease modifying effects in slowly progressive diseases using disease progression analysis. *Pharm. Stat.* 8, 225–238. doi: 10.1002/pst.355

Poirier, J., Davignon, J., Bouthillier, D., Kogan, S., Bertrand, P., and Gauthier, S. (1993). Apolipoprotein E polymorphism and Alzheimer's disease. *Lancet* 342, 697–699. doi: 10.1016/0140-6736(93)91705-Q

Pressler, R., and Auvin, S. (2013). Comparison of brain maturation among species: an example in translational research suggesting the possible use of bumetanide in newborn. *Front. Neurol.* 4:36. doi: 10.3389/fneur.2013.00036

Prestia, F. A., Galeano, P., Martino Adami, P. V., Do Carmo, S., Castano, E. M., Cuello, A. C., et al. (2018). Platelets bioenergetics screening reflects the impact of brain abeta plaque accumulation in a rat model of alzheimer. *Neurochem. Res.* doi: 10.1007/s11064-018-2657-x [Epub ahead of print].

Puzzo, D., Gulisano, W., Palmeri, A., and Arancio, O. (2015). Rodent models for Alzheimer's disease drug discovery. *Expert Opin. Drug Discov.* 10, 703–711. doi: 10.1517/17460441.2015.1041913

Qi, Y., Klyubin, I., Cuello, A. C., and Rowan, M. J. (2018). NLRP3-dependent synaptic plasticity deficit in an Alzheimer's disease amyloidosis model in vivo. *Neurobiol. Dis.* 114, 24–30. doi: 10.1016/j.nbd.2018.02.016

Qi, Y., Klyubin, I., Harney, S. C., Hu, N., Cullen, W. K., Grant, M. K., et al. (2014). Longitudinal testing of hippocampal plasticity reveals the onset and maintenance of endogenous human Ass-induced synaptic dysfunction in individual freely behaving pre-plaque transgenic rats: rapid reversal by anti-Ass agents. *Acta Neuropathol. Commun.* 2:175. doi: 10.1186/s40478-014-0175-x

Rajavashisth, T. B., Kaptein, J. S., Reue, K. L., and Lusis, A. J. (1985). Evolution of apolipoprotein E: mouse sequence and evidence for an 11-nucleotide ancestral unit. *Proc. Natl. Acad. Sci. U.S.A.* 82, 8085–8089. doi: 10.1073/pnas.82.23.8085

Rocchi, A., Pellegrini, S., Siciliano, G., and Murri, L. (2003). Causative and susceptibility genes for Alzheimer's disease: a review. *Brain Res. Bull.* 61, 1–24. doi: 10.1016/S0361-9230(03)00067-4

Rogers, J. (2018). Principles for central nervous system inflammation research: a call for a consortium approach. *Alzheimers Dement.* 14, 1553–1559. doi: 10.1016/j.jalz.2018.01.008

Roses, A. D., Strittmatter, W. J., Pericak-Vance, M. A., Corder, E. H., Saunders, A. M., and Schmechel, D. E. (1994). Clinical application of apolipoprotein E genotyping to Alzheimer's disease. *Lancet* 343, 1564–1565. doi: 10.1016/S0140-6736(94)92960-2

Ryman, D. C., Acosta-Baena, N., Aisen, P. S., Bird, T., Danek, A., Fox, N. C., et al. (2014). Symptom onset in autosomal dominant Alzheimer disease: a systematic review and meta-analysis. *Neurology* 83, 253–260. doi: 10.1212/WNL.0000000000000596

Saito, T., Matsuba, Y., Mihira, N., Takano, J., Nilsson, P., Itohara, S., et al. (2014). Single App knock-in mouse models of Alzheimer's disease. *Nat. Neurosci.* 17, 661–663. doi: 10.1038/nn.3697

Sasaguri, H., Nilsson, P., Hashimoto, S., Nagata, K., Saito, T., De Strooper, B., et al. (2017). APP mouse models for Alzheimer's disease preclinical studies. *EMBO J.* 36, 2473–2487. doi: 10.15252/embj.201797397

Schenk, D., Barbour, R., Dunn, W., Gordon, G., Grajeda, H., Guido, T., et al. (1999). Immunization with amyloid-beta attenuates Alzheimer-disease-like pathology in the PDAPP mouse. *Nature* 400, 173–177. doi: 10.1038/22124

Seabrook, T. J., Jiang, L., Maier, M., and Lemere, C. A. (2006). Minocycline affects microglia activation, Abeta deposition, and behavior in APP-tg mice. *Glia* 53, 776–782. doi: 10.1002/glia.20338

Seblova, D., Quiroga, M. L., Fors, S., Johnell, K., Lovden, M., de Leon, A. P., et al. (2018). Thirty-year trends in dementia: a nationwide population study of Swedish inpatient records. *Clin. Epidemiol.* 10, 1679–1693. doi: 10.2147/CLEP.S178955

Sharma, A., Gerbarg, P., Bottiglieri, T., Massoumi, L., Carpenter, L. L., Lavretsky, H., et al. (2017). S-adenosylmethionine (SAMe) for neuropsychiatric disorders: a clinician-oriented review of research. *J. Clin. Psychiatry* 78, e656–e667. doi: 10.4088/JCP.16r11113

Smith, A. R., Smith, R. G., Condliffe, D., Hannon, E., Schalkwyk, L., Mill, J., et al. (2016). Increased DNA methylation near TREM2 is consistently seen in the superior temporal gyrus in Alzheimer's disease brain. *Neurobiol. Aging* 47, 35–40. doi: 10.1016/j.neurobiolaging.2016.07.008

Snyder, J. S., Choe, J. S., Clifford, M. A., Jeurling, S. I., Hurley, P., Brown, A., et al. (2009). Adult-born hippocampal neurons are more numerous, faster maturing, and more involved in behavior in rats than in mice. *J. Neurosci.* 29, 14484–14495. doi: 10.1523/JNEUROSCI.1768-09.2009

Spires, T. L., and Hyman, B. T. (2005). Transgenic models of Alzheimer's disease: learning from animals. *NeuroRx* 2, 423–437. doi: 10.1602/neurorx.2.3.423

Strittmatter, W. J., Saunders, A. M., Schmechel, D., Pericak-Vance, M., Enghild, J., Salvesen, G. S., et al. (1993). Apolipoprotein E: high-avidity binding to beta-amyloid and increased frequency of type 4 allele in late-onset familial Alzheimer disease. *Proc. Natl. Acad. Sci. U.S.A.* 90, 1977–1981. doi: 10.1073/pnas.90.5.1977

Terao, T., Nakano, H., Inoue, Y., Okamoto, T., Nakamura, J., and Iwata, N. (2006). Lithium and dementia: a preliminary study. *Prog. Neuropsychopharmacol. Biol. Psychiatry* 30, 1125–1128. doi: 10.1016/j.pnpbp.2006.04.020

Tosto, G., and Reitz, C. (2013). Genome-wide association studies in Alzheimer's disease: a review. *Curr. Neurol. Neurosci. Rep.* 13:381. doi: 10.1007/s11910-013-0381-0

Tran, T. N., Kim, S. H., Gallo, C., Amaya, M., Kyees, J., and Narayanaswami, V. (2013). Biochemical and biophysical characterization of recombinant rat apolipoprotein E: similarities to human apolipoprotein E3. *Arch. Biochem. Biophys.* 529, 18–25. doi: 10.1016/j.abb.2012.10.007

Villard, V., Espallergues, J., Keller, E., Vamvakides, A., and Maurice, T. (2011). Anti-amnesic and neuroprotective potentials of the mixed muscarinic receptor/sigma 1 (sigma1) ligand ANAVEX2-73, a novel aminotetrahydrofuran derivative. *J. Psychopharmacol.* 25, 1101–1117. doi: 10.1177/0269881110379286

West, R. L., Lee, J. M., and Maroun, L. E. (1995). Hypomethylation of the amyloid precursor protein gene in the brain of an Alzheimer's disease patient. *J. Mol. Neurosci.* 6, 141–146. doi: 10.1007/BF02736773

Whishaw, I. Q., Metz, G. A., Kolb, B., and Pellis, S. M. (2001). Accelerated nervous system development contributes to behavioral efficiency in the laboratory mouse: a behavioral review and theoretical proposal. *Dev. Psychobiol.* 39, 151–170. doi: 10.1002/dev.1041

Wilson, E. N., Abela, A. R., Do Carmo, S., Allard, S., Marks, A. R., Welikovitch, L. A., et al. (2017a). Intraneuronal amyloid beta accumulation disrupts hippocampal CRTC1-dependent gene expression and cognitive function in a rat model of Alzheimer disease. *Cereb. Cortex* 27, 1501–1511. doi: 10.1093/cercor/bhv332

Wilson, E. N., Do Carmo, S., Iulita, M. F., Hall, H., Ducatenzeiler, A., Marks, A. R., et al. (2017b). BACE1 inhibition by microdose lithium formulation NP03 rescues memory loss and early stage amyloid neuropathology. *Transl. Psychiatry* 7:e1190. doi: 10.1038/tp.2017.169

Wilson, E. N., Do Carmo, S., Iulita, M. F., Hall, H., Austin, G. L., Jia, D. T., et al. (2018). Microdose lithium NP03 diminishes pre-plaque oxidative damage and neuroinflammation in a rat model of Alzheimer's-like amyloidosis. *Curr. Alzheimer Res.* 15, 1220–1230. doi: 10.2174/1567205015666180904154446

Wood, S. L., Beyer, B. K., and Cappon, G. D. (2003). Species comparison of postnatal CNS development: functional measures. *Birth Defects Res. B Dev. Reprod. Toxicol.* 68, 391–407. doi: 10.1002/bdrb.10037

Yoshiyama, Y., Higuchi, M., Zhang, B., Huang, S. M., Iwata, N., Saido, T. C., et al. (2007). Synapse loss and microglial activation precede tangles in a P301S tauopathy mouse model. *Neuron* 53, 337–351. doi: 10.1016/j.neuron.2007.01.010

Zhang, C., Wang, Y., Wang, D., Zhang, J., and Zhang, F. (2018). NSAID exposure and risk of Alzheimer's disease: an updated meta-analysis from cohort studies. *Front. Aging Neurosci.* 10:83. doi: 10.3389/fnagi.2018.00083

Zhang, D., Qi, Y., Klyubin, I., Ondrejcak, T., Sarell, C. J., Cuello, A. C., et al. (2017). Targeting glutamatergic and cellular prion protein mechanisms of amyloid beta-mediated persistent synaptic plasticity disruption: longitudinal studies. *Neuropharmacology* 121, 231–246. doi: 10.1016/j.neuropharm.2017.03.036

Zhao, J., Zhu, Y., Yang, J., Li, L., Wu, H., De Jager, P. L., et al. (2017). A genome-wide profiling of brain DNA hydroxymethylation in Alzheimer's disease. *Alzheimers Dement.* 13, 674–688. doi: 10.1016/j.jalz.2016.10.004

Zhao, L., Gong, N., Liu, M., Pan, X., Sang, S., Sun, X., et al. (2014). Beneficial synergistic effects of microdose lithium with pyrroloquinoline quinone in an Alzheimer's disease mouse model. *Neurobiol. Aging* 35, 2736–2745. doi: 10.1016/j.neurobiolaging.2014.06.003

Zimmer, E. R., Parent, M. J., Cuello, A. C., Gauthier, S., and Rosa-Neto, P. (2014). MicroPET imaging and transgenic models: a blueprint for Alzheimer's disease clinical research. *Trends Neurosci.* 37, 629Ű641. doi: 10.1016/j.tins.2014.07.002

15

Inhibition of TRIB3 Protects Against Neurotoxic Injury Induced by Kainic Acid in Rats

Jing Zhang[1], Ying Han[1], Yang Zhao[1], Qinrui Li[1], Hongfang Jin[1] and Jiong Qin[2]**

[1]Department of Pediatrics, Peking University First Hospital, Beijing, China, [2]Department of Pediatrics, Peking University People's Hospital, Beijing, China

***Correspondence:**
Ying Han
hanying1568@126.com
Jiong Qin
qinjiong@pkuph.edu.cn

Epilepsy refers to a group of neurological disorders of varying etiologies characterized by recurrent seizures, resulting in brain dysfunction. Endoplasmic reticulum (ER) stress is highly activated in the process of epilepsy-related brain injury. However, the mechanisms by which ER stress triggers neuronal apoptosis remain to be fully elucidated. Tribbles pseudokinase 3 (TRIB3) is a pseudokinase that affects a number of cellular functions, and its expression is increased during ER stress. Here, we sought to clarify the role of TRIB3 in neuronal apoptosis mediated by ER stress. In the kainic acid (KA) (10 mg/kg)-induced rat seizure model, we characterized neuronal injury and apoptosis after KA injection. KA induced an ER stress response, as indicated by elevated expression of glucose-regulated protein 78 (GRP78) and C/EBP homologous protein (CHOP). TRIB3 protein was upregulated concomitantly with the downregulation of phosphorylated-protein kinase B (p-AKT) in rats following KA administration. In rat cortical neurons treated with KA, TRIB3 knockdown by siRNA reduced the number of dying neurons, decreased the induction of GRP78 and CHOP and the activation of caspase-3, and blocked the dephosphorylation of AKT after KA treatment. Our findings indicate that TRIB3 is involved in neuronal apoptosis occurring after KA-induced seizure. The knockdown of TRIB3 effectively protects against neuronal apoptosis *in vitro*, suggesting that TRIB3 may be a potential therapeutic target for the treatment of epilepsy.

Keywords: epilepsy, endoplasmic reticulum stress, tribbles pseudokinase 3, neuronal apoptosis, kainic acid

INTRODUCTION

Epilepsy is one of the most common neurological disorders in children. More than 70% of patients successfully respond to the therapy with antiepileptic drugs, but a large number of resistant patients continue to experience recurrent seizures, leading to severe incapacitation and cognitive dysfunction (Jensen, 2014). Increasing evidence has revealed that neuronal apoptosis is a prominent feature in epileptogenesis and may contribute to the impairment of cognitive function (Hopkins et al., 2000; Henshall and Simon, 2005). Therefore, the possibility of reducing neuronal apoptosis has potentially important implications in the treatment of epilepsy.

Endoplasmic reticulum (ER) stress can induce neuronal apoptosis in association with many neurological diseases (Imai et al., 2001; Takahashi and Imai, 2003; Rao and Bredesen, 2004; Wang et al., 2005; Han et al., 2015), such as epilepsy, febrile seizures, and Alzheimer's and Parkinson's diseases. ER stress occurs under various stressors that provoke the accumulation of unfolded proteins and disturb calcium homeostasis (Rutkowski and Kaufman, 2004; Walter and Ron, 2011). Cells initially respond to ER stress through the activation of the unfolded protein response (UPR) (Walter and Ron, 2011), which in turn elicits an adaptive and restorative effect mainly through the activation of the protein kinase RNA-like ER kinase (PERK), inositol-requiring protein 1α (IRE1α), and transcription factor 6 (ATF6) pathways (Gorman et al., 2012; Sano and Reed, 2013). However, if stressors are persistent or severe, the UPR leads to an execution phase consisting of C/EBP homologous protein (CHOP)-mediated apoptosis (Oyadomari and Mori, 2004; Szegezdi et al., 2006). CHOP is upregulated in human epilepsy and is important for neuronal survival after status epilepticus (SE) (Engel et al., 2013; Sheedy et al., 2014). Although the mechanisms by which CHOP targets apoptosis are not completely understood, it has been shown that ER stress promotes the expression of tribbles pseudokinase 3 (TRIB3), a novel stress-inducible gene induced *via* the ATF4-CHOP pathway, causing cell death (Ohoka et al., 2005).

TRIB3 is a pseudokinase molecule that affects a number of cellular functions (Hegedus et al., 2007; Yokoyama and Nakamura, 2011). TRIB3 has been reported to be highly activated in the presence of a variety of stressors, including the deprivation of neurotrophic factors, hypoxia, and ER stress (Mayumi-Matsuda et al., 1999; Ord et al., 2007; Avery et al., 2010). The induction of TRIB3 can play a detrimental role in the ER stress response of cardiac myocytes by antagonizing cardiac glucose metabolism (Avery et al., 2010), as well as in ER stress-related neuronal apoptosis of PC 12 cells (Zou et al., 2009). TRIB3 is elevated and mediates cell death in Parkinson's disease (Aime et al., 2015). TRIB3 has also been reported to be an important regulatory protein involved in insulin resistance and tumorigenesis through interfering with AKT activation (Du et al., 2003; Prudente et al., 2012; Salazar et al., 2015a). However, the role of TRIB3 in epilepsy and epilepsy-related brain injury remains controversial. Here, we sought to clarify the role of TRIB3 in neuronal apoptosis mediated by ER stress after seizures. KA activates excitatory glutamate receptors and triggers a delayed type of excitotoxic cell death in various brain regions, including hippocampus, cerebral cortex, and amygdala, which is recognized as an important underlying mechanism in neurodegenerative disorders, such as epilepsy (Wang et al., 2005; Sokka et al., 2007). The seizures in pediatric patients arise frequently in the neocortical structures, which are different from the hippocampal part often seen in adult epilepsy (Wong and Yamada, 2001). In the present study, we used a kainic acid (KA) (10 mg/kg)-induced rat seizure model to investigate the role of TRIB3 and the relationship between TRIB3 and AKT in childhood epilepsy-related neuronal apoptosis of the cortex.

Abbreviations: AKT, protein kinase B; ATF4 transcription factor 4; ATF6, transcription factor 6; CHOP, C/EBP homologous protein; ER stress, endoplasmic reticulum stress; GRP78, glucose-regulated protein 78; KA, kainic acid; PERK, protein kinase RNA-like ER kinase; SE, status epilepticus; TRIB3, tribbles pseudokinase 3; UPR, unfolded protein response.

MATERIALS AND METHODS

Experimental Model of SE

Three-week-old male Sprague-Dawley rats (n = 120) were obtained from the Laboratory Animal Center. Care and experimental protocols used in this study were approved by the Animal Research Ethics Committee of Peking University First Hospital. All efforts were made to minimize the number of animals used and their suffering. The experimental animals were randomly divided into the normal control group (n = 60) and the epileptic model group (n = 60). Each group was randomly divided into the following subgroups: 6, 12, 24, and 72 h subgroups (n = 15 per subgroup). Rats in the epileptic model group were systemically administered KA (10 mg/kg, i.p., Sigma, USA) (Vincent and Mulle, 2009). Then, animal behavior was observed over a period of 3 h. Rats exhibited standing and jumping behavior, such as wet dog shakes similar to limbic seizures, followed by tonic and generalized seizures observed at 30 min to 3 h after KA application. Onset of SE was determined by the presence of stage 3 to 5 level seizures according to Racine's scale (Racine, 1972). In the present study, only one rat died after KA application, and 83.3% of the KA-injected rats developed SE. Rats in the control group were injected i.p. with the same volume of physiological saline and divided into the same four time-point subgroups. The animals were euthanized at various time points after KA application. One set of rats (n = 6 per subgroup) was perfused through the heart with 0.9% saline to remove blood components for Western blot analysis. The second set (n = 6 per subgroup) was perfused transcardially with phosphate-buffered saline (PBS) followed by the 4% paraformaldehyde (PFA) for 30 min, and then brain samples of rats were collected and fixed in 4% PFA for 20 h, transferred to 20% sucrose in PBS overnight at 4°C following the fixation, the brains were subsequently kept in 30% sucrose in PBS until they sank 3 or 4 days later, frozen in liquid nitrogen, and stored at −70°C for further analysis. Fixed brains were ultimately sliced into 10-μm thick sections using a freezing microtome for TUNEL assay and immunofluorescence staining. The brain of rats in the third set (n = 3 per subgroup) was used for electronic microscopy, and the rats were transcardially perfused with 0.9% saline followed by 3% PFA and 1% glutaraldehyde in PBS.

Neuronal Cultures and Transfection of siRNA

Cortical neurons were prepared from embryonic gestation day 18 rat embryos and cultured for 4 days in Neurobasal medium with B27-supplement (GIBCO) on dishes coated with poly-ornithine (Sigma). For the transfection experiments, neurons were transfected with 75 pmol siRNA (TRIB3 or non-targeting control) using Lipofectamine 3000 (Life Technologies) according to the manufacturer's protocol. At 48 h after transfection, KA (Sigma) was added to the cells to a final concentration of 100 μM for 24 h. Then, the neurons were subjected to the TUNEL assay, immunofluorescence staining, Western blot, and qPCR analysis. The target sequence used for TRIB3 siRNA knockdown was 5′-GAAGAAACCGUUGGAGUUTT-3′ (Biolino).

Synthetic siRNA targeting rat TRIB3 (Gene ID: 57761) and non-targeting control siRNA were obtained from Beijing Biolino Inc.

Electron Microscopy

Cortical tissues were removed, immersed in 3% glutaraldehyde in PBS, and cut into semi-thin sections of approximately 1 mm^3. Sections were then cut into semi-thin sections of 1-μm and ultrathin sections of 100-nm thickness, all in the coronal plane. The changes of cortex ultrastructure were observed by transmission electronic microscopy (JEM-100CX, JEOL, Japan).

Tunel Assay

About 10 μm sections of brain tissue were used to evaluate apoptosis, and sections of the temporal lobe of the cortex were selected for examination (Defazio et al., 2015). The number of apoptotic neurons was determined using TUNEL staining with an *in situ* cell death detection kit (Roche Applied Science, Germany) according to the protocol provided by the manufacturer. Nuclear staining with DAPI and apoptotic cells labeled with TUNEL (green) were examined under a fluorescence microscope. Six sections were conducted in each group. In each section, the number of TUNEL-positive cells was counted in six counting frames that were randomly selected on images of 400× magnification.

Western Blotting

Cortical tissues and cultured neurons were lysed using ice-cold radioimmunoprecipitation assay buffer (RIPA) supplemented with a protease inhibitor mixture. Equal amounts of protein were subjected to SDS-PAGE and blotted onto nitrocellulose membranes (Pall). Subsequently, membranes were first incubated for 1 h in 5% skimmed milk and then overnight at 4°C with the following primary antibodies: anti-GRP78 (1:1000; Sigma, USA), anti-CHOP (1:250; Santa Cruz Biotechnology), anti-TRIB3 (1:500; LifeSpan BioSciences, USA), anti-phosphorylated (p)-AKT (1:500) and anti-AKT (1:500; both from Cell Signaling), anti-caspase-3 (1:1000; Cell Signaling), anti-Bax (1:1000; Abcam), and anti-β-actin (1:1000; Zhong Shan Golden Bridge Biotechnology, China). The following day, after being washed three times (TBST, 10 min each), the filters were incubated with horseradish peroxidase-conjugated secondary antibodies (1:5000; Zhong Shan Golden Bridge Biotechnology, China) for 1 h and washed with TBST three times (10 min each), followed by detection using enhanced chemiluminescence. Quantification was performed using ImageJ software. The relative amount of GRP78, CHOP, TRIB3, and p-AKT in control group was arbitrarily assigned as 1 for comparison.

Immunofluorescence Staining

Frozen sections were immersed in acetone at 4°C for 20 min. Next, the samples were washed with PBS three times (5 min each) and permeabilized with 0.3% Triton X-100. Then, sections were heated in a microwave oven for 10 min in citrate buffer (0.1 M, pH 6.0) for antigen retrieval. Sections were subsequently washed with PBS and blocked with 3% bovine serum albumin (BSA) and 20% normal goat serum for 30 min. Sections were then co-incubated with mouse anti-CHOP (Santa Cruz) and rabbit anti-TRIB3 (LifeSpan, LS-C1535841) or a mixture of mouse anti-TRIB3 (Santa Cruz, sc-390242) and rabbit anti-phospho-AKT (Ser473) (Cell Signaling) and NeuN (Abcam 104224 and 104225) at 4°C overnight. The next day, following three washes in PBS, sections were co-incubated with Alexa Fluor®594 (goat anti-rabbit IgG, red) and Alexa Fluor®488 (goat anti-mouse IgG, green) secondary antibody (Life Technologies) in the dark for 1 h at 37°C and then washed in PBS three times. Next, sections were counterstained with DAPI. Laser scanning confocal microscopy was performed to examine fluorescence.

In vitro, neurons were fixed for 20 min using 4% paraformaldehyde. They were then washed three times in PBS and incubated for 1 h in 5% BSA/0.1% Triton X-100. Then, the samples were incubated with antibodies against active caspase-3 (Abcam) and NeuN (Abcam 104224) or co-incubated with mouse anti-TRIB3 (Santa Cruz, sc-390,242) and rabbit anti-phosphor-AKT (Ser473) (Cell Signaling) and then stained with secondary antibody as above.

Quantitative PCR

RNA was prepared from cultured neurons and cDNA synthesized using 50 U of SuperScript II reverse transcriptase and components given by the vendor (Invitrogen). Primers used in qPCR included: 5′-CGGAGTCAACGGATTTGGTCGTAT-3′ (sense) and 5′-AG CCTTCTCCATGGTGGTGAAGAC-3′ (antisense) for GAPDH cDNA and 5′-CACATCTCTGGCTGCTTCTG-3′ (sense), and 5′-CAGTTGCCTTGCTCTCGTTC-3′ (antisense) for TRIB3 cDNA. Real-time PCR amplification was performed using a SYBR Green PCR Master Mix Kit (Invitrogen). Cycling conditions included denaturation at 95°C for 10 min, followed by 40 cycles of 95°C for 15 s, and extension at 58°C for 1 min. The relative quantity of mRNA was normalized to GAPDH and calculated using the delta-delta method from threshold cycle numbers. On the basis of exponential amplification of the target gene as well as a calibrator, the amount of amplified cDNA at the threshold cycle was given by $2^{-\Delta\Delta Ct}$.

Statistical Analyses

Quantitative results are expressed as the mean ± SEM. Statistical comparisons were performed using one-way ANOVA, followed by a post hoc analysis (Bonferroni's test). For each time point *in vivo*, six rats were used, and the *in vitro* assays were repeated more than three times. A $p < 0.05$ was considered significant.

RESULTS

Excitotoxic Neuronal Injury and Apoptosis in Rats With KA-Induced Seizure

A TUNEL assay and the activation of caspase-3 and Bax were used to assess the level of neuronal injury and apoptosis in the cortex induced by KA. The number of TUNEL-NeuN-positive cells increased by 24 h after KA administration compared with the control group (**Figure 1A**). Expressions of active caspase-3 and Bax were increased by 12 h post-KA administration

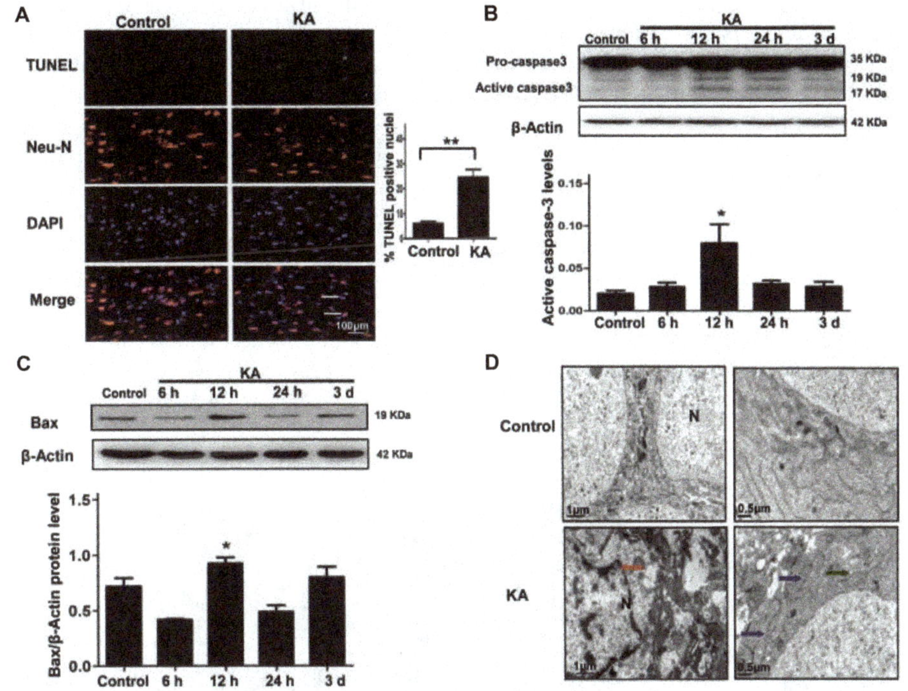

FIGURE 1 | Excitotoxic neuronal cell death is induced by addition of KA. **(A)** TUNEL assay showing apoptotic neurons in rat cortex samples. TUNEL-NeuN-positive cells are indicated by an arrow. Scale bar = 100 μm in all images. Western blot was performed for evaluation of active caspase-3 **(B)** and Bax **(C)** protein levels. $^{*}p < 0.05$ vs. control ($n = 6$). **(D)** Neuron ultrastructure. Control group: Normal ultrastructure of neurons. KA group: Disrupted or shrunken nuclei (red arrow); swollen mitochondria (blue arrow), with dissolved and ruptured ridges; and dilated rough endoplasmic reticulum (RER) lumens (green narrow). KA, KA group; N, nucleus.

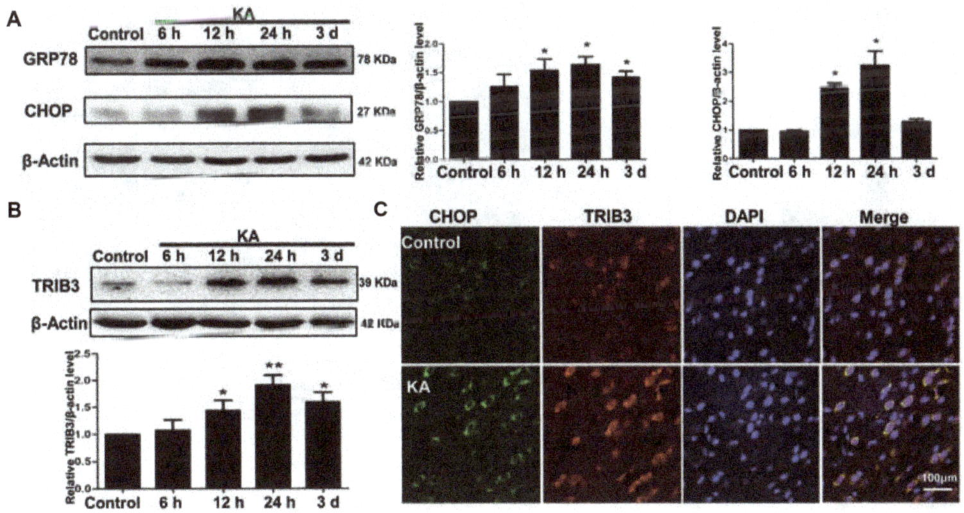

FIGURE 2 | ER stress and the induction of TRIB3 following KA-induced excitotoxicity. Western blots for GRP78 and CHOP **(A)** and TRIB3 **(B)** at various times after KA. **(C)** Double immunofluorescence staining for TRIB3 and CHOP, and the relative amount of GRP78, CHOP, and TRIB3 in the control group was arbitrarily assigned a value of 1 for comparison. $^{*}p < 0.05$ vs. control ($n = 6$). KA, KA group.

and detected by Western blotting (**Figures 1B,C**). These results suggest that KA administration results in the apoptosis of cortical neurons *in vivo*.

Ultrastructural changes of cortical neurons were observed by electron microscopy. Neurons in the control group showed a normal neuronal structure, including an intact and defined nuclear membrane, normally distributed basic nuclear chromatin, and a normal quantity of organelles. Compared with the changes observed in the control group, striking alterations in ultrastructural changes were manifested in coronal sections of cortical neurons 24 h after KA injection, including nuclear pyknosis and shrinkage of the perikarya, swollen dendrites and mitochondria, rough ER with a swollen lumen, and decreased numbers of ribosomes (**Figure 1D**).

ER Stress and the Induction of TRIB3 in Rats With KA-Induced Seizure

Protein expression of ER chaperones following KA administration was detected by Western blot. Alterations in the ER stress markers GRP78 and CHOP were used to determine whether ER stress occurred following KA-induced seizure. GRP78 was elevated in the rat cortex, beginning at 12 h after KA administration and remained increase until 3 days (**Figure 2A**). The results also showed that the expression of CHOP in rat cortex increased at 12 h and decreased to control level at 3 days after KA injection. These results indicate that cells within the cortex were undergoing ER stress.

To determine whether TRIB3, a novel ER stress-inducible gene, was involved in neuronal apoptosis, we measured TRIB3 expression by Western blot analysis and then investigated the relationship between CHOP and TRIB3 through double staining. Interestingly, similar to ER stress markers, TRIB3 protein was clearly upregulated by 12 h post-KA and persisted at elevated levels for at least 3 days (**Figure 2B**). Double immunofluorescence staining for TRIB3 and CHOP showed that the expression levels of TRIB3 and CHOP were increased in cortical neurons 24 h after KA, whereas their expression

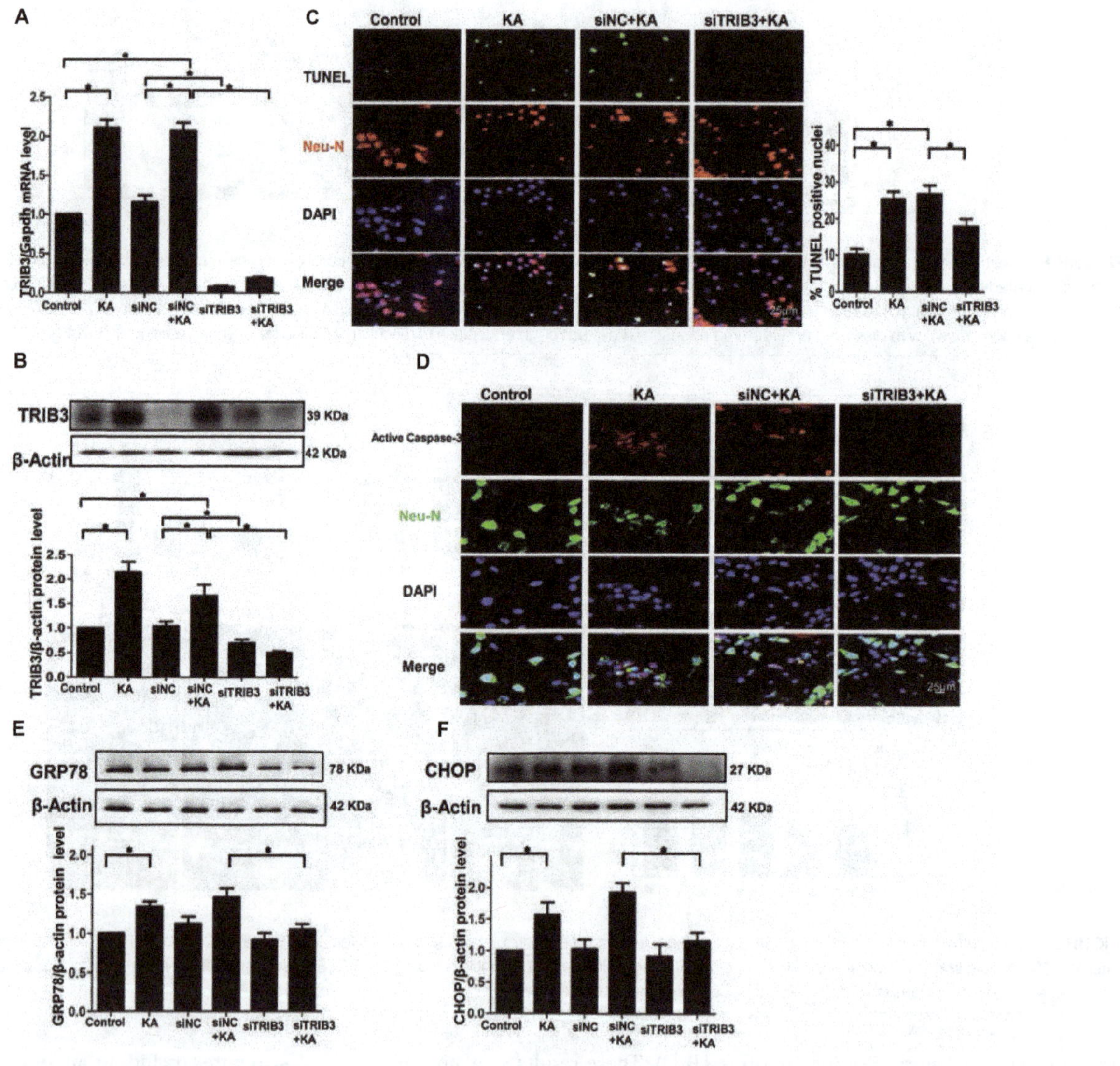

FIGURE 3 | TRIB3 downregulation reduces KA-induced excitotoxic neuronal death *in vitro*. TRIB3 total mRNA **(A)** and protein **(B)** were detected after transfection with siTRIB3. **(C)** Apoptosis of cultured cortical neurons (positive NeuN) was analyzed using the TUNEL assay. **(D)** Activated caspase-3 was detected by immunofluorescence. Expression of GRP78 **(E)** and CHOP **(F)** in cultured neurons was detected by Western blot. *$p < 0.05$ vs. control. Control, control group; KA, KA-treated group; siNC+KA, siNC+KA-treated group; siTRIB3 + KA, siTRIB3 + KA-treated group.

was barely detectable in the control rat cortex (**Figure 2C**), similar to our Western blot results.

TRIB3 Downregulation Reduces KA-Induced Neuronal Apoptosis and ER Stress *in vitro*

To explore whether ER stress-induced TRIB3-mediated neuronal apoptosis following KA-induced excitotoxicity, we used three different TRIB3 siRNAs to downregulate TRIB3 in primary cultures of rat cortical neurons treated with or without KA. Downregulation of TRIB3 mRNA and protein was confirmed through qPCR and Western blot analysis, respectively (**Figures 3A,B**). TUNEL staining revealed an increase in the number of TUNEL-NeuN-positive cells in the KA and siNC+KA group, whereas the targeted downregulation of the TRIB3 (siTRIB3 + KA) group decreased the number of apoptotic cells in cultures compared with the number in the siNC+KA group (**Figure 3C**). As in the rat cortex, we also detected the activated caspase-3 *in vitro*. Immunofluorescence staining for activated caspase-3 indicated a significant increase in the KA and siNC+KA groups, compared with the level in the untreated control group, and TRIB3 knockdown reduced the activation of caspase-3 caused by KA (**Figure 3D**).

TRIB3 knockdown has been shown to confer resistance against ER stress in HEK293 and HeLa cells (Ohoka et al., 2005). Therefore, we measured ER stress and TRIB3 expression in KA-treated neuronal cultures. The activation of the ER stress chaperones GRP78 and CHOP was increased following KA exposure, but decreased in the siTRIB3 + KA-treated cells compared with the level in the siNC+KA group (**Figures 3E,F**).

TRIB3 Downregulation Inhibits the KA-Mediated Reduction of Phospho-AKT

Levels of p-AKT (Ser473) were decreased by 12 h following KA administration, whereas total AKT remained unchanged compared with the level in the control (**Figure 4A**). Double immunofluorescence labeling for TRIB3 and p-AKT in rat cortices isolated at 24 h post-KA revealed that p-AKT was expressed at very low levels in cortical neurons expressing TRIB3. Conversely, in control cortices, TRIB3 expression was seldom observed in neurons immunoreactive for p-AKT (**Figure 4B**). Therefore, *in vivo*, TRIB3 was upregulated after KA injection, and in the same neurons, p-AKT levels were decreased.

The above results suggest that TRIB3 promotes neuronal apoptosis possibly by interacting with and inhibiting AKT activity in rats with KA-induced seizures. To determine the causal relationship between TRIB3 and p-AKT in excitotoxic neuronal injury, we measured p-AKT (S473) in cultured neurons by immunofluorescence staining. Phosphorylated AKT was rarely detected in KA- and siNC+KA-treated cells, whereas TRIB3 was induced. Importantly, increased p-AKT was observed in the siTRIB3 + KA group (**Figure 4C**). It is likely that TRIB3 downregulation may at least partially block the decrease in p-AKT caused by KA addition.

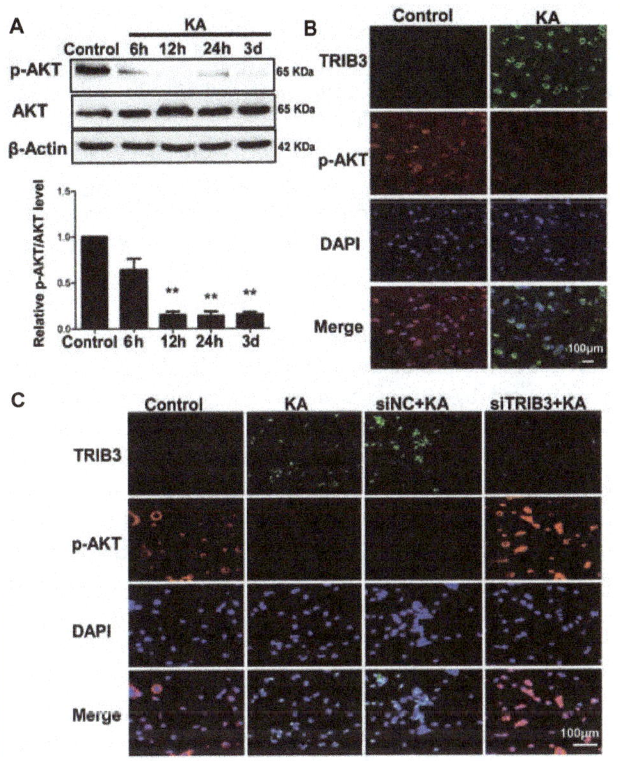

FIGURE 4 | TRIB3 downregulation inhibits the KA-mediated reduction of phospho-AKT. **(A)** Total AKT and phospho-AKT (Ser473) were detected by Western blotting. **(B)** Double immunofluorescence staining for TRIB3 and phospho-AKT. **(C)** Double immunofluorescence staining for TRIB3 and phospho-AKT *in vitro*. $^{**}p < 0.05$. Control, control group; KA, KA-treated group; siNC+KA, siNC+KA-treated group; siTRIB3 + KA, siTRIB3 + KA-treated group.

DISCUSSION

In the present study, our data demonstrate that TRIB3 is elevated after KA-induced excitotoxicity *in vivo* and *in vitro*; inhibition of TRIB3 attenuates the neuronal apoptosis observed after kainate *in vitro*; and the targeted downregulation of TRIB3 partially reverses the KA-mediated decrease in phospho-AKT levels *in vitro*. Overall, we show that TRIB3 plays a crucial role in mediating ER stress-induced neuronal apoptosis, possibly by interacting with AKT.

Neuronal apoptosis plays an important role in brain injury after seizures and the formation of chronic epilepsy. Unlike adult epilepsy originating in the hippocampus, in infants and children epilepsy originates in the cerebral cortex (Wong and Yamada, 2001). Neuronal damage involving excitatory glutamate receptors is recognized as an important underlying mechanism in epilepsy; KA-mediated excitotoxicity as a seizure model has been widely used to study the mechanisms of neuronal injury in epileptic disease (Diaz-Ruiz et al., 2013; Liu et al., 2015). ER stress, activation of caspase-3, and changes in the pro-apoptotic protein Bax have been suggested to be involved in neuronal cell death following excitotoxicity induced by KA administration (Sperk et al., 1983; Henshall et al., 2000; Djebaili et al., 2001; Wang et al., 2005; Sokka et al., 2007; Tokuhara et al., 2007;

Liu et al., 2009; Urino et al., 2010). A diverse time course of neuronal death has been noted in the KA-lesion rat model, with degenerating neurons being detected at 4 and 6 h, and massive neuronal damage being observed at 1 to 4 days after SE (Hopkins et al., 2000). Understanding the pathological changes in the brain and the mechanism for neuronal damage could further contribute to determining the most suitable time to treat chronic epilepsy. In our study, we used an animal model of childhood epilepsy in which the patients are vulnerable to seizures during the phase of development of the nervous system. We also characterized excitotoxic neuronal injury in the rat cortex following KA administration. We observed the damage of the ultrastructure of the cortex by 24 h after KA injection, as manifested by shrunken nuclei and swollen mitochondria. In addition, the number of dying cells increased by 24 h following KA administration, as determined using the TUNEL assay. Both activation of caspase-3 and protein Bax upregulation occurred in the rat cortex beginning 12 h after KA administration. We also showed that ER stress was involved in excitotoxic neuronal injury induced by KA, as indicated by the upregulation of GRP78 and CHOP. In this study, the ER stress markers GRP78 and CHOP were chosen because they both were involved in each of the three branches of the ER stress pathway (Szegezdi et al., 2006). In addition, the results showed that the increased GRP78 was maintained until 3 days after KA administration, whereas CHOP was significantly decreased at 3 days after KA administration. The study by Sokka et al. showed that CHOP was increased at 24 h and restored to normal level at 48 h in rat after KA administration (Sokka et al., 2007). The study by Irma et al. reported the acute, sub-acute, and chronic changes induced by SE in the immature rat hippocampus. The acute changes included the neuronal death process that mainly occurred within 3 days after SE in the immature rat hippocampus, and then, the activation of inflammatory process and synaptic plasticity triggered the sub-acute changes (Holopainen, 2008). CHOP is known to be involved in ER stress-induced apoptosis (Oyadomari and Mori, 2004), and the expression of CHOP was decreased at 3 days after KA injection, consistent with the change at acute response. The studies by Engel et al. showed that the functions of CHOP in neuronal death induced by seizures might be context-dependent (Engel et al., 2013), and according to Lin's study, the effects of CHOP may depend on differences in parallel signaling pathways or the duration of activity of individual branches of the unfolded protein response (Lin et al., 2007). Therefore, it might be likely that the different signals activated downstream of ER stress in neuronal damage, neurogenesis, and cellular reorganization in the developing brain after seizures.

Several studies have demonstrated that prolonged ER stress overwhelms UPR survival mechanisms to initiate pro-apoptotic pathways by activating transcription factors (e.g., ATF4 and CHOP), which leads to the overexpression of TRIB3. Furthermore, TRIB3 promotes cellular dysfunction and ultimately results in apoptosis (Ohoka et al., 2005; Bromati et al., 2011; Prudente et al., 2012). ER stress has been shown to be involved in β-cell apoptosis after expression of TRIB3, and TRIB3 is a downstream effector of ER stress and is induced *via* the ATF4-CHOP pathway (Bromati et al., 2011). Cardiomyocyte apoptosis induced by stretching is also mediated by TRIB3 (Cheng et al., 2015). Overexpression of TRIB3 is sufficient to promote neuronal apoptosis even in the presence of nerve growth factor (Zareen et al., 2013) and increased chronic glucose-induced apoptosis in INS-TRIB3 cells (Qian et al., 2008). TRIB3 induction also occurs in response to neurotrophic factor (NGF) deprivation, Parkinson's disease, and metabolic stress (Mayumi-Matsuda et al., 1999; Du et al., 2003; Hua et al., 2011). However, little information on the effects of TRIB3 in KA-mediated neuronal apoptosis has been previously reported. In the present study, we explored the role of TRIB3 in an epilepsy paradigm. Our data show that TRIB3 is elevated post-KA administration *in vivo* and *in vitro*. Furthermore, TRIB3 upregulation occurs in cortical cells, as observed using immunofluorescence staining following KA administration. *In vitro*, we found that the targeted downregulation of TRIB3 partially reduces the number of apoptotic neurons and decreases the activation of caspase-3 in cortical neurons treated with KA. This suggests that TRIB3 is highly activated in the rat cortex in response to neuronal injury following KA-induced seizure, while TRIB3 mediates neuronal apoptosis and inhibition of TRIB3 protects against neurotoxic injury induced by kainic acid in rats. These findings indicate that TRIB3 could be important for the translation of novel therapeutic approaches in epilepsy.

Under mild or transient ER stress, previous investigators suggested that TRIB3 was primarily regulated by ATF4 and CHOP, and TRIB3 also acted *via* a negative feedback mechanism to inhibit ATF4 and CHOP, thereby promoting cell survival (Rzymski et al., 2008; Su and Kilberg, 2008; Bromati et al., 2011). In the present study, we showed that TRIB3 downregulation attenuated the ER stress response by reducing KA-mediated increase in GRP78 and CHOP. These results suggest that there might be a feedback relationship between TRIB3 and CHOP. TRIB3 plays a crucial role in balancing neuronal survival and death in rats with KA-induced seizures.

Studies have shown that TRIB3 can bind to numerous molecules and regulate their biological functions. Thus, TRIB3 plays a crucial function at the juncture of homeostasis, metabolic disease, and cancer (Humphrey et al., 2010; Hua et al., 2011; Mondal et al., 2016). AKT is known to maintain cell survival by inhibiting apoptosis and promoting cell cycle progression (Song et al., 2005). TRIB3 has been reported to be a negative modulator of AKT (Du et al., 2003) and has been shown to suppress cell survival by interacting with and inhibiting the activation of AKT (Zareen et al., 2013). Loss of TRIB3 enables AKT-driven tumorigenesis *via* forkhead box class O (FoxO) inactivation, and TRIB3 knockdown provides prolonged protection from NGF deprivation, protects axons, and maintains overall neuronal morphology (Zhang et al., 2011; Prudente et al., 2012; Salazar et al., 2015b). Therefore, we explored the level of active AKT [p-AKT (S473)] in the rat cortex. In this study, our data reveal that the levels of active AKT are suppressed in the cortex from 12 h post-KA to 3 days post-KA. Importantly, we found that p-AKT is deficient in cells overproducing TRIB3 in rats following KA-induced seizures. Moreover, we also show that targeted downregulation of TRIB3 partially reverses the decrease in phospho-AKT caused by KA application in cortical cultures, and the deactivation of phospho-AKT corresponds with the induction of TRIB3 in the cortex, supporting the hypothesis that TRIB3 may be responsible for the inhibition of AKT in rats following KA administration. These findings suggest that neuronal apoptosis induced by ER stress is regulated by TRIB3-mediated suppression of AKT in rats with KA-induced seizures. Collectively, epilepsy induces ER stress and overexpression of TRIB3. Additionally, TRIB3 decreases the levels of activated AKT, ultimately resulting in an activation of caspase-3 and upregulation of Bax to mediate neuronal apoptosis. Inhibition of TRIB3 is effective in protecting against neurotoxic injury induced by KA *via* maintaining levels of activated Akt.

Several studies have shown that the expression of TRIB3 and its subcellular localization varied in different tissues, as well as in different disease models. TRIB3 expression was documented in both cytoplasm and nucleus (Prudente et al., 2012; Mondal et al., 2016). In agreement with other researchers, the expression of TRIB3 was observed both in the nucleus and cytoplasm in KA group by using immunofluorescence staining, while the expression of TRIB3 in control group was located in the cytoplasm relatively more than in KA group. Furthermore, it is interesting to explore the mechanisms underlying the changes of intracellular localization of TRIB3 in the KA group.

As shown by our data, targeted downregulation of TRIB3 effectively protects against neuronal injury caused by KA, although the extent of protection is not complete. It is likely that cross-talk with other parallel signaling pathways is fine-tuned at the juncture of neuronal apoptosis in rats with KA-induced seizures. TRIB3 can inhibit AKT phosphorylation and suppress the PI3K/AKT/mTOR pathway (Du et al., 2003), and there is cross-talk between MAPK, NF-κB, and TRIB3 (Okamoto et al., 2007; Rzymski et al., 2008). TRIB3 regulates multiple stress response pathways and fine-tunes stress-inducing and stress-adaptive mechanisms (Mondal et al., 2016). A study by Wei implied that the downregulation of TRIB3 attenuated endoplasmic reticulum stress, enhanced Akt phosphorylation, and protected neuron from apoptosis by stereotaxic injection of TRB3 shRNA lentivirus in the global cerebral ischemia and reperfusion injury in rats (Wei et al., 2017). Erazo's study showed that the new antitumor drug (ABTL0812) mediated cell death by upregulating the expression of TRIB3 (Erazo et al., 2016). Given the evolving roles and cellular functions of TRIB3 in diseases and biology, it may provide an attractive opportunity for drug design (Eyers et al., 2017). In the present study, we demonstrated the crucial role of TRIB3 in the neuronal apoptosis induced by KA *in vitro*. Further studies would be of help in clarifying the mechanisms for the role of TRIB3 in neuronal apoptosis for a better understanding of the molecular mechanisms underlying epilepsy-related brain damage *in vivo*.

In conclusion, we show that TRIB3 is upregulated in rats with KA-induced seizures and that the induction of TRIB3 and TRIB3-mediated suppression of AKT facilitate neuronal apoptosis in rats following KA-induced seizures. Inhibition of TRIB3 is effective in protecting against neurotoxic injury induced by KA. Our findings suggest that TRIB3 and its regulatory pathways be considered potential and promising therapeutic targets for the treatment of epilepsy.

AUTHOR CONTRIBUTIONS

JQ and YH conceived and designed the experiments. JZ conducted the experiments. YZ and QL participated in the completion of the experiments. JZ, HJ, and YH analyzed the data. JZ wrote the paper. YH and JQ revised the manuscript. All the authors read and approved the final paper.

FUNDING

The present study was supported by grants from the National Natural Science Foundation of China (81200998), Beijing Natural Science Foundation (7092105 and 7112131), Key Clinical Project from the Ministry of Public Health (2010-12), and National Key Technology R & D Program (2012BAI03B02).

REFERENCES

Aime, P., Sun, X., Zareen, N., Rao, A., Berman, Z., Volpicelli-Daley, L., et al. (2015). Trib3 is elevated in Parkinson's disease and mediates death in Parkinson's disease models. *J. Neurosci.* 35, 10731–10749. doi: 10.1523/JNEUROSCI.0614-15.2015

Avery, J., Etzion, S., Debosch, B. J., Jin, X., Lupu, T. S., Beitinjaneh, B., et al. (2010). TRB3 function in cardiac endoplasmic reticulum stress. *Circ. Res.* 106, 1516–1523. doi: 10.1161/CIRCRESAHA.109.211920

Bromati, C. R., Lellis-Santos, C., Yamanaka, T. S., Nogueira, T. C., Leonelli, M., Caperuto, L. C., et al. (2011). UPR induces transient burst of apoptosis in islets of early lactating rats through reduced AKT phosphorylation via ATF4/CHOP stimulation of TRB3 expression. *Am. J. Physiol. Regul. Integr. Comp. Physiol.* 300, R92–R100. doi: 10.1152/ajpregu.00169.2010

Cheng, W. P., Wang, B. W., Lo, H. M., and Shyu, K. G. (2015). Mechanical stretch induces apoptosis regulator TRB3 in cultured cardiomyocytes and volume-overloaded heart. *PLoS One* 10:e0123235. doi: 10.1371/journal.pone.0145422

Defazio, R., Criado, A., Zantedeschi, V., and Scanziani, E. (2015). Neuroanatomy-based matrix-guided trimming protocol for the rat brain. *Toxicol. Pathol.* 43, 249–256. doi: 10.1177/0192623314538345

Diaz-Ruiz, A., Mendez-Armenta, M., Galvan-Arzate, S., Manjarrez, J., Nava-Ruiz, C., Santander, I., et al. (2013). Antioxidant, anticonvulsive and neuroprotective effects of dapsone and phenobarbital against kainic acid-induced damage in rats. *Neurochem. Res.* 38, 1819–1827. doi: 10.1007/s11064-013-1087-z

Djebaili, M., Lerner-Natoli, M., Montpied, P., Baille, V., Bockaert, J., and Rondouin, G. (2001). Molecular events involved in neuronal death induced in the mouse hippocampus by in-vivo injection of kainic acid. *Brain Res. Mol. Brain Res.* 93, 190–198. doi: 10.1016/S0169-328X(01)00197-8

Du, K., Herzig, S., Kulkarni, R. N., and Montminy, M. (2003). TRB3: a tribbles homolog that inhibits Akt/PKB activation by insulin in liver. *Science* 300, 1574–1577. doi: 10.1126/science.1079817

Engel, T., Sanz-Rodgriguez, A., Jimenez-Mateos, E. M., Concannon, C. G., Jimenez-Pacheco, A., Moran, C., et al. (2013). CHOP regulates the p53-MDM2 axis and is required for neuronal survival after seizures. *Brain* 136, 577–592. doi: 10.1093/brain/aws337

Erazo, T., Lorente, M., Lopez-Plana, A., Munoz-Guardiola, P., Fernandez-Nogueira, P., Garcia-Martinez, J. A., et al. (2016). The new antitumor drug ABTL0812 inhibits the Akt/mTORC1 axis by upregulating Tribbles-3 pseudokinase. *Clin. Cancer Res.* 22, 2508–2519. doi: 10.1158/1078-0432.CCR-15-1808

Eyers, P. A., Keeshan, K., and Kannan, N. (2017). Tribbles in the 21st century: the evolving roles of tribbles pseudokinases in biology and disease. *Trends Cell Biol.* 27, 284–298. doi: 10.1016/j.tcb.2016.11.002

Gorman, A. M., Healy, S. J., Jager, R., and Samali, A. (2012). Stress management at the ER: regulators of ER stress-induced apoptosis. *Pharmacol. Ther.* 134, 306–316. doi: 10.1016/j.pharmthera.2012.02.003

Han, Y., Yi, W., Qin, J., Zhao, Y., Zhang, J., and Chang, X. (2015). Carbon monoxide offers neuroprotection from hippocampal cell damage induced by recurrent febrile seizures through the PERK-activated ER stress pathway. *Neurosci. Lett.* 585, 126–131. doi: 10.1016/j.neulet.2014.11.040

Hegedus, Z., Czibula, A., and Kiss-Toth, E. (2007). Tribbles: a family of kinase-like proteins with potent signalling regulatory function. *Cell. Signal.* 19, 238–250. doi: 10.1016/j.cellsig.2006.06.010

Henshall, D. C., Chen, J., and Simon, R. P. (2000). Involvement of caspase-3-like protease in the mechanism of cell death following focally evoked limbic seizures. *J. Neurochem.* 74, 1215–1223. doi: 10.1046/j.1471-4159.2000.741215.x

Henshall, D. C., and Simon, R. P. (2005). Epilepsy and apoptosis pathways. *J. Cereb. Blood Flow Metab.* 25, 1557–1572. doi: 10.1038/sj.jcbfm.9600149

Holopainen, I. E. (2008). Seizures in the developing brain: cellular and molecular mechanisms of neuronal damage, neurogenesis and cellular reorganization. *Neurochem. Int.* 52, 935–947. doi: 10.1016/j.neuint.2007.10.021

Hopkins, K. J., Wang, G., and Schmued, L. C. (2000). Temporal progression of kainic acid induced neuronal and myelin degeneration in the rat forebrain. *Brain Res.* 864, 69–80. doi: 10.1016/S0006-8993(00)02137-5

Hua, F., Mu, R., Liu, J., Xue, J., Wang, Z., Lin, H., et al. (2011). TRB3 interacts with SMAD3 promoting tumor cell migration and invasion. *J. Cell Sci.* 124, 3235–3246. doi: 10.1242/jcs.082875

Humphrey, R. K., Newcomb, C. J., Yu, S. M., Hao, E., Yu, D., Krajewski, S., et al. (2010). Mixed lineage kinase-3 stabilizes and functionally cooperates with TRIBBLES-3 to compromise mitochondrial integrity in cytokine-induced death of pancreatic beta cells. *J. Biol. Chem.* 285, 22426–22436. doi: 10.1074/jbc.M110.123786

Imai, Y., Soda, M., Inoue, H., Hattori, N., Mizuno, Y., and Takahashi, R. (2001). An unfolded putative transmembrane polypeptide, which can lead to endoplasmic reticulum stress, is a substrate of Parkin. *Cell* 105, 891–902. doi: 10.1016/S0092-8674(01)00407-X

Jensen, F. E. (2014). Epilepsy in 2013: progress across the spectrum of epilepsy research. *Nat. Rev. Neurol.* 10, 63–64. doi: 10.1038/nrneurol.2013.277

Lin, J. H., Li, H., Yasumura, D., Cohen, H. R., Zhang, C., Panning, B., et al. (2007). IRE1 signaling affects cell fate during the unfolded protein response. *Science* 318, 944–949. doi: 10.1126/science.1146361

Liu, J., Naegele, J. R., and Lin, S. L. (2009). The DNA-PK catalytic subunit regulates Bax-mediated excitotoxic cell death by Ku70 phosphorylation. *Brain Res.* 1296, 164–175. doi: 10.1016/j.brainres.2009.07.101

Liu, H., Song, Z., Liao, D., Zhang, T., Liu, F., Zhuang, K., et al. (2015). Neuroprotective effects of trans-caryophyllene against kainic acid induced seizure activity and oxidative stress in mice. *Neurochem. Res.* 40, 118–123. doi: 10.1007/s11064-014-1474-0

Mayumi-Matsuda, K., Kojima, S., Suzuki, H., and Sakata, T. (1999). Identification of a novel kinase-like gene induced during neuronal cell death. *Biochem. Biophys. Res. Commun.* 258, 260–264. doi: 10.1006/bbrc.1999.0576

Mondal, D., Mathur, A., and Chandra, P. K. (2016). Tripping on TRIB3 at the junction of health, metabolic dysfunction and cancer. *Biochimie* 124, 34–52. doi: 10.1016/j.biochi.2016.02.005

Ohoka, N., Yoshii, S., Hattori, T., Onozaki, K., and Hayashi, H. (2005). TRB3, a novel ER stress-inducible gene, is induced via ATF4-CHOP pathway and is involved in cell death. *EMBO J.* 24, 1243–1255. doi: 10.1038/sj.emboj.7600596

Okamoto, H., Latres, E., Liu, R., Thabet, K., Murphy, A., Valenzeula, D., et al. (2007). Genetic deletion of Trb3, the mammalian drosophila tribbles homolog, displays normal hepatic insulin signaling and glucose homeostasis. *Diabetes* 56, 1350–1356. doi: 10.2337/db06-1448

Ord, D., Meerits, K., and Ord, T. (2007). TRB3 protects cells against the growth inhibitory and cytotoxic effect of ATF4. *Exp. Cell Res.* 313, 3556–3567. doi: 10.1016/j.yexcr.2007.07.017

Oyadomari, S., and Mori, M. (2004). Roles of CHOP/GADD153 in endoplasmic reticulum stress. *Cell Death Differ.* 11, 381–389. doi: 10.1038/sj.cdd.4401373

Prudente, S., Sesti, G., Pandolfi, A., Andreozzi, F., Consoli, A., and Trischitta, V. (2012). The mammalian tribbles homolog TRIB3, glucose homeostasis, and cardiovascular diseases. *Endocr. Rev.* 33, 526–546. doi: 10.1210/er.2011-1042

Qian, B., Wang, H., Men, X., Zhang, W., Cai, H., Xu, S., et al. (2008). TRIB3 [corrected] is implicated in glucotoxicity- and endoplasmic reticulum-stress-induced [corrected] beta-cell apoptosis. *J. Endocrinol.* 199, 407–416. doi: 10.1677/JOE-08-0331

Racine, R. J. (1972). Modification of seizure activity by electrical stimulation. II. Motor seizure. *Electroencephalogr. Clin. Neurophysiol.* 32, 281–294. doi: 10.1016/0013-4694(72)90177-0

Rao, R. V., and Bredesen, D. E. (2004). Misfolded proteins, endoplasmic reticulum stress and neurodegeneration. *Curr. Opin. Cell Biol.* 16, 653–662. doi: 10.1016/j.ceb.2004.09.012

Rutkowski, D. T., and Kaufman, R. J. (2004). A trip to the ER: coping with stress. *Trends Cell Biol.* 14, 20–28. doi: 10.1016/j.tcb.2003.11.001

Rzymski, T., Paantjens, A., Bod, J., and Harris, A. L. (2008). Multiple pathways are involved in the anoxia response of SKIP3 including HuR-regulated RNA stability, NF-kappaB and ATF4. *Oncogene* 27, 4532–4543. doi: 10.1038/onc.2008.100

Salazar, M., Lorente, M., Garcia-Taboada, E., Gomez, E. P., Davila, D., Zuniga-Garcia, P., et al. (2015a). TRIB3 suppresses tumorigenesis by controlling mTORC2/AKT/FOXO signaling. *Mol. Cell. Oncol.* 2:e980134. doi: 10.4161/23723556.2014.980134

Salazar, M., Lorente, M., Garcia-Taboada, E., Perez Gomez, E., Davila, D., Zuniga-Garcia, P., et al. (2015b). Loss of Tribbles pseudokinase-3 promotes Akt-driven tumorigenesis via FOXO inactivation. *Cell Death Differ.* 22, 131–144. doi: 10.1038/cdd.2014.133

Sano, R., and Reed, J. C. (2013). ER stress-induced cell death mechanisms. *Biochim. Biophys. Acta* 1833, 3460–3470. doi: 10.1016/j.bbamcr.2013.06.028

Sheedy, C., Mooney, C., Jimenez-Mateos, E., Sanz-Rodriguez, A., Langa, E., Mooney, C., et al. (2014). De-repression of myelin-regulating gene expression after status epilepticus in mice lacking the C/EBP homologous protein CHOP. *Int. J. Physiol. Pathophysiol. Pharmacol.* 6, 185–198.

Sokka, A. L., Putkonen, N., Mudo, G., Pryazhnikov, E., Reijonen, S., Khiroug, L., et al. (2007). Endoplasmic reticulum stress inhibition protects against excitotoxic neuronal injury in the rat brain. *J. Neurosci.* 27, 901–908. doi: 10.1523/JNEUROSCI.4289-06.2007

Song, G., Ouyang, G., and Bao, S. (2005). The activation of Akt/PKB signaling pathway and cell survival. *J. Cell. Mol. Med.* 9, 59–71. doi: 10.1111/j.1582-4934.2005.tb00337.x

Sperk, G., Lassmann, H., Baran, H., Kish, S. J., Seitelberger, F., and Hornykiewicz, O. (1983). Kainic acid induced seizures: neurochemical and histopathological changes. *Neuroscience* 10, 1301–1315. doi: 10.1016/0306-4522(83)90113-6

Su, N., and Kilberg, M. S. (2008). C/EBP homology protein (CHOP) interacts with activating transcription factor 4 (ATF4) and negatively regulates the stress-dependent induction of the asparagine synthetase gene. *J. Biol. Chem.* 283, 35106–35117. doi: 10.1074/jbc.M806874200

Szegezdi, E., Logue, S. E., Gorman, A. M., and Samali, A. (2006). Mediators of endoplasmic reticulum stress-induced apoptosis. *EMBO Rep.* 7, 880–885. doi: 10.1038/sj.embor.7400779

Takahashi, R., and Imai, Y. (2003). Pael receptor, endoplasmic reticulum stress, and Parkinson's disease. *J. Neurol.* 250(Suppl. 3), Iii25–Iii29. doi: 10.1007/s00415-003-1305-8

Tokuhara, D., Sakuma, S., Hattori, H., Matsuoka, O., and Yamano, T. (2007). Kainic acid dose affects delayed cell death mechanism after status epilepticus. *Brain Dev.* 29, 2–8. doi: 10.1016/j.braindev.2006.05.003

Urino, T., Hashizume, K., Maehara, M., Kato, K., Okada, Y., Hori, T., et al. (2010). Epileptic focus stimulation and seizure control in the rat model of kainic acid-induced limbic seizures. *Neurol. Med. Chir. (Tokyo)* 50, 355–360. doi: 10.2176/nmc.50.355

Vincent, P., and Mulle, C. (2009). Kainate receptors in epilepsy and excitotoxicity. *Neuroscience* 158, 309–323. doi: 10.1016/j.neuroscience.2008.02.066

Walter, P., and Ron, D. (2011). The unfolded protein response: from stress pathway to homeostatic regulation. *Science* 334, 1081–1086. doi: 10.1126/science.1209038

Wang, Q., Yu, S., Simonyi, A., Sun, G. Y., and Sun, A. Y. (2005). Kainic acid-mediated excitotoxicity as a model for neurodegeneration. *Mol. Neurobiol.* 31, 3–16. doi: 10.1385/MN:31:1-3:003

Wei, K., Wan, L., Liu, J., Zhang, B., Li, X., Zhang, Y., et al. (2017). Downregulation of TRB3 protects neurons against apoptosis induced by global cerebral ischemia and reperfusion injury in rats. *Neuroscience* 360, 118–127. doi: 10.1016/j.neuroscience.2017.07.062

Wong, M., and Yamada, K. A. (2001). Developmental characteristics of epileptiform activity in immature rat neocortex: a comparison of four in vitro seizure models. *Brain Res. Dev. Brain Res.* 128, 113–120. doi: 10.1016/S0165-3806(01)00149-3

Yokoyama, T., and Nakamura, T. (2011). Tribbles in disease: signaling pathways important for cellular function and neoplastic transformation. *Cancer Sci.* 102, 1115–1122. doi: 10.1111/j.1349-7006.2011.01914.x

Zareen, N., Biswas, S. C., and Greene, L. A. (2013). A feed-forward loop involving Trib3, Akt and FoxO mediates death of NGF-deprived neurons. *Cell Death Differ.* 20, 1719–1730. doi: 10.1038/cdd.2013.128

Zhang, J., Wen, H. J., Guo, Z. M., Zeng, M. S., Li, M. Z., Jiang, Y. E., et al. (2011). TRB3 overexpression due to endoplasmic reticulum stress inhibits AKT kinase activation of tongue squamous cell carcinoma. *Oral Oncol.* 47, 934–939. doi: 10.1016/j.oraloncology.2011.06.512

Zou, C. G., Cao, X. Z., Zhao, Y. S., Gao, S. Y., Li, S. D., Liu, X. Y., et al. (2009). The molecular mechanism of endoplasmic reticulum stress-induced apoptosis in PC-12 neuronal cells: the protective effect of insulin-like growth factor I. *Endocrinology* 150, 277–285. doi: 10.1210/en.2008-0794

16

Attenuation of Novelty-Induced Hyperactivity of *Gria1*−/− Mice by Cannabidiol and Hippocampal Inhibitory Chemogenetics

Teemu Aitta-aho[1†], Milica Maksimovic[1†], Kristiina Dahl[1], Rolf Sprengel[2] and Esa R. Korpi[1]*

[1] Department of Pharmacology, Faculty of Medicine, University of Helsinki, Helsinki, Finland, [2] Research Group of the Max Planck Institute for Medical Research at the Institute of Anatomy and Cell Biology, Heidelberg University, Heidelberg, Germany

***Correspondence:**
Esa R. Korpi
esa.korpi@helsinki.fi

† These authors have contributed equally to this work

Gene-targeted mice with deficient AMPA receptor GluA1 subunits (*Gria1*−/− mice) show robust hyperlocomotion in a novel environment, suggesting them to constitute a model for hyperactivity disorders such as mania, schizophrenia and attention deficit hyperactivity disorder. This behavioral alteration has been associated with increased neuronal activation in the hippocampus, and it can be attenuated by chronic treatment with antimanic drugs, such as lithium, valproic acid, and lamotrigine. Now we found that systemic cannabidiol strongly blunted the hyperactivity and the hippocampal c-Fos expression of the *Gria1*−/− mice, while not affecting the wild-type littermate controls. Acute bilateral intra-dorsal hippocampal infusion of cannabidiol partially blocked the hyperactivity of the *Gria1*−/− mice, but had no effect on wild-types. The activation of the inhibitory DREADD receptor hM4Gi in the dorsal hippocampus by clozapine-*N*-oxide robustly inhibited the hyperactivity of the *Gria1*−/− mice, but had no effect on the locomotion of wild-type mice. Our results show that enhanced neuronal excitability in the hippocampus is associated with pronounced novelty-induced hyperactivity of GluA1 subunit-deficient mice. When this enhanced response of hippocampal neurons to novel stimuli is specifically reduced in the hippocampus by pharmacological treatment or by chemogenetic inhibition, *Gria1*−/− mice recover from behavioral hyperactivity, suggesting a hippocampal dysfunction in hyperactive behaviors that can be treated with cannabidiol.

Keywords: AMPA receptors, cannabidiol, DREADD, hippocampus, c-Fos, hyperactivity, novelty, hM4Gi

INTRODUCTION

Neurological and psychiatric brain diseases cause vast harm and excessive costs to affected individuals and the society at large (DiLuca and Olesen, 2014). There are many clinical evidence-based pharmacological and non-pharmacological treatment options (Millan et al., 2015a,b), but their efficacy should be greatly improved. Unfortunately, there has been a slow progress in neuropsychiatric drug development, especially for schizophrenia, schizoaffective disorder and bipolar disorder, justifying further efforts in finding testable mechanisms, drug candidates and novel targets (Vazquez et al., 2017).

Animal models play an important role in testing mechanisms how neuronal modulations and drug effects are mediated into behavioral responses (Cryan and Slattery, 2007; Forrest et al., 2014), even if they cannot reproduce a full repertoire of symptoms in often heterogeneous brain diseases. Especially difficult are the models of psychosis, since in animals the behavioral outcomes are usually related to motor functions as they are most easily quantifiable. In addition to lithium therapy, presently there are no specific drugs for the treatment of bipolar disorder with mania (Millan et al., 2015b). A simple symptom in that illness is the mania-like hyperactivity, which can be habituated in a constant environment. A mouse line with deficient AMPA-type glutamate receptor GluA1 subunits [the *Gria1−/−* mouse line (Zamanillo et al., 1999)] has been proposed as an animal model for hyperactive disorders, including schizoaffective disorder and bipolar disorder with mania (Fitzgerald et al., 2010; Barkus et al., 2011; Procaccini et al., 2011). This is based on (1) robust novelty-induced hyperactivity that is eventually habituated, leading to unaltered diurnal home-cage activity in the *Gria1−/−* mice (Vekovischeva et al., 2001; Fitzgerald et al., 2010; Sanderson et al., 2010; Procaccini et al., 2011), (2) consistent attenuation of this behavior by chronic treatment with drugs having antimanic efficacy in patients (Maksimovic et al., 2014a,b), and (3) linkage equilibrium of *GRIA1*-gene polymorphisms in psychotic disorders (Ripke et al., 2013, 2014; Devor et al., 2017).

The basic characteristics of *Gria1−/−* mice do not deviate from *Gria1+/+* wild-type littermates (WT). Physical health, body weight, food consumption, nociception, neurological, motor, sexual, sensory functions, and circadian rhythm appear normal (Vekovischeva et al., 2001, 2004; Bannerman et al., 2004; Hartmann et al., 2004; Feyder et al., 2007; Chourbaji et al., 2008; Fitzgerald et al., 2010; Procaccini et al., 2011). Extensive behavioral comparison of *Gria1−/−* and *Gria1+/+* mice suggests a schizophrenia- and depressive-like phenotype. Deficiency in prepulse inhibition of an acoustic startle reflex is indicative of psychosis-related properties (Wiedholz et al., 2008) and increased learned helplessness as deficits in coping skills in aversive situations indicative of depressive phenotype of *Gria1−/−* mice (Chourbaji et al., 2008). Short term spatial working memory of *Gria1−/−* mice is disrupted (Reisel et al., 2002; Sanderson et al., 2009). However, despite the prominent role of GluA1-type AMPA receptors in hippocampal synaptic plasticity *Gria1−/−* mice can form spatial reference memory (Zamanillo et al., 1999).

The most striking and reproducible behavioral response of *Gria1−/−* mice has been hyperactivity provoked by a novel environment. They have normal locomotion compared to their WT littermates in a familiar home-cage environment (Wiedholz et al., 2008; Procaccini et al., 2011), but when transferred to novel environment, they double their locomotor activity (Vekovischeva et al., 2001; Bannerman et al., 2004; Chourbaji et al., 2008; Fitzgerald et al., 2010; Procaccini et al., 2011) and fail to habituate (Barkus et al., 2011; Sanderson and Bannerman, 2012).

This increased activity is sustained, and it takes 30 to 40 min before the *Gria1−/−* mice show signs of habituation to the novelty. Thus, any confrontation with a novel signal, such as a new object or littermate, induce an aberrant reaction in *Gria1−/−* mice due to the lack of habituation (Wiedholz et al., 2008). Similarly, in sociability and resident-intruder tests *Gria1−/−* mice show remarkably low level of intermale aggression, suggesting poor ability to adapt to social encounters (Vekovischeva et al., 2004).

We have recently found that *Gria1−/−* mice react to novel environment by increased neuronal activation of the hippocampi, as shown by the enhanced immediate early gene expression (Procaccini et al., 2011). In the present study, we used *Gria1−/−* mice to analyze the effect of systemic application and acute hippocampal infusion of the non-psychoactive phytocannabinoid cannabidiol (CBD) (Izzo et al., 2009) on the hyperactivity and hippocampal c-Fos expression in *Gria1−/−* and controls. CBD has been shown potential as treatment for schizophrenia (Schubart et al., 2014). We also tested whether selective inhibition of the dorsal hippocampal principal neurons is sufficient to down-regulate the hyperactivity by using the activation of the virus-mediated, cell-type specific expression of an inhibitory designer receptors exclusively activated by designer drug (DREADD) (Roth, 2016), the hM4Gi receptor (Armbruster et al., 2007).

In our experiments, both the CBD and DREADD approaches attenuated the behavioral response to novelty of *Gria1−/−* mice, indicating that the paradoxical hippocampal activation is associated with hyperactivity of this mouse model. Importantly, acute infusion of CBD specifically into the hippocampus reduced the abnormal hyperactivity of the *Gria1−/−* knockout mice but did not affect the spontaneous activity of the wild-type littermates.

MATERIALS AND METHODS

Animals

Gria1−/− mice (*Gria1*$^{-/-}$, *Gria1*^{tm1Rsp}; MGI:2178057) and their *Gria1+/+* wild-type littermate controls (WT) were from heterozygous breeding, generated by inactivation of the *Gria1* gene (Zamanillo et al., 1999) and genotyped as described (Vekovischeva et al., 2001). The *Gria1−/−* mouse line is available at the Jackson Laboratory (B6N.129-*Gria1*^{tm1Rsp}/J, stock number: 019011). Mice were group-housed under standard laboratory conditions (12-h light-dark cycle; lights on at 6:00 A.M.; temperature 20–23°C; relative humidity 50–60%; aspen chip beddings). For locomotor activity, a total of 24 *Gria1−/−* (14.12 ± 0.92 weeks; 24.58 ± 1.03 g) and 23 WT mice (11.14 ± 0.66 weeks; 24.63 ± 0.92 g) were used.

All experimental procedures were approved by the State Provincial Government of Southern Finland (ESAVI-0010026/041003/2010). All efforts were made to minimize the number and suffering of animals.

Novelty-Induced Locomotor Activity

Locomotor activity in a novel environment after acute systemic cannabidiol treatments was observed in plastic cages (40 cm × 30 cm × 20 cm) as described in detail (Procaccini et al., 2011; Maksimovic et al., 2014b). At least 1 h before the tests was allowed for the animals to habituate to the experimental room. Horizontal movements of eight mice, placed in visually isolated cages in a sound-attenuated room at the light intensity of 175 lx, were simultaneously recorded for 2 h using EthoVision Color-Pro 3.0 video tracking software (Noldus Information Technology, Wageningen, Netherlands). The same method, but only during 30-min recordings, was used to assess the effects of intrahippocampal CBD infusions and chemogenetic inhibition of hippocampal neurons (see below).

c-Fos Immunostaining

The animals were quickly decapitated after 2-h novelty-exploration, the brains dissected, frozen on dry ice and stored at −80°C. Fourteen-μm thick sections were cut on a cryostat (Leica CM 3050 S; Leica Microsystem, Nußloch, Germany), thaw-mounted on Fisher Superfrost Plus slides (Menzel-Glaeser, Braunschweig, Germany) and stored at −80°C. To obtain sections of the ventral hippocampi, we changed the plane of cutting to horizontal one after we had collected the coronal sections until Bregma −2.4 mm (Franklin and Paxinos, 2008) as described earlier (Procaccini et al., 2013; Maksimovic et al., 2014b).

In immunohistochemistry, the protocol described in Procaccini et al. (2011) was followed. In brief, the sections were thawed, air-dried, marked with hydrophobic pen (Daido Sangyo, Tokyo, Japan) and all incubations performed using so-called liquid bubble technique. The sections were fixed with ice-cold 4% paraformaldehyde in Tris-buffered saline (TBS; in mM: Tris, 50; NaCl, 150; pH 7.4) for 10 min. As a washing medium, we used TBS supplemented with 0.05% Tween 20 (TBST) between incubations. Endogenous peroxidases were blocked by 0.3% H_2O_2 in methanol. Endogenous proteins were blocked with 10% normal horse serum (Sigma-Aldrich) and avidin blocking solution (Avidin/Biotin blocking kit; Vector Laboratories, Burlingame, CA, United States) diluted in TBST containing 1% bovine serum albumin (BSA; Sigma-Aldrich). Sections were incubated with goat anti-c-Fos antibody (1:1000; Santa Cruz Biotechnology, Santa Cruz, CA, United States) in TBST/1% BSA and biotin blocking solution (Avidin/Biotin blocking kit) overnight at 4°C, followed by 30 min in biotinylated horse anti-goat secondary antibody (1:200; Vector Laboratories). Avidin–biotin peroxidase complex (Vectastain Standard Elite; Vector Laboratories) and diaminobenzidine with nickel sulfate intensification (DAB Substrate kit; Vector Laboratories) were used for visualization. Then, the sections were dehydrated in gradual ethanol solutions (70, 96, and 99.5%), rinsed in Histoclear (National Diagnostic, Atlanta, GA, United States) and finally coverslipped with DPX mounting medium (BHD Chemicals, Poole, United Kingdom).

In quantifying the c-Fos-positive cells, photomicrographs from anatomically-matched sections were captured using a light microscope with a 10× objective (Leica DMR, Leica Microsystems, Wetzlar, Germany) and a CCD camera (Leica DC 300). The analysis was carried out blind to the treatment and genotype. Detection of c-Fos-positive cells was automatic, using ImageJ software (National Institutes of Health, Bethesda, MD, United States), by setting a constant threshold and 'region of interest' area based on brain atlas (Franklin and Paxinos, 2008). Analysis comprised bilaterally-obtained values from one or two sections (for dorsal and ventral hippocampi) of 12 brain areas (as shown in **Figure 2** and **Supplementary Table S1**). Apart from the hippocampus, expression of c-Fos protein was studied in those regions that may have a role in explorative locomotor task or where relatively high c-Fos expression is observed (Montag-Sallaz et al., 1999).

Intrahippocampal Injections of CBD

The hippocampus was targeted with CBD injections by microinjection cannulae. Mice were anesthetized with isoflurane (induction 5%, 2% maintenance; Vetflurane, Virbac, Carros, France), and implanted with bilateral 26-gauge stainless steel guide cannulae (Plastics One, Roanoke, VA, United States) into the dorsal dentate gyrus using a stereotactic device (David Kopf Instruments, Tujunga, CA, United States). Dental cement (Simplex Rapid, Associated Dental Products, Ltd., Swindon, United Kingdom) and two stainless steel screws were used to secure the cannula placement. The coordinates used were 1.9 mm posterior to bregma, 1.0 mm lateral to midline, and 1.0 mm ventral to skull level. Stainless steel obturators were inserted to keep cannulae unobstructed during the 1-week recovery period. Animals' recovery was monitored daily and none showed signs of distress. Prior to experiments, the mice were gently handled and CBD was injected through the guide cannulae by using 31-gauge internal stainless-steel injectors protruding an additional 1.0 mm below the guide cannulae. The injectors were connected to a microsyringe (Hamilton, Bonaduz, Switzerland) via polyethylene tubing. CBD (5 μg/side) or vehicle was injected in a volume of 0.2 μL at 0.1 μL/min by an infusion pump (kDScientific, Holliston, MA, United States). After the injection, the injectors remained in place for 1 min to allow solutions to diffuse into the tissue. The measurement of novelty-induced locomotor activity was recorded immediately after the injections as described above. After the experiments, the injector tip placements were confirmed histologically.

Chemogenetics

Dorsal hippocampal dentate gyrus was stereotactically targeted in isoflurane anesthesia as described above for CBD infusions. To each mouse, a total volume of 0.15 μL of AAV5-CaMKIIα-hM4Gi-mCherry viral vector (3.4 × 10^{12} genome copies/mL, University of North Carolina, Gene Therapy Center, Chapel Hill, NC, United States) was injected through a 31-gauge injection cannula using a microsyringe and an injection pump as described above. The animals recovered for 3 weeks. Thirty minutes prior to behavioral experiments the animals were administered clozapine-*N*-oxide (CNO) at 3 mg/kg i.p. in home cage. Non-DREADD-transduced mice acted as controls to test for DREADD receptor-non-specific effects of CNO. The measurement of novelty-induced locomotor activity was recorded immediately after the injections. After the experiments, the animals were deeply anesthetized with pentobarbital (Mebunat, Orion Pharma, Espoo, Finland), transcardially perfused with 0.1 M phosphate-buffered saline (PBS) followed by 4% paraformaldehyde in PBS. Brains were removed, post-fixed overnight at 4°C, and cryoprotected in 30% sucrose in PBS at 4°C until sunk. Forty-μm-thick coronal sections were cut by cryostat (Leica CM 3050 S; Leica Microsystem, Nußloch, Germany). To visualize the DREADD receptors, mCherry tag immunohistochemistry was performed. In brief, brain sections were washed at RT in 0.1 M PBS, blocked with 1% BSA (Merck, Darmstadt, Germany) supplemented with 0.3% Triton X-100 (Fisher Scientific, Fair Lawn, NJ, United States) in 0.1 M PBS. Sections were then incubated overnight at RT in primary antibody (rabbit anti-mCherry, 1:800, ab167453, Abcam, Cambridge, United Kingdom) diluted in blocking buffer, washed in PBS, incubated in secondary antibody (donkey anti-rabbit AlexaFluor 594, 1:1000, ab150076, Abcam) for 2 h at RT, washed in PBS, and mounted on microscope slides and coverslipped. Digital images were captured with a Zeiss Axioimager Z1 microscope using Apotome optical sectioning (Zeiss, Oberkochen, Germany) and Hamamatsu Orca R2 CCD camera (Hamamatsu, Japan).

Drugs

The doses of cannabidiol (CBD, from THC Pharm GmbH, Frankfurt, Germany) were based on literature (Zuardi et al., 1991; Moreira and Guimaraes, 2005; Long et al., 2006, 2010, 2012; Gururajan et al., 2011, 2012) and on preliminary dose–response experiments. The drug was dissolved in a mixture of ethanol:Tween 80:saline (1:1:18, which was used as a vehicle for controls) (Todd and Arnold, 2016) and injected (i.p.) in a volume of 10 ml/kg. For intrahippocampal injection, CBD was dissolved in 1% Tween 80 and 10% DMSO in sterile saline. Clozapine-*N*-oxide (CNO, Sequoia Research Products, Ltd., Pangbourne, United Kingdom) was dissolved in 0.5% DMSO in saline.

Statistical Analyses

Data are expressed as means ± standard errors of the mean (SEM). Statistical analyses were carried out using IBM SPSS Statistics 21 software (IBM SPSS, Inc., Somers, NY, United States) using (repeated measures) two-way ANOVA (genotype, treatment) followed by a Bonferroni *post hoc* test. Statistical significance was set at $P < 0.05$.

RESULTS

Effect of Acute Systemic Cannabidiol (CBD) Treatment on Novelty-Induced Locomotor Activity

In keeping with our previous results (Procaccini et al., 2013; Maksimovic et al., 2014b), the *Gria1−/−* mice showed robust

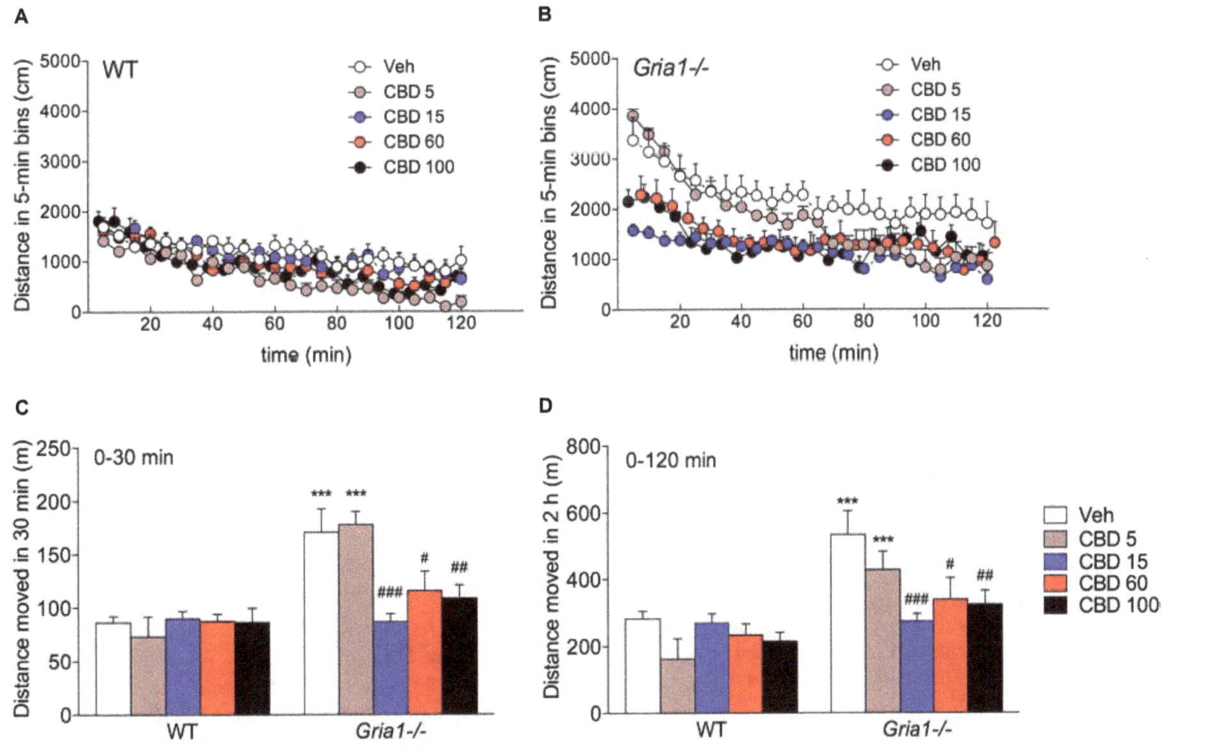

FIGURE 1 | Dose–response analysis of cannabidiol on novelty-induced hyperlocomotion of *Gria1−/−* mice. **(A,B)** Distance traveled in a novel environment in 5-min periods after treatment with vehicle and doses of cannabidiol (mg/kg, i.p.). **(C)** Distance traveled from the beginning of the trial until 30 min. **(D)** Total distance traveled during the whole 2 h test trial. Means ± SEMs are shown for 5–6 mice per group. ***$P < 0.001$ for the significances of the differences between WT and *Gria1−/−* mice after vehicle treatment; #$P < 0.05$, ##$P < 0.01$, and ###$P < 0.001$ between vehicle and CBD within the same genotype (Bonferroni post-test). Veh, vehicle; CBD, cannabidiol.

hyperlocomotion as compared to the WT mice, when placed into an unfamiliar environment (**Figures 1A,B**, ANOVA for genotype effect, $F_{1.49}$ = 33.09, $P < 0.001$). They gradually habituated over the observation period of 2 h (time effect $F_{23,1127}$ = 56.89, $P < 0.001$), although not down to the average level of WT mice (time × genotype interaction $F_{23,1127}$ = 2.23, $P < 0.01$), as determined by the comparison of the mean path length of the last three timebins (genotype effect, $F_{1,10}$ = 6.48, $P < 0.05$). CBD treatment dose-dependently attenuated the novelty-induced hyperlocomotion of *Gria1−/−* mice (treatment effect, $F_{4.49}$ = 4.16, $P < 0.01$; genotype effect, $F_{1.49}$ = 33.09, $P < 0.001$), while the locomotor activity of WT mice remained unaltered (treatment × genotype interaction, $F_{4.49}$ = 3.74, $P < 0.01$; **Figure 1**, Bonferroni post-test, vehicle vs. CBD, $P > 0.05$). *Post hoc* comparisons showed that all doses of CBD (15, 60, and 100 mg/kg), except for the lowest dose (5 mg/kg), brought the hyperactivity of *Gria1−/−* mice back to the level of WT mice (**Figure 1C**, locomotor activity analyzed from the beginning of the trial until 30 min, and **Figure 1D**, locomotor activity analyzed over the whole 2 h trial, Bonferroni post-test, $P > 0.05$ for the genotype difference within all doses, except for 5 mg/kg, when it was $P < 0.001$). The 5 mg/kg dose seemed to fail to rescue the hyperactivity of the *Gria1−/−* mice in the beginning of the trial, but to facilitate the habituation in the later stage of the trial (**Figures 1A,B**, time × genotype × treatment interaction $F_{92,1127}$ = 1.85, $P < 0.001$).

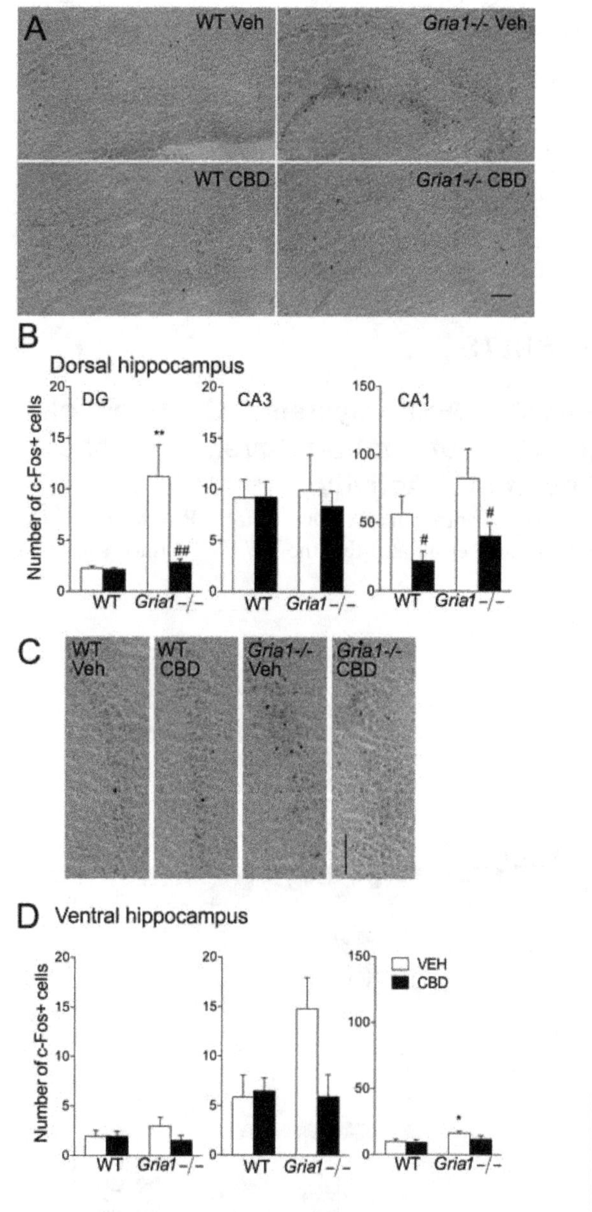

FIGURE 2 | Expression of c-Fos protein in hippocampal subregions of the *Gria1−/−* and WT mice after a 2-h exposure to a novel environment with pre-treatment with vehicle or cannabidiol (15 mg/kg). **(A)** Representative images of the dorsal hippocampus. **(B)** Counts of c-Fos+ cells in the subregions of the dorsal hippocampus. Open bars for the vehicle- (VEH) treated and closed bars for cannabidiol- (CBD) treated groups. **(C)** Representative images of the ventral hippocampus. **(D)** Counts of c-Fos+ cells in the subregions of the ventral hippocampus. Means ± SEMs are shown for 4–6 mice per group. *$P < 0.5$, **$P < 0.01$ for the significances of the differences between genotypes after the same treatment, #$P < 0.05$, ##$P < 0.01$ for the difference from the vehicle within the same genotype (Bonferroni post-test). Scale bar: 100 μm.

Effects of Acute Cannabidiol Treatment on c-Fos Expression

As the lowest effective dose of cannabidiol to block the novelty-induced hyperactivity in *Gria1−/−* mice was 15 mg/kg (**Figures 1A,B**), we analyzed the brain regional c-Fos protein expression after this dose (**Figure 2**). In the dentate gyrus granule cell layer of the dorsal hippocampus, the number of c-Fos-positive cells of the vehicle-treated *Gria1−/−* mice was significantly increased compared to the number of c-Fos positive cells in WT mice (**Figure 2A**, genotype effect, $F_{1,20}$ = 9.32, $P < 0.01$). The CBD treatment of WT mice did not alter the number of c-Fos positive cells in the dentate gyrus, but CBD normalized the number of c-Fos positive cells in that of *Gria1−/−* mice (**Figure 2B**, treatment effect $F_{1,20}$ = 7.34, $P < 0.05$; genotype × treatment interaction $F_{1,20}$ = 6.90, $P < 0.05$). However, in the CA1 subfield, CBD treatment decreased c-Fos-positive cell counts in both *Gria1−/−* and WT mice (treatment effect, $F_{1,20}$ = 7.35, $P < 0.05$). The c-Fos cell count in CA3 was equal between the genotypes ($F_{1,20}$ = 0.001, $P > 0.05$) and not affected by the CBD treatment ($F_{1,20}$ = 0.12, $P > 0.05$).

In the ventral hippocampus (**Figures 2C,D**), novelty-induced hyperactivity did not change the number of c-Fos positive cells in dentate gyrus subfield (genotype effect for DG, $F_{1,19}$ = 0.24, $P > 0.05$). In the CA1 subfield, *Gria1−/−* mice had slightly higher number of c-Fos positive cells (genotype effect, $F_{1,19}$ = 5.04, $P < 0.05$), but CBD treatment failed to reduce the cell count significantly (treatment effect $F_{1,19}$ = 1.76, $P > 0.05$; genotype × treatment interaction $F_{1,19}$ = 1.00, $P > 0.05$). In the CA3 subfield, novelty-induced hyperactivity did not change the number of c-Fos positive cells, although a non-significant trend was detected (genotype effect, $F_{1,19}$ = 3.22, $P > 0.05$; genotype × treatment interaction, $F_{1,19}$ = 4.13, P = 0.056).

The numbers of c-Fos-positive cells after treatment with CBD in extra-hippocampal brain regions are summarized in **Supplementary Table S1**. In the basolateral amygdala, CBD treatment reduced the number of c-Fos-positive cells in WT animals only (genotype × treatment interaction $F_{1,20} = 4.74$, $P < 0.05$). In the lateral septum, the number of c-Fos-positive cells increased in WT mice after CBD treatment (genotype × treatment interaction $F_{1,19} = 8.54$, $P < 0.01$). In the prelimbic cortex, the greater number of c-Fos-positive cells was observed in WT mice than in *Gria1−/−* mice, a difference that disappeared after CBD treatment (genotype × treatment interaction, $F_{1,20} = 4.72$, $P < 0.05$). Thus, compared to the hippocampus, extra-hippocampal brain areas of wild-type mice were hardly affected by the CBD. Only in the lateral septal nucleus of *Gria1−/−* mice the c-Fos response to CBD injection was opposite.

Effect of Intrahippocampal Cannabidiol Treatment on Novelty-Induced Hyperactivity

The c-Fos-based neuronal activation mapping revealed the hippocampal complex as a main locus of novelty-induced hyperactivity in *Gria1−/−* mice (**Figure 2** and Procaccini et al., 2011). Because systemic CBD both decreased the novelty-induced hyperactivity and re-adjusted the c-Fos positive cell score in the hippocampal dentate gyrus of *Gria1−/−* mice (**Figures 1, 2**), we sought to determine whether infusion of CBD into the dorsal hippocampus is sufficient to down-regulate the hyperactivity. We found that the intrahippocampal CBD microinjection (**Figure 3A**) significantly decreased, but did not completely reverse, the novelty-induced hyperactivity of *Gria1−/−* mice (**Figures 3B,C**), while not changing locomotor activity of WT mice (genotype effect, $F_{1,16} = 49.08$, $P < 0.001$; genotype × treatment interaction, $F_{1,16} = 9.39$, $P < 0.01$), supporting our hypothesis that the attenuation of the hyperactivity by CBD of *Gria1−/−* mice is mainly mediated by its action in the hippocampus.

Chemogenetic Inhibition of Novelty-Induced Hyperactivity

The c-Fos-based neuronal activation mapping has revealed the hippocampal complex as a main locus of novelty-induced overactivity in *Gria1−/−* mice (**Figure 2** and Procaccini et al., 2011). We used the clozapine-*N*-oxide (CNO) activation of the Gi-DREADD receptors (hM4Gi; Armbruster et al., 2007) to inhibit neuronal activity in the dorsal hippocampus of *Gria1−/−* mice and to reveal the anatomical and cellular substrate for the hyperlocomotion phenotype of the *Gria1−/−* mice (**Figures 4A,B**). *Gria1−/−* mice that received these bilateral AAV5-CaMKIIα-hM4Gi-mCherry injections in the dorsal hippocampus, CNO-induced DREADD inhibition of hippocampal CaMKIIα-expressing, excitatory cells decreased hyperlocomotion of *Gria1−/−* mice to the level of WT littermates (**Figures 4C,D**). In the WTs, CNO-induced DREADD inhibition in the same cell population had no modifying effect on the locomotor activity (treatment effect, $F_{1,16} = 5.61$, $P < 0.05$; genotype effect, $F_{1,16} = 12.11$, $P < 0.01$; genotype × treatment interaction, $F_{1,16} = 10.27$, $P < 0.01$). The effect persisted

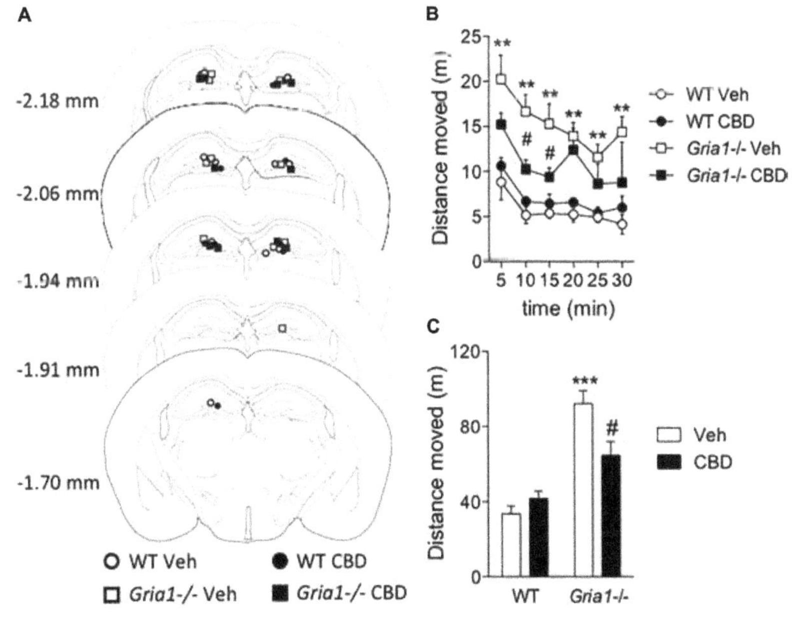

FIGURE 3 | Intrahippocampal infusion of cannabidiol decreases novelty-induced hyperlocomotion of *Gria1−/−* mice. Animals were given an infusion with vehicle or cannabidiol (5 μg/side) followed by recording of distance moved for 30 min. **(A)** Injector tip placements within the dorsal hippocampus for all experimental groups. The brain images were modified with permission from Paxinos and Franklin (2001). **(B)** Distance traveled in a novel environment in 5-min periods. **(C)** Total distance traveled during 30-min trials. $^{**}P < 0.01$ and $^{***}P < 0.001$ for the significances of the differences between the genotypes after vehicle; $^{\#}P < 0.05$ between vehicle and CBD within the same genotype (Bonferroni post-test). $N = 10$ for both genotypes. Veh, vehicle; CBD, cannabidiol.

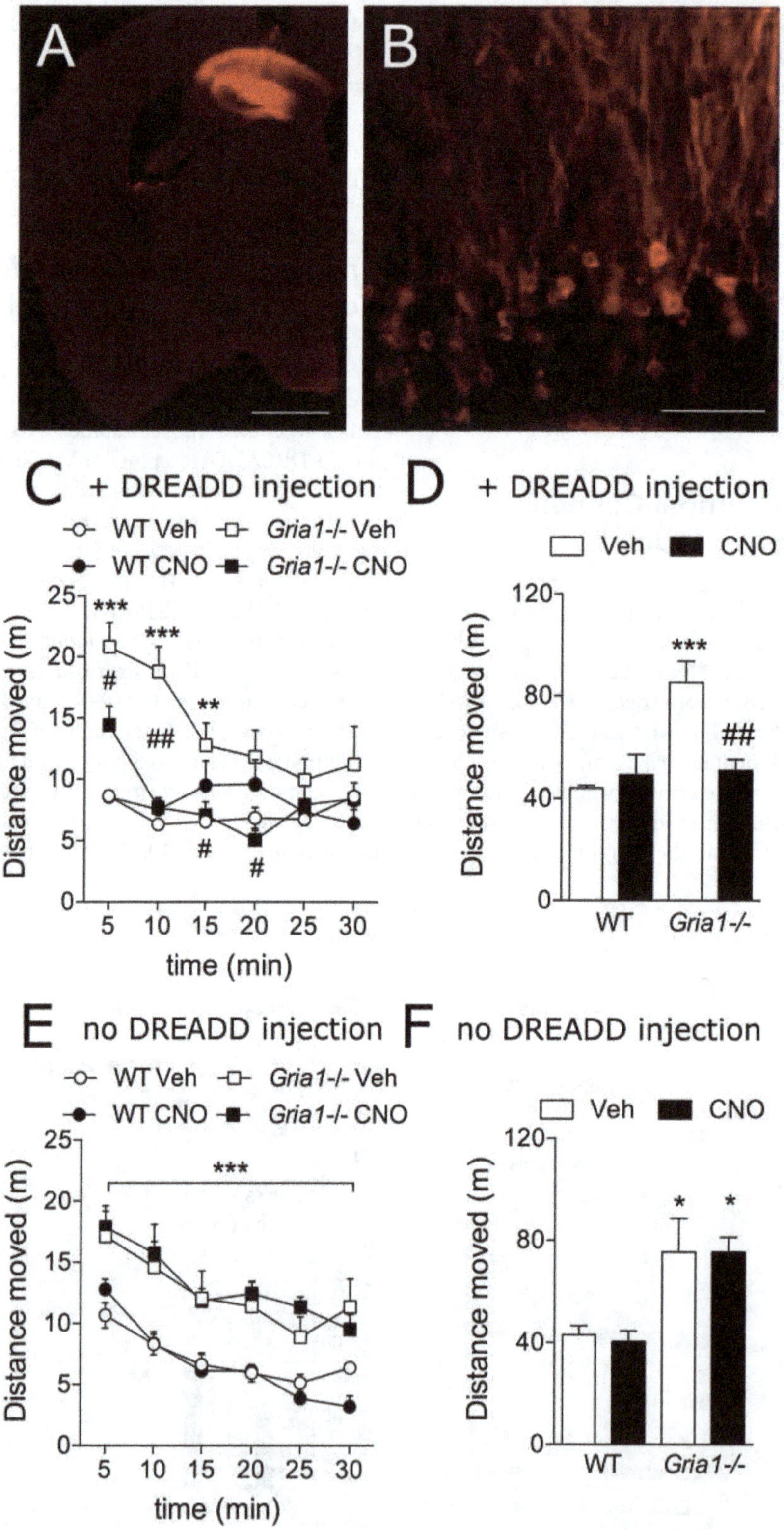

FIGURE 4 | Chemogenetic inhibition of novelty-induced hyperlocomotion in *Gria1−/−* mice. **(A)** Virus injection resulted in hM4Gi-mCherry expression in the dorsal hippocampus. Hb, habenula; fi, fimbria; scale bar: 1 mm. **(B)** A close-up photograph displaying transduced neurons and neurites in the dentate gyrus. No transduced neurites were observed outside the hippocampus (not shown). Gr, granule cell layer; Mol, molecular layer; scale bar: 50 μm. **(C)** Distance traveled in a novel environment in 5-min periods in mice transduced with DREADDs. **(D)** Total distance traveled during the 30-min trial in mice transduced with DREADDs.

(Continued)

FIGURE 4 | Continued
$^{**}P < 0.01$ and $^{***}P < 0.001$ for the significances of the differences between the genotypes after vehicle; $^{\#}P < 0.05$ and $^{\#\#}P < 0.01$ between vehicle and CNO treatments within the same genotype (Bonferroni post-test), $n = 10$ for both genotypes. **(E)** Distance traveled in a novel environment in 5-min periods in non-DREADD expressing WT and *Gria1−/−* control mice. $^{***}P < 0.001$ for the significances within drug treatment and between genotypes (ANOVA). **(F)** Total distance traveled during the 30-min trial in non-DREADD-expressing control mice. $^{*}P < 0.05$ between genotypes and within drug treatment (Bonferroni post-test). $n = 11–14$. Veh, vehicle; CNO, clozapine-*N*-oxide.

until the *Gria1−/−* mice habituated to the locomotor activity level of the WT mice (**Figure 4C**, time effect, $F_{5,80} = 9.63$, $P < 0.001$; time × genotype interaction, $F_{5,80} = 7.46$, $P < 0.001$; time × genotype × treatment interaction, $F_{5,80} = 3.26$, $P < 0.01$). In contrast, in DREADD-non-expressing mice, the drug CNO did not change the locomotor activity of either genotype (treatment effect, $F_{1,17} = 0.47$, $P > 0.05$; treatment × genotype interaction, $F_{1,17} = 0.49$, $P > 0.05$) and the *Gria1−/−* mice displayed hyperlocomotion (genotype effect, $F_{1,17} = 15.61$, $P < 0.001$) irrespective of the CNO treatment (**Figures 4E,F**).

DISCUSSION

Increased novelty-induced hyperactivity has been the most consistent and robust behavioral phenotypic alteration in mice with deficient AMPA-type glutamate receptor GluA1 subunits (for review see, Sanderson et al., 2008). In the present study, *Gria1−/−* mice again reproduced the hyperactive phenotype, also after stresses of the surgeries and intracerebral infusions, indicating that the model is stable for these kinds of experimental scrutiny.

The hippocampus is considered a most important brain area for spatial learning and adaptation (Bannerman et al., 2014; Moser et al., 2017). Inhibition of hippocampal principal neurons by DREADD receptors after CNO strongly blocked the novelty-induced hyperactivity in *Gria1−/−* mice, without affecting the locomotor activity of wild-type mice, indicating that the hippocampus is abnormally activated in the mutants during extensive exploration of novel environments. Such an increased hippocampal activity of *Gria1−/−* mice can be visualized by increased numbers of c-Fos expressing cells during exposure to unfamiliar surroundings [the present study (Procaccini et al., 2011)]. Both acute and chronic drug treatments have reduced both hippocampal c-Fos expression and behavioral hyperactivity (Procaccini et al., 2013; Maksimovic et al., 2014a,b).

Our data, using hippocampus specific Gi-DREADD and hippocampal infusion of CBD indicate that the hippocampal dysfunction is responsible for the impaired habituation of GluA1 deficient mice to new environments or situations. This view finds support by an inducible hippocampal deletion of GluA1 subunits from principal neurons during late adolescence which phenocopied the hyperactivity as seen in mice with global reduction of GluA1 (Inta et al., 2014). Since the DREADD system targeted mainly the dentate gyrus granule cells but was detected also in *cornu ammonis* regions (**Figure 4A**), it is likely that the DREADD-driven inhibition recruited more extensively the hippocampal formation leading to complete normalization of the novelty-induced hyperactivity in *Gria1−/−* mice. Similarly, the restoration of GluA1 in the hippocampus had attenuates the open field hyperactivity of *Gria1−/−* mice (Freudenberg et al., 2016). In our critical control experiment (MacLaren et al., 2016), the drug used to activate the DREADD receptors, clozapine-*N*-oxide (CNO) at the dose of 3 mg/kg, did not alter locomotor activities of the mouse lines without the DREADD expression (**Figures 4E,F**). This result is in line with the recent report that showed only higher than 5 mg/kg doses of CNO having partial clozapine-like effects in mice (Manvich et al., 2018).

Although hyperactivity and responses to novelty are often linked to increased dopaminergic mechanisms (Boekhoudt et al., 2016) and the *Gria1−/−* mice have been suggested to show hyperdopaminergic phenotype (Wiedholz et al., 2008), our previous experiments failed to find differential c-Fos expression between the *Gria1−/−* and WTs in the midbrain and striatal dopaminergic regions after exposure to a novel environment (Procaccini et al., 2011) and the hyperactive, hippocampally restricted GluA1 subunit-deficient mice had normal striatal dopamine levels (Inta et al., 2014). However, pharmacological antagonism of dopamine D2 receptors has been shown to non-selectively reduce hyperactivity in both *Gria1−/−* and WT mice (Wiedholz et al., 2008), making it difficult to fully exclude the role of putatively enhanced dopamine mechanisms in the *Gria1−/−* mice. Furthermore, recent neuronal pathway modulation on regulation of habituation and novelty preference in mice has indicated important interactive roles of the medial habenula and interpeduncular nucleus with the VTA, with the habenula activating the interpeduncular nucleus to recognize familiarity and the VTA inhibiting the interpeduncular nucleus to promote novelty seeking (Molas et al., 2017).

Despite that the dopaminergic dysfunction has a recognized role in schizoaffective disorders and might play a role in *Gria1−/−* mice, there is evidence rather pointing to indirect effects of cannabinoids on dopamine cell firing, by altering glutamate neurotransmission (Colizzi et al., 2016). The *Gria1−/−* mouse model has been sensitive to drugs that downregulate glutamate neurotransmission including several antiepileptic drugs and AMPA antagonists (Procaccini et al., 2013; Maksimovic et al., 2014a,b). CBD shows little target selectivity and has multiple actions on various receptors and ion channels (Izzo et al., 2009; Ibeas Bih et al., 2015). While our data on attenuation of locomotor hyperactivity by silencing glutamatergic neurons via G_i-coupled DREADDs could imply the involvement of the inhibitory CB_1 receptors, the inhibition of the presynaptic glutamate release via CBD action on the cannabinoid receptors have been largely dismissed (Ibeas Bih et al., 2015). One of the most interesting and relevant CBD actions is the inhibition of the G protein-coupled receptor 55 (GPR55). Hippocampally expressed G-protein-coupled receptor 55 (GPR55) induces Ca^{2+} release from presynaptic stores leading to increased synaptic neurotransmitter release (Sylantyev et al., 2013; Hurst et al., 2017). As GPR55 colocalizes presynaptically with the vesicular glutamate transporter 1 (Sylantyev et al., 2013), glutamate is the likely neurotransmitter for the GPR55-induced increase of excitatory transmitter release. Importantly, CBD inhibits GPR55-mediated excitatory drive in hippocampal synapses (Sylantyev et al., 2013), which may suggest a pharmacological significance in damping overactivated network within the hippocampal circuits (Kaplan et al., 2017). While a direct measurement of glutamate release in response to novelty-induced hyperactivity in *Gria1−/−* mice needs to be established, previous data suggest a role for glutamate release in novel environments (Bianchi et al., 2003). Therefore, the GPR55-regulated glutamate release provides a possible mechanism for the CBD-mediated downregulation of hippocampal excitatory activity and behavioral hyperactivity in *Gria1−/−* mice.

In addition to the activation of GPR55, CBD appears also to possess agonistic properties at serotonergic G_i-coupled 5-HT_{1A} receptors, through which it can induce anxiolytic-like effects and mediate adaptation to stress (Joca et al., 2003; Russo et al., 2005; Rock et al., 2012). These receptors are localized at presynaptic terminals of glutamatergic synapses and their activation suppresses glutamatergic signaling (Cai et al., 2002). Thus, CBD actions on 5-HT_{1A} receptors might have contributed to the decrease in hippocampal neuronal overactivation in *Gria1−/−* mice.

The intrahippocampal CBD injection partially rescued the novelty-induced hyperactive phenotype in the *Gria1−/−* mice. Similar doses as in our study (bilaterally 5 μg/side) have been previously injected into the brain parenchyma, although not into the hippocampus. A 10-fold lower dose of CBD (0.4 μg/side) facilitated fear extinction, when injected bilaterally to rat infralimbic cortex (Do Monte et al., 2013). A higher unilateral periaqueductal CBD dose of 10 μg was required to produce an anxiolytic-like effect in rats, while 20 μg dose failed to affect the behavioral output (Campos and Guimaraes, 2008). In a summary, these studies suggest that bilateral 5 μg/side dose of CBD reaches appropriate concentration intrahippocampally to have an effect on various hippocampally expressed CBD targets, although the affinity of CBD to them might vary (Ibeas Bih et al., 2015).

Overall, our data suggest that silencing hippocampal glutamatergic neurons and systemic and intrahippocampal pharmacological treatment with CBD alleviate behavioral hyperactivity in *Gria1−/−* mice. CBD in this study has reproduced the effects of glutamate-modulating drug-treatments in blunting the excessive hyperlocomotion and the hyperactivity of the dorsal hippocampus in *Gria1−/−* mice (Procaccini et al., 2013; Maksimovic et al., 2014a,b). Although the precise brain circuitry and pharmacological targets involved in the CBD effect require further elucidation, our data contribute to the possibility that CBD actions on glutamatergic transmission in the hippocampus could be therapeutically applied to dampen hyperexcitable hippocampal and other brain circuitries.

AUTHOR CONTRIBUTIONS

TA-a, MM, and ERK originated the study and wrote the first draft of the manuscript. TA-a, MM, and KD performed the experiments and statistical analyses. RS provided some mouse cohorts. All authors contributed to manuscript revision, read and approved the submitted version.

FUNDING

The study was partially supported by the Academy of Finland, The Finnish Foundation for Alcohol Studies and the Sigrid Juselius Foundation (TA-a, ERK), the Emil Aaltonen Foundation (MM) and by the Ingeborg-Ständer Foundation (RS). The one access publication fee is paid by the Library of the University of Helsinki.

REFERENCES

Armbruster, B. N., Li, X., Pausch, M. H., Herlitze, S., and Roth, B. L. (2007). Evolving the lock to fit the key to create a family of G protein-coupled receptors potently activated by an inert ligand. *Proc. Natl. Acad. Sci. U.S.A.* 104, 5163–5168. doi: 10.1073/pnas.0700293104

Bannerman, D. M., Deacon, R. M., Brady, S., Bruce, A., Sprengel, R., Seeburg, P. H., et al. (2004). A comparison of GluR-A-deficient and wild-type mice on a test battery assessing sensorimotor, affective, and cognitive behaviors. *Behav. Neurosci.* 118, 643–647. doi: 10.1037/0735-7044.118.3.643

Bannerman, D. M., Sprengel, R., Sanderson, D. J., McHugh, S. B., Rawlins, J. N., Monyer, H., et al. (2014). Hippocampal synaptic plasticity, spatial memory and anxiety. *Nat. Rev. Neurosci.* 15, 181–192. doi: 10.1038/nrn3677

Barkus, C., Feyder, M., Graybeal, C., Wright, T., Wiedholz, L., Izquierdo, A., et al. (2011). Do GluA1 knockout mice exhibit behavioral abnormalities relevant to the negative or cognitive symptoms of schizophrenia and schizoaffective disorder? *Neuropharmacology* 62, 1263–1272. doi: 10.1016/j.neuropharm.2011.06.005

Bianchi, L., Ballini, C., Colivicchi, M. A., Della Corte, L., Giovannini, M. G., and Pepeu, G. (2003). Investigation on acetylcholine, aspartate, glutamate and GABA extracellular levels from ventral hippocampus during repeated exploratory activity in the rat. *Neurochem. Res.* 28, 565–573. doi: 10.1023/A:1022881625378

Boekhoudt, L., Omrani, A., Luijendijk, M. C., Wolterink-Donselaar, I. G., Wijbrans, E. C., van der Plasse, G., et al. (2016). Chemogenetic activation of dopamine neurons in the ventral tegmental area, but not substantia nigra, induces hyperactivity in rats. *Eur. Neuropsychopharmacol.* 26, 1784–1793. doi: 10.1016/j.euroneuro.2016.09.003

Cai, X., Gu, Z., Zhong, P., Ren, Y., and Yan, Z. (2002). Serotonin 5-HT1A receptors regulate AMPA receptor channels through inhibiting Ca2+/calmodulin-dependent kinase II in prefrontal cortical pyramidal neurons. *J. Biol. Chem.* 277, 36553–36562. doi: 10.1074/jbc.M203752200

Campos, A. C., and Guimaraes, F. S. (2008). Involvement of 5HT1A receptors in the anxiolytic-like effects of cannabidiol injected into the dorsolateral periaqueductal gray of rats. *Psychopharmacology* 199, 223–230. doi: 10.1007/s00213-008-1168-x

Chourbaji, S., Vogt, M. A., Fumagalli, F., Sohr, R., Frasca, A., Brandwein, C., et al. (2008). AMPA receptor subunit 1 (GluR-A) knockout mice model the glutamate hypothesis of depression. *FASEB J.* 22, 3129–3134. doi: 10.1096/fj.08-106450

Colizzi, M., McGuire, P., Pertwee, R. G., and Bhattacharyya, S. (2016). Effect of cannabis on glutamate signalling in the brain: a systematic review of human and animal evidence. *Neurosci. Biobehav. Rev.* 64, 359–381. doi: 10.1016/j.neubiorev.2016.03.010

Cryan, J. F., and Slattery, D. A. (2007). Animal models of mood disorders: recent developments. *Curr. Opin. Psychiatry* 20, 1–7. doi: 10.1097/YCO.0b013e3280117733

Devor, A., Andreassen, O. A., Wang, Y., Maki-Marttunen, T., Smeland, O. B., Fan, C. C., et al. (2017). Genetic evidence for role of integration of fast and slow neurotransmission in schizophrenia. *Mol. Psychiatry* 22, 792–801. doi: 10.1038/mp.2017.33

DiLuca, M., and Olesen, J. (2014). The cost of brain diseases: a burden or a challenge? *Neuron* 82, 1205–1208. doi: 10.1016/j.neuron.2014.05.044

Do Monte, F. H., Souza, R. R., Bitencourt, R. M., Kroon, J. A., and Takahashi, R. N. (2013). Infusion of cannabidiol into infralimbic cortex facilitates fear extinction via CB1 receptors. *Behav. Brain. Res.* 250, 23–27. doi: 10.1016/j.bbr.2013.04.045

Feyder, M., Wiedholz, L., Sprengel, R., and Holmes, A. (2007). Impaired associative fear learning in mice with complete loss or haploinsufficiency of AMPA GluR1 receptors. *Front. Behav. Neurosci.* 1:4. doi: 10.3389/neuro.08.004.2007

Fitzgerald, P. J., Barkus, C., Feyder, M., Wiedholz, L. M., Chen, Y. C., Karlsson, R. M., et al. (2010). Does gene deletion of AMPA GluA1 phenocopy features of schizoaffective disorder? *Neurobiol. Dis.* 40, 608–621. doi: 10.1016/j.nbd.2010.08.005

Forrest, A. D., Coto, C. A., and Siegel, S. J. (2014). Animal models of psychosis: current state and future directions. *Curr. Behav. Neurosci. Rep.* 1, 100–116. doi: 10.1007/s40473-014-0013-2

Franklin, K. B. J., and Paxinos, G. (2008). *The Mouse Brain in Stereotaxic Coordinates*, 3rd Edn, Amsterdam: Elsevier.

Freudenberg, F., Resnik, E., Kolleker, A., Celikel, T., Sprengel, R., and Seeburg, P. H. (2016). Hippocampal GluA1 expression in Gria1(-/-) mice only partially restores spatial memory performance deficits. *Neurobiol. Learn. Mem.* 135, 83–90. doi: 10.1016/j.nlm.2016.07.005

Gururajan, A., Taylor, D. A., and Malone, D. T. (2011). Effect of cannabidiol in a MK-801-rodent model of aspects of schizophrenia. *Behav. Brain Res.* 222, 299–308. doi: 10.1016/j.bbr.2011.03.053

Gururajan, A., Taylor, D. A., and Malone, D. T. (2012). Cannabidiol and clozapine reverse MK-801-induced deficits in social interaction and hyperactivity in Sprague-Dawley rats. *J. Psychopharmacol.* 26, 1317–1332. doi: 10.1177/0269881112441865

Hartmann, B., Ahmadi, S., Heppenstall, P. A., Lewin, G. R., Schott, C., Borchardt, T., et al. (2004). The AMPA receptor subunits GluR-A and GluR-B reciprocally modulate spinal synaptic plasticity and inflammatory pain. *Neuron* 44, 637–650. doi: 10.1016/j.neuron.2004.10.029

Hurst, K., Badgley, C., Ellsworth, T., Bell, S., Friend, L., Prince, B., et al. (2017). A putative lysophosphatidylinositol receptor GPR55 modulates hippocampal synaptic plasticity. *Hippocampus* 27, 985–998. doi: 10.1002/hipo.22747

Ibeas Bih, C., Chen, T., Nunn, A. V., Bazelot, M., Dallas, M., and Whalley, B. J. (2015). Molecular targets of cannabidiol in neurological disorders. *Neurotherapeutics* 12, 699–730. doi: 10.1007/s13311-015-0377-3

Inta, D., Vogt, M. A., Elkin, H., Weber, T., Lima-Ojeda, J. M., Schneider, M., et al. (2014). Phenotype of mice with inducible ablation of GluA1 AMPA receptors during late adolescence: relevance for mental disorders. *Hippocampus* 24, 424–435. doi: 10.1002/hipo.22236

Izzo, A. A., Borrelli, F., Capasso, R., Di Marzo, V., and Mechoulam, R. (2009). Non-psychotropic plant cannabinoids: new therapeutic opportunities from an ancient herb. *Trends Pharmacol. Sci.* 30, 515–527. doi: 10.1016/j.tips.2009.07.006

Joca, S. R., Padovan, C. M., and Guimaraes, F. S. (2003). Activation of post-synaptic 5-HT(1A) receptors in the dorsal hippocampus prevents learned helplessness development. *Brain Res.* 978, 177–184. doi: 10.1016/S0006-8993(03)02943-3

Kaplan, J. S., Stella, N., Catterall, W. A., and Westenbroek, R. E. (2017). Cannabidiol attenuates seizures and social deficits in a mouse model of Dravet syndrome. *Proc. Natl. Acad. Sci. U.S.A.* 114, 11229–11234. doi: 10.1073/pnas.1711351114

Long, L. E., Chesworth, R., Huang, X. F., McGregor, I. S., Arnold, J. C., and Karl, T. (2010). A behavioural comparison of acute and chronic Delta9-tetrahydrocannabinol and cannabidiol in C57BL/6JArc mice. *Int. J. Neuropsychopharmacol.* 13, 861–876. doi: 10.1017/S1461145709990605

Long, L. E., Chesworth, R., Huang, X. F., Wong, A., Spiro, A., McGregor, I. S., et al. (2012). Distinct neurobehavioural effects of cannabidiol in transmembrane domain neuregulin 1 mutant mice. *PLoS One* 7:e34129. doi: 10.1371/journal.pone.0034129

Long, L. E., Malone, D. T., and Taylor, D. A. (2006). Cannabidiol reverses MK-801-induced disruption of prepulse inhibition in mice. *Neuropsychopharmacology* 31, 795–803. doi: 10.1038/sj.npp.1300838

MacLaren, D. A., Browne, R. W., Shaw, J. K., Krishnan Radhakrishnan, S., Khare, P., Espana, R. A., et al. (2016). Clozapine N-oxide administration produces behavioral effects in long-evans rats: implications for designing DREADD experiments. *eNeuro* 3:ENEURO.0219-16.2016. doi: 10.1523/eneuro.0219-16.2016

Maksimovic, M., Aitta-Aho, T., and Korpi, E. R. (2014a). Reversal of novelty-induced hippocampal c-Fos expression in GluA1 subunit-deficient mice by chronic treatment targeting glutamatergic transmission. *Eur. J. Pharmacol.* 745, 36–45. doi: 10.1016/j.ejphar.2014.10.005

Maksimovic, M., Vekovischeva, O. Y., Aitta-aho, T., and Korpi, E. R. (2014b). Chronic treatment with mood-stabilizers attenuates abnormal hyperlocomotion of GluA1-subunit deficient mice. *PLoS One* 9:e100188. doi: 10.1371/journal.pone.0100188

Manvich, D. F., Webster, K. A., Foster, S. L., Farrell, M. S., Ritchie, J. C., Porter, J. H., et al. (2018). The DREADD agonist clozapine N-oxide (CNO) is reverse-metabolized to clozapine and produces clozapine-like interoceptive stimulus effects in rats and mice. *Sci. Rep.* 8:3840. doi: 10.1038/s41598-018-22116-z

Millan, M. J., Goodwin, G. M., Meyer-Lindenberg, A., and Ogren, S. O. (2015a). 60 years of advances in neuropsychopharmacology for improving brain health, renewed hope for progress. *Eur. Neuropsychopharmacol.* 25, 591–598. doi: 10.1016/j.euroneuro.2015.01.015

Millan, M. J., Goodwin, G. M., Meyer-Lindenberg, A., and Ove Ogren, S. (2015b). Learning from the past and looking to the future: emerging perspectives for improving the treatment of psychiatric disorders. *Eur. Neuropsychopharmacol.* 25, 599–656. doi: 10.1016/j.euroneuro.2015.01.016

Molas, S., Zhao-Shea, R., Liu, L., DeGroot, S. R., Gardner, P. D., and Tapper, A. R. (2017). A circuit-based mechanism underlying familiarity signaling and the preference for novelty. *Nat. Neurosci.* 20, 1260–1268. doi: 10.1038/nn.4607

Montag-Sallaz, M., Welzl, H., Kuhl, D., Montag, D., and Schachner, M. (1999). Novelty-induced increased expression of immediate-early genes c-fos and arg 3.1 in the mouse brain. *J. Neurobiol.* 38, 234–246. doi: 10.1002/(SICI)1097-4695(19990205)38:2<234::AID-NEU6>3.0.CO;2-G

Moreira, F. A., and Guimaraes, F. S. (2005). Cannabidiol inhibits the hyperlocomotion induced by psychotomimetic drugs in mice. *Eur. J. Pharmacol.* 512, 199–205. doi: 10.1016/j.ejphar.2005.02.040.

Moser, E. I., Moser, M. B., and McNaughton, B. L. (2017). Spatial representation in the hippocampal formation: a history. *Nat. Neurosci.* 20, 1448–1464. doi: 10.1038/nn.4653

Paxinos, G., and Franklin, K. B. J. (2001). *The Mouse Brain in Stereotaxic Coordinates.* New York, NY: Academic Press

Procaccini, C., Aitta-aho, T., Jaako-Movits, K., Zharkovsky, A., Panhelainen, A., Sprengel, R., et al. (2011). Excessive novelty-induced c-Fos expression and altered neurogenesis in the hippocampus of GluA1 knockout mice. *Eur. J. Neurosci.* 33, 161–174. doi: 10.1111/j.1460-9568.2010.07485.x

Procaccini, C., Maksimovic, M., Aitta-Aho, T., Korpi, E. R., and Linden, A. M. (2013). Reversal of novelty-induced hyperlocomotion and hippocampal c-Fos expression in GluA1 knockout male mice by the mGluR2/3 agonist LY354740. *Neuroscience* 250, 189–200. doi: 10.1016/j.neuroscience.2013.07.010

Reisel, D., Bannerman, D. M., Schmitt, W. B., Deacon, R. M., Flint, J., Borchardt, T., et al. (2002). Spatial memory dissociations in mice lacking GluR1. *Nat. Neurosci.* 5, 868–873. doi: 10.1038/nn910

Ripke, S., Neale, B. M., Corvin, A., Walters, J. T., Farh, K. H., Holmans, P. A., et al. (2014). Biological insights from 108 schizophrenia-associated genetic loci. *Nature* 511, 421–427. doi: 10.1038/nature13595.

Ripke, S., O'Dushlaine, C., Chambert, K., Moran, J. L., Kahler, A. K., Akterin, S., et al. (2013). Genome-wide association analysis identifies 13 new risk loci for schizophrenia. *Nat. Genet.* 45, 1150–159. doi: 10.1038/ng.2742

Rock, E. M., Bolognini, D., Limebeer, C. L., Cascio, M. G., Anavi-Goffer, S., Fletcher, P. J., et al. (2012). Cannabidiol, a non-psychotropic component of cannabis, attenuates vomiting and nausea-like behaviour via indirect agonism of 5-HT(1A) somatodendritic autoreceptors in the dorsal raphe nucleus. *Br. J. Pharmacol.* 165, 2620–2634. doi: 10.1111/j.1476-5381.2011.01621.x

Roth, B. L. (2016). DREADDs for neuroscientists. *Neuron* 89, 683–694. doi: 10.1016/j.neuron.2016.01.040

Russo, E. B., Burnett, A., Hall, B., and Parker, K. K. (2005). Agonistic properties of cannabidiol at 5-HT1a receptors. *Neurochem. Res.* 30, 1037–1043. doi: 10.1007/s11064-005-6978-1

Sanderson, D. J., and Bannerman, D. M. (2012). The role of habituation in hippocampus-dependent spatial working memory tasks: evidence from GluA1 AMPA receptor subunit knockout mice. *Hippocampus* 22, 981–994. doi: 10.1002/hipo.20896

Sanderson, D. J., Good, M. A., Seeburg, P. H., Sprengel, R., Rawlins, J. N., and Bannerman, D. M. (2008). The role of the GluR-A (GluR1) AMPA receptor subunit in learning and memory. *Prog. Brain Res.* 169, 159–178. doi: 10.1016/S0079-6123(07)00009-X

Sanderson, D. J., Good, M. A., Skelton, K., Sprengel, R., Seeburg, P. H., Rawlins, J. N., et al. (2009). Enhanced long-term and impaired short-term spatial memory in GluA1 AMPA receptor subunit knockout mice: evidence for a dual-process memory model. *Learn. Mem.* 16, 379–386. doi: 10.1101/lm.1339109

Sanderson, D. J., McHugh, S. B., Good, M. A., Sprengel, R., Seeburg, P. H., Rawlins, J. N., et al. (2010). Spatial working memory deficits in GluA1 AMPA receptor subunit knockout mice reflect impaired short-term habituation: evidence for Wagner's dual-process memory model. *Neuropsychologia* 48, 2303–2315. doi: 10.1016/j.neuropsychologia.2010.03.018

Schubart, C. D., Sommer, I. E., Fusar-Poli, P., de Witte, L., Kahn, R. S., and Boks, M. P. (2014). Cannabidiol as a potential treatment for psychosis. *Eur. Neuropsychopharmacol.* 24, 51–64. doi: 10.1016/j.euroneuro.2013.11.002

Sylantyev, S., Jensen, T. P., Ross, R. A., and Rusakov, D. A. (2013). Cannabinoid- and lysophosphatidylinositol-sensitive receptor GPR55 boosts neurotransmitter release at central synapses. *Proc. Natl. Acad. Sci. U.S.A.* 110, 5193–5198. doi: 10.1073/pnas.1211204110

Todd, S. M., and Arnold, J. C. (2016). Neural correlates of interactions between cannabidiol and Delta(9) -tetrahydrocannabinol in mice: implications for medical cannabis. *Br. J. Pharmacol.* 173, 53–65. doi: 10.1111/bph.13333

Vazquez, G. H., Camino, S., Tondo, L., and Baldessarini, R. J. (2017). Potential novel treatments for bipolar depression: ketamine, fatty acids, anti-inflammatory agents, and probiotics. *CNS Neurol. Disord. Drug. Targets* 16, 858–869. doi: 10.2174/1871527316666170728165648

Vekovischeva, O. Y., Aitta-Aho, T., Echenko, O., Kankaanpaa, A., Seppala, T., Honkanen, A., et al. (2004). Reduced aggression in AMPA-type glutamate receptor GluR-A subunit-deficient mice. *Genes Brain Behav.* 3, 253–265. doi: 10.1111/j.1601-1848.2004.00075.x

Vekovischeva, O. Y., Zamanillo, D., Echenko, O., Seppala, T., Uusi-Oukari, M., Honkanen, A., et al. (2001). Morphine-induced dependence and sensitization are altered in mice deficient in AMPA-type glutamate receptor-A subunits. *J. Neurosci.* 21, 4451–4459. doi: 10.1523/JNEUROSCI.21-12-04451.2001

Wiedholz, L. M., Owens, W. A., Horton, R. E., Feyder, M., Karlsson, R. M., Hefner, K., et al. (2008). Mice lacking the AMPA GluR1 receptor exhibit striatal hyperdopaminergia and 'schizophrenia-related' behaviors. *Mol. Psychiatry* 13, 631–640. doi: 10.1038/sj.mp.4002056

Zamanillo, D., Sprengel, R., Hvalby, O., Jensen, V., Burnashev, N., Rozov, A., et al. (1999). Importance of AMPA receptors for hippocampal synaptic plasticity but not for spatial learning. *Science* 284, 1805–1811. doi: 10.1126/science.284.5421.1805

Zuardi, A. W., Rodrigues, J. A., and Cunha, J. M. (1991). Effects of cannabidiol in animal models predictive of antipsychotic activity. *Psychopharmacology* 104, 260–264. doi: 10.1007/BF02244189

17

Beyond the Activity-Based Anorexia Model: Reinforcing Values of Exercise and Feeding Examined in Stressed Adolescent Male and Female Mice

Imane Hurel[1,2†], *Bastien Redon*[1,2†], *Amandine Scocard*[1,2], *Meryl Malezieux*[1,2‡], *Giovanni Marsicano*[1,2] *and Francis Chaouloff*[1,2*]

[1] *Endocannabinoids and NeuroAdaptation, NeuroCentre INSERM U1215, Bordeaux, France,* [2] *University of Bordeaux, Bordeaux, France*

***Correspondence:**
Francis Chaouloff
francis.chaouloff@inserm.fr

†These authors have contributed equally to this work.

‡Present Address:
Meryl Malezieux,
Synaptic Circuits of Memory,
IINS CNRS UMR5297,
Bordeaux, France

Anorexia nervosa (AN), mostly observed in female adolescents, is the most fatal mental illness. Its core is a motivational imbalance between exercise and feeding in favor of the former. The most privileged animal model of AN is the "activity-based anorexia" (ABA) model wherein partly starved rodents housed with running wheels exercise at the expense of feeding. However, the ABA model bears face and construct validity limits, including its inability to specifically assess running motivation and feeding motivation. As infant/adolescent trauma is a precipitating factor in AN, this study first analyzed post-weaning isolation rearing (PWIR) impacts on body weights and wheel-running performances in female mice exposed to an ABA protocol. Next, we studied through operant conditioning protocols i) whether food restriction affects in a sex-dependent manner running motivation before ii) investigating how PWIR and sex affect running and feeding drives under *ad libitum* fed conditions and food restriction. Besides amplifying ABA-elicited body weight reductions, PWIR stimulated wheel-running activities in anticipation of feeding in female mice, suggesting increased running motivation. To confirm this hypothesis, we used a cued-reward motivated instrumental task wherein wheel-running was conditioned by prior nose poke responses. It was first observed that food restriction increased running motivation in male, but not female, mice. When fed grouped and PWIR mice were tested for their running and palatable feeding drives, all mice, excepted PWIR males, displayed increased nose poke responses for running over feeding. This was true when rewards were proposed alone or within a concurrent test. The increased preference for running over feeding in fed females did not extend to running performances (time, distance) during each rewarded sequence, confirming that motivation for, and performance during, running are independent entities. With food restriction, mice displayed a sex-independent increase in their preference for feeding over running in both group-housed and PWIR conditions. This study shows that the ABA model does not specifically capture running and feeding drives, i.e. components known to be affected in AN.

Keywords: restrictive anorexia nervosa, post-weaning isolation rearing, wheel-running, palatable food, food anticipatory activity, operant conditioning, motivation, reward choice

INTRODUCTION

Anorexia nervosa (AN), which mainly affects older adolescent and young adult females (with a sex ratio of 8 for 1 male), is a psychiatric disorder where self-starvation and hence dramatic underweight is a core symptom (Kaye et al., 2009; Zipfel et al., 2015). As opposed to a general belief, it is unlikely that socio/cultural influences play a major, if not unique, role as AN was already reported centuries ago (Casper, 2006). Its lifetime prevalence in high-income countries is ~1–4% (Smink et al., 2012; Zipfel et al., 2015; Keski-Rahkonen and Mustelin, 2016), with a constant increase in that percentage over recent years (Smink et al., 2012). However, AN, whether restrictive or associated with purgative behavior, is not solely accounted for by a decreased drive for feeding. In many cases, especially in restrictive anorexia, this decrease is associated, and often preceded by, motor restlessness and/or an increased drive for another reward, i.e. exercise, mostly running (Brewerton et al., 1995; Davis, 1997; Klein et al., 2004; Meyer et al., 2011; Casper, 2018). Reinforcing the hypothesis that increased exercise is at the core of AN are the reports that i) exercise dependence might be one cause of altered eating behavior (Cook and Hausenblas, 2008), ii) remitted AN patients still display craving for exercise (Shroff et al., 2006), and that iii) the latter amplifies the anhedonic profile of these patients (Davis and Woodside, 2002). It is this imbalance between energetic supply and energy consumption rates that provides AN with severe and often lethal consequences. Although AN etiology is ill-defined (Clarke et al., 2012), family and twin studies have indicated that AN patients are at risk to transmit the disease to their progeny (Bulik et al., 2007; Zipfel et al., 2015). However, the identification of AN genetic defects is rendered complex as this disease is not accounted for by one single gene (Bulik et al., 2007). Besides familial causes, environmental risk factors have also been delineated. Among these, perinatal (e.g., prematurity, imbalanced maternal control) and/or childhood trauma have been underlined (Leung et al., 2000; Romans et al., 2001; Canetti et al., 2008; Pike et al., 2008; Zipfel et al., 2015). This might explain why patients suffering AN display comorbidity with mood disorders, including major depression, anxiety, and obsessive-compulsive disorders (Kaye et al., 2009; Zipfel et al., 2015). With respect to childhood trauma, physical abuse, sexual abuse and parental neglect are the more documented forms of social stress that might, in combination with genetic or other environmental factors, precipitate AN (Yackobovitch-Gavan et al., 2009; Jaite et al., 2012; Racine and Wildes, 2015). The negative impact of childhood trauma is further illustrated by the report that post-traumatic stress disorder and AN might actually co-occur (Reyes-Rodríguez et al., 2011). The observation that early traumatic events provide a long-term psychoneuroendocrine vulnerability to future stressors in laboratory rodents (Lupien et al., 2009; McCormick et al., 2016) provides support for an etiological role of early trauma in AN.

To date, the model considered to be the most pertinent for AN—although it is unlikely that a single model recapitulates such a complex pathology—is the so-called "activity-based anorexia (ABA)" paradigm (Boakes, 2007; Scheurink et al., 2010; Kim, 2012; Mequinion et al., 2015). Thus, rodents housed with a running wheel and placed under a severe restricted feeding regimen (i.e., a single time- or quantity-limited access to food per day) display a progressive increase in running activity at the expense of feeding. Such an increase is mainly accounted for by high wheel-running activity prior to food delivery (namely food anticipatory activity, FAA). After several days, body weight loss is so pronounced (up to 30%) that death might occur, especially in rats (Routtenberg and Kuznesof, 1967). Beyond methodological limits that might question the causal relationship between food scarcity and physical hyperactivity (Dwyer and Boakes, 1997; Rowland et al., 2018), the validity of the ABA paradigm as an animal model of AN might be discussed with regard to the construct, face, and predictive validity criteria thought to define any model of human (psycho)pathology (see Willner, 1984). This is especially true for the construct criterium in which factors thought to be of etiological significance in AN pathology should thus logically bear consequences in the ABA model. In keeping with the data reported above, genetics, sex (female *vs.* males), age (adolescence *vs.* adulthood), and early traumatic stimuli are expected to have significant impacts in the ABA model. As opposed to genetic studies, which provide thorough evidence that the consequences of the exposure to the ABA model depend on the rat/mouse line tested therein (Pjetri et al., 2012; Klenotich et al., 2012), studies aimed at investigating the respective impacts of sex and age in this model have provided contradictory results (Mequinion et al., 2015; Rowland et al., 2018). As opposed to genetics, sex, and age, available data on the impact of early traumatic stimuli in the ABA paradigm are somewhat scarce. Prenatal stress (Boersma et al., 2016; Schroeder et al., 2018), early weaning (Glavin and Pare, 1985) or postnatal separation (Carrera et al., 2009; Hancock and Grant, 2009) have shown diverse effects, including when considering the animal sex. Although these studies addressed the consequences of prenatal and perinatal stress manipulations that might bear translational value with respect to AN, the question of the impact of stress during childhood and early adolescence should be considered. As mentioned above, physical and/or sexual insults during these periods have long-lasting psychological consequences, especially in females where such stressors increase the propensity to develop affective disorders (Bale and Epperson, 2015). Of major relevance to the present focus, childhood and early adolescence trauma can be modeled in rodents through the so-called post-weaning isolation rearing (PWIR) stress paradigm. Actually, rodents housed individually immediately after weaning (21 days in rodents), and thus deprived of social contacts, display long-lasting emotional disturbances (e.g., anxiety, cognitive rigidity, aggression, proneness to drug self-administration; Fone and Porkess, 2008; Walker et al., 2019) that might be translationally relevant to AN in humans.

Herein, we first studied the consequences of PWIR on wheel-running performances in an ABA paradigm wherein food-restricted female mice were provided a limited amount of food at the onset of the dark cycle. Because the core of AN is an imbalance between the respective motivation drives for exercise and feeding (Klein et al., 2004; Casper, 2006; Keating, 2010; Keating et al., 2012), we next asked whether the impact of PWIR in the ABA found its origin at the motivation level. To do so, we shifted to an operant conditioning procedure wherein mice needed to nose-poke to unbrake a running wheel (Muguruza et al., 2019). This procedure allowed us to examine how i) food restriction and ii) PWIR respectively affected running motivation. As AN involves decreased motivation for feeding, we finally asked the question of i) the impact of PWIR on motivation for palatable food before ii) examining the respective drives for wheel-running and palatable feeding under *ad libitum* and food restricted conditions when these rewards were made concurrent (Muguruza et al., 2019).

MATERIALS AND METHODS

Animals

All protocols, which complied with the French (Décret 2013–118) and European (2010/63/EU) rules on animal experimentation, were approved by the local Ethic Committee (Comité d'Ethique 50) with agreement numbers DIR13111, 13649, 33-063-69 (F.C.) and A33-063-098 (animal facilities) provided under authority of the Préfecture de Gironde and the Ministry of Agriculture. Accordingly, the 3R-rules were followed, including through the use of the minimal number of animals per series of experiments that was required to reach conclusions. In addition, in keeping with the procedures used in this study (see the methodological outline), and which could have long-lasting consequences, all animals were only used once and sacrificed thereafter.

This study mainly used 3-week-old male and female C57BL/6N mice (Elevage Janvier, Le Genest Saint Isle, France). Upon arrival in our animal facilities, these mice were housed either singly (PWIR) or in three to four (group-housed). This study also involved 8-week-old male and female C57BL/6N mice, all individually housed (to avoid inter-individual aggression). All animals were housed in a thermoregulated room (21–22°C) placed under a partly inverted 12-h light/12-h dark cycle with lights off at 2:00 PM (free wheel-running experiments) or at 10:00 AM (operant conditioning experiments). Excepted for experiments involving restriction feeding regimen (see below), mice were provided with food and water *ad libitum*.

Methodological Outline

A first series of experiments involved group-housed and PWIR female mice provided with wheels in their home cages under *ad libitum* fed conditions before being food-restricted (ABA protocol; **Figure 1A**). A second series of experiments involved individually-housed fed and food-restricted male and female mice, these mice being conditioned to nose poke for access to running wheels located in operant chambers (wheel-running motivation; **Figure 1B**). A third series of experiments used group-housed and PWIR male and female mice which were conditioned to nose poke for access to wheel-running or palatable food, these rewards being first proposed alone before being proposed in competition under fed and, then, food-restricted conditions (**Figure 1C**).

Activity-Based Anorexia Protocol

At the age of 5 weeks, group-housed mice and mice singly-housed after weaning were singly placed in cages housing a running wheel (25-cm diameter, Intellibio, Seichamps, France). Following a 7-day period of habituation to their new environment during which food intakes, body weights and daily running activity were monitored, mice were then placed under a food-restriction procedure for another 7-day period (**Figure 1A**). This restriction procedure consisted in the daily placement of a limited amount of food (50% of the mean daily intake measured during the preceding week) in each cage, this amount being provided (after having checked for the absence of food crumbs) at the onset of the dark part of the light/dark cycle. Body weights were monitored daily while wheel-running performances were recorded on an hourly basis.

Operant Conditioning Set-Up

Motivation for wheel-running and/or food intake was studied in 12 individual operant chambers (28 cm long × 26 cm wide × 38 cm high) located in a room adjacent to the animal housing room, as previously described (Muguruza et al., 2019). These chambers were placed inside wooden casings (60 cm long × 62 cm wide × 49 cm high) that were ventilated to guarantee air circulation and to provide background noise (Imetronic, Pessac, France). For operant running experiments, lateral walls were made of gray Perspex while the rear wall had a central hollow for mounting the 20-cm-diameter wheel, the release trigger of which was connected to a circuit enabling the wheel to be locked or unlocked (by means of a brake-pad) in accordance with predefined experimental conditions (**Figure 1D**, operant running configuration). A cue-light placed above the wheel indicated the wheel unlocking. The wheel was flanked by two small ports (2.5 cm above the chamber grilled floor with cue lights located above) set into the rear wall to allow the animal to "poke" its nose through. For operant feeding, the rear side (running wheel, nose poke ports, cue-lights) was covered by gray Perspex whereas the left panel of the chamber housed in its center a recessed pellet tray surrounded by two nose poke (nose poke) ports (**Figure 1D**, operant feeding configuration). Cue-lights were placed above the nose poke ports and the feeder to indicate respectively effectiveness of the nose poke and pellet distribution. For reward choice sessions, the above-mentioned Perspex walls were removed to allow conditioned wheel-running or conditioned feeding (**Figure 1D**, running/feeding choice configuration). Nose poke performance could be either "active" (leading to cue-light illumination and wheel unlocking or cue-light illumination and pellet distribution) or "inactive" (having no consequence). Left/right allocation of active/inactive nose poke ports was counterbalanced between animals during experiments. All devices in the operant chambers were linked to a computer which recorded both the number of active/inactive nose poke, the number of running sequences, and the running duration/distance covered during each rewarded sequence (wheel-running configuration), and the number of active/inactive nose pokes, the number of pellets distributed, and the number of entries into the feeder (feeding configuration). Food

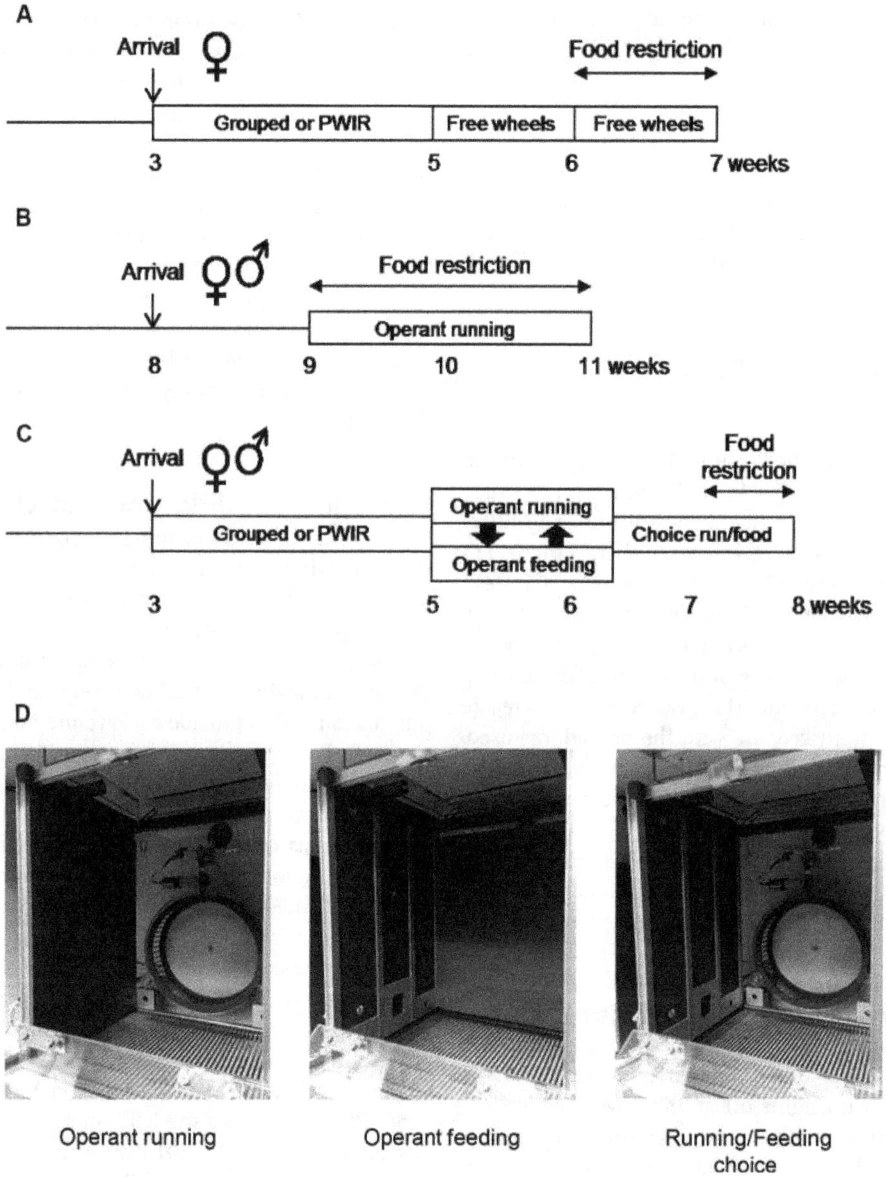

FIGURE 1 | Experimental protocols and operant chamber set-ups. **(A–C)** Protocol schemes for the three series of experiments aimed respectively at investigating the effects of post-weaning isolation rearing (PWIR) on free wheel-running in food-restricted mice **(A)**, of the mouse sex on running motivation under fed and food restriction conditions **(B)**, and of the mouse sex and of PWIR on the choice between running and feeding under fed and food restriction conditions **(C)**. **(D)** Operant chamber set-up for the study of running motivation alone (left), palatable feeding motivation alone (center), and the preference between running and feeding in a concurrent choice design (right).

pellets were 20-mg chocolate-flavored pellets composed of 59.1% glucids, 18.4% proteins, 5.5% lipids, 6.5% minerals and 4.6% fibers (72 cal per 20-mg F05301 BioServ pellet; Plexx, Elst, The Netherlands).

Operant Conditioning Protocols

All protocols were similar to those already reported (Muguruza et al., 2019). In one series of experiments aimed at assessing the respective influences of the animal sex and of food restriction on wheel-running motivation (see above), operant conditioning procedures involved training under fixed-ratio 1 (FR1) and FR3 schedules of wheel-running reinforcement followed by a progressive ratio (PR) schedule of reinforcement. In a second series of experiments aimed at assessing the respective influences of the animal sex, of PWIR and of food restriction on wheel-running motivation and on feeding motivation in a choice paradigm, operant conditioning procedures first involved training under FR1 and FR3 schedules of wheel-running or palatable food intake reinforcements, each reward being available alone. These training procedures were then followed by a PR schedule of reinforcement for each reward. Mice were then returned to one session of FR3 schedule reinforcement with wheel-running and palatable food intake being reinforced separately. Thereafter, mice were placed under additional FR3 schedules of reinforcement with both rewards being provided in a choice paradigm. The selection of one reward temporarily excluded any possibility to obtain the second reward. In all experiments, food-restricted mice, whether tested for running motivation or for palatable food motivation, were provided their daily chow at least 1 h after their operant session. Daily food provision, which was calculated as to promote a 10% reduction in initial body weights, took into account the amount of food eaten during the preceding test session. The time schedule that we chose, i.e., motivation tests 1–2 h before feeding, thus allowed to examine running and feeding drives at time periods corresponding to those during which FAA was observed in the ABA protocol.

For the first series of experiments (**Figure 1B**), male and female mice singly housed for a week, and aged 9 weeks old, underwent one daily habituation session in the operant chambers for two consecutive days. Mice were placed in the operant chambers with the cue light above the unlocked running wheel remaining illuminated while the two nose poke ports were covered-up by metal pieces. These two 60-min sessions were aimed at habituating the mice to both the operant chamber, the wheel and the cue indicating wheel-unlocking. When learning sessions began (**Figure 1D**, operant running configuration), the wheel locking/unlocking mechanism and the nose poke ports were fully operational. The wheel was unlocked for 60 s (wheel brake release) following nose pokes the mouse executed in its allocated active nose poke port. In the FR1 condition, a single active nose poke was sufficient to simultaneously illuminate the cue-light above the port for 10 s, unlock the running wheel for 60 s and illuminate a light above the wheel. Nose pokes in the other port were counted but were without functional consequence. When the 60-s period had elapsed, the wheel-light extinguished and the brake applied, so that the mouse had to step down from the wheel and execute a further nose poke in order to unlock it again. Nose pokes made in the active port while the wheel was already unlocked, counted as uncorrect responses, were without consequence. Habituation and FR1 sessions were run once daily and lasted for 60 min. After completing six FR1 sessions, mice moved on to the FR3 condition, i.e., a 60-s wheel-running period was contingent on three consecutive nose pokes in the active port. The day after the last FR3 session mice were tested under a linear PR schedule of reinforcement where i) the number of active nose pokes required to free the running wheel was incremented by three between each rewarded step (three, six, nine ... etc: PR3), with ii) a time limit of 15 min between two successive steps.

For the second series of experiments (**Figure 1C**), group-housed mice and PWIR mice were first habituated to the 20-mg food pellets by providing them 3 to 5 pellets/day in their home cages for the 3 days that preceded their first day of exposure to the operant chambers. On this first day of habituation to the chambers, mice were exposed to two consecutive 30-min sessions with the running wheel being unlocked during the first session (**Figure 1D**, operant running configuration) while during the second session, the feeder distributed 17 chocolate pellets (**Figure 1D**, operant feeding configuration). In between, mice were returned for 5 min in their home cages (with drinking water) as to allow operant chamber configuration changes (wheel to food or *vice versa*). During these two sessions, whose reward order was counterbalanced, cue lights above the unlocked running wheel or the pellet tray remained illuminated while nose poke ports were covered-up by metal pieces for each configuration. These habituation periods were followed by a conditioning phasis wherein animals learned the contingency between the introduction of the muzzle into the "active" nose poke port and the access to the related reward. For this purpose, nose poke holes were not masked anymore as to allow the mouse to "poke" its nose through. As for habituation, two consecutive sessions per day (30 min/session) were performed: one for food (50% of the individuals in each mouse group) and the second for wheel-running (the remining 50% of the individuals in each mouse group), the order between the sessions being daily alterned. To facilitate the learning of the contingency for food (and hence running), mice were first food-restricted (as to display a stable 10% body weight reduction) for the first two to three FR1 sessions, i.e., sessions during which a single nose poke was sufficient to illuminate the cue light above the wheel or the food port for 5 s. Simultaneously the cue light above the wheel was activated for 20 s (indicating the possibility to run) while that above the food magazine was activated for 15 s (indicating the distribution of one food pellet). Although mice consumed their food pellet rapidly, we decided not to shorten the rewarding periods as i) to allow sufficient time for running and ii) to avoid rapid food satiety. Wheel unlocking or pellet distribution was respectively followed by 20- and 15-s time-out periods during which nose poke activity was inefficient. Five sessions of FR1 for each reward were sufficient to ensure that all animals learned and expressed stable performance over days. Then, animals were placed for another 5-day period under a FR3 schedule wherein three consecutive nose pokes in the active port were required to get one reward (i.e., 20-s wheel running or one chocolate pellet). All mice had a minimal discrimination index of 80% between active and inactive nose pokes. On the two consecutive days that followed the last FR3 session, mice were tested under PR 3 schedule of reinforcements where the number of consecutive active nose pokes required to free the running wheel or to trigger the distribution of one pellet was incremented by three between each rewarded step (three, six, nine...). Half of the mice within each mouse group were tested for wheel-running reinforcement on the first day, the second half being tested for food reinforcement, and vice versa on the second day PR session. PR schedules of reinforcement, by allowing an estimation of the maximal number of consecutive nose pokes performed (and hence the last rewarded step that was reached, i.e., the so-called "breakpoint" level), provide an index of the appetitive motivation for each reward.

Preference for Wheel-Running Over Palatable Food Consumption

The day after the last PR session, mice from the second series of experiments were returned to FR3 schedules of wheel and food reinforcement as to indicate to the mice that the rewards were again available following a fixed number of active nose pokes. Then, animals were placed in a choice condition (**Figure 1D**, running/feeding choice configuration) with either wheel unlocking or food distribution being accessible under an FR3 schedule (Muguruza et al., 2019). However, choosing one reward excluded the possibility to obtain simultaneously the second reward. The respective durations of activation of the wheel (20 s) and the feeder (15 s) cue-lights remained as in the preceding sessions. However, to further indicate to the mice that might run during the entire 20-s sequence that the reward choice was mutually exclusive, we added a 5-s period during which a green ceiling light was switched on while none of the nose poke ports was active. Five daily consecutive choice sessions were performed to establish food and wheel preferences, each session being 60-min long. To explore how PWIR affected the impact of food restriction on the preference between wheel-running and feeding (as under ABA conditions; see above), these choice sessions were followed by five choice sessions during which the mice were food-restricted (to extents similar to those measured during the first two to three FR1 sessions; see above).

Data Analyses and Statistics

Measures of wheel-running performances (ABA experiments) were gathered using the ActiviWheel software (Intellibio, France) while operant running and/or feeding data were obtained using the PolyWheel software (Imetronic, France). To evaluate wheel-running consumption during FR/PR sessions in the operant protocols, we divided the total running duration (or the total distance covered) within each session over the number of rewarded events during that session. Additionally, wheel preference (%) in the choice sessions was quantified by dividing the number of active nose pokes that led access to the wheel by the total number of active nose pokes performed for both rewards (food + wheel). Scores above 50% thus indicates a preference for wheel-running while scores below 50% indicates a preference for food.

All data are shown as means ± standard errors of the mean. Two-group (treatment or genotype) comparisons of the data gathered during the PR sessions were achieved by means of two-tailed Student t-tests. Multiple data comparisons were performed through multiple (two- or three-way) analyses of variance (with/without repeated factor), data being log-transformed to achieve variance homogeneity if needed. *Post hoc* comparisons (Tukey test) were only performed if interactions between main variables were significant. In choice experiments, preference scores were compared to non-preference (50% preference for one reward) by one-tailed Student's t-tests. All analyses were achieved using the GB-Stat 10.0 software (Dynamic Microsystems, USA).

RESULTS

PWIR Female Mice Display Increased Food Anticipatory Wheel-Running Activity

Food-restricted grouped and PWIR mice displayed a progressive session-dependent shift of wheel-running activity from the dark part of the nycthemeral cycle to its light part (**Figure 2A**). This shift, which was mainly observed during the hours that preceded food availability (i.e., FAA), concerned to a higher extent the PWIR mice, compared to their grouped counterparts (**Figure 2A**). The overall analysis of wheel-running performances confirmed the latter observation. Thus, food restriction, which decreased body weights in all mice ($F_{7,91} = 119.92$, $p < 0.0001$), this decrease being larger in PWIR mice ($F_{1,13} = 24.84$, $p = 0.0002$; **Figure 2B**), inhibited wheel-running activity in both mouse groups ($F_{7,91} = 18.26$, $p < 0.0001$; **Figure 2C**). However, this overall inhibition was associated with an increased wheel-running activity during the light part of the cycle, hence reflecting increased FAA ($F_{7,91} = 7.07$, $p < 0.0001$), the amplitude of which was more pronounced in PWIR females, compared to their controls ($F_{7,91} = 4.33$, $p = 0.0004$ for the time × mouse group interaction; **Figure 2D**).

Sex-Dependent Effects of Food Restriction on Wheel-Running Motivation

Taken together, the above-mentioned results indicated that PWIR amplified the stimulatory impact of food restriction on FAA in female mice. To examine whether this impact of PWIR in food-restricted mice was accounted for by specific changes in wheel-running motivation, and if so, whether these changes were sex-specific, we shifted from "free" wheel-running experiments to "effort-based" wheel-running experiments. Using operant conditioning, we first examined how food restriction affected running motivation in male and female mice before we analyzed the extent to which PWIR in male and female mice affected their motivation for i) wheel-running and ii) food intake under fed and food-restricted conditions. Food restriction did not affect male (**Figure 3A**) and female (**Figure 3B**) nose poke responses for wheel-running under FR1/FR3 schedules of reinforcement. Beside, the overall analysis of nose pokes in (fed and food-restricted) male and female mice revealed higher scores in females, as compared to males ($F_{1,44} = 20.74$, $p < 0.0001$; **Figure 3A** and **B**). As opposed to its lack of effect on nose poke responses, food-deprivation increased both the running duration per rewarded sequence ($F_{1,23} = 11.82$, $p = 0.0022$; **Figure 3C**) and the distance ran per rewarded sequence ($F_{1,23} = 12.83$, $p = 0.0016$; **Figure 3E**) in male mice, but not in female mice (**Figure 3D** and **F**). When tested under a PR schedule of reinforcement, fed and food-restricted females were found to perform better than their fed and food-restricted male counterparts ($F_{1,44} = 10.42$, $p = 0.0024$; **Figure 3G** and **H**), indicating higher motivation in the former mouse groups. However, when focusing on the effects of the feeding regimen on running motivation, males (**Figure 3G**), but not females (**Figure 3H**), proved sensitive to the stimulatory impact of food restriction although the latter bore sex-independent body weight-reducing effects (**Figure 3G** and **H**). Sex- and food restriction-dependent influences on wheel-running performances during the FR sessions extended to PR sessions as running durations per rewarded sequences (39.74 ± 2.83 s) and running distances per rewarded sequences (10.04 ± 1.22 m) were respectively increased by food restriction (47.91 ± 1.96 s and 14.81 ± 1.11 m; $p = 0.031$ and $p = 0.011$, respectively) in males, but not in females (data not shown). Taken together, these results revealed that although females displayed higher running motivation than males, their drive proved insensitive to food restriction, as opposed to that of males.

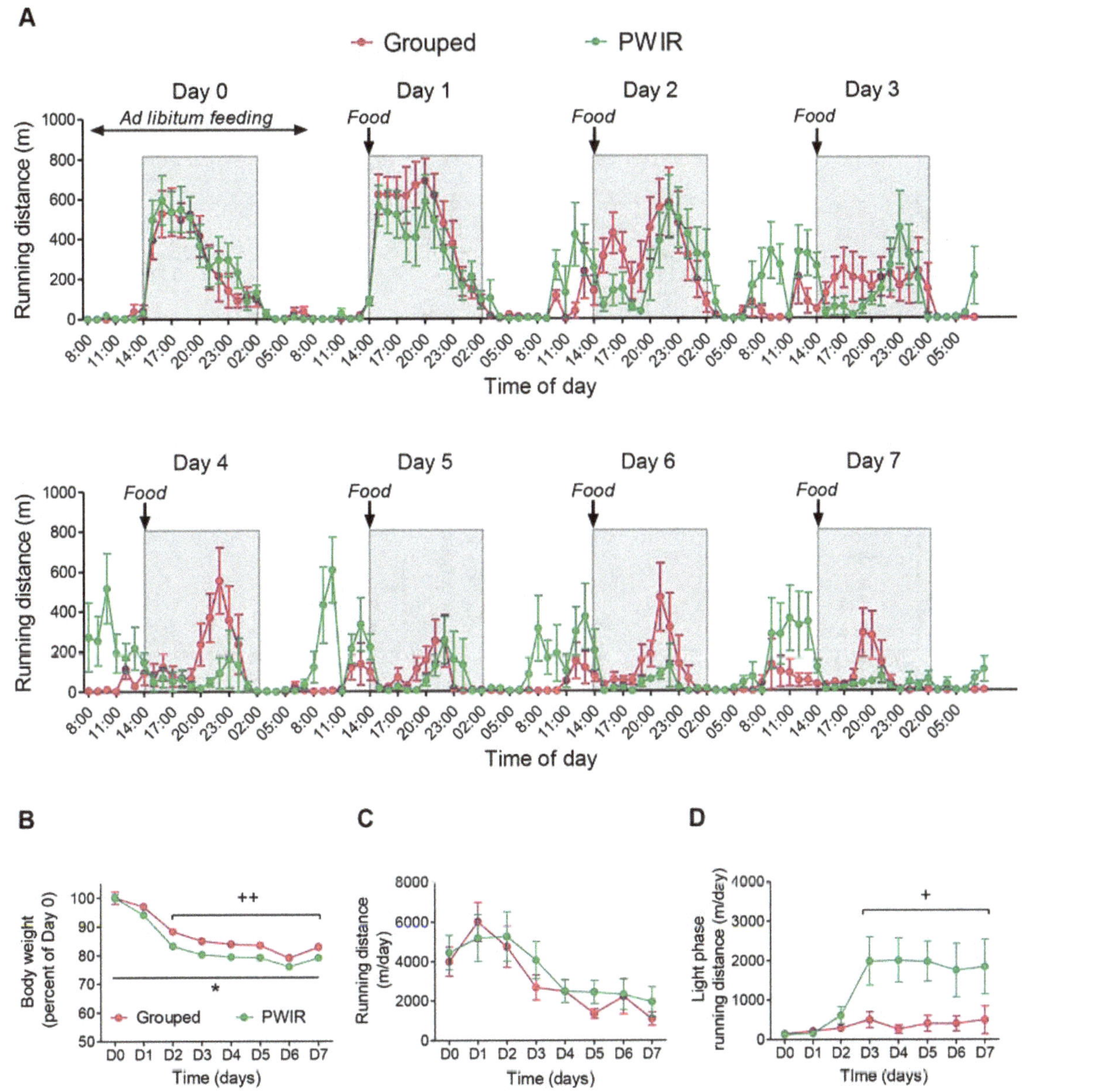

FIGURE 2 | Wheel-running performances of grouped and post-weaning isolation reared (PWIR) female mice submitted to a restricted feeding protocol. **(A)** Hourly wheel-running activities before and during repeated food restriction (days 1–7). A limited amount of food (50% of the food quantity consumed during *ad libitum* feeding conditions) was provided at the daily onset of the dark period of the light/dark cycle. **(B)** Food restriction-elicited body weight reductions in grouped and PWIR mice. **(C,D)** Food restriction effects on daily running distances **(C)** and on daily distances ran during the light part of the light/dark cycle **(D)**. The values are the mean ± standard error of the mean of n = 7–8 mice. * $p < 0.05$ for the impact of PWIR (multiple-way analysis of variance). + $p < 0.05$ and ++ $p < 0.01$ for the difference with D0 (*post hoc* Tukey test following a significant day × mouse group interaction in the multiple-way analyses of variance). D0–D7 refer to day 0–day 7.

Sex-Dependent Effects of PWIR on Nose-Poke Responding Reinforced by Wheel-Running or Palatable Food

The results gathered in the two preceding series of experiments rose the hypothesis that PWIR might increase nose poke responses for wheel-running in food-restricted females while possibly amplifying those evoked by food restriction in males. To test this hypothesis, we however had first to document i) the specificity of the effects of PWIR with regard to the nutritional status of the animals (*ad libitum* fed vs. food restricted), and ii) measure whether these wheel-running responses were associated with PWIR- and/or sex-dependent changes in nose poke responses for food with/without food restriction. Accordingly, we measured the respective influences of PWIR, food restriction, and sex on nose poke responses for wheel-running and palatable feeding, each reward being provided alone. Grouped (**Figure 4A**), but not PWIR (**Figure 4B**), males displayed higher nose poke responses for wheel-running than

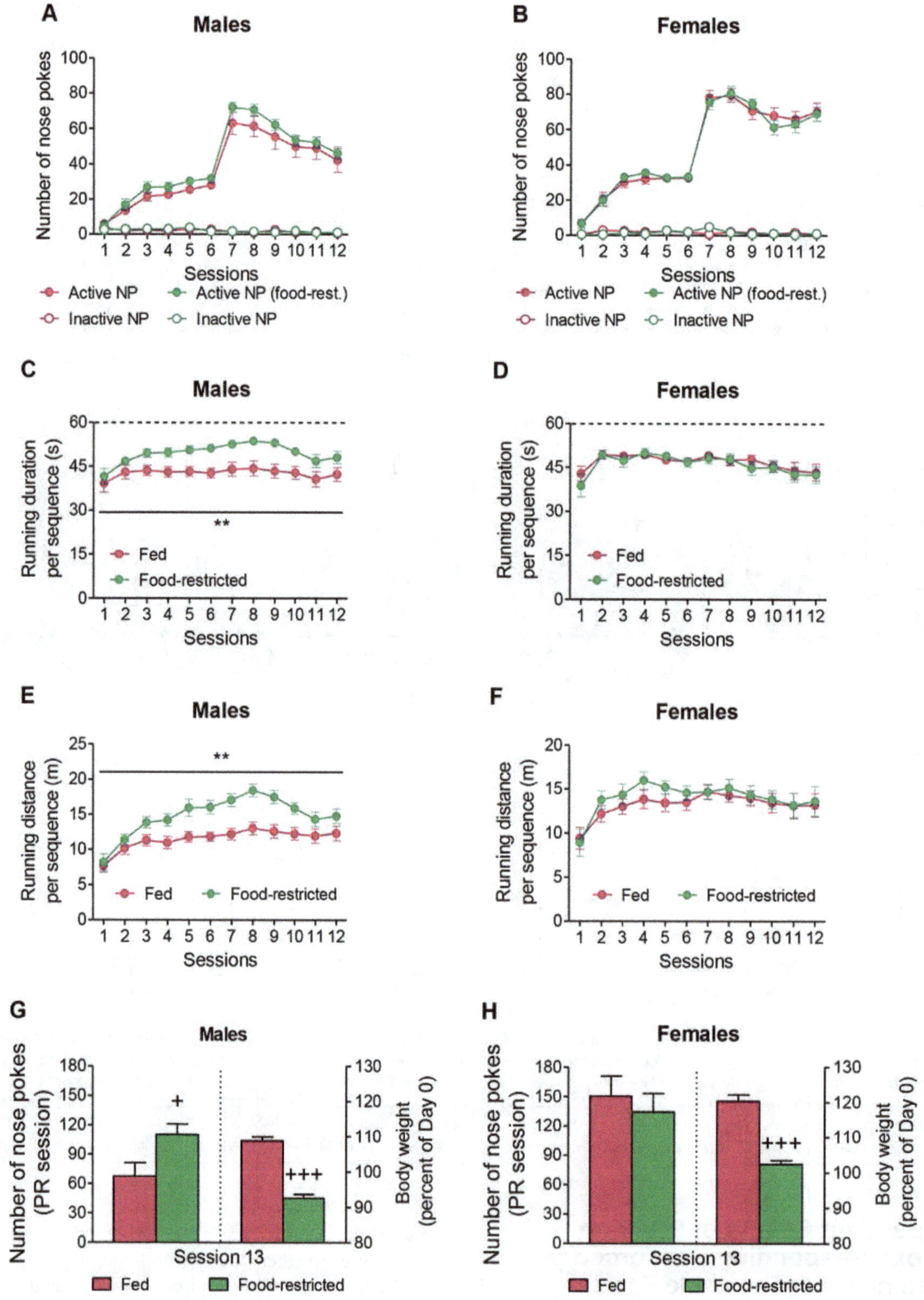

FIGURE 3 | Sex-dependent effects of food restriction on running motivation and running performances. **(A,B)** Neither male mice **(A)** nor female mice **(B)** displayed changes in their nose poke responses for wheel-running with food restriction when placed under FR1/FR3 schedules of reinforcement. **(C,D)** Food restriction increased the running duration per rewarded sequence in male mice **(C)**, but not in female mice **(D)**. **(E,F)** Food restriction increased the distance ran per rewarded sequence in male mice **(E)**, but not in female mice **(F)**. **(G,H)** A food restriction regimen leading to a 15–16% reduction in body weight amplified male **(G)**, but not female **(H)** nose poke responses for wheel-running during a PR session. The values are the mean ± standard error of the mean of n = 11–14 mice. ** $p < 0.01$ for the impact of food restriction (multiple-way analysis of variance). + $p < 0.05$ and +++ $p < 0.001$ for the effect of food restriction during the PR session (Student t-test).

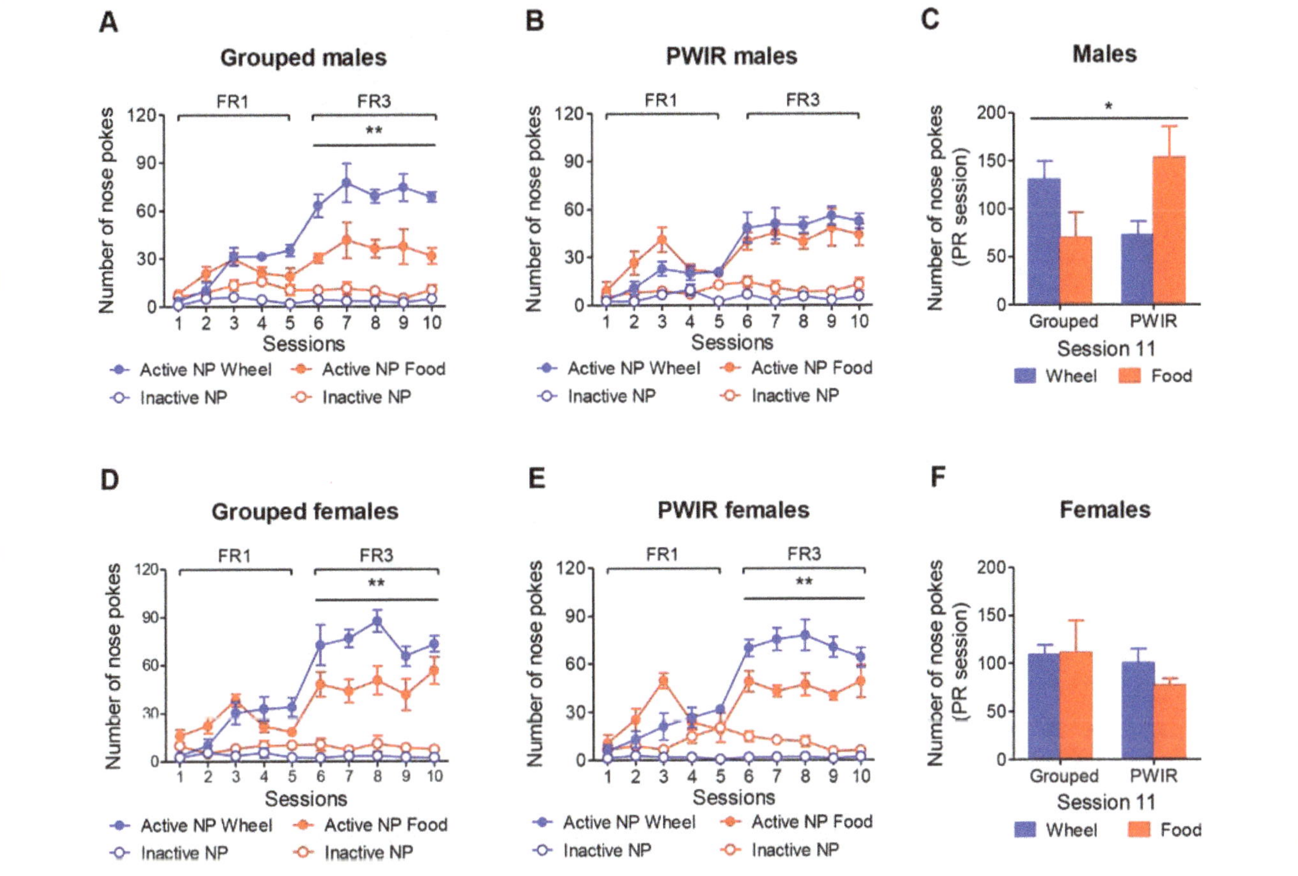

FIGURE 4 | Sex-dependent effects of post-weaning isolation rearing (PWIR) on running motivation and palatable feeding motivation (each reward provided separately). **(A,B)** Grouped **(A)**, but not PWIR **(B)**, males displayed higher nose poke responses for wheel-running than for palatable food under FR3 schedules of reinforcement. **(C)** Grouped and PWIR male mice showed opposed profiles of nose poke responses for running and feeding during a PR session. **(D,E)** Both grouped **(D)** and PWIR **(E)** females displayed a higher number of nose poke responses for running, compared to feeding, under FR3 schedules of reinforcement. **(F)** Neither PWIR nor the reward nature exerted influences on the number of nose responses displayed by female mice for reward access during a PR session. The values are the mean ± standard error of the mean of n = 5–6 mice. * $p < 0.05$ for the PWIR x reward interaction during the PR session, and ** $p < 0.01$ for the overall difference between rewards under FR3 schedules of reinforcement (multiple-way analyses of variance).

for palatable food under an FR3 schedule of reinforcement ($F_{1,8} = 17.19$, $p = 0.0031$). Examination of these responses under a PR schedule of reinforcement revealed a reward x housing interaction ($F_{1,9} = 5.86$, $p = 0.0385$) that was mainly accounted for by increased motivation for palatable food over wheel-running in isolated animals (**Figure 4C**). As opposed to males, both group-housed ($F_{1,8} = 12.21$, $p = 0.008$; **Figure 4D**) and PWIR ($F_{1,10} = 13.49$, $p = 0.0043$; **Figure 4E**) female mice responded more for wheel-running than for food under FR3 schedules of reinforcement. However, these trends did not translate into higher responses for wheel-running in the PR sessions whether nose poke numbers (**Figure 4F**) or breakpoint levels (data not shown) were considered.

Sex-Dependent Effects of PWIR on the Choice Between Wheel-Running and Palatable Food

The aforementioned experiments alternatively used wheel-running or palatable feeding as reinforcers. To examine whether the conclusions raised by these experiments extended to a reward choice situation (as daily encountered by humans, including AN patients), we performed one series of experiments wherein mice placed under an FR3 schedule of reinforcement could select one of the two rewards, this choice being temporarily exclusive. Moreover, as PWIR affected the amplitudes of the respective impacts of food restriction on body weight losses and FAA in female mice (**Figure 2B** and **D**), these experiments involved mice initially provided food *ad libitum* before being placed under a food restriction regimen. The analysis of the respective nose poke responses for wheel-running and palatable feeding revealed significant reward × food regimen × session interactions on nose poke responses in grouped males ($F_{4,32} = 8.23$, $p = 0.0001$; **Figure 5A**) and in PWIR males ($F_{4,40} = 22.31$, $p < 0.0001$; **Figure 5B**). However, while nose poke responses for wheel-running exceeded those for feeding during *ad libitum* feeding conditions—a difference which vanished during food restriction—in grouped males (**Figure 5A**), nose poke responses for each reward were similar in their PWIR counterparts (**Figure 5B**). Comparisons of the

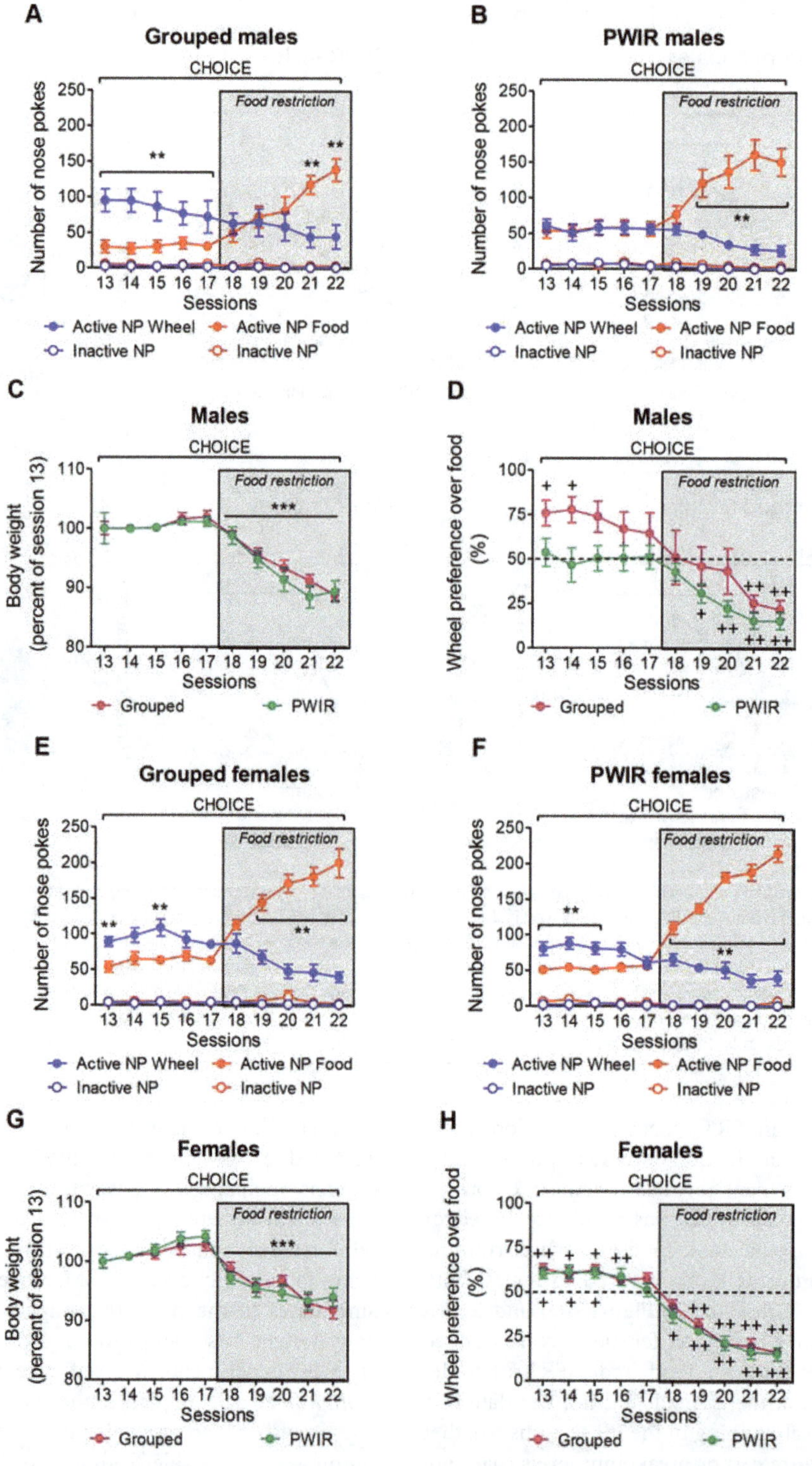

FIGURE 5 | Sex-dependent effects of post-weaning isolation rearing (PWIR) on the preference between running and palatable feeding (choice sessions). **(A)** The difference in nose poke responses for running over feeding in grouped males was progressively inversed with food restriction. **(B)** Fed PWIR males displayed equal numbers of nose responses for running and feeding. **(C)** Grouped and PWIR male mice showed similar body weight losses during food restriction. **(D)** Grouped, but not PWIR, mice displayed time-dependent preferences for wheel-running over feeding. **(E,F)** The difference in nose poke responses for running over feeding in grouped and PWIR females was progressively inversed with food restriction. **(G)** Identical body weight losses in food-restricted grouped and PWIR female mice during the choice sessions. **(H)** Similar profiles of wheel-running preference over feeding in grouped and PWIR females during the choice sessions. The values are the mean ± standard error of the mean of n = 5–6 mice. ** $p < 0.01$ for the time-dependent differences between nose poke responses for wheel-running and feeding (*post hoc* Tukey tests following significant session x reward interaction in the multiple-way analyses of variance), and *** $p < 0.001$ for the overall impacts of food restriction on body weights (multiple-way analyses of variance). $^{+}$ $p < 0.05$ and $^{++}$ $p < 0.01$ for the differences with the non-preference (50%) level (one-tailed Student t-tests).

respective reward preference ratios in grouped males and in PWIR males ($F_{4,36} = 4.90$, $p = 0.0029$) confirmed these trends based on absolute nose poke responses for each reward (**Figure 5D**). Actually, the slopes of the session-dependent decreases in body weights ($F_{1,9} = 67.07$, $p < 0.0001$; **Figure 5C**) and wheel preference (**Figure 5D**) were similar in food-restricted grouped and PWIR males. As in males, PWIR in female mice did not affect the amplitude of body weight losses following food restriction ($F_{1,9} = 54.88$, $p < 0.0001$; **Figure 5G**). However, as opposed to *ad libitum* fed males, PWIR proved ineffective on the amplitude of the preference for wheel-running over feeding during *ad libitum* feeding. This was true whether absolute nose poke responses for wheel-running and palatable feeding ($F_{4,32} = 20.81$, $p < 0.0001$ and $F_{4,40} = 19.28$, $p < 0.0001$ in group-housed mice and in PWIR mice, respectively; **Figure 5E** and **F**) or reward preference ratios ($F_{4,36} = 14.25$, $p = 0.0001$; **Figure 5H**) were considered. Lastly, it is worthy of mention that the mean running preference ratio, although over 50% in grouped males (**Figure 5D**) and grouped females (**Figure 5H**), showed a sex-dependent heterogeneity of responses. Hence, in males, this heterogeneity was partly, but not fully, accounted for by one male (over five) which displayed 88–100% preference for wheel-running over feeding under *ad libitum* fed conditions before showing delayed preference for feeding, compared to the other males, under restricted conditions.

PWIR Decreases Wheel-Running Performances in Male Mice

The aforementioned observation that PWIR reduced the wheel preference over food in male mice might have been biased by an increased wheel-running performance during each rewarded sequence. If so, "consumption" of the reward would have compensated for decreased reward motivation in this mouse group. Analyses of wheel-running performances during each rewarded sequence argued against such a possibility. Thus, either the running duration ($F_{1,9} = 10.57$, $p = 0.01$; **Figure 6A**) or the running distance ($F_{1,9} = 5.85$, $p = 0.039$; **Figure 6C**) per rewarded sequence proved sensitive to PWIR, PWIR mice displaying decreased performances compared to group-housed mice. Indeed, these two performance indices were affected to a similar extent by PWIR, an observation which accounted for the lack of influence of that stressor on the mouse mean speed (data not shown). The impact of PWIR on wheel-running performances was sex-specific as it proved ineffective in female mice (**Figure 6B** and **D**).

DISCUSSION

AN bears the highest mortality rate among psychiatric diseases (Kaye et al., 2009), which is accounted for by our poor knowledge of its neurobiological underpinnings and hence a lack of efficient therapy for the most dramatic cases. Our ignorance of AN neurobiology lies on both its complex etiology and the translational limits of AN animal models. Although different animal models of AN exist (Mequinion et al., 2015), the one that has gained much audience is the ABA model. However, the great majority of ABA studies uses "free" wheel-running (i.e. costless access to running wheels) in their quest to elucidate the bases of AN. This can be questionned on the basis of former evidence for a motivation conflict between exercise and feeding in AN (Klein et al., 2004; Casper, 2006; Keating, 2010; Keating et al., 2012). Actually, recent observations strengthen the hypothesis of a general alteration in reward pathways in AN, whether brain responses to losses in monetary gambling tasks or therapeutic responses to the deep brain stimulation of the nucleus accumbens—a key node in brain reward pathways—are concerned (Bischoff-Grethe et al., 2013; Lipsman et al., 2017; Bernardoni et al., 2018). To date, only one study addressed the role of these pathways in the ABA model. Thus, selective chemogenetic stimulation of the dopaminergic mesoaccumbal pathway increased the percent survival to the ABA protocol, doing so by increasing food intakes and FAA-induced body weight loss in female rats (Foldi et al., 2017). An additional concern with the use of the ABA model relates to the observation that it provides neither an index of feeding motivation nor an analysis of the balance between running motivation and feeding motivation when both are available (as in the daily life of anorectics). By comparing the respective results provided by the ABA on the one hand, and reward-motivated instrumental responses on the other hand, this study provides evidence that conclusions based on the former are not valid when motivation-driven responses are considered.

As indicated above, the wide use of the ABA model is accounted for by the seminal observation that rats undergoing a food restriction regimen, i.e., a unique (time- or quantity-restricted) daily access to food, progressively increase their running performances when housed with running wheels. Actually, such an increase in performance mainly relates to FAA, a behavior classically observed in food-restricted animals prior to food presentation. The negative balance between energy intake and energy expenditure in favor of the latter thus accounts for the widespread use of ABA as an animal model of AN (although species-dependent sensitivities must be considered; Rowland et al., 2018). If so, it is expected that AN precipitating factors, such as perinatal and postnatal trauma (see Introduction), amplify such an imbalance. Actually, the use of prenatal stress, early weaning or repeated maternal separation has indicated that ABA symptomatology might be exacerbated by these procedures, albeit not necessarily in a sex-dependent manner (Glavin and Pare, 1985; Hancock and Grant, 2009; Schroeder et al., 2018). In the present study, we selected PWIR as the infant trauma. Thus, social isolation at the onset of the post-weaning period and throughout adolescence is endowed with long-lasting behavioral disturbances (e.g. anxiety, alterations in impulse control, deficit in social interactions, increased drug preference, efficient acquisition of drug self-administration; Burke et al., 2017; Walker et al., 2019) that are relevant to the scope of this study. The origins of these disturbances are likely due to the inability to express social play behavior, a highly rewarding activity that contributes to a major extent to the normal development of emotional processes (Vanderschuren et al., 2016).

As indicated above, ABA relies on a unique time- or quantity-restricted daily access to food. In most cases, a short time-window is privileged for daily food access. In our hands, preliminary observations using a daily 3-h access to food indicated that this protocol was too severe for the animals, as illustrated by precipitated

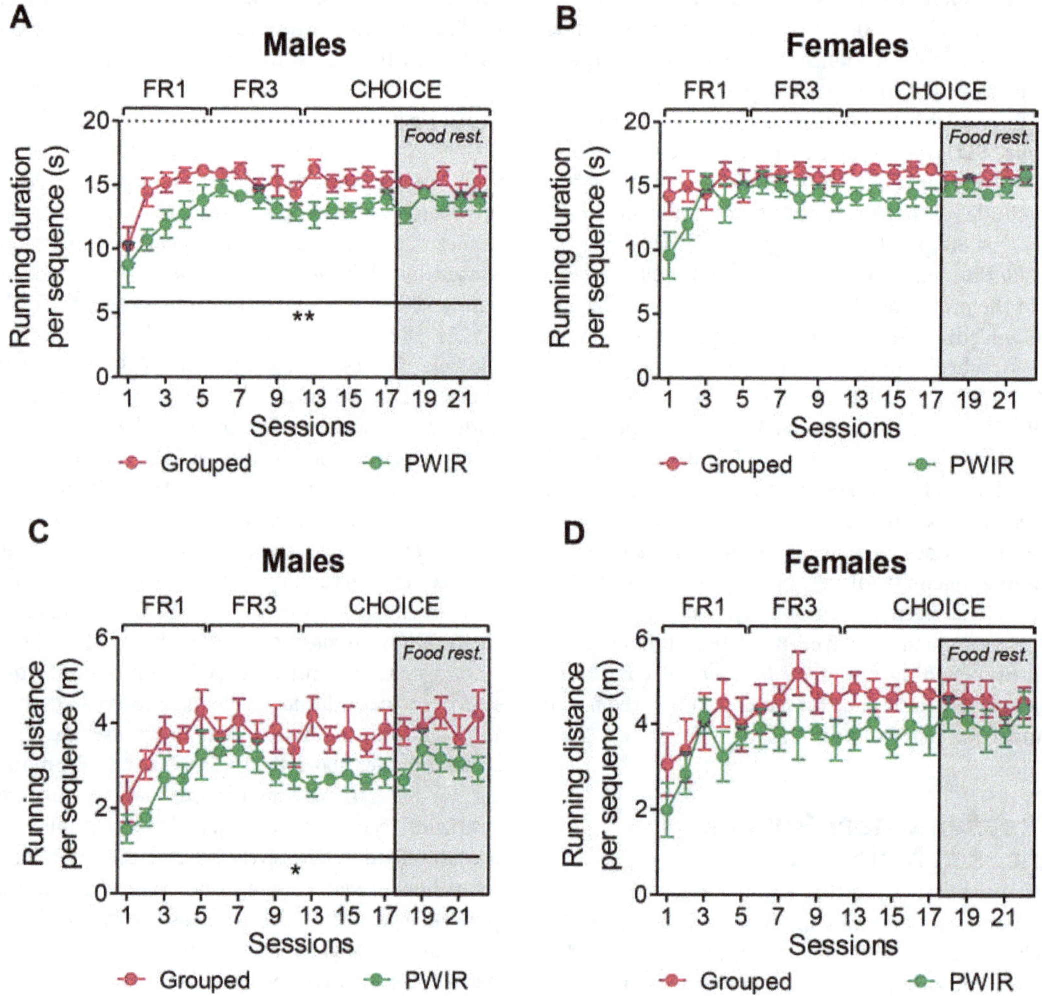

FIGURE 6 | Impaired nose poke responses for wheel-running were associated with decreased running performances in PWIR males. **(A,B)** PWIR decreased the running duration per rewarded sequence in males **(A)**, but not in females **(B)**. **(C,D)** PWIR males **(C)**, but not females **(D)**, ran less distance per rewarded sequence, compared to their respective grouped controls. The values are the mean ± standard error of the mean of n = 5–6 mice. * $p < 0.05$ and ** $p < 0.01$ for the overall impacts of PWIR throughout test sessions (multiple-way analyses of variance).

and important body weight decreases that led to the discontinuation of wheel-running activity after 4 days in several animals (and hence interruption of the study for welfare reasons). Accordingly, we chose a quantity-restricted paradigm that allowed to observe significant wheel-running activity in all animals. In keeping with the aforementioned prevalence of woman suffering AN, as compared to males, we first tested whether PWIR was endowed with a significant impact in female mice exposed to an ABA paradigm. The observation that PWIR amplified the food restriction-elicited decrease in body weight—extending data in male rats (Ness et al., 1995)—while amplifying FAA, but not postprandial activity, argues against the proposal that the latter is directly related to weight loss (Wu et al., 2014). Besides putative species differences (mice vs. rats), one likely explanation for this discrepancy lies on the fact that in the latter study food-restricted animals were provided food during the light phase of the light/dark cycle (as in many other ABA studies), and not at the onset of the dark phase (present study), i.e., when rodents normally begin eating. Actually, such a time-dependent importance of food delivery, with respect to the light/dark cycle, has been documented elsewhere (Dwyer and Boakes, 1997). Thus, body weight losses, besides being of lower amplitude if food is provided at the onset of the dark period, were found to stabilize more rapidly when feeding occurred within the dark period than within the light period (Dwyer and Boakes, 1997). Noteworthy is the additional finding that the comparison between animals only allowed FAA (i.e., by unblocking the wheels during the hours preceding food provision) and animals allowed to run throughout the light/dark cycle indicated that ABA was fully accounted for by FAA (Dwyer and Boakes, 1997).

Our finding that FAA was increased in PWIR females, as compared to group-housed females, suggested that wheel-running motivation might be exacerbated in the former animals. Besides indicating the crucial need to shift to a paradigm allowing to specifically measure running motivation (Collier and Hirsch, 1971; Iversen, 1993; Belke, 1997; Muguruza et al., 2019)—doing so through the quantitation of the efforts the mice accept to provide to unlock a running wheel—this result raised two issues. The first was related to the impact of sex, if any, on running motivation in PWIR mice. The second issue involved the need to measure feeding motivation as to appreciate how PWIR might affect the balance between running and feeding drives. To explore these issues, we exposed fed/food-restricted group-housed/PWIR mice to operant protocols that specifically allow to estimate wheel-running and feeding drives as well as running performances (Muguruza et al., 2019). However, before focusing on these issues, we asked two preliminary, albeit important, questions within the present context, i.e. does food-restriction increase wheel-running motivation, and if so, is the amplitude of that increase sex-dependent? Thus, although the stimulatory impacts of either food restriction or complete fasting on wheel-running performance are known since almost 70 years (Finger, 1951), only one study, which used rats, compared males and females with respect to wheel-running motivation under fed and food-restricted conditions (Pierce et al., 1986). It was observed that the relationship between the amplitude of food restriction and running motivation, as estimated during a PR session, followed an inverted U-shaped curve with females responding to food restriction with seemingly higher running motivation than males (albeit the low number of animals impedes any conclusion; Pierce et al., 1986). The observation that food-restriction might increase running motivation fits with the finding that motivation for wheel-running under food-limited conditions is food-related, hence increasing performance, at least under "free" wheel-running conditions (Belke and Pierce, 2016). To our surprise, our female mice, albeit responding more than males for wheel-running under both constant (FR) and progressive (PR) reinforcement schedules, proved insensitive to food restriction. Conversely, food restriction stimulated male nose poke responses during the PR, but not the FR, sessions, indicating increased motivation. Interestingly, the lack of impact of food restriction on male nose poke responses during FR sessions did not extend to wheel-running performances at each rewarded sequence, as illustrated by the increased running duration/distance throughout these sessions. In keeping with our previous observation that mice bearing a deletion of the cannabinoid type-1 (CB1) receptor display decreased nose poke responses for wheel-running during FR/PR sessions without any alteration in running duration/distance at each rewarded sequence (Muguruza et al., 2019), the present study reinforces the belief that running motivation and running "consumption" (as assessed from running performances) are different entities (Belke and Garland, 2007; Muguruza et al., 2019).

That food restriction did not stimulate running motivation in our female mice although ABA-induced FAA, albeit of weak amplitude, could be observed in these animals suggested that FAA is not an index of running motivation. If so, this in turn would indicate that the aforementioned stimulatory impact of PWIR on FAA occurs without any change in running motivation. At first sight, this possibility might appear counterintuitive in keeping with the aforementioned report that chemogenetic stimulation of the mesolimbic pathway, which plays a key role in motivation for rewards, slightly, but significantly, amplifies FAA (Foldi et al., 2017). Accordingly, we analyzed wheel-running motivation in PWIR and grouped females, extending this investigation to males as running motivation was stimulated in a sex-dependent manner by food restriction. Moreover, as AN associates high exercise motivation with low feeding motivation under circumstances during which both rewards are in competition, we took advantage of our recently developed operant paradigm wherein the reinforcing values of these two rewards can be assessed separately in fed animals before being compared within a choice paradigm under fed and food-restricted conditions (Muguruza et al., 2019). Under fed conditions, whether the rewards were provided separately or within a choice paradigm, PWIR males responded to similar extents for wheel-running and for palatable food when all other mouse groups displayed increased responding for wheel-running. The negative impact of PWIR on male nose poke responding for wheel-running, compared to that measured in the other mouse groups, extended to running performance. Thus, when analyzed when wheel-running was proposed either solely or in concurrence with palatable food, the running duration/distance per rewarded sequence was decreased in PWIR males, compared to grouped males. This suggests that PWIR bears negative consequences on both wheel-running motivation and wheel-running "consumption". Considering the finding mentioned above that wheel-running motivation is under tight control by CB1 receptors (Rasmussen and Hillman, 2011; Muguruza et al., 2019), the observation that PWIR decreases CB1 receptor activity in rats (Zamberletti et al., 2012) and mice (Muguruza et al., in preparation) might provide a route of investigation to unravel the neurobiological underpinnings of decreased running motivation in PWIR males. As concerns the reduced wheel-running performance in these animals, the finding that opioid receptors, the density of which is reduced by PWIR (Schenk et al., 1982), might control wheel-running performance without impacting on running motivation (Rasmussen and Hillman, 2011), provides another promising route of investigation. Confirmingly, opiate receptor blockade has been reported to alleviate, through decreased wheel-running, ABA severity (Boer et al., 1990). Using a food restriction protocol similar to that used in animals which were only tested for their running motivation (see above), motivation for food overpassed progressively that for running in all groups (with females reaching higher levels than males). In sharp contrast with the above-mentioned higher FAA in PWIR females, compared to grouped females, motivation for wheel-running proved insensitive to PWIR. Besides running protocol differences, the fact that another reward, namely palatable food, was accessible might explain this differential effect of PWIR. Indeed, studies from Ahmed's group have shown that the rank of motivation for one of two rewards provided separately might be reversed when both rewards are proposed in concurrence (Cantin et al., 2010).

Taken together, the results from this study show that changes in "free" wheel-running performances, including FAA, in an ABA protocol by no means reflect alterations in the drive for running (as assessed through an effort-based protocol). Because AN imbalances in the respective drives for exercise and feeding are at the core of the pathology, our results question the translational usefulness of ABA. There are of course limits to the present study. One limit relates to the low numbers of animals which might have underpowered our analyses. Although this possibility must be taken into account, the data gathered in the present study clearly show that the measurement of FAA in the ABA protocol does not provide information on running motivation. The second limit is linked to our use of palatable food, instead of normal chow food, to assess the impact of PWIR on feeding motivation. Thus, adding food palatability to normal (i.e., chow) feeding behavior likely recruits additional central circuit components, including those projecting to the mesocorticolimbic dopaminergic system (Fulton, 2010). However, because i) only food-restricted mice do work to a significant extent to get access to normal chow food, and ii) this study wished to assess the respective impacts of PWIR on feeding drives under both *ad libitum* fed and food restriction conditions, the sole option was to use palatable food although we acknowledge the fact that such a use amplified PR nose poke responses, at least in fed animals, compared to normal chow. A third limit relates to the fact that this study involved animals tested daily for 30–60 min, hence increasing the objective value of each reward. Thus, AN patients are confronted throughout their daily life to the choice between these two rewards. A fourth limit is in keeping with former evidence for the oestrous cycle stage impacting on reward motivation (oestrus > dioestrus), at least for cocaine (Calipari et al., 2017). Although we cannot exclude that cycle variations contributed to the differential impacts of PWIR in the present study, it should be noted that its respective effects on FAA and nose poke responses under an FR3 schedule of reinforcement were studied through a successive number of days that encompassed the duration of the oestrus cycle. The fact that we did not include genetics in our study—although these are involved in AN etiology (see above)—might be considered another key limit. Hence, it might be that testing mouse lines different from the one used herein would have provided a female-specific increase in running motivation at the expense of that for feeding after PWIR. Another important limit stems from our procedure which only compared the respective drives for running and feeding under one schedule of reinforcement (i.e., FR3). Although the purpose of this study was not to compare the intrinsic rewarding values of running and feeding, a procedure which would have required different schedules of reinforcement (Hursh et al., 1988; Hursh and Silberberg, 2008), we cannot exclude that increasing the costs for each reward would have led to results differing from the present ones. As rightly proposed by Rowland et al., 2018 in their use of a cost-based anorexia model, increasing the cost to access food would mimic the high cost AN patients feel with regard to food. Accordingly, using a cost-based anorexia model wherein mice would be proposed food at progressively higher costs in their living environment (Atalayer and Rowland, 2011), and adding to that model increasing costs for running, could help to disentangle the neurobiologial grounds of AN. Such a model would prove useful for the development of pharmacological agents aimed at specifically altering the exercise/food drive balance (in either direction) for therapeutic goals.

AUTHOR CONTRIBUTIONS

BR, IH, GM, and FC designed the research. BR, IH, AS, MM, and FC performed research. BR, IH, AS, MM, and FC analyzed the data. FC wrote the first version of the manuscript before it was edited and approved by all authors.

FUNDING

This work was supported by Institut National de la Santé et de la Recherche Médicale (to GM), la Région Aquitaine (to GM), the University of Bordeaux (to GM), the European Research Council (ERC-2017-AdG-786467 to GM), l'Agence Nationale de la Recherche (to GM and FG), l'Agence Française de Lutte contre le Dopage (to FC), and the LabEx-Bordeaux Région Aquitaine Initiative for Neuroscience (to GM and FC).

ACKNOWLEDGMENTS

The reviewers of this publication are thanked for their constructive criticisms. We also thank all the personnel from the Animal Facility and the Genotyping platform of the NeuroCentre Magendie, Virginie Morales and the other members of Marsicano's laboratory for their daily support and for useful discussions, and Dr Serge Ahmed (IMN, CNRS UMR 5293, Bordeaux) for his help in setting the choice paradigm.

REFERENCES

Atalayer, D., and Rowland, N. E. (2011). Structure of motivation using food demand in mice. *Physiol. Behav.* 104, 15–19. doi: 10.1016/j.physbeh.2011.04.042

Bale, T. L., and Epperson, C. N. (2015). Sex differences and stress across the lifespan. *Nat. Neurosci.* 18, 1413–1420. doi: 10.1038/nn.4112

Belke, T. W. (1997). Running and responding reinforced by the opportunity to run: effect of reinforcement duration. *J. Exp. Anal. Behav.* 67, 337–351. doi: 10.1901/jeab.1997.67-337

Belke, T. W., and Garland, T., Jr. (2007). A brief opportunity to run does not function as a reinforcer for mice selected for high daily wheel-running rates. *J. Exp. Anal. Behav.* 88, 199–213. doi: 10.1901/jeab.2007.62-06

Belke, T. W., and Pierce, W. D. (2016). Wheel-running reinforcement in free-feeding and food-deprived rats. *Behav. Processes.* 124, 1–9. doi: 10.1016/j.beproc.2015.11.018

Bernardoni, F., Geisler, D., King, J. A., Javadi, A. H., Ritschel, F., Murr, J., et al. (2018). Altered medial frontal feedback learning signals in anorexia nervosa. *Biol. Psychiatry* 83, 235–243. doi: 10.1016/j.biopsych.2017.07.024

Bischoff-Grethe, A., McCurdy, D., Grenesko-Stevens, E., Irvine, L. E., Wagner, A., Yau, W. Y., et al. (2013). Altered brain response to reward and punishment in adolescents with anorexia nervosa. *Psychiatry Res.* 214, 331–340. doi: 10.1016/j.pscychresns.2013.07.004

Boakes, R. A. (2007). Self-starvation in the rat: running versus eating. *Span. J. Psychol.* 10, 251–257. doi: 10.1017/S113874160000651X

Boer, D. P., Epling, W. F., Pierce, W. D., and Russell, J. C. (1990). Suppression of food deprivation-induced high-rate wheel running in rats. *Physiol. Behav.* 48, 339–342. doi: 10.1016/0031-9384(90)90324-W

Boersma, G. J., Liang, N. C., Lee, R. S., Albertz, J. D., Kastelein, A., Moody, L. A., et al. (2016). Failure to upregulate Agrp and Orexin in response to activity based anorexia in weight loss vulnerable rats characterized by passive stress coping and prenatal stress experience. *Psychoneuroendocrinology* 67, 171–181. doi: 10.1016/j.psyneuen.2016.02.002

Brewerton, T. D., Stellefson, E. J., Hibbs, N., Hodges, E. L., and Cochrane, C. E. (1995). Comparison of eating disorder patients with and without compulsive exercising. *Int. J. Eat. Disord.* 17, 413–416. doi: 10.1002/1098-108X(199505)17:4<413::AID-EAT2260170414>3.0.CO;2-0

Bulik, C. M., Slof-Op't Landt, M. C., van Furth, E. F., and Sullivan, P. F. (2007). The genetics of anorexia nervosa. *Annu. Rev. Nutr.* 27, 263–275. doi: 10.1146/annurev.nutr.27.061406.093713

Burke, A. R., McCormick, C. M., Pellis, S. M., and Lukkes, J. L. (2017). Impact of adolescent social experiences on behavior and neural circuits implicated in mental illnesses. *Neurosci. Biobehav. Rev.* 76, 280–300. doi: 10.1016/j.neubiorev.2017.01.018

Calipari, E. S., Juarez, B., Morel, C., Walker, D. M., Cahill, M. E., Ribeiro, E., et al. (2017). Dopaminergic dynamics underlying sex-specific cocaine reward. *Nat. Commun.* 10, 13877. doi: 10.1038/ncomms13877

Canetti, L., Kanyas, K., Lerer, B., Latzer, Y., and Bachar, E. (2008). Anorexia nervosa and parental bonding: the contribution of parent-grandparent relationships to eating disorder psychopathology. *J. Clin. Psychol.* 64, 703–716. doi: 10.1002/jclp.20482

Cantin, L., Lenoir, M., Augier, E., Vanhille, N., Dubreucq, S., Serre, F., et al. (2010). Cocaine is low on the value ladder of rats: possible evidence for resilience to addiction. *PLoS ONE* 5, e11592. doi: 10.1371/journal.pone.0011592

Carrera, O., Cerrato, M., Sanchez, A., and Gutierrez, E. (2009). Long maternal separation has protective effects in rats exposed to activity-based anorexia. *Dev. Psychobiol.* 51, 616–624. doi: 10.1002/dev.20396

Casper, R. C. (2006). The 'drive for activity' and "restlessness" in anorexia nervosa: potential pathways. *J. Affect. Disord.* 92, 99–107. doi: 10.1016/j.jad.2005.12.039

Casper, R. C. (2018). Not the function of eating, but spontaneous activity and energy expenditure, reflected in "restlessness" and a "drive for activity" appear to be dysregulated in anorexia nervosa: treatment implications. *Front. Psychol.* 9, 2303. doi: 10.3389/fpsyg.2018.02303

Clarke, T. K., Weiss, A. R., and Berrettini, W. H. (2012). The genetics of anorexia nervosa. *Clin. Pharmacol. Ther.* 91, 181–188. doi: 10.1038/clpt.2011.253

Collier, G. H., and Hirsch, E. (1971). Reinforcing properties of spontaneous activity in the rat. *J. Comp. Physiol. Psychol.* 77, 155–160. doi: 10.1037/h0031588

Cook, B. J., and Hausenblas, H. A. (2008). The role of exercise dependence for the relationship between exercise behavior and eating pathology: mediator or moderator? *J. Health. Psychol.* 13, 495–502. doi: 10.1177/1359105308088520

Davis, C. (1997). Eating disorders and hyperactivity: a psychobiological perspective. *Can. J. Psychiatry* 42, 168–175. doi: 10.1177/070674379704200207

Davis, C., and Woodside, D. B. (2002). Sensitivity to the rewarding effects of food and exercise in the eating disorders. *Compr. Psychiatry* 43, 189–194. doi: 10.1053/comp.2002.32356

Dwyer, D. M., and Boakes, R. A. (1997). Activity-based anorexia in rats as failure to adapt to a feeding schedule. *Behav. Neurosci.* 111, 195–205. doi: 10.1037/0735-7044.111.1.195

Finger, F. W. (1951). The effect of food deprivation and subsequent satiation upon general activity in the rat. *J. Comp. Physiol. Psychol.* 44, 5575–5564. doi: 10.1037/h0055692

Foldi, C. J., Milton, L. K., and Oldfield, B. J. (2017). The role of mesolimbic reward neurocircuitry in prevention and rescue of the activity-based anorexia (ABA) phenotype in rats. *Neuropsychopharmacology* 42, 2292–2300. doi: 10.1038/npp.2017.63

Fone, K. C., and Porkess, M. V. (2008). Behavioural and neurochemical effects of post-weaning social isolation in rodents-relevance to developmental neuropsychiatric disorders. *Neurosci. Biobehav. Rev.* 32, 1087–1102. doi: 10.1016/j.neubiorev.2008.03.003

Fulton, S. (2010). Appetite and reward. *Front. Neuroendocrinol.* 31, 85–103. doi: 10.1016/j.yfrne.2009.10.003

Glavin, G. B., and Pare, W. P. (1985). Early weaning predisposes rats to exacerbated activity-stress ulcer formation. *Physiol. Behav.* 34, 907–909. doi: 10.1016/0031-9384(85)90012-5

Hancock, S., and Grant, V. (2009). Early maternal separation increases symptoms of activity-based anorexia in male and female rats. *J. Exp. Psychol. Anim. Behav. Process.* 35, 394–406. doi: 10.1037/a0014736

Hursh, S. R., Raslear, T. G., Shurtleff, D., Bauman, R., and Simmons, L. (1988). A cost-benefit analysis of demand for food. *J. Exp. Anal. Behav.* 50, 419–440. doi: 10.1901/jeab.1988.50-419

Hursh, S. R., and Silberberg, A. (2008). Economic demand and essential value. *Psychol. Rev.* 115, 186–198. doi: 10.1037/0033-295X.115.1.186

Iversen, I. H. (1993). Techniques for establishing schedules with wheel-running as reinforcement in rats. *J. Exp. Anal. Behav.* 60, 219–238. doi: 10.1901/jeab.1993.60-219

Jaite, C., Schneider, N., Hilbert, A., Pfeiffer, E., Lehmkuhl, U., and Salbach-Andrae, H. (2012). Etiological role of childhood emotional trauma and neglect in adolescent anorexia nervosa: a cross-sectional questionnaire analysis. *Psychopathology* 45, 61–66. doi: 10.1159/000328580

Kaye, W. H., Fudge, J. L., and Paulus, M. (2009). New insights into symptoms and neurocircuit function of anorexia nervosa. *Nat. Rev. Neurosci.* 10, 573–584. doi: 10.1038/nrn2682

Keating, C. (2010). Theoretical perspective on anorexia nervosa: the conflict of reward. *Neurosci. Biobehav. Rev.* 34, 73–79. doi: 10.1016/j.neubiorev.2009.07.004

Keating, C., Tilbrook, A. J., Rossell, S. L., Enticott, P. G., and Fitzgerald, P. B. (2012). Reward processing in anorexia nervosa. *Neuropsychologia* 50, 567–575. doi: 10.1016/j.neuropsychologia.2012.01.036

Keski-Rahkonen, A., and Mustelin, L. (2016). Epidemiology of eating disorders in Europe: prevalence, incidence, comorbidity, course, consequences, and risk factors. *Curr. Opin. Psychiatry* 29, 340–345. doi: 10.1097/YCO.0000000000000278

Kim, S. F. (2012). Animal models of eating disorders. *Neuroscience* 211, 2–12. doi: 10.1016/j.neuroscience.2012.03.024

Klein, D. A., Bennett, A. S., Schebendach, J., Foltin, R. W., Devlin, M. J., and Walsh, B. T. (2004). Exercise "addiction" in anorexia nervosa: model development and pilot data. *CNS Spectr.* 9, 531–537. doi: 10.1017/S1092852900009627

Klenotich, S. J., Seiglie, M. P., McMurray, M. S., Roitman, J. D., Le Grange, D., Dugad, P., et al. (2012). Olanzapine, but not fluoxetine, treatment increases survival in activity-based anorexia in mice. *Neuropsychopharmacology* 37, 1620–1631. doi: 10.1038/npp.2012.7

Leung, N., Thomas, G., and Waller, G. (2000). The relationship between parental bonding and core beliefs in anorexic and bulimic women. *Br. J. Clin. Psychol.* 39, 205–213. doi: 10.1348/014466500163220

Lipsman, N., Lam, E., Volpini, M., Sutandar, K., Twose, R., Giacobbe, P., et al. (2017). Deep brain stimulation of the subcallosal cingulate for treatment-refractory anorexia nervosa: 1 year follow-up of an open-label trial. *Lancet Psychiatry* 4, 285–294. doi: 10.1016/S2215-0366(17)30076-7

Lupien, S. J., McEwen, B. S., Gunnar, M. R., and Heim, C. (2009). Effects of stress throughout the lifespan on the brain, behaviour and cognition. *Nat. Rev. Neurosci.* 10, 434–445. doi: 10.1038/nrn2639

McCormick, C. M., Green, M. R., and Simone, J. J. (2016). Translational relevance of rodent models of hypothalamic-pituitary-adrenal function and stressors in adolescence. *Neurobiol. Stress* 6, 31–43. doi: 10.1016/j.ynstr.2016.08.003

Mequinion, M., Chauveau, C., and Viltart, O. (2015). The use of animal models to decipher physiological and neurobiological alterations of anorexia nervosa patients. *Front. Endocrinol. (Lausanne)* 6, 68. doi: 10.3389/fendo.2015.00068

Meyer, C., Taranis, L., Goodwin, H., and Haycraft, E. (2011). Compulsive exercise and eating disorders. *Eur. Eat. Disord. Rev.* 19, 174–189. doi: 10.1002/erv.1122

Muguruza, C., Redon, B., Fois, G. R., Hurel, I., Scocard, A., Nguyen, C., et al. (2019). The motivation for exercise over palatable food is dictated by cannabinoid type-1 receptors. *JCI Insight* 4, 1–4. doi: 10.1172/jci.insight.126190. eCollection 2019 Mar 7.

Ness, J. W., Marshall, T. R., and Aravich, P. F. (1995). Effects of rearing condition on activity-induced weight loss. *Dev. Psychobiol.* 28, 165–173. doi: 10.1002/dev.420280304

Pierce, W. D., Epling, W. F., and Boer, D. P. (1986). Deprivation and satiation: the interrelations between food and wheel running. *J. Exp. Anal. Behav.* 46, 199–210. doi: 10.1901/jeab.1986.46-199

Pike, K. M., Hilbert, A., Wilfley, D. E., Fairburn, C. G., Dohm, F. A., Walsh, B. T., et al. (2008). Toward an understanding of risk factors for anorexia nervosa: a case-control study. *Psychol. Med.* 38, 1443–1453. doi: 10.1017/S0033291707002310

Pjetri, E., de Haas, R., de Jong, S., Gelegen, C., Oppelaar, H., Verhagen, L. A., et al. (2012). Identifying predictors of activity based anorexia susceptibility in diverse genetic rodent populations. *PLoS One* 7, e50453. doi: 10.1371/journal.pone.0050453

Racine, S. E., and Wildes, J. E. (2015). Emotion dysregulation and anorexia nervosa: an exploration of the role of childhood abuse. *Int. J. Eat. Disord.* 48, 55–58. doi: 10.1002/eat.22364

Rasmussen, E. B., and Hillman, C. (2011). Naloxone and rimonabant reduce the reinforcing properties of exercise in rats. *Exp. Clin. Psychopharmacol.* 19, 191–197. doi: 10.1037/a0024142

Reyes-Rodríguez, M. L., Von Holle, A., Ulman, T. F., Thornton, L. M., Klump, K. L., Brandt, H., et al. (2011). Posttraumatic stress disorder in anorexia nervosa. *Psychosom. Med.* 73, 491–497. doi: 10.1097/PSY.0b013e31822232bb

Romans, S. E., Gendall, K. A., Martin, J. L., and Mullen, P. E. (2001). Child sexual abuse and later disordered eating: a New Zealand epidemiological study. *Int. J. Eat. Disord.* 29, 380–392. doi: 10.1002/eat.1034

Routtenberg, A., and Kuznesof, A. W. (1967). Self-starvation of rats living in activity wheels on a restricted feeding schedule. *J. Comp. Physiol. Psychol.* 64, 414–421. doi: 10.1037/h0025205

Rowland, N. E., Atalayer, D., Cervantez, M. R., Minaya, D. M., and Splane, E. C. (2018). Cost-based anorexia: a novel framework to model anorexia nervosa. *Appetite.* 130, 50–58. doi: 10.1016/j.appet.2018.07.034

Schenk, S., Britt, M. D., Atalay, J., and Charleson, S. (1982). Isolation rearing decreases opiate receptor binding in rat brain. *Pharmacol. Biochem. Behav.* 16, 841–842. doi: 10.1016/0091-3057(82)90245-3

Scheurink, A. J., Boersma, G. J., Nergårdh, R., and Södersten, P. (2010). Neurobiology of hyperactivity and reward: agreeable restlessness in anorexia nervosa. *Physiol. Behav.* 100, 490–495. doi: 10.1016/j.physbeh.2010.03.016

Schroeder, M., Jakovcevski, M., Polacheck, T., Drori, Y., Ben-Dor, S., Röh, S., et al. (2018). Sex dependent impact of gestational stress on predisposition to eating disorders and metabolic disease. *Mol. Metab.* 17, 1–16. doi: 10.1016/j.molmet.2018.08.005

Shroff, H., Reba, L., Thornton, L. M., Tozzi, F., Klump, K. L., Berrettini, W. H., et al. (2006). Features associated with excessive exercise in women with eating disorders. *Int. J. Eat. Disord.* 39, 454–461. doi: 10.1002/eat.20247

Smink, F. R., van Hoeken, D., and Hoek, H. W. (2012). Epidemiology of eating disorders: incidence, prevalence and mortality rates. *Curr. Psychiatry Rep.* 14, 406–414. doi: 10.1007/s11920-012-0282-y

Vanderschuren, L. J., Achterberg, E. J., and Trezza, V. (2016). The neurobiology of social play and its rewarding value in rats. *Neurosci. Biobehav. Rev.* 70, 86–105. doi: 10.1016/j.neubiorev.2016.07.025

Walker, D. M., Cunningham, A. M., Gregory, J. K., and Nestler, E. J. (2019). Long-term behavioral effects of post-weaning social isolation in males and females. *Front. Behav. Neurosci.* 13, 66. doi: 10.3389/fnbeh.2019.00066

Willner, P. (1984). The validity of animal models of depression. *Psychopharmacology (Berl)* 83, 1–16. doi: 10.1007/BF00427414

Wu, H., van Kuyck, K., Tambuyzer, T., Luyten, L., Aerts, J. M., and Nuttin, B. (2014). Rethinking food anticipatory activity in the activity-based anorexia rat model. *Sci. Rep.* 4, 3929. doi: 10.1038/srep03929

Yackobovitch-Gavan, M., Golan, M., Valevski, A., Kreitler, S., Bachar, E., Lieblich, A., et al. (2009). An integrative quantitative model of factors influencing the course of anorexia nervosa over time. *Int. J. Eat. Disord.* 42, 306–317. doi: 10.1002/eat.20624

Zamberletti, E., Viganò, D., Guidali, C., Rubino, T., and Parolaro, D. (2012). Long-lasting recovery of psychotic-like symptoms in isolation-reared rats after chronic but not acute treatment with the cannabinoid antagonist AM251. *Int. J. Neuropsychopharmacol.* 15, 267–280. doi: 10.1017/S1461145710001185

Zipfel, S., Giel, K. E., Bulik, C. M., Hay, P., and Schmidt, U. (2015). Anorexia nervosa: aetiology, assessment, and treatment. *Lancet Psychiatry* 2, 1099–1111. doi: 10.1016/S2215-0366(15)00356-9

Permissions

All chapters in this book were first published by Frontiers; hereby published with permission under the Creative Commons Attribution License or equivalent. Every chapter published in this book has been scrutinized by our experts. Their significance has been extensively debated. The topics covered herein carry significant findings which will fuel the growth of the discipline. They may even be implemented as practical applications or may be referred to as a beginning point for another development.

The contributors of this book come from diverse backgrounds, making this book a truly international effort. This book will bring forth new frontiers with its revolutionizing research information and detailed analysis of the nascent developments around the world.

We would like to thank all the contributing authors for lending their expertise to make the book truly unique. They have played a crucial role in the development of this book. Without their invaluable contributions this book wouldn't have been possible. They have made vital efforts to compile up to date information on the varied aspects of this subject to make this book a valuable addition to the collection of many professionals and students.

This book was conceptualized with the vision of imparting up-to-date information and advanced data in this field. To ensure the same, a matchless editorial board was set up. Every individual on the board went through rigorous rounds of assessment to prove their worth. After which they invested a large part of their time researching and compiling the most relevant data for our readers.

The editorial board has been involved in producing this book since its inception. They have spent rigorous hours researching and exploring the diverse topics which have resulted in the successful publishing of this book. They have passed on their knowledge of decades through this book. To expedite this challenging task, the publisher supported the team at every step. A small team of assistant editors was also appointed to further simplify the editing procedure and attain best results for the readers.

Apart from the editorial board, the designing team has also invested a significant amount of their time in understanding the subject and creating the most relevant covers. They scrutinized every image to scout for the most suitable representation of the subject and create an appropriate cover for the book.

The publishing team has been an ardent support to the editorial, designing and production team. Their endless efforts to recruit the best for this project, has resulted in the accomplishment of this book. They are a veteran in the field of academics and their pool of knowledge is as vast as their experience in printing. Their expertise and guidance has proved useful at every step. Their uncompromising quality standards have made this book an exceptional effort. Their encouragement from time to time has been an inspiration for everyone.

The publisher and the editorial board hope that this book will prove to be a valuable piece of knowledge for researchers, students, practitioners and scholars across the globe.

List of Contributors

Sebastiano Alfio Torrisi, Gian Marco Leggio, Filippo Drago and Salvatore Salomone
Department of Biomedical and Biotechnological Sciences, University of Catania, Catania, Italy

Ioanna Prionisti
Division of Digestive and Transplantation Surgery, Geneva University Hospitals, Geneva, Switzerland Lemanic Neuroscience Doctoral School, Geneva, Switzerland

Léo H. Bühler
Division of Digestive and Transplantation Surgery, Geneva University Hospitals, Geneva, Switzerland

Paul R. Walker
Center for Translational Research in Onco-Hematology, Division of Oncology, Geneva University Hospitals – University of Geneva, Geneva, Switzerland

Renaud B. Jolivet
Département de Physique Nucléaire et Corpusculaire (DPNC), University of Geneva, Geneva, Switzerland European Organization for Nuclear Research (CERN), Geneva, Switzerland

Hui Zhao and Tiejun Li
Department of Pharmacy, Punan Hospital, Shanghai, China College of Pharmacology, Anhui University of Chinese Medicine, Hefei, China

Junqin Mao
Department of Pharmacy, Shanghai Pudong New Area People's Hospital, Shanghai, China

Yuan Yuan, Jingjing Feng and Hao Cheng
College of Pharmacology, Anhui University of Chinese Medicine, Hefei, China

Guorong Fan
Department of Clinical Pharmacy, Shanghai General Hospital, Shanghai JiaoTong University School of Medicine, Shanghai, China

Yuefan Zhang
Department of Clinical Pharmacy, Shanghai General Hospital, Shanghai JiaoTong University School of Medicine, Shanghai, China Department of Pharmacology, College of Pharmacy,Second Military Medical University, Shanghai, China

Bin Liu, Jing Liu, Jiangong Wang, Fengjiao Sun, Shujun Jiang, Fengai Hu, Dan Wang, Dunjiang Liu, Cuilan Liu and Haijing Yan
Institute for Metabolic and Neuropsychiatric Disorders, Binzhou Medical University Hospital, Binzhou, China

Christine Ibrahim
Translational Addiction Research Laboratory, Centre for Addiction and Mental Health, Toronto, ON, Canada Department of Pharmacology, University of Toronto, Toronto, ON, Canada

Dafna S. Rubin-Kahana
Translational Addiction Research Laboratory, Centre for Addiction and Mental Health, Toronto, ON, Canada Department of Psychiatry, Faculty of Medicine, University of Toronto, Toronto, ON, Canada

Abhiram Pushparaj
Qunuba Sciences, Toronto, ON, Canada Ironstone Product Development, Toronto, ON, Canada

Martin Musiol
Ironstone Product Development, Toronto, ON, Canada

Daniel M. Blumberger and Zafiris J. Daskalakis
Department of Psychiatry, Faculty of Medicine, University of Toronto, Toronto, ON, Canada Temerty Centre for Therapeutic Brain Intervention, Campbell Family Mental Health Research Institute, Centre for Addiction and Mental Health, Toronto, ON, Canada

Abraham Zangen
Department of Life Sciences and the Zlotowski Centerfor Neuroscience, Ben-Gurion University of the Negev, Beer-Sheva, Israel

Bernard Le Foll
Translational Addiction Research Laboratory, Centre for Addiction and Mental Health, Toronto, ON, Canada Department of Pharmacology, University of Toronto, Toronto, ON, Canada Department of Psychiatry, Faculty of Medicine, University of Toronto, Toronto, ON, Canada Addictions Division, Campbell Family Mental Health Research Institute, Centre for Addiction and Mental Health, Toronto, ON, Canada Institute of Medical Sciences, University of Toronto, Toronto, ON, Canada Alcohol Research and Treatment Clinic, Centre for Addiction and Mental Health, Toronto, ON, Canada Department of Family and Community Medicine, University of Toronto, Toronto, ON, Canada

Gustavo Balbinot
Brain Institute, Universidade Federal do Rio Grande do Norte, Natal, Brazil

Clarissa Pedrini Schuch
Graduate Program in Rehabilitation Sciences, Universidade Federal de Ciências da Saúde de Porto Alegre (UFCSPA), Porto Alegre, Brazil

Shivani C. Kharod and Seok Kyu Kang
Neuroscience Laboratory, Hugo W. Moser Research Institute at Kennedy Krieger, Baltimore, MD, United States

Shivani C. Kharod and Seok Kyu Kang
Neuroscience Laboratory, Hugo W. Moser Research Institute at Kennedy Krieger, Baltimore, MD, United States

Kyle Malone and Christian Waeber
Department of Pharmacology and Therapeutics, School of Pharmacy, University College Cork, Cork, Ireland

Sylvie Amu
Cancer Research UCC, University College Cork, Cork, Ireland

Anne C. Moore
School of Biochemistry and Cell Biology, University College Cork, Cork, Ireland

D. Mango
Laboratory of Neuropharmacology, European Brain Research Institute, Rita Levi Montalcini Foundation, Rome, Italy

R. Nisticò
Laboratory of Neuropharmacology, European Brain Research Institute, Rita Levi-Montalcini Foundation, Rome, Italy Department of Biology, School of Pharmacy, University of Rome Tor Vergata, Rome, Italy

Charles Chavkin, Joshua H. Cohen and Benjamin B. Land
Department of Pharmacology, University of Washington, Seattle, WA, United States

Yanhui Lu and Ruiyi Zhang
Department of Neurology, The First Affiliated Hospital of Zhengzhou University, Zhengzhou, China Academy of Medical Sciences, Zhengzhou University, Zhengzhou, China

Yan Zhou
Department of Radiology, The First Affiliated Hospital of Zhengzhou University, Zhengzhou, China

Lulu Wen, Kaimin Wu, Yanfei Li, Yaobing Yao, Ranran Duan and Yanjie Jia
Department of Neurology, The First Affiliated Hospital of Zhengzhou University, Zhengzhou, China

Federica Geraci, Maria Rosaria Tropea, Giulia Sanfilippo, Agostino Palmeri
Department of Biomedical and Biotechnological Sciences, University of Catania, Catania, Italy

Margherita Grasso and Filippo Caraci
Department of Drug Sciences, University of Catania, Catania, Italy Oasi Research Institute—IRCCS, Troina, Italy

Giuseppe Caruso
Oasi Research Institute—IRCCS, Troina, Italy

Annamaria Fidilio
Department of Drug Sciences, University of Catania, Catania, Italy

Nicolò Musso
Bio-nanotech Research and Innovation Tower (BRIT), University of Catania, Catania, Italy

Fabio Tascedda
Department of Life Sciences and Center for Neuroscience and Neurotechnology, University of Modena and Reggio Emilia, Modena, Italy

Daniela Puzzo
Department of Biomedical and Biotechnological Sciences, University of Catania, Catania, Italy Oasi Research Institute—IRCCS, Troina, Italy

Harald Hampel, Simone Lista and Andrea Vergallo
AXA Research Fund & Sorbonne University Chair, Paris, France Sorbonne University, GRC n 21, Alzheimer Precision Medicine (APM), AP HP, Pitié-Salpêtrière Hospital, Paris, France Brain & Spine Institute (ICM), INSERM U 1127, CNRS UMR 7225, Boulevard de l'Hôpital, Paris, France Department of Neurology, Institute of Memory and Alzheimer's Disease (IM2A), Pitié-Salpêtrière Hospital, AP-HP, Boulevard de l'Hôpital, Paris, France

Edward J. Goetzl
Department of Medicine, University of California, San Francisco, San Francisco, CA, United States

Dimitrios Kapogiannis
Laboratory of Neurosciences, Intramural Research Program, National Institute on Aging, Baltimore, MD, United States

A. Claudio Cuello
Department of Pharmacology and Therapeutics, McGill University, Montreal, QC, Canada Department of Neurology and Neurosurgery, McGill University, Montreal, QC, Canada Department of Anatomy and Cell Biology, McGill University, Montreal, QC, Canada

Hélène Hall and Sonia Do Carmo
Department of Pharmacology and Therapeutics, McGill University, Montreal, QC, Canada

Jing Zhang, Ying Han, Yang Zhao, Qinrui Li and Hongfang Jin
Department of Pediatrics, Peking University First Hospital, Beijing, China

Jiong Qin
Department of Pediatrics, Peking University People's Hospital, Beijing, China

Teemu Aitta-aho, Milica Maksimovic, Kristiina Dahl and Esa R. Korpi
Department of Pharmacology, Faculty of Medicine, University of Helsinki, Helsinki, Finland

Rolf Sprengel
Research Group of the Max Planck Institute for Medical Research at the Institute of Anatomy and Cell Biology, Heidelberg University, Heidelberg, Germany

Imane Hurel, Bastien Redon, Amandine Scocard, Meryl Malezieux, Giovanni Marsicano and Francis Chaouloff
Endocannabinoids and Neuro Adaptation, Neuro Centre INSERM U 1215, Bordeaux, FrancUniversity of Bordeaux, Bordeaux, France

Index

www.ingramcontent.com/pod-product-compliance
Lightning Source LLC
LaVergne TN
LVHW082220200926
848484LV00008B/2280